An Introduction to
THE PRINCIPLES OF DISEASE

John B. Walter, M.D.

*Department of Pathology and
Department of Medicine
(Division of Dermatology)
University of Toronto
Toronto, Ontario, Canada*

W. B. SAUNDERS COMPANY
Philadelphia, London, Toronto

W. B. Saunders Company: West Washington Square
Philadelphia, PA 19105

1 St. Anne's Road
Eastbourne, East Sussex BN21 3UN, England

1 Goldthorne Avenue
Toronto, Ontario M8Z 5T9, Canada

An Introduction to the Principles of Disease   ISBN   0-7216-9114-5

Last digit is the print number: 9   8   7   6   5   4

To Elizabeth

PREFACE

The aim of *An Introduction to the Principles of Disease* is to initiate the student into clinical medicine via the study of pathology. In the past such an approach has been successful in the training of physicians; recently, attempts to deviate from this course have not been particularly popular or successful. Although pathology has often been likened to the basis or roots of medicine, efforts to make students study it in great detail before venturing into clinical medicine have also been unpopular. This lack of enthusiasm for an in-depth study of pathology is quite understandable: Does any tree develop a full root system before embarking on the exciting experiment of sending a shoot toward the sky? Pathology and clinical medicine must be closely associated: This introduction to disease is intended to be no more than a primer in the study of medicine. No prior knowledge of medicine is assumed, but the reader should have had some instruction in biology, chemistry, human anatomy, and physiology.

Part I of this book describes the general principles of disease and the disorders that affect the body as a whole. Part II concentrates on diseases of individual organs. The objective has been to describe important mechanisms of diseases in considerable detail and to omit any reference to rare conditions. This book is not a synopsis of pathology; consequently, readers who are aiming for a degree in medicine will have to graduate to the larger texts of clinical medicine and pathology before attaining their objective.

The complexity and ever-increasing cost of providing medical care has led to a reappraisal of the role of the medical doctor. In the past, it was expected that physicians would assume absolute responsibility for the diagnosis and treatment of their patients. No longer can this view be upheld. Physicians must now rely on the competence of coworkers not trained as medical practitioners, but whose specialized knowledge is of vital importance in the diagnosis and treatment of patients. Nurses, midwives, physical therapists, pharmacists, and medical technologists are among this group of workers in the allied health sciences for whom this book has been written.

When studying medicine for the first time, the student meets many new words and concepts. An attempt has been made in this book to define these items when they are first introduced so that learning can proceed by a series of progressive steps. Little attempt has been made to avoid the specialized terminology of medicine, because this technical language is widely used in medical practice. If used correctly, it acts as a type of shorthand by which medical personnel can express their ideas by either the spoken or the written word. Without learning the language of medicine, one finds it difficult to converse with a physician or to comprehend the medical literature. The medical student and allied health worker must be able to do both. In an effort to encourage independent thought by the reader, each chapter ends with a list of selected readings in which further details or different views can be found.

ACKNOWLEDGMENTS

The production of this book would have been greatly delayed and extremely difficult without the cooperation of Churchill Livingstone of Edinburgh; Mr Robert Duncan has generously allowed me to use material from their publication *General Pathology*, which I coauthored with Dr. Martin Israel. Over 40 illustrations have been taken from this source. Dr. Israel reviewed the manuscript, and I am deeply indebted to him for his many valuable suggestions. A number of illustrations are taken from *Principles of Pathology for Dental Students*, also published by Churchill Livingstone. I thank my other coauthor, Margaret Grundy (née Hamilton), for permitting me to use this material as well as for her assistance in the section devoted to disorders of the mouth.

I owe special gratitude to those who have given me pictorial material or who have allowed me to modify their original published work. The source of material is detailed in the caption of each figure. I am particularly grateful to the following: Dr. Y. C. Bedard, for providing many electron micrographs; Dr. J. B. Cullen, for his help in providing pictures of autopsy and surgical material from the Toronto General Hospital; Dr. P. Stuart, for pictures of intestinal parasites; Dr. N. B. Rewcastle, for many of the illustrations in the chapter on the nervous system; and Micheline Fauvel, for her excellent electron micrographs of viruses.

A number of figures (also appearing in *General Pathology*) are of specimens from the Welcome Museum of Pathology, Royal College of Surgeons of England, London; I am grateful to the President and the Council of the Royal College of Surgeons of England for permission to reproduce these illustrations. In accordance with the wishes of the council, each specimen is acknowledged at the end of the caption and the catalogue number of each is indicated. Some specimens are from the Boyd Museum, University of Toronto, and I thank Dr. E. Farber of that institution for permission to use these.

I am indebted to a number of colleagues for providing valuable criticism and for assisting in the areas of their particular expertise: Dr. G. T. Simone (electron microscopy), Dr. Agnes Reicher (diseases of the skin), Dr. Susan Ritchie (diseases of the kidney and liver), Dr. J. S. Speakman (diseases of the eye), and Dr. A. W. P. Van Nostrand (diseases of the ear).

I owe special gratitude to Mrs. Sonja Duda, librarian at the Banting Institute, for valuable help in checking and obtaining references, and to several secretaries, particularly Barbara Demchyshyn and Sandra Cox, for expert secretarial assistance. Members of the photographic department of the Toronto General Hospital as well as Harold Lane of the North York General Hospital have provided valuable photographic assistance. Margot Mackay and other members of the Department of Art as Applied to Medicine, University of Toronto, have provided most of the diagrams that appear in this book.

As with many other authors, my greatest debt is to my family. My wife Elizabeth, my son Anthony, and my daughter Susan, between them have read most of the proofs and have provided ideas and diagrams when most needed.

Finally, it is a pleasure to acknowledge the help of W. B. Saunders Company: in particular, Walter Bailey, who stimulated me to write this book; Brian C. Decker, who guided it to completion in record time; and Theresa M. Linietsky, whose skillful editing is apparent on every page.

JOHN B. WALTER
Toronto, Ontario, Canada

CONTENTS

Part II.
DISEASES OF INDIVIDUAL ORGANS

INTRODUCTION

Chapter 1

After studying this chapter the student should be able to:

- Define the terms *sign, symptom, lesion, etiology, pathogenesis, syndrome, idiopathic, biopsy, thoracotomy,* and *laparotomy.*
- List the units of measurement used in microscopy.
- Compare and contrast the techniques and value of light microscopy with those of electron microscopy with respect to (a) resolution, (b) magnification, (c) ease of studying living cells, (d) thickness of tissue sections used, and (e) methods of staining.
- Describe the major steps in the preparation of a paraffin-wax section and the appearance of cells when stained with hematoxylin and eosin (H & E).
- Describe the main uses in pathology of phase contrast and dark ground illumination in microscopy.
- Discuss the advantages that the frozen section technique has over the paraffin-wax technique.
- Give examples of the use of radioactive isotopes in clinical medicine and in experimental pathology.
- Distinguish between cell culture and organ culture.

2

Introduction

The majority of persons seeking medical help do so because of some abnormality causing them distress. Often such *symptoms* can be dispelled by simple remedies—quite often by reassurance. Much of medicine is an art, which its practitioners—whether they be doctors, dentists, nurses, or physical therapists—must learn. Nevertheless, there have always been individuals who were not content simply to observe disease and the effects of time-honored remedies upon it. They have attempted to describe and record the abnormalities in their patients in an objective manner; by introducing measurements, they initiated the science called *pathology.*

Disease itself is as difficult to define as is the normal, from which it is a departure. As generally used, the term "disease" is employed to describe a state in which there is a sufficient departure from the normal for *signs* or *symptoms* to be produced. A symptom is an abnormality noted by the patient. A sign is one noted by another observer. The objective variations from the normal are called *lesions*, and although the term generally refers to structural changes, it may also be used to describe functional abnormalities, such as biochemical lesions (see Chapter 4). The theory of the cause of a disease is its *etiology,* and the development of the lesions is its *pathogenesis.* When used strictly, these two terms are quite separate entities, but in practice they are often used interchangeably. Thus, it is commonly said that the cause of a heart attack is blockage of a diseased coronary artery (arteriosclerosis). Nevertheless, the cause of this may be some genetic defect or an abnormality in the diet. Thus, the coronary disease is merely part of the pathogenesis of the whole picture.

The great advances in bacteriology that started at the end of the nineteenth century fostered the concept that each disease had a single cause. To state that the common wart is always caused by a particular virus is true; nevertheless, this is an incomplete statement. It is known that some patients with multiple warts have a deficient immunity that either can be inherited or can be acquired by administration of drugs. Which is the cause of the warts—the virus or the impaired immunity? Present doctrine would still favor the organism, but the genetic or acquired immunological deficiency would be labeled a major predisposing factor. Multiple causes are probably much more common than we think. The doctrine of one cause for one disease has certainly failed to be a profitable concept in the search for the etiology of many common diseases such as cancer, arteriosclerosis, emphysema, and chronic bronchitis. Nevertheless, the concept that each disease is an entity implies a specific cause for each.

To avoid the difficulty of defining disease the term *syndrome* has been introduced. A syndrome is a condition having a defined collection of lesions,

3

signs, or symptoms that are not necessarily always due to the same agent. Thus, Raynaud's syndrome is a condition in which the hands are unduly susceptible to cold, and on exposure become pale and finally blue and painful. This syndrome can be found in patients with systemic lupus erythematosus (see Chapter 27), it may be seen in workers who use pneumatic hammers, and finally it can occur for no apparent reason. When the cause is unknown, the condition is said to be *idiopathic.* Clearly, those conditions that are commonly labeled "diseases," and in which the cause is not known, are difficult to distinguish from syndromes. Indeed, the terms "syndrome" and "disease" are frequently used quite indiscriminately and interchangeably.

Pathology is thus the scientific study of disease. It describes the cause, course, and termination of disease as well as the nature of its lesions. In almost all diseases the lesions are of varying nature and may be morphological, chemical, or functional. Nevertheless, anything that can be measured is within the domain of pathology. The height of the blood pressure, the rate of the heart beat, and the temperature of the patient are all valued measurements. If they are accurately recorded, they are as scientific as measurements of the size of a nucleus or of the amount of DNA that it contains. The remainder of this chapter is devoted to a brief account of the methods of investigation that can be employed.

Microscopy

THE LIGHT MICROSCOPE

The application of the compound light microscope to the examination of biological material was one of the most important steps ever taken in scientific medicine. From it stemmed the concept that all living organisms are composed of cells and cell products. The light microscope is now routinely used in the examination of diseased tissue; *histopathology* is the study of changes in diseased tissue.

The ability to distinguish two closely placed points is called the *resolving power* of the microscope. When light is used, it is limited by the wavelength of the light beam used. With the light microscopes currently available, the resolving power is about 250 nm.* One of the great advantages of the electron microscope is that its resolution is much greater; in fact, it is about 0.5 nm. The maximum magnification obtainable with light microscopes of current design is about 1200. Further magnification is useless, since it merely produces a large but indistinct image that is due to the limited resolution obtainable.

Living tissue is transparent, and the homogeneity in optical density of its components hides its detailed structure. Staining techniques must therefore be employed. Unfortunately, staining almost invariably means that the cells must be dead. Nevertheless, there are two special techniques, having limited specific uses, which can be employed to visualize living cells.

---

*1 mm = 1000 μm (micrometers or microns); 1 μm = 1000 nm; 1 nm = 10Å (Ångström units). The present tendency is to dispense with the Ångström unit and use the nanometers (nm) instead. It is useful to remember that most cocci (*e.g., Staphylococcus aureus*) are about 1 μm in diameter, a normal red cell is about 7 μm in diameter, and most nuclei are 5 to 10 μm in diameter.

Dark ground illumination relies upon the fact that objects placed in a beam of light may be seen by the light they reflect in much the same way that dust particles are rendered visible by a shaft of sunlight. Using a special sub-stage condenser, this method finds particular application in the demonstration of the organism responsible for syphilis, *Treponema pallidum,* which is regularly demonstrated in venereal disease clinics by this method.

Phase contrast microscopy takes advantage of the different refractive indices of various parts of the cell. These differences are converted into differences in optical density. In this way, living cells can be examined, and the method may be applied in virology where thin sheets of cells in culture can be seen and the effect of viruses on them examined (Figs. 12–4, 12–7, and 12–8).

For the routine examination of tissue, the material must be processed and then sectioned into thin slices. The two methods available, the paraffin section technique and the frozen section technique, are described later in this chapter. Human tissue for histopathological studies is obtained in three ways:

1. SIMPLE BIOPSY. This entails the removal of a small piece of living tissue for examination. With skin lesions, this can be done easily under the anesthesia produced by the local injection of 1 or 2 per cent Xylocaine solution. Biopsy through an endoscope is an extension of this method, *e.g.,* bronchoscopy for lung lesions, and cystoscopy for bladder lesions. Solid tissues like liver, spleen, and tumors can be examined by needle biopsy; a core of tissue is obtained with this technique.

2. BIOPSY AT OPERATION. An operation is occasionally performed specifically to obtain a biopsy. Thus *thoracotomy* (opening the chest wall) is used to diagnose some diffuse lung lesions not readily examined by needle biopsy. *Laparotomy* (opening the peritoneal cavity) is a necessary prelude to the biopsy of abdominal lesions and is generally followed by some definitive treatment.

3. NECROPSY. Necropsy provides abundant tissue for histopathological study, but unfortunately postmortem autolysis (Chapter 4) often limits detailed examination.

Paraffin Section Technique. This is the most commonly used routine method of examination. Fresh tissue is placed as soon as possible in *fixative,* generally a 10 per cent solution of formalin. It can remain in this solution for many months without deteriorating. Fixation renders many cell constituents insoluble, and it also inhibits enzymatic action. Blocks no thicker than 2 mm are prepared, *dehydrated* in graded alcohol, *cleared* in xylol, chloroform, or some other solvent that is miscible in both alcohol and wax, *impregnated* with molten paraffin wax, and finally when cooled, are blocked out or *embedded* in paraffin wax. From the block obtained in this way 5-μm sections are *cut* on a microtome (Fig. 1–1).

When mounted on glass slides the sections must be stained to render tissue components visible. The commonly used stains are *hematoxylin and eosin* (H & E). Hematoxylin is a blue basic dye obtained from the bark of a South American tree. It is taken up by acidic substances in the cell. Hence, the nucleus with its nucleic acid content is stained blue. Eosin is a red synthetic acidic dye that binds to basic proteins found for the most part in cytoplasm. H & E stained sections are used routinely for diagnostic purposes.

FIGURE 1-1. *The rotary microtome.*

When the wheel (W) is rotated, the chuck holding the paraffin-embedded tissue (T) moves up and down against the knife. With each rotation the tissue advances 5 μm, and a thin section is obtained. Each section adheres to the previous one so that a ribbon of sections is formed.

Histochemistry. H & E and many other staining techniques used in histopathology have been discovered empirically (Fig. 1–2). Others have been developed with the intention of demonstrating specific chemicals in tissue. The technique is called *histochemistry,* and the Prussian blue reaction for hemosiderin may be cited as an example (Fig. 1–3). Acid is applied to a section and releases Fe^{+++} from hemosiderin, a breakdown product of hemoglobin. Next potassium ferrocyanide is applied; this reacts with the Fe^{+++} to form blue insoluble ferric ferrocyanide. Other methods have been devised for detecting enzymes in cells.

Frozen Section Technique. The *cryostat* is an instrument consisting of a microtome within a refrigerator. Tissue is frozen and cut in this solid state when embedded in a block of ice. The technique has several advantages over the paraffin-wax technique:

1. Frozen sections can be prepared and stained within two or three

FIGURE 1-3. *Section stained for hemosiderin by the prussian blue method.*

The section shows massive deposition of hemosiderin in liver cells. The pigment is stained brilliant blue by this method but appears black in the photograph. The detailed structure of the liver cells is not well shown. This tissue was from a patient with hemochromatosis, a type of cirrhosis of the liver associated with deposition of iron pigments (× 600).

FIGURE 1–2. *Detection of calcification in tissue sections.*

This section of kidney has been stained by the von Kóssa method, which employs silver nitrate. Black insoluble metallic silver is precipitated at sites of phosphate and carbonate deposition. In practice these are always laid down as calcium salts, and the method is used to detect areas of calcification. Other deposits (e.g., urates) are sometimes stained; the method, although useful, is somewhat empirical. The tissue is from a patient with a high blood level of calcium (hypercalcemia). Note the deposits of calcium in the wall of an arteriole (Art) entering a functioning glomerulus (G), in a shrunken glomerulus (g), and in the basement membrane (Bm) of many of the renal tubules.

FIGURE 1–3. *See legend on opposite page.*

minutes. Hence, a diagnosis can be given rapidly during the course of an operation. Some hospital laboratories use this method routinely, so that all surgical material can be examined immediately and the surgeon advised as to the nature of the lesions he encounters and the extent of any disease process, *e.g.*, the extent of the spread of a cancer. The quality of frozen sections does not equal that of the routine paraffin sections, but the technique provides for a rapid diagnosis and often saves the patient from having to be operated on a second time.

2. The paraffin-wax technique removes lipids from cells and tissues. These substances are retained in the frozen section technique and can be stained specifically.

3. Frozen sections contain the active enzymes present in the cell, and these can be detected histochemically.

4. The frozen section technique causes little protein denaturation. Specific proteins, such as antigens and immunoglobulins, can be detected by immunological procedures (Fig. 9–13).

THE ELECTRON MICROSCOPE

Transmission Electron Microscope. This instrument resembles the ordinary microscope except that a stream of electrons is used instead of light, and electromagnetic fields replace the glass lenses. The theoretical resolving power is in the order of 0.005 nm. In practice, most instruments have a working resolving power of approximately 0.5 nm and magnifications of up to 500,000 are possible. The electron microscope has revealed cell structure in minute detail, but it has many disadvantages. It is expensive and needs constant expert maintenance. The blocks of tissue for electron microscopy must be small (1 to 2 mm in size) and embedded in an epoxy resin. Sections that are 50 to 60 nm thick are cut on a microtome with a glass or diamond knife; the technique is not easy. Finally, the sections are placed on a copper grid and examined in the vacuum of the column of the electron microscope (Fig. 1–4). The tremendous magnification available is impressive, but it does cut down the field of view by

FIGURE 1–4. *Transmission electron micrograph showing the medulla of a hemolymph node of a rat.*

The tissue was fixed in osmium tetroxide solution, and the section was then treated with lead hydroxide. Since these metals are electron-dense, they are used as stains in electron microscopy.

Hemolymph nodes differ from the usual type of lymph node present in humans in that red cells are present in the sinuses. This picture shows two sinuses, S_1 and S_2, which are separated by a thin medullary cord (MC) containing a capillary (Cap) and macrophages (Ma) to which many red blood cells (rbc) are adherent. In the cytoplasm of the macrophages there are many phagosomes representing degradation products of red cells. In S_1, red cells in groups appear to be free. On closer examination, however, they are partially surrounded by pseudopods of macrophages (large arrows). The medullary cords are covered by sinus endothelial cells (E) between which the macrophages push out pseudopodia to entrap the red cells. The macrophages and lymphocyte (Lym) seen at the top of the picture are in one of the trabeculae that cross the sinus (× 2400). (From Nopajaroonsri, C., Luk, S. C., and Simon, G. T.: The structure of the hemolymph node—a light, transmission, and scanning electron microscopic study. Journal of Ultrastructure Research, *48*:325–341, 1974.)

FIGURE 1–4. *See legend on opposite page.*

a similar dimension. In addition, although the image in the electron microscope can be seen on a fluorescent screen, any detailed examination must be done by taking photographic pictures. Electron microscopy therefore is a highly specialized technique that is very time consuming. It can be used for specific research or diagnostic purposes, but not for routine tissue examination.

Viruses can be seen with ease by the electron microscope; it is in this field that the instrument has really great diagnostic capability. Thus, occasionally cases are encountered in which the clinician cannot on clinical grounds distinguish between a diagnosis of chickenpox and smallpox. If the patient has recently returned from an area where smallpox is endemic, the possibility of this disease is a very real one, and the distinction is of vital importance for the health of the community. An electron microscopist can distinguish between the two diseases within a few minutes of receiving tissue from the skin lesions (see Chapter 12).

Scanning Electron Microscope. This instrument works on a different principle from the conventional transmission electron microscopy: a very fine beam of electrons is focused to a point and made to scan the surface of a specimen. Secondary electrons scattered from the surface are collected and amplified. The current so generated is used to modulate the brightness of a television tube that is scanned in synchronicity with the electron beam scanning the object. With this method for examining the surfaces of objects, the pictures so

FIGURE 1–5. *Scanning electron micrograph of a hemolymph node of the rat.*

Trabeculae (arrow) are seen crossing a sinus. Grapelike groups of red cells (asterisks) are present around macrophages in the medullary sinus. Compare this picture with Figure 1–4, noting the difference in magnification (× 1300). (From Luk, S. C., Nopajaroonsri, C., and Simon, G. T.: The architecture of the normal lymph node and hemolymph node. Laboratory Investigation, *29*:258–265, 1973. © 1973 U.S.-Canadian Division of the International Academy of Pathology.)

obtained have a remarkable three-dimensional appearance (Fig. 1–5). Microorganisms, red cells, the lung, sinuses of the spleen, and the surface of the intestinal mucosa have all been studied with advantage by this technique.

Radioactive Isotopes

Radioactive isotopes are treated by living cells in the same way as the normal elements. Their radiation can be detected by suitable counters, and they may usefully be employed as labels in a wide range of fields. Clinically, the greatest breakthrough in this area has been the introduction of the man-made

FIGURE 1–6. *Bone scan showing tumor of the right tibia in a 15-year-old boy.*

See Case History 1 for complete description of case.

element *technetium.* This element emits gamma radiation only, and is therefore safer to use than isotopes that emit other more damaging radiation. It has a half-life of six hours. When injected intravenously with pyrophosphate, technetium is selectively taken up by bone, probably by the osteoid tissue. Using this technique, the whole skeleton can be surveyed, and the method now augments radiography in the detection of bony lesions, particularly tumors (Fig. 1–6). If the technetium is attached to aggregated albumin, it becomes concentrated in the lung; an estimate of blood flow through this organ is then obtained. By various techniques, it is now possible to scan many other organs. It is particularly useful in investigating lesions of the liver and thyroid. In the past, thyroid function has been investigated by estimating the distribution of an administered dose of radioactive iodine, but this has now been replaced by the technetium technique. Many other radioactive techniques are used in medicine; for example, radioactive chromium can be attached to red cells and the length of their survival estimated (see Chapter 26).

Case History I (See Figure 1–6).   The patient was a 15-year-old boy who complained of pain and swelling of the right leg. About one year prior to seeking medical aid he noticed aching of the leg after skiing or skating. He paid little attention to this, but he noticed the aching gradually became severe and continuous. About three months previously he first noticed a swelling. On examination a slightly tender swelling over the midshaft of the right tibia was the only abnormality detected. A radiograph revealed a bony defect in the region; a provisional diagnosis of primary bone tumor was made. Secondary cancer could have produced a similar picture, but this condition is very uncommon at this age. The figure shows a technetium bone scan; the increased activity in the region of the tumor is obvious. Note also the increased activity over the ends of the long bones, particularly at the knee, wrist, and upper ends of the humeri. This is due to epiphyseal bone growth in this 15-year-old boy. A chest radiograph and a liver scan revealed no evidence of metastatic tumor (see Chapter 17). A biopsy of the tumor revealed osteosarcoma. An above-knee amputation was performed. The boy adapted well to the procedure but shortly afterwards developed a wound infection from *Staphylococcus aureus.* Three months after the amputation a sinus was excised, and a 2-inch section of femur was removed so that a better stump could be fashioned. The wound healed well, and the patient was able to walk. He remains well 14 months after diagnosis. Nevertheless, the prognosis must be guarded, since less than 20 per cent of patients survive for more than five years following treatment. This case illustrates two other important features: (1) Noninvasive investigations such as a bone scan are carried out before invasive procedures such as biopsy; and (2) radical surgery for malignant disease should never be undertaken without first obtaining a definite tissue diagnosis.

AUTORADIOGRAPHY

Radioactive isotopes can be used at a microscopic level. If a section of tissue is placed on a photographic film for a suitable time, subsequent photographic development will reveal the site of isotope localization as a series of black grains. This principle is often applied in experimental pathology; for example, it is found that tritiated thymidine (thymidine containing tritium, the radioactive isotope of hydrogen) is incorporated into DNA in the same way as ordinary thymidine. DNA synthesis and therefore mitotic activity can be investigated by this technique (Fig. 1–7).

A

B

FIGURE 1–7. *Autoradiograph of a mitotic figure in a squash preparation of the root tip of an onion fed with tritiated thymidine.*

A, Photographed at the level of the section to show the chromosomes. *B,* The same cell photographed at the level of the photographic emulsion. The labeled thymidine has been taken up by the cell and incorporated into DNA. Note how the silver dots correspond to the chromosomes. This technique is used to locate the sites of DNA synthesis during the period when the labeled thymidine was available (× 3200). (Photographs courtesy of Dr. P. B. Gahan.)

Tissue Culture

Tissues of various types can be cultured outside the body with comparative ease. Growth commonly occurs on the surface of glass or plastic, and tissues can be grown in test tubes, medicine-flat bottles, or the surface of a coverslip.

There are two types of tissue culture:

Cell Culture. If isolated cells of an organ or tissue (or portions of a tissue) are placed in a tissue culture medium, individual cells grow as a flat sheet on the surface of the container. This is an extremely important technique in virology, because viruses can be grown in the cultivated cells (see Chapter 12). Its use for other purposes, such as in cancer research, has proved disappointing, because the cells are growing in a highly artificial medium and often do not carry out the specific functions of the organ from which they were isolated. Sometimes enzyme studies on human cells have shed light on genetic enzyme defects seen in some diseases (see Chapter 3).

Organ Culture.   A fragment of tissue is grown on a grid, so that there is no cellular outgrowth, but histologically the organ is kept as normal as possible. Limb buds, eye rudiments, and bones have been studied while growing in an artificial medium, and their differentiation has been observed.

Chemical and Physical Analysis of Biological Materials

Chemical technology has now advanced to the stage at which it is possible to analyze substances as complex as the insulin molecule and the ribonuclease molecule, the latter containing 124 amino acid residues. X-ray diffraction techniques have revealed the complex folded structure of a large molecule such as myoglobin. Apart from these research applications, modern methods of chemical analysis combined with automation now make it possible to estimate a large number of chemical substances in the small quantity of body fluids, *e.g.*, blood. With the SMA-12 AutoAnalyzer, which is routinely used, it is currently possible to estimate 12 substances from a single sample of blood, *e.g.*, sodium, potassium, chloride, blood urea nitrogen, glucose, etc.* In many centers, this biochemical analysis *(biochemical profile)* is now performed routinely in much the same way that the pulse has been taken and the blood pressure recorded for many years.

The separation and identification of proteins have been greatly facilitated by the technique of electrophoresis, which is illustrated in Figure 25–1.

As more and more complex techniques become available and adapted to medical use, there is a tendency to regard patients as objects for the academic exercise of investigation and scientific treatment. Batteries of investigations are ordered and abnormalities are treated. This can lead to disastrous results, because every test has its limitations: experimental errors, biological variations, and significance under particular circumstances, all of which must be taken into consideration. The patient must be treated as an individual and not dehumanized by the modern medical center. Too often one hears of a patient failing to respond to treatment and then dying. The truth is that the wrong treatment was applied through miscalculations on the part of the medical attendants. Alternatively, no effective treatment was available. Blame the practice of medicine but not the patient!

Review Questions

1. Describe the basis for the use of hematoxylin and eosin as histological stains. How would you expect the following cells to appear when stained with H & E?
   (a) Mature red cells, which have no nuclei, and cytoplasm that contains basic proteins.
   (b) Reticulocytes, which are young red cells but differ in that the cytoplasm also contains threads or strands rich in ribonucleic acid (RNA).

---

*The others usually estimated are serum glutamic-oxaloacetic transaminase (SGOT), lactic dehydrogenase (LDH), alkaline phosphatase, bilirubin, calcium, phosphate, and uric acid.

(c) Plasma cells, which are nucleated, and whose cytoplasm contains basic protein as well as some RNA.

(d) Thyroid cells whose cytoplasm contains basic protein but very little RNA.

2. The fate of ingested potassium iodide is to be investigated. A number of rats are given a dose of radioactive iodine in the form of potassium iodide. How would you attempt to follow the absorption, utilization, and excretion of the labeled iodine?

3. The frozen section technique is an essential component of a modern laboratory service. Discuss the use of this technique from the viewpoint of the surgeon, the patient, and the pathologist.

4. Define the following terms: (a) biochemical profile, (b) histopathology, (c) histochemistry, (d) resolution, as applied to microscopy.

Selected Readings

Champion, R. H., Gillman, T., Rook, A. J., and Sims, R. T.: An Introduction to the Biology of the Skin. Oxford, Blackwell, 1970. Note, in particular, Chapter 4, "Some Tinctorial and Cytochemical Methods," which is a simple account of the principles underlying the action of common fixatives and stains.

Ham, A. W.: Histology. 7th ed. Philadelphia, J. B. Lippincott Company, 1974. Chapters 1 and 2 elaborate on many of the topics covered in this chapter.

Leeson, C. R., and Leeson, T. S.: Histology. 3rd ed. Philadelphia, W. B. Saunders Company, 1976. Note, in particular, Chapter 1, which provides basic information on microscopy, tissue preparation, examination of sections and stains.

Chapter 2

After studying this chapter the student should be able to:

- Distinguish epithelial cells from connective tissue cells with respect to their structure and function.
- Describe the structure of the plasma membrane and list its functions.
- Draw a diagram of a typical epithelial cell and include its nucleus, nucleolus, mitochondria, lysosomes, glycogen granules, endoplasmic reticulum, and Golgi apparatus.
- Describe the important functions of each of the organelles.
- Relate the structure of DNA to chromosomes and genes.
- Draw a diagram to show how the information of DNA is utilized in the formation of protein.

NORMAL STRUCTURE AND FUNCTION

- ● Describe how gene action is controlled.
- ● List the kinds of information that can be learned about the chromosomes and their arrangement from an examination of:
    - (a) nuclear morphology
    - (b) nuclear function
    - (c) the Barr body
    - (d) the Y body.
- ● Describe the two components of the endoplasmic reticulum and relate them to lysosomes and the Golgi apparatus in terms of both structure and function.
- ● Describe the components of the ground substance.
- ● Describe collagen fibers with respect to their
    - (a) distribution in the body
    - (b) appearances under the light microscope and the transmission electron microscope
    - (c) relationship to reticulin
    - (d) chemical composition
    - (e) formation.
- ● Describe the cell cycle and the phases of mitosis.

Introduction

The human body is formed from the division of the fertilized ovum. The process of division, *mitosis*, is described later in this chapter. It results in the formation of two daughter cells, each of which closely resembles the original. Nevertheless, as division follows division, the daughter cells can exhibit new or altered structure and function. This process is called *differentiation* or *maturation*. The first evidence of differentiation in the mass of cells of the developing embryo is the formation of three distinct germ layers. An outer layer of cells forms the *ectoderm*, while a tube develops within the mass and the cells lining it form the *endoderm*. This tube forms the basis of the future alimentary canal and organs that bud from it — lungs, liver, pancreas, and others. The *mesoderm* consists of cells lying between the ectoderm and the endoderm.

The primitive cells of each germ layer can differentiate along two separate lines — forming either epithelium or connective tissue.

Epithelial cells cover surfaces (*e.g.*, skin) or line cavities (*e.g.*, the mouth); in these situations they are essentially protective in function. Covering epithelia may also perform a secretory function: the intestinal and respiratory epithelia, for instance, secrete mucus (Figs. 2–1 and 2–2).

FIGURE 2–1. *Small intestine.*

This photomicrograph shows part of the muscle coat (M) covered by the mucosa. Between the muscle coat and the mucosa there is a layer of loose connective tissue called the submucosa (Sm). The picture is typical of a slide prepared by the paraffin-wax technique and stained with hematoxylin and eosin (× 50).

In addition to covering surfaces, the secretory type of epithelium may be arranged to form solid glands. Thus, hollow buds of endodermal cells form masses that subsequently differentiate into liver, pancreas, salivary gland, and other similar structures. Likewise, buds from the ectoderm form sweat glands and breast tissue. The secretory cells are arranged around a central cavity to form acini into which the secretion is poured (Fig. 2–3). From here the secretion passes into collecting ducts and reaches the epithelial surface from which the gland originated. In some glands the connection with the epithelial surface is lost, the duct disappears, and secretion takes place directly into the blood stream. Such secreting organs are the *endocrine glands;* even in these, although no secretion is collected into ducts, acinar spaces may be formed. This effect is clearly seen in the normal thyroid (Fig. 39–3). A feature common to all epithelial cells is that they are closely contiguous with one another. This struc-

FIGURE 2–2. *Mucosa of the small intestine.*

The mucosa is covered by an epithelium composed of a single layer of tall columnar cells, some of which secrete mucus. More detail of these cells is shown in Figures 2–7 and 2–8. The absorptive surface is increased by the folds, or villi, which project into the lumen of the gut. Simple tubular glands (G) open into the crypts (Cy). Beneath the epithelium, the mucosa consists of connective tissue containing thin fibers of collagen, associated fibroblasts, and blood vessels. There is a sparse infiltration by small round cells, most of which are lymphocytes or plasma cells. It is not possible to identify individual cells at this magnification. The thin layer of muscle of the mucosa, the muscularis mucosae (MM), is seen in the lower part of the picture (× 200).

FIGURE 2–3. *Normal pancreas.*

The exocrine portion of the gland is composed of secretory epithelial cells arranged in groups or acini (Ac), each of which has a central lumen into which the secretion is poured (the lumina cannot be seen at this magnification). Secretion is collected into small ducts, and these drain into larger ducts and finally into a main pancreatic duct. The endocrine portion of the gland forms a small portion of the pancreas and is represented in this figure by one islet of Langerhans, which has no acini or duct. The connective tissue of the gland is represented by small blood vessels (Bv) and a collagenous stroma, scanty between the acini, but more obvious around the duct (Col) (× 250).

tural feature is evident on light microscopy, and even under the electron microscope the cells appear to be separated by only a thin layer of electron-dense material that is about 15 nm in width.

Connective tissue cells are the other cell type present in the body. They are usually widely separated from each other by a zone containing ground substance in which fibers are embedded. *Collagen fibers* are the most abundant, but in some areas (*e.g.*, the walls of large arteries) *elastic fibers* are also present. This type of connective tissue—typified by tendon, bone, cartilage, and fibrous tissue—is primarily supportive in function. Other connective tissue cells have been endowed with specialized cytoplasm either for *contraction* (muscle fibers) or for *conduction* (nerve cells). It should be noted that while much of the body's connective tissue is derived from mesodermal cells, the mesoderm is also capable of differentiating into epithelium. The kidney and the gonads are mesodermal in origin, and yet they are epithelial in structure. The ectoderm and endoderm tend to differentiate into epithelia; even here, however, there are exceptions. Some of the muscle of the eye is of ectodermal origin. Most of the nervous system, including its glial connective tissue, is derived from ectoderm. Only the microglia are mesodermal.*

The study of the embryological origin of cells and tissues is of some importance in pathology in explaining certain curious phenomena. Thus, in some diseases of the breast, gland structures are found that closely resemble those of the apocrine sweat gland (see Chapter 38). Both sweat glands and breast tissue have a common ectodermal origin. Likewise, tumors can be found in the anterior lobe of the pituitary that closely resemble those found normally in the jaw or skin. The pituitary gland, teeth, and epidermis all have a common ectodermal origin.

The process of differentiation, by which cells become highly specialized, is sometimes accompanied by loss of ability to divide. Thus, neurons are highly specialized and are quite incapable of mitosis as they become differentiated. Nevertheless, in other tissues—liver cells, for instance—the power to divide is never lost. What is lost during the process of maturation is the ability to differentiate along different lines. The fertilized ovum is *totipotent, i.e.*, capable

---

*Because nervous tissue and muscle are so different from ordinary connective tissue, some authorities describe four basic tissues: epithelial, connective, nervous, and muscular. This further subdivision serves little purpose in pathology.

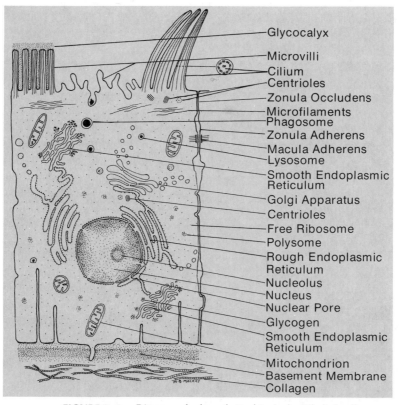

FIGURE 2–4. *Diagram of a hypothetical typical epithelial cell.*

Drawn by Margot Mackay, Department of Art as Applied to Medicine, University of Toronto.)

of producing all the tissues of the body, and its immediate daughter cells have a similar capability. Separation of cells at this early stage results in multiple fetuses with consequent identical twins, triplets, and other such multiple births.

The cells of the body show considerable diversity of structure and function, yet each is remarkably independent. Each receives a supply of oxygen and foodstuff from the blood stream, with which it must produce its own structural components and secretions. Each cell must also release the energy required for mechanical, chemical, or electrical work. It is therefore not surprising that all cells are built upon a similar plan (Fig. 2–4).

The number of chemical reactions known to occur inside the cell is so great that it would be difficult to understand how these could proceed in a structure that appears, under the light microscope, to be so simple. The electron microscope has changed all this; the cell's appearance has been changed from a barren wilderness to that of a structure resembling a large industrial city with its factories, warehouses, streets, and powerhouses (Fig. 2–5).

STRUCTURE OF THE NORMAL CELL

The Plasma Membrane

Each cell is surrounded by a *plasma membrane*, which is composed of a complex protein-lipid combination (Fig. 2–6). The plasma membrane is not a rigid structure and its movement allows for phagocytosis,* a process whereby prolongations of the cell surround particles and envelop them to form a vacuole in which the contents are digested. Likewise, motility of cells is a function of plasma-membrane movement. This is well illustrated by the ameboid movement of the white blood cells.

At an electron microscopic level, small invaginations of the cell membrane can become nipped off to form vesicles. In this way, small quantities of fluid may be imbibed by a process known as micropinocytosis* (Figs. 2–7 and 2–8).

The plasma membrane has other important functions. It contains specific antigens by which the body is able to *recognize* its own cells and tolerate them. The cells from another individual are regarded as aliens and are attacked (see Chapter 9). The cell membrane (another term for "plasma" membrane) is also concerned with *adhesiveness,* which is a factor that induces cells of like constitution to stick together. This property can be well demonstrated experimentally: if the cells of an embryo are separated from each other and then are allowed to come together again under suitable conditions, like cells tend to aggregate to reform organs and tissues. This affinity that cells have for their own kind must be an important mechanism in the development and maintenance of the architecture of multicellular animals. But not all cells behave in this manner. The mature cells of the blood do not stick to each other, and the lack of adhesiveness exhibited by cancer cells allows them to wander off and infiltrate freely into the surrounding tissues. This characteristic allows cancer cells to spread and kill.

---

*It is now common practice to group the processes of "phagocytosis" and "micropinocytosis" under the term "endocytosis."

FIGURE 2-5. *Survey of normal human liver.* (Courtesy of Dr. Y. C. Bedard.)

Parts of six cells are shown (× 10,000). Compare this with Figure 2–4. See Review Questions, No. 4.

FIGURE 2-6. *Diagrammatic representation of the plasma membrane.*

The membrane is shown as a double layer of phospholipid molecules with their hydrophilic (water-loving) ends pointing outward and their hydrophobic (water-hating) ends facing inward. Globular proteins are partially or completely embedded in the lipid. This concept of a fluid lipid bilayer with embedded protein was described by Singer and Nicolson (Science, *175*:720, 1972). It is believed that the carbohydrate side-chains of the protein molecules form the glycocalyx, which is illustrated in Figure 2–8. (Drawn by Margot Mackay, Department of Art as Applied to Medicine, University of Toronto.)

FIGURE 2–7. *Radioautograph of mouse jejunum.*

The mouse was killed one hour after the instillation of radioactive iron in its stomach. The silver grains (arrows) represent radioactive iron that has been absorbed into the cell. The course of this radioactive material can be followed by examining animals killed at different times after being fed with labeled iron. Note the regular arrangement of the microvilli, which form the brush border of light microscopy. This arrangement appears to be adapted for absorption. An endocytotic vesicle is clearly shown (end). A junctional complex with its desmosome (des) is seen near the free border of the two epithelial cells depicted in this illustration. Figure 2–8 shows details of this complex. Mitochondria (m) and rough endoplasmic reticulin (rer) can be identified but are shown more clearly in other figures ($\times$ 28,000). (From Bedard, Y. C.: Ultrastructural and Radiographic Studies on Iron Absorption in the Mouse. University of Toronto Ph.D. Thesis, 1972.)

The cell membrane acts as an *exchange surface* across which cell constituents are interchanged with those of the extracellular fluids. Thus, the cell membrane acts as a chemical barrier as well as a mechanical one, and it is this function which is responsible for the maintenance of the characteristic chemical composition of the interior of the cell. Potassium, magnesium, and phosphate ions are present in high concentration in the cytoplasm. In contrast, the

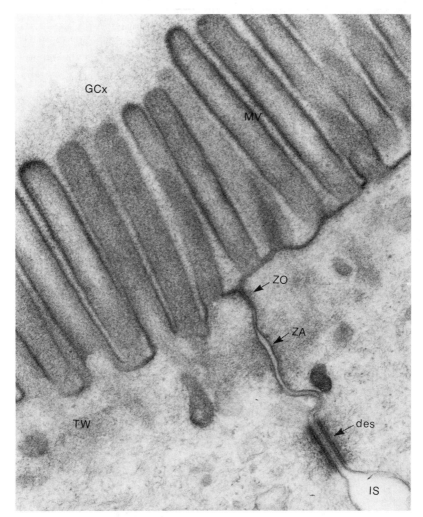

FIGURE 2–8. *Details of the luminal surface of an absorptive cell of the human small intestine.*

The apical cell membrane is thrown into regular microvilli (MV). There is a fuzzy covering, which is termed a *glycocalyx* (GCx). One junctional complex is shown. It consists of three parts: (1) The tight junction, or *zonula occludens* (ZO), which is an area where the plasma membranes of the two adjacent cells appear to fuse. "Zonule" means an encircled band or girdle; the zone forms an effective seal between adjacent cells. It is an area where one cell can communicate with adjacent ones. (2) The *zonula adherens* (ZA), which is an area where the cell membranes are closely applied to each other but are not fused. Filaments of the terminal web are concentrated at this area. (3) The desmosomes or macula adherens (des), which are complex structures and are button-shaped. Numerous microfilaments converge on the desmosomes. Where junctional complexes are not present there is often a space between adjacent cells (IS = intercellular space). (× 112,000). (Photograph courtesy of Dr. Y. C. Bedard.)

extracellular fluids are rich in sodium, chloride, and bicarbonate ions. The cell membrane is able to extrude sodium ions and thereby allows potassium to accumulate within the cell. This mechanism, which is sometimes known as the *sodium pump*, requires energy. The integrity and normal functions of the plasma membrane are therefore important factors in maintaining this special chemical composition of the cell substance. Another interesting feature of the cell membrane is the presence of areas of so-called *cell*, or *surface*, *receptors*. It is to these areas that viruses become attached, and it is at these sites that many substances such as drugs and toxins act. An interesting application of the receptor concept is the supposition that many hormones react with specific receptors on their target cells. The interaction appears to activate an enzyme that leads to the formation of adenosine 3′:5′-cyclic monophosphate, usually referred to as *cyclic AMP*. This substance triggers a sequence of events specific for that cell and leads to its response associated with the hormone. Cyclic AMP is therefore regarded as a *second messenger* acting within the cell (Fig. 2–9).

The Cytoplasm

The *cytoplasm* is that part of the protoplasm not included in the nucleus. It is subdivided into many compartments by membranes that closely resemble the plasma membrane in structure. The most extensive subdivision is effected by the endoplasmic reticulum. The cytoplasm also contains other membrane-bound structures or *organelles, e.g.*, mitochondria and lysosomes.

FIGURE 2–9. *The second-messenger concept.*

Many hormones act first by becoming attached to specific receptor sites on the membranes of target cells. Thus, adrenal cells have receptors that "recognize" adrenocorticotropin. The enzyme adenylate cyclase is activated in the cell membrane and passes into the cytoplasm where it catalyzes the formation of cyclic AMP, which acts as a second messenger. In some cells it leads to enzyme activation. Thus, in the liver, phosphorylase is activated and leads to the formation of glucose from glycogen. This is a mechanism by which epinephrine causes the release of glucose from the liver cell. Cyclic AMP appears to act also by stimulating the expression of genetic information. It may therefore be regarded as a type of chemical switch that turns on the cell to perform specific functions. (Drawn by Anthony J. Walter.)

FIGURE 2–10. *Liver cell showing part of its nucleus (Nuc) and cytoplasmic organelles.*

Mitochondria (m) with their cristae (Cr) are shown along with rough endoplasmic reticulum (rer) to which are attached ribosomes (r). Smooth endoplasmic reticulum (Ser) is associated with glycogen granules (Gly). Some ribosomes appear free in the cytoplasm and are forming rosettes (rr). Note also the nuclear membrane (NucM) surrounding the nucleus ($\times$ 40,000). (Photograph courtesy of Dr. Y. C. Bedard.)

ENDOPLASMIC RETICULUM

This consists of a series of membranes that enclose an intercommunicating series of tubes and vesicles (Fig. 2–10). In most areas, ribosomes are attached to the endoplasmic reticulum, which therefore appears rough; this part is known as the granular or *rough endoplasmic reticulum.* Ribosomes appear as granules 15 nm in diameter, contain ribonucleic acid (RNA), and play a very important part in cell metabolism; it is in relation to them that protein synthesis occurs. Some of the ribosomes are seen lying free within the cytoplasm, and their activity leads to the formation of protein that is retained within the cell for its own requirements. Protein produced for export is synthesized in the rough endoplasmic reticulum. It passes into the Golgi apparatus and leaves the cell as a secretion.

The endoplasmic reticulum and its associated ribosomal granules cannot be distinguished in the ordinary "paraffin" sections used in routine pathology. The ribonucleoprotein content, however, can be distinguished by its basophilia (cells having an affinity for basic dyes) with hematoxylin. It follows that the cytoplasm of cells actively engaged in protein synthesis appears mauve or blue in H & E sections.

In some cells the endoplasmic reticulum also forms a complex lattice of tubules that have no attached ribosomes and therefore appear smooth (Fig. 2–10). The functions of this part of the cell are less clearly defined, but *smooth endoplasmic reticulum* appears to be related to detoxification of drugs as well as to the synthesis of steroid hormones. It should be noted that the membranes of the smooth and rough endoplasmic reticulum are continuous with each other, with the outer lamina of the nuclear membrane, and perhaps also with the plasma membrane.

MITOCHONDRIA

These rod-shaped bodies have a characteristic appearance (Fig. 2–10); their complex internal structure is a reflection of their function. They contain all the enzymes of the Krebs cycle and of the terminal electron transport system. The Krebs cycle, illustrated in Figure 2–11, is a system whereby the prod-

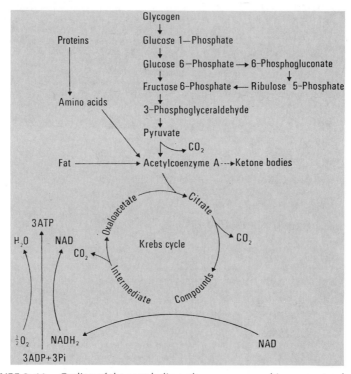

FIGURE 2–11. *Outline of the metabolic pathways concerned in energy production.*

The entire process in the oxidation of glycogen to CO_2 and H_2O can be considered as occurring in two phases. The first, which requires no oxygen (anaerobic), results in the formation of pyruvate and is known as *glycolysis*. The second phase, which requires oxygen (aerobic), is known as the *Krebs cycle*. Products of carbohydrate, fat, and protein metabolism are fed into the Krebs cycle, and the energy generated ultimately appears in the form of ATP. The hexose monophosphate shunt is shown on the right as an alternate pathway and results in the formation of ribulose 5-phosphate. This is an aerobic process and is important in the metabolism of white cells and red cells. Various genetic defects are known that result in hemolytic anemia or incompetent polymorphs, which are unable to destroy bacteria. (Key: NAD, nicotinamide adenine dinucleotide; $NADH_2$, dihydronicotinamide adenine dinucleotide; Pi, inorganic phosphate; ADP, adenosine diphosphate; ATP, adenosine triphosphate.)

FIGURE 2–12. *Liver showing bile canaliculi.*

Parts of three adjacent liver cells are shown; between them are the bile canaliculi, which ultimately drain into the bile duct. Short, irregular microvilli are seen projecting into the lumen. This illustrates how the morphology of the cell surface reflects its function. Compare the microvilli with those of small intestine, where absorption is the major function. One liver cell contains numerous lysosomes (Ly). Also shown are parts of one nucleus (Nuc) with the double-layered nuclear membrane (NucM), glycogen granules (Gly), and mitochondria (m) (×17,500). (Photograph courtesy of Dr. Y. C. Bedard.)

ucts of carbohydrate, fat, and protein metabolism are oxidized to produce energy. The energy is stored in the form of high-energy bonds of adenosine triphosphate (ATP) and is utilized whenever the cell performs any kind of work. The mitochondria are therefore the powerhouses of the cell and are among the first structures to be affected when adverse conditions prevail. An interesting feature of mitochondrial structure is that these bodies also contain some DNA, which appears to replicate during cell division. Some people have held it to indicate that mitochondria originated from symbiotic bacteria.

LYSOSOMES

These are round, membrane-bound bodies containing lytic enzymes that are active at a low pH (Fig. 2–12). Acid phosphatase and various proteolytic enzymes come into this group. The lysosomes cannot normally be seen in paraffin sections, but in certain cells (polymorphonuclear leukocytes, for instance) the lysosomes are visible as the characteristic granules. Particles ingested by a cell during the process of phagocytosis appear as membrane-bound bodies, and fusion with lysosomes results in these vacuoles' acquiring digested enzymes. Lysosomes are therefore important as a source of the enzymes necessary for digestion of phagocytosed material. Likewise, when parts of a cell wear out or are damaged, they also are enclosed in lysosomal bodies. Such lysosomes containing remnants of degenerate cell structure are called *cytolysosomes,* or *autophagocytic vacuoles.* Release of lysosomal enzymes from dead cells plays an important part in the digestion of dead material. Under some circumstances these enzymes can damage living tissue (see Chapter 5).

GOLGI COMPLEX (GOLGI APPARATUS)

The Golgi complex, which is best developed in glandular cells and is usually situated close to the nucleus on the side nearest to the lumen, consists of a series of flattened sacs and small vesicles. The Golgi complex appears to be responsible for packaging proteins in membrane-bound vacuoles. Thus, in secreting cells, such as those in the pancreas, secretions formed in the endoplasmic reticulum collect in the Golgi complex, and the vesicles so formed are then discharged onto the cell surface. Likewise, lysosomes are probably assembled in the Golgi complex, and the completed packages of enzymes are pinched off as membrane-bound organelles (Fig. 2–13).

Lipoprotein synthesis occurs in the Golgi complex, and its vacuoles can migrate to the cell surface and fuse with the plasma membrane. Damaged membrane can be replaced and new membrane formed.

OTHER STRUCTURES

High-resolution electron microscopy has revealed many other structures in the cell cytoplasm. Among these are small tubular structures called *microtubules,* which in some cells appear to act as an internal skeleton and to give the cell rigidity. These structures are called *neurotubules* in the axons of nerve cells; possibly, these microtubules act as means of transport from one part of the cell to another. Microtubules form the spindle in mitosis and are components of cilia. Thus, they are concerned with movement. *Microfilaments* are thin filaments found in all cells and are adapted for special function in certain situations. They form the *tonofilaments* of epidermal cells and the *myofilaments* of muscle. Other structures seen in cells are glycogen granules, fat droplets, and specialized granules in secreting cells. As refinements in the electron microscope have allowed for increased resolution further structures have been described. In many instances their function is poorly understood, but there is little doubt that in due course, the ultrastructure of cells will prove to be very complex—as complex as life itself.

The Nucleus

Situated within the cell and enclosed by a membrane is the nucleus, an important structure because it contains in chemical form the coded information

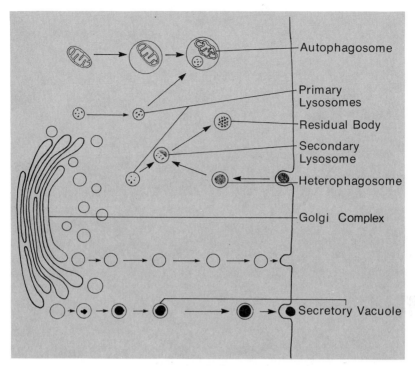

FIGURE 2-13. *The Golgi complex (Golgi apparatus) and its possible functions.*

This diagram depicts the Golgi complex as a series of flattened sacs from which numerous vacuoles arise. Some vacuoles contain secretory material that has been synthesized in the endoplasmic reticulum. Some vacuoles appear to be empty and travel to the cell surface where their membranes fuse with the cell membrane. Other vacuoles contain lytic enzymes and become primary lysosomes. These fuse with autophagosomes or heterophagosomes to form secondary lysosomes. Undigested material remains in residual bodies. (Drawn by Margot Mackay, Department of Art as Applied to Medicine, University of Toronto.)

that is handed down from one cell to its progeny and from one generation to the next. The chemical that performs this function is deoxyribonucleic acid (DNA). Like the RNA of the cytoplasm, this substance is basophilic in H & E–stained sections, and the nucleus invariably stains deep blue. This blue material was named *chromatin* before the discovery of DNA, and the term is still convenient and in common use.

CHEMICAL STRUCTURE OF DNA

The chemical structure of DNA is well known. It is a polymer composed of a long chain of monounits or nucleotides. Each nucleotide consists of a base combined with deoxyribose sugar and phosphate. The common bases are either purines (adenine and guanine) or pyrimidines (cytosine and thymine). As a result of x-ray diffraction studies, Watson and Crick proposed a structure that fits remarkably well with our concept of DNA as a self-replicating genetic material (Fig. 2–14).

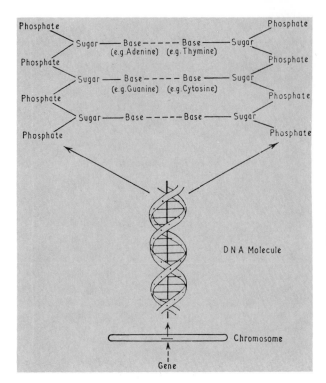

FIGURE 2–14. *Suggested chemical structure of DNA.*

The two polynucleotide chains are united by their bases, the order of which constitutes the genetic code. (After Watson, J. D., and Crick, F. H. C.: Nature (London), *171*:737, 1953.)

ROLE OF NUCLEIC ACIDS AS GENETIC MATERIAL

It is believed that the DNA of the nucleus contains genetic information that is passed via RNA into the cytoplasm where it is used in the manufacture of proteins—often enzymes—of exact composition. The word *gene* is used to describe a hypothetical unit of heredity for any single characteristic. Genes are an expression of the information contained within the DNA molecule. The order of the bases in DNA constitutes the genetic code, a sequence of three bases designating a single amino acid. A type of RNA (messenger RNA, or "mRNA") is manufactured in the nucleus in the presence of DNA-dependent RNA polymerase. This process is called *transcription,* and the mRNA is modeled after one of the polynucleotide chains of DNA, which acts as a template. The base sequence of the RNA is complementary to that of DNA, *i.e.,* cytosine corresponds with guanine, uracil corresponds with adenine, etc.* This mRNA passes into the cytoplasm and becomes associated with a group of ribosomes (a polysome). Here protein synthesis occurs. Each triplet, or codon, of the RNA base order codes for one amino acid. As the ribosomes "read along" the RNA molecule, successive amino acids are added to an ever-increasing polypeptide chain. In this way, a protein of exact composition is built up. The actual addition of each amino acid is effected by another type of RNA (transfer RNA, or "tRNA"), a separate form of which exists for each of the amino acids. This process is described as *translation,* for the code of the DNA finally appears legible in the form of a polypeptide chain (Fig. 2–15).

---

*When DNA replicates, the double helix unwinds and each strand acts as a template for the formation of a new strand. Thus, cytosine pairs with guanine, and adenine pairs with thymine. In the formation of single-stranded mRNA, thymine is replaced by uracil.

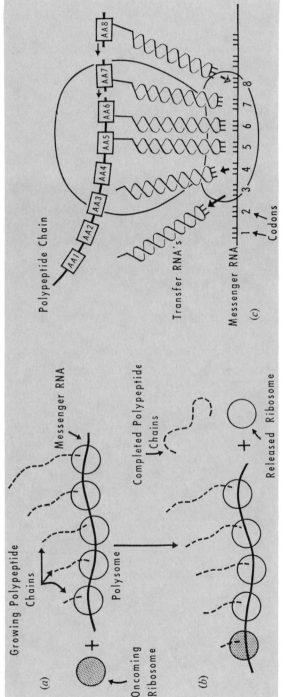

FIGURE 2–15.

Schematic model of protein synthesis. In (a) and (b) a long single-stranded molecule of messenger RNA (mRNA) is seen associated with a group of ribosomes to form a polysome. As each ribosome moves along the mRNA, an ever-growing polypeptide chain is produced. In (c) a single ribosome is depicted as a combination of two particles of unequal size. The sequence of bases of the mRNA forms triplets, or codons, which for the sake of clarity are drawn as groups of three upright lines. Each molecule of transfer RNA (tRNA) is composed of a long thread bent on itself to form a helical structure. At one end of the molecule there is a particular amino acid (AA1, AA2, etc.), and at the other end, where it is bent on itself, there are three unpaired bases that form an anticodon. Each codon of the mRNA is "recognized" by a corresponding anticodon of a tRNA. In this way specific amino acids are added to the polypeptide chain in a specific linear sequence determined by the mRNA which is itself modeled on the nuclear DNA. (Drawn by the Department of Art as Applied to Medicine, University of Toronto, after Warner, J. R., and Soeiro, R.: New England Journal of Medicine, 276:613, 1967 and Nirenberg, M. W.: The Living Cell. San Francisco, W. H. Freeman & Company, 1965. Reprinted by permission from the New England Journal of Medicine.)

Thus, the genetic code of DNA consists of codons that determine the insertion of particular amino acids in the peptide chain. The sequence of the codons is colinear with the sequence of amino acids. Codons responsible for an entire peptide chain form a group called a *cistron*. It is believed that a number of cistrons are grouped together to form a larger unit, the *operon*, which is described below. The actual code has been investigated by various means. Synthetic polyribonucleotides have been prepared and can act like mRNA in cell-free preparations containing ribosomes, suitable substrates, and a source of energy. Thus, a polynucleotide containing only uridine (poly U) leads to the formation of a polypeptide containing only phenylalanine. Hence the code for this amino acid is "UUU."

CONTROL OF GENE ACTION

It is evident that each newly created cell of the body contains the necessary information for the manufacture of every protein of which the body is composed. That all cells do not do so at all times is evidence that there is some very adequate control mechanism. By example, erythroid cells manufacture hemoglobin, and plasma cells form immunoglobulin. Nevertheless, it is not surprising that under abnormal circumstances cells produce substances that are alien to their accustomed products. It is for this reason that a tumor of the lung can produce hormones normally produced only by the pituitary. Many examples of this phenomenon will be seen later.

Some genes lead to the production of either enzymes or proteins used in the metabolism of the cell. These are termed *structural genes*. It has been found that a group of genes can be closely linked together and can either function together or be completely repressed, *i.e.*, no mRNA is produced. Figure 2–16 illustrates a simple scheme based on the hypothesis of Jacob and Monod. Each group of genes, or operon, is controlled by a closely associated gene called the *operator gene*. This itself is regulated by another gene, the *regulator gene*, which through its own mRNA leads to the formation in the cytoplasm of a

FIGURE 2–16. *The regulator-operator hypothesis.*

A, The regulator gene (R) forms a repressor substance that acts through the cytoplasm to repress the operator gene (O). When O is thus inhibited, the structural genes (S1 and S2) in its operon cannot form mRNA. *B,* If the regulator gene cannot form repressor substance, or if the repressor does not reach the operator gene, the operator is *derepressed* and S1 and S2 are then able to produce mRNA. (Redrawn from Thompson, J. S., and Thompson, M. W.: Genetics in Medicine. 2nd ed. Philadelphia, W. B. Saunders Company, 1973. The hypothesis is that of Jacob, F., and Monod, J.: Journal of Molecular Biology, 3:318, 1961.)

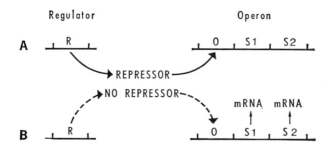

protein (repressor substance), which suppresses the operator gene. The regulator gene may itself be inhibited, and in that event, the operator is derepressed, the genes of the operon are allowed to act, mRNA is produced, and protein synthesis proceeds. The complexity of gene action is apparent when it is appreciated that in every cell, every gene is under continuous control and is so regulated that the requirements of the body are met. This applies not only during adult life but also during the complex processes of development. The ovum provides an excellent example of how protein synthesis can be inhibited, only to be switched on suddenly by the event of fertilization.

CHROMOSOMES

The DNA molecules are not lying free in the nucleus but are contained in long threads called *chromosomes*. Each resting somatic cell contains a definite number of chromosomes, the diploid or 2N number. This corresponds to the normal amount of DNA. In humans, the diploid number is 46; of these, 23 are derived from each parent. Two chromosomes, which are related specifically to sex, are called the *sex chromosomes*. One is considerably larger than the other and is called an X chromosome, whereas the smaller one is the Y chromosome. Females have two X chromosomes; males have one X and one Y. The remaining 22 pairs are identical in appearance in both sexes, and are called the *autosomes*.

Each resting somatic nucleus contains a constant number of chromosomes (the diploid number, which is twice the haploid number). Certain exceptions to this condition are found. As a person ages, some cells of the liver contain more chromosomes than normal. When a cell contains three or more times the haploid number of chromosomes, the condition is termed *polyploidy*. Thus, some liver cells have large nuclei containing 92 chromosomes. A similar event occurs in tumor cells.

During the period between cell divisions, the chromosomes are present in the nucleus as long, drawn-out threads. These are not visible as such when the light microscope is used, but in some areas along the thread there is sufficient coiling for the condensation of material to render these areas visible as basophilic chromatin dots in the nucleus. Such chromatin is thought to represent regions of the chromosomes that are condensed and relatively inert metabolically. The remainder of the nucleus is lightly stained and the chromatin appears dispersed. The actual morphology of the nucleus varies considerably from one cell to another, and an assessment of function can be made from nuclear structure. Thus in active cells, *e.g.*, cancer and nerve cells, the nucleus contains little condensed chromatin and is described as "vesicular." In inactive cells, such as small lymphocytes and spermatozoa, the condensed chromatin occupies much of the nucleus, which consequently is deeply basophilic and small.

Some very large cells, *e.g.*, megakaryocytes of the bone marrow, contain many nuclei and are called *multinucleate giant cells*.

Apart from DNA, the nucleus contains RNA, and some of this may appear as a separate structure called the *nucleolus*. This structure is particularly prominent in cells that are active metabolically. Nucleoli are therefore prominent features in nerve cells and in many cancer cells.

The Barr Body.   Dr. Murray Barr first noticed a discrete mass of chromatin in the nuclei of cells from a female animal—a mass that was not present in the nuclei of the male. This can be easily demonstrated in the human by examining suitably stained cells scraped from the buccal mucosa; it appears as a demilune on the nuclear membrane (Fig. 2–17). This chromatin can be shown to be formed by an X chromosome that is tightly condensed and mostly inactive. The normal female has two X chromosomes, and one of these is extended and active, while the other forms the Barr body. This hypothesis was first proposed by Dr. Mary Lyon, and it appears that the inactivation of one of the X chromosomes is random and occurs in each cell in early embryonic life. Hence, in the normal female about one half of the cells carry an active maternal X chromosome, while the other half carry an active paternal X chromosome. The inactive chromosome divides later than other chromosomes during cell division, and its descendants follow the same pattern. It occasionally happens that an individual has more than two X chromosomes, and in these cases the number of Barr bodies seen in a cell is equal to the total number of X chromosomes less one. Examination of the buccal smear is an important investigation in cases of chromosomal abnormality. Cells possessing a Barr body are also called *chromatin positive.*

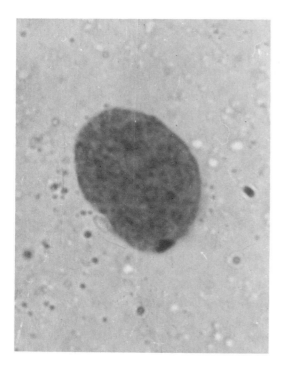

FIGURE 2–17.   *The Barr body.*

Nucleus of a cell from female buccal mucosal smear showing the sex chromatin mass on the nuclear membrane. (Photograph courtesy of Dr. Nigel H. Kemp.)

FIGURE 2-18. *The Y body.*

Nucleus from a normal male cell stained with quinacrine hydrochloride and examined under ultra-violet light. The bright fluorescent dot represents the Y chromosome. (Photograph courtesy of Dr. Peter K. Lewin.)

The Y Body.   The Y chromosome selectively takes up the dye quinacrine hydrochloride, which has the property of fluorescing strongly under ultraviolet light. If the smear of buccal mucosal scraping or peripheral blood is stained with this dye, a bright fluorescent dot in the nucleus indicates the presence of a Y chromosome (Fig. 2–18).

THE RETICULOENDOTHELIAL SYSTEM

This system of cells is found widely scattered throughout the body, and its components all share an ability to become phagocytic. Not only do they phagocytose coarse particles but they also are able to abstract highly diluted dyes when injected into the blood stream. It was by using this technique that the reticuloendothelial (RE) system was first delineated by Aschoff. The RE cells are closely associated with lymphocytes, and they are sometimes considered together as the *lymphoreticular system.*

There are two groups of RE cells:

FIXED CELLS.   These comprise cells that line the sinuses of certain organs, notably the liver (Kupffer cells), spleen, bone marrow, and lymph nodes (sinus-lining, or littoral, cells), and also the resting histiocytes that lie in the various connective tissues of the body. Those in the central nervous system are called microglia. The fixed reticuloendothelial cells are supported by and closely associated with thin fibers called *reticulin fibers,* which are described later in this chapter. Whether the reticulin fibers are actually formed by RE cells or by specialized reticulum cells is a moot point. In practice, it is difficult to distinguish between these two types of cells, and they are probably interchangeable.

In most tissues it is assumed that there are primitive multipotential cells that when suitably stimulated can differentiate into reticulum cells, reticuloendothelial cells, hematopoietic cells, and probably other more specialized connective tissue cells such as fibroblasts. These *stem cells* are poorly defined morphologically, and indeed they may differ in appearance in different organs. In the bone marrow they are believed to resemble lymphocytes.

FIGURE 2–19. *Macrophages.*

Section from an area of brain damage showing many macrophages that are engaged in removing dead brain tissue. The cells have abundant cytoplasm (×500).

MOBILE OR WANDERING CELLS.   These are the blood monocytes.

Whenever there is a local pathological process in a tissue, such as an infection or tissue damage, reticuloendothelial cells migrate to the area, become phagocytic, and in this form are called *macrophages* (Fig. 2–19). The majority of these cells are derived from the blood monocytes, but a variable number are probably also derived from local tissue histiocytes. It should be noted that the other phagocytic cells of the body, the neutrophil granulocytes of the blood, are not included in the RE system by definition. This is because they cannot perform the same type of phagocytosis generally associated with the RE system. The name "reticuloendothelial system" derives from the situation of the sinus-lining (endothelial) cells that are found in close relationship to reticulin fibers. Since the sinus-lining cells are quite different from normal vascular endothelial cells, the name is unfortunate. An alternative term, the *mononuclear phagocytic system,* has been suggested.

THE INTERCELLULAR SPACE

THE GROUND SUBSTANCE

The ground substance varies in consistency from an amorphous gel forming the translucent material of hyaline cartilage to the glairy fluid found in the synovial joint cavities. It is in the molecular meshes of the ground substance that the extracellular, or interstitial, fluid is contained. This fluid constitutes about one third of the total body water and lies between the blood vessels and the cells. It contains many electrolytes in a concentration similar to that of plasma as well as small uncharged solute materials such as oxygen, carbon dioxide, urea, and glucose, which are being conveyed either for cellular metabolism or for excretion. In addition, the ground substance contains the following:

GLYCOPROTEINS. These are proteins that contain a firmly bound component of carbohydrate.

MUCOPROTEINS. These are loose combinations of protein with acid mucopolysaccharides; the latter consists of polymers of hexose sugars containing amino groups. The best-known acid mucopolysaccharide is hyaluronic acid. The mucoproteins are largely responsible for the viscosity of the intercellular ground substance. The enzyme hyaluronidase, which is produced by streptococci, depolymerizes hyaluronic acid and renders the ground substance more watery. This may play some part in the spread of infection by streptococci. The special property of hyaluronidase can be used in therapy. If fluid has to be injected into the subcutaneous tissues, *e.g.*, in a young child, the addition of hyaluronidase facilitates the penetration of saline as well as its subsequent absorption.

COLLAGEN

Collagen fibers constitute about one third of the body's protein. They form the scaffold in all tissues and are the chief component of such tissues as fascia, dermis, cornea, and tendon. They give these structures tensile strength. Collagen accounts for about 90 per cent of the organic matrix of bone, and in this situation is adapted for the deposition of bone salts.

The collagen and ground substance are synthesized by fibroblasts and by similar cells such as are found in tendon, cornea, bone, and cartilage.

Light-Microscopic Appearance of Collagen. The first formed collagen consists of fine branching fibers called reticulin (Fig. 2–20). These fibers are demonstrated by silver impregnation methods and are not seen in ordinary H & E sections. In many organs of the body, collagen formation stops at this stage, and the reticulin forms a scaffold for the parenchyma (*e.g.*, liver, spleen, and lymph nodes). In the connective tissues proper, the fibers become enlarged and are then called collagen fibers. They lose their affinity for silver but readily take up eosin and can be stained specifically with aniline dyes combined with phosphotungstic acid (Mallory's trichrome stain).

Under the electron microscope both reticulin and collagen fibers are seen to be composed of fibrils having a characteristic cross-banding with a periodicity of about 64 nm (Fig. 2–21).

Composition of Collagen. The basic unit of collagen is a molecule called *tropocollagen*. This consists of three polypeptide chains, each coiled on itself. The three coiled chains are wound around a common axis like a three-stranded rope. It is thus a coiled coil! The tropocollagen molecules are bound to their lateral neighbors with a quarter overlap, so that the periodicity so characteristic of collagen is produced (Fig. 2–22).

FIGURE 2–20.   *Reticulin fibers in liver.*

This section of liver has been stained by a silver technique; only reticulin fibers, which are stained black, can be seen clearly. The spaces between the reticulin fibers are occupied by hepatocytes and sinusoids that drain blood into a venule (Ven).

FIGURE 2–21. *Section of collagen fibrils in a peripheral nerve.*

The fibrils show the characteristic cross-banding (arrow), which is best seen where the fibrils are cut longitudinally. Part of the cytoplasm of a Schwann cell (Sch) is also shown (×12,000). (Photograph courtesy of Dr. N. B. Rewcastle.)

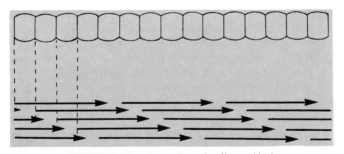

FIGURE 2–22. *Formation of collagen fibril.*

Diagram to illustrate how the lateral arrangement of tropocollagen molecules, depicted as arrows, results in the formation of banded collagen fibril. (Drawn by Anthony J. Walter.)

Collagen is characterized by its high content of glycine (33 per cent), proline, and hydroxyproline (the latter two together constituting about 22 per cent). Hydroxyproline is an amino acid that is not found to any extent in other proteins; an estimation of the amount of it in hydrolysates of tissue may therefore be used to measure the amount of collagen present.

The formation of collagen is a complex affair involving the formation of the three polypeptide chains in the rough endoplasmic reticulum, and the subsequent winding together to produce mature tropocollagen. For this process to take place, vitamin C is necessary. The tropocollagen finally passes into the extracellular tissues and a variety of bonds are formed so that the collagen, from being a soluble solution of tropocollagen, is converted first into reticulin fibers, then into collagen fibers, and finally into adult, mature, tough collagen tissue.

ELASTIC FIBERS

Elastic fibers are found in large blood vessels, in the lung, and to a lesser extent in many other tissues. On light microscopy they stain deep red with eosin and can be specifically demonstrated by staining with orcein, which renders them black. Elastic fibers are quite different from collagen; they have a different electron microscopic appearance and a different chemical composition. There is some debate as to how elastic fibers are formed as well as evidence that they can be produced by both fibroblasts and smooth muscle cells.

CELL DIVISION

MITOSIS

Before cell division occurs, the DNA molecules unwind, and each half acts as a template for the manufacture of the corresponding half. In this way, the amount of DNA is doubled. The chromosomes divide and become double structures called *chromatids;* these are joined together by a single *centromere.* The chromosomes become coiled along their whole length, thereby becoming shorter, thicker, and therefore visible. The cell has now entered the first phase of mitosis—*prophase.* Meanwhile, two centrioles have migrated, one to each pole of the cell, and microtubules develop in association with them. Each centriole looks like an *aster,* or star (Fig. 2–23).

The nucleoli and the nuclear membrane disappear next, and the cell enters into *metaphase.* By this time, the centrioles are at opposite poles of the cell, and their associated microtubules enter the nuclear region where the split chromosomes become arranged along an imaginary equatorial plate that bisects the cells. The microtubules are attached to the centromeres, and in this way the spindle is formed.

During the next phase, *anaphase,* each set of chromatids, now again called chromosomes, is pulled by the microtubules of the spindle to either pole of the cell. The final stage *(telophase)* involves division of the cytoplasm of the cell, and reconstitution of the nuclear membrane of each daughter cell.

It can readily be understood how during mitosis each chromosome reduplicates itself exactly, and the two daughter cells contain an identical quota of

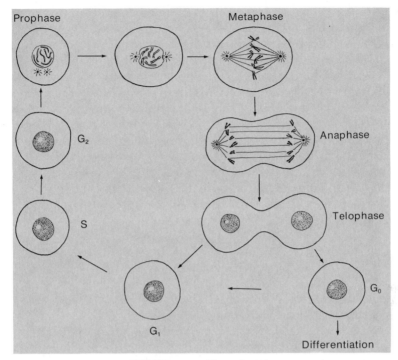

FIGURE 2–23. *The cell cycle.*

DNA reduplication occurs during the synthesis (S stage). This is followed by a short resting stage (G_2) before the cell enters mitosis. Following division the daughter cells may enter the second resting stage (G_1) before recommencing DNA synthesis. Other daughter cells can pass into a resting phase (G_0) and after a period can either re-enter the cell cycle or become differentiated and cease to be capable of mitosis.

nuclear material. Each DNA molecule is also reduplicated exactly. Should an error occur during mitosis such that an abnormality of the DNA is produced, the process is called a *somatic mutation.* Presumably, this is related to an abnormal sequence of the bases in the DNA molecule.

MEIOSIS

In the testis and ovary, the process of cell division is more complex and is called meiosis. The process results in cells containing only half the number of chromosomes (the "N", or haploid number, *i.e.,* 23 in man) and half the amount of DNA. These cells develop into gametes—either sperm or ova. With fertilization the diploid number of chromosomes (46) is restored.

During meiosis, the chromosomes become paired off into 23 pairs, with one of each moving into each of the daughter cells. Which chromosome of each pair migrates into which daughter cell is random; thus, the total number of possible combinations is extremely great. Furthermore, during the complex process of meiosis, portions of one chromosome sometimes move and are replaced by corresponding portions of the homologous chromosome. This crossing over and the random distribution of each of the pairs of chromosomes within a single gamete are responsible for the tremendous variation that is seen in the progeny of individuals produced by sexual reproduction.

It sometimes happens that during meiosis, a pair of chromosomes fail to separate and both are drawn into one daughter cell. This is called *nondisjunction*, and it results in one gamete having an extra chromosome while the other is deficient. Sometimes fragments of chromosomes are lost (by a process called *deletion*), or become attached to another chromosome (by a process called *translocation*). If two breaks occur in the same chromosome, the ends may join together to form a ring chromosome. Chromosomal breaks that result in deletion, translocation, or the formation of ring chromosomes can be induced by the action of ionizing radiation, by certain drugs, and by viruses. It is of interest that it is these same agents that are capable of causing cancer.

The next chapter deals with some of the effects of genetic errors and chromosomal abnormalities.

Review Questions

1. How would you attempt to determine the number of cells in a whole liver? How could its total content of collagen be estimated?
2. Apart from fertilizing ova, spermatozoa have only one major function: to travel several centimeters as fast as possible with their inactive genetic material. Can you relate this function to their structure?
3. Write a brief account of the formation and functions of ATP in a cell.
4. Name the structures numbered 1–10 in Figure 2–5.
5. Examine Figure 2–2. The epithelial cells covering the villi are thought to arise in the crypts by mitosis. From there they migrate along the surface of the villi and are cast off finally from the tip. How would you attempt to confirm this movement, and to measure the time taken for a cell to migrate from the crypt to the tip?
6. How many types of RNA are there in a cell? Indicate their main functions.
7. The genes that control the formation of the enzyme glucose 6-phosphate dehydrogenase (GPD) are situated on the X chromosome. If you were able to culture cells from various parts of a normal human female, would you expect every cell to manufacture GPD? Explain the reasoning behind your answer.

Selected Readings

Bucher, N. L. R.: Microtubules. New England Journal of Medicine, *287*:195–196, 1972.
Fawcett, D. W.: The Cell: Its Organelles and Inclusions. Philadelphia, W. B. Saunders Company, 1966.
Fox, C. F.: The structure of cell membranes. Scientific American, *226*:30–38, 1972.
Grant, M. E., and Prockop, D. J.: The biosynthesis of collagen, Parts I, II, and III. New England Journal of Medicine, *286*:194–199; 242–249; 291–300; 1972.
Ham, A. W.: Histology. 7th ed. Philadelphia, J. B. Lippincott Company, 1974, Chapters 2–5.
Leeson, C. R., and Leeson, T. S.: Histology. 3rd ed. Philadelphia, W. B. Saunders Company, 1976. Note, in particular, Chapters 2 to 6.
Pastan, I.: Cyclic AMP. Scientific American, *227*:97–105, 1972.
Ross, L. M.: The cell. *In* Clinical Symposia (Ciba), *26*:4–35, 1974.
Weinstein, R. S., and McNutt, N. C.: Cell junctions. New England Journal of Medicine, *286*:521–524, 1972.

GENETIC CAUSES OF DISEASE

Chapter 3

After studying this chapter the student should be able to:

- Define the terms gene, locus, allele, heterozygote, penetrance, expressivity, homozygote, phenotype, genotype, and polymorphism.
- Draw diagrams to illustrate the mode of inheritance of a disease inherited as
  - (a) an autosomal dominant
  - (b) an autosomal recessive
  - (c) an X-linked dominant
  - (d) an X-linked recessive.

  Give at least one example of each type of inheritance.
- Describe the biochemical defect, the effects of the abnormality, and the mode of inheritance of the following genetic diseases:
  - (a) galactosemia
  - (b) phenylketonuria
  - (c) sickle cell disease.
- Describe the chromosomal abnormality and the outstanding clinical features of each of the following:
  - (a) the most common type of Down's syndrome
  - (b) Klinefelter's syndrome
  - (c) ovarian dysgenesis
  - (d) cri du chat syndrome.
- List the investigations that can be performed on amniotic fluid to detect fetal abnormality. Give examples of the types of defects that may be found.

GENETIC CAUSES OF DISEASE

The study of medicine has largely revolved around the effects of adverse external agents. The great discoveries made in bacteriology, virology, and immunology at the end of the last century strengthened the belief that each disease had a specific cause and that often this cause was a particular external agent—frequently a living organism. As diseases of obviously infective origin have been recognized and brought under control, it has become clear that some diseases have no simple cause and are probably due to many agents acting simultaneously. Inherited diseases were certainly recognized in the past, but they were often regarded as being uncommon. Inherited traits were believed to result from a merging of parental traits, and in this climate of thought the discoveries of Gregor Mendel were passed over and ignored for 25 years. Mendel himself followed the course of many other successful yet frustrated investigators: he abandoned research and became an administrator.

Today we realize that disease has two major bases. It is the result of the interplay between inherited genetic constitution on the one hand and the environment on the other. This chapter is mainly concerned with the first of these components.

THE GENETIC BASIS OF DISEASE

Mendel's laws of inheritance have laid the foundations of the science of genetics and are of great importance in the understanding of many disease processes. He postulated that a particular characteristic is determined by a pair of factors, now called *genes,* each of which is situated at a particular site (or *locus)* on one of a pair of chromosomes. Such genes, forming a pair, are called *alleles.* An individual with a pair of similar genes is called *homozygous,* whereas if the genes are dissimilar, he is *heterozygous.* The genetic make-up of an individual is called the *genotype,* and the effect that is produced is called the *phenotype.*

It is basic in modern genetics to assume that genes occur in pairs, that one of each pair is received from each parent, and that the genes remain unchanged through many generations. The simplest approach to the mode of inheritance of a particular characteristic—for example, a disease—is to consider that genes may be either dominant or recessive. A dominant gene produces its effect both in the heterozygote and in the homozygote. Recessive genes, on the other hand, produce their effects only in the homozygous condition. Genes occupying an intermediate position are described later. Sometimes a particular locus on a chromosome can be occupied by one of many possible genes. An example of this type is illustrated below with the explanation of ABO blood grouping.

DOMINANT GENES

A simple example of inheritance of a dominant gene is shown by reference to the ABO blood grouping. The allelic genes that can occupy one locus are "A," "B," or "O."

A homozygous individual who has two A genes (genotype AA) has on his red cells the blood group substance "A" (phenotype group A). Likewise, the heterozygote AO is also phenotypically blood group A because A gene is dominant, whereas O is recessive. The B gene, like the A gene, is dominant, and both are described as *codominant*. The possible blood groups in this system are shown below.*

GENOTYPE	PHENOTYPE
AA	A
AO	A
OO	O
BB	B
BO	B
AB	AB

Thus, the six genotypes produce only four recognizable blood groups. A person of blood group "A" may be genotype AA or AO. It is not easy to distinguish between these two genotypes by an examination of the individual himself, but the genotype can be deduced from the family pedigree. It should be noted that the occurrence of two or more genetically different classes of individuals with respect to a single trait is known as *polymorphism*. The blood groups provide an excellent example of this, but many others are known. For example, there are many genetically determined variants of plasma proteins, hemoglobin, and enzymes.

The mode of inheritance of a dominant disease is illustrated in Figure 3–1. It should be noted that:

1. The disease appears in every generation or else it dies out. The occasional instance of poor penetrance (discussed later in this chapter) and the occurrence of a new mutant provide exceptions to this rule. If the disease greatly reduces the breeding potential of the affected person, it follows that most cases encountered will be sporadic and due to new mutations.

2. Unaffected members do not pass on the disease (see "Penetrance and Expressivity" later in this chapter).

3. The affected members are usually heterozygous, and if the breeding partner is normal, the chances of his offspring being affected are 50 per cent.

4. Males and females are equally liable to be affected.

---

*The ABO blood groups are more complicated than this. For example, O is an amorph, and subgroups of A are known.

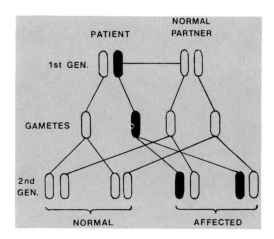

FIGURE 3–1. *Transmission of a disease inherited as a dominant trait.*

One pair of chromosomes is shown for each individual, the black chromosome being the one carrying the defective gene. Each person inheriting the defective gene will have the disease. The probability of passing the disease on to each member of the next generation is 50 per cent.

Huntington's chorea, achondroplasia, osteogenesis imperfecta, and multiple neurofibromatosis (Fig. 3–2) are examples of diseases inherited as a dominant trait.

DISEASES INHERITED AS A RECESSIVE TRAIT

Frequently, these are severe and reduce the breeding potential of the affected person. The mode of transmission is shown diagrammatically in Figure 3–3. The following features should be noted:

FIGURE 3–2. *Multiple neurofibromatosis (von Recklinghausen's disease).*

This patient appeared normal at birth except for the presence of several irregularly shaped pigmented macules (café-au-lait spots). The skin lesions shown in the picture began to appear at about 13 years of age. The patient, who is now 60, has thousands of soft skin nodules, many of which are pedunculated. Microscopically these show neurofibromas. The disease is named after von Recklinghausen, who gave the first good account of the disease in 1882. The patient was an orphan and has three children. One daughter is similarly affected, the others apparently have escaped the disease.

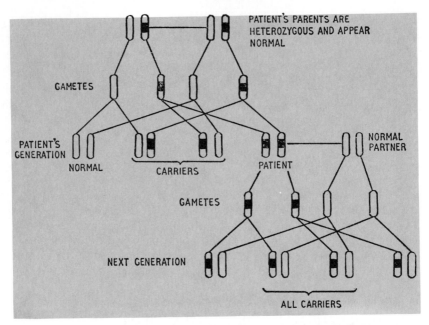

FIGURE 3–3. *Transmission of a disease inherited as a recessive factor.*

The patient is homozygous and therefore expresses the disease. Both parents are heterozygous and consequently appeared normal. All the patient's offspring are heterozygotes and thus carriers of the trait.

1. The birth of an abnormal child is usually the first indication of the condition.

2. As with other Mendelian characters, the chances of additional members of the family being affected or passing on the trait can be calculated. Thus, the chances of the next child being affected are one in four. One half of the offspring will be heterozygous and carriers of the trait. If the affected individual mates with a normal partner, all of the progeny will be carriers.

3. The seriousness of producing carriers should not be overemphasized. It has been estimated that we all carry harmful genes that usually remain hidden for generations. A particular gene is liable to be more frequent in a particular family; the danger of close intermarriage is therefore evident. The incidence of defective offspring is much higher in consanguineous matings (those between close relatives) than when the parents are not related.

Some of the best-known diseases inherited as recessive traits are galactosemia, albinism,* phenylketonuria, and cystic fibrosis of the pancreas (see Fig. 30–8).

Sex-Linked Genes. A gene is said to be sex-linked when it is localized on an 'X' or 'Y' chromosome. Usually the gene is recessive and is situated on the X

---

*In albinism the pigment-producing cells (melanocytes) are defective and fail to produce pigment. The transparency of the irides combined with the lack of retinal pigment causes the eyes to appear pink. The hair is white and the skin pale. The white mouse is an example of the typical albino. In the human counterpart there is some pigment formed, so that the hair is a very pale yellow and the eyes are blue.

chromosome. The most famous disease to be inherited as a sex-linked recessive is hemophilia, which is illustrated in Figure 3–4.

Sex-linked dominant traits are recognized but are rare. Affected females convey the gene to half their sons and daughters, whereas affected males transmit it only to their daughters. Since there can be no male-to-male transmission, there is therefore an excess of female victims. Hemolytic anemia due to glucose 6-phosphate dehydrogenase deficiency is an example of this type of inheritance.

OTHER FEATURES OF GENE EXPRESSION

Not all human inherited disease can be explained in terms of simple dominant or recessive gene action. There are many complicating factors:

PENETRANCE AND EXPRESSIVITY. It may happen that a trait, although apparently dominant, occasionally misses a generation. The trait is said to exhibit *reduced penetrance*. Another complication is seen in some families in which a dominant gene produces a variable effect. Some individuals who possess it have a severe disease, whereas others have a minor defect (known as *forme fruste*) of the disease. In this instance the trait is said to exhibit *variable expressivity*. Clearly, penetrance and expressivity are closely related, but while penetrance is defined in terms of an all-or-none effect, expressivity is variable.

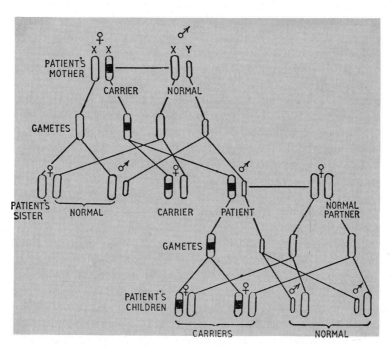

FIGURE 3–4. *Mode of transmission of a disease inherited as an X-linked recessive Mendelian factor.*

A common example of such a disease is hemophilia. The abnormal gene is situated on an X chromosome and therefore produces its effect in the male but not in the female except in the very rare event of her being homozygous. The patient's daughters are all carriers of the disease, and his sons are all normal. There is never any direct male-to-male transmission; the disease is perpetuated by the females in the family.

INTERMEDIATE INHERITANCE.   When the heterozygote differs from either homozygote, the inheritance is described as *intermediate*. A good example is sickle cell disease. The homozygote who has two sickle cell genes has the fully developed sickle cell anemia, whereas the heterozygote carrying one defective allele and one normal allele has the mild sickle cell trait—a state intermediate between the disease and the normal. This condition is described in more detail later in the chapter.

Other complicating factors are recognized in human disease. Sometimes several nonallelic genes interact in complex ways; in other instances, a particular trait appears to be the result of many genes acting in various ways. Thus, in the inheritance of intelligence and height there is no simple explanation of the means of inheritance, and it is assumed that many genes are involved. Likewise, some diseases, such as systemic hypertension and diabetes mellitus, appear to fall into this group. Additional complicating factors are the effect of environmental agents acting in concert with the inherited tendency.

MODE OF GENE ACTION

With the discovery of chromosomes and DNA it was logical that attempts should be made to equate genes with segments of the DNA molecule. The first clue came with the description of some diseases characterized by a deficiency of a single enzyme. These genetically determined biochemical lesions, or *inborn errors of metabolism*, to use a term coined by Sir Archibald Garrod over 50 years ago, are a group of diseases in which the individual lacks one particular enzyme. An excellent example of this is the disease *galactosemia*. Babies with this defect lack an enzyme that converts galactose to glucose. The galactose or its metabolites, derived from the lactose in milk, accumulate in the blood and interfere with the development of the brain, the eye, and the liver. Mental defect, cataracts, and cirrhosis of the liver are the results of this simple biochemical defect. It should be noted that the effects of this enzyme deficiency can be averted by eliminating lactose from the diet. If a child with galactosemia is fed a lactose-free diet, development proceeds normally. The ethics of condemning a person to a lifelong artificial diet might, however, be questioned. Nevertheless, this example illustrates the inter-relationship between a genetic defect and an external agent—in this instance, a particular chemical in the diet.

A second example of this type of disease is *phenylketonuria*. Between 3 and 5 persons per 100,000 of the population exhibit this condition, which commences shortly after birth, and is characterized by retardation of mental development. The disease is due to the absence of an enzyme that converts the amino acid phenylalanine to tyrosine. Hence, with a normal diet an affected baby develops a high blood level of phenylalanine and its keto derivatives. These are the cause of brain damage, which can be largely averted by the administration of a diet low in phenylalanine. Early diagnosis, by finding phenylalanine or its derivatives in the urine, is therefore very important. The condition is inherited as a mendelian autosomal recessive trait; 1 per cent of the population are heterozygotes, and the condition can be detected by the administration of a test dose of phenylalanine, when the blood level rises. This does not occur in a normal individual. This detection of heterozygotes has a practical value. If a married couple are both carriers, their chance of producing an affected child is 25 per cent. They can be warned of this risk. This is just one example of the kind of information offered in *genetic counseling*.

Hemoglobinopathies. The translation of the mysterious gene action into concrete chemical terms was first achieved successfully with a group of diseases in man known as the hemoglobinopathies, in which an abnormal form of hemoglobin is manufactured. The globin of the hemoglobin molecule is a protein of known amino acid sequence. In certain individuals, usually of African ancestry, the hemoglobin contains an abnormal globin in which valine replaces the usual glutamic acid in the sixth position of one of the two polypeptide chains of the molecule. Presumably, this is due to an error in one codon of one section of the DNA molecule. Homozygous individuals manufacture the abnormal hemoglobin S, which renders their red cells liable to distort to a sickle shape at low oxygen tensions. These abnormally shaped red cells are easily removed from the circulation and are quickly destroyed, with the result that the patient becomes severely ill with sickle cell anemia. Heterozygous individuals suffer from a mild anemia and are said to have the sickle cell trait. Their red cells contain both normal hemoglobin A and the abnormal hemoglobin S.

Many other diseases are known in which the body synthesizes an abnormal form of a protein — either a structural protein such as hemoglobin or an enzyme. These diseases are grouped together as the *molecular diseases.* Presumably these have arisen by mutations. If the product of the mutant gene differs little from the previous substance, the gene probably becomes part of the gene pool of the population. This is probably the mechanism whereby genetic polymorphism arises. Thus, there are 22 variants of the enzyme glucose 6-phosphate dehydrogenase and at least 150 variants of hemoglobin. Sometimes the mutant provides a definite advantage over the pre-existing gene and presumably will eventually replace the original. In the case of the sickle cell gene, it is believed that those who have the sickle cell trait possess an increased immunity to infection with malaria. It is evident that although sickle cell anemia is a lethal disease, the sickle cell trait provides an advantage to those who possess it and live in a tropical climate where malaria is endemic.

Diseases Associated With Genetic Constitution

In spite of the recent great advances in genetics, there are many diseases in which the mode of inheritance is not understood. Some, which are more common in certain families, are spoken of as *familial disease;* their occurrence and distribution cannot be predicted. High blood pressure, obesity, and heart disease seem to fall into this group.

Sometimes particular characteristics are associated with certain diseases, although they are not themselves the obvious cause. The association of a particular disease with a particular ethnic group, *e.g.*, diabetes mellitus and pemphigus vulgaris with Jews, or with sex, *e.g.*, goiter in women and cancer of the lung in men, is an example of this. In addition, innate immunity to infection is

FIGURE 3–5. *Human chromosomes at metaphase.*

Lymphocytes from the blood of a normal woman were grown in culture for 72 hours before colcemid (a colchicine derivative) was added. This chemical inhibits spindle formation so that mitoses are halted at metaphase. Two hours later a hypotonic solution was added to make the cells swell. The dispersed chromosomes were then stained with Giemsa after they had been pretreated with trypsin. This technique brings out the banding of the chromosomes.

The mitosis shown contains 46 chromosomes, each of which is a divided structure joined by a centromere. The individual chromosomes can be cut out with scissors and arranged in pairs as shown in Figure 3–6. Such an arrangement is called a karyotype. (Photograph courtesy of Dr. H. A. Gardner, Division of Cytogenetics, Toronto General Hospital.)

an inherited characteristic, as is the inherited liability to develop atopic disease (see Chapter 9). The association of certain diseases with particular blood groups has also been recognized. Thus, cancer of the stomach is more frequent in persons of phenotype "A," while duodenal ulceration is more frequently associated with those of phenotype "O." More recently, tissue typing has revealed a similar association. People with tissue type HL-A 27 are more prone to develop ankylosing spondylitis (see Chapter 40). We are quite ignorant of the mechanisms involved in these associations, but undoubtedly this type of coincidence was noted by the great clinicians of the past who often referred to a characteristic disease diathesis.

Diseases Associated With Gross Chromosomal Abnormalities

The techniques described in Figure 3–5 have made it possible to study the chromosomes as a routine investigation. Certain individuals have been found to have more than 46 chromosomes, while others have fewer. Abnormalities in shape or form of individual chromosomes have also been noted. These abnormalities may be considered under two headings: (1) alteration in *number* of chromosomes and (2) alteration in *structure* of chromosomes.

Although the finding of chromosomal abnormality is regarded as uncommon, it is now apparent that those cases detected in postnatal life represent only the residue of a much larger group of abnormal zygotes. About one half of the fetuses spontaneously aborted in the first three months of pregnancy have chromosomal abnormalities, one of the commonest being *triploidy* (the cells having 69 chromosomes). It has been estimated that about one third of the results of conception are aborted spontaneously and that gross genetic errors are a major cause of this (Fig. 3–6).

FIGURE 3–6. *Karyotype showing trisomy 18 from a stillborn male with cyclopia.*

The karyotype is that of a cell with 47 chromosomes. It is evidently from a male, since there is a Y chromosome. The anomaly must therefore be of fetal origin, since the mother had a normal 46,XX karyotype. The additional chromosome No. 18 arose by nondisjunction; its manifestations were incompatible with postuterine life. (From Lang, A. P., Schlager, M., and Gardner, H. A.: Trisomy 18 and cyclopia. Teratology, *14*:195–203, 1976.) For a more complete description, see Case History I.

Case History I. (See Figure 3–6.) A 26-year-old woman gave birth to a stillborn male child at 41 weeks of gestation. Before birth there was clinical evidence of a small head, which was confirmed at ultrasonic examination. No fetal heart was heard during the three days prior to delivery.

The infant showed many abnormalities, the most striking of which was a single eye, containing two lenses, in the center of the forehead. The brain was underdeveloped and exhibited many severe abnormalities. An attempt was made to culture fetal skin cells, but no growth could be obtained. This was not unexpected, since the fetus showed obvious signs of autolysis. However, placental tissue was viable and grew well in culture; photographs of several mitoses were obtained. One of these was arranged as shown in Figure 3–6. The chromosomes are arranged in pairs and are numbered 1 to 22 in order of length, position of the centromere, and banding characteristics. With good technique it is possible to identify each chromosome. When this identification is not possible, the pairs of chromosomes are then arranged into seven groups, A to G, excluding the X and Y chromosomes.

ALTERATION IN NUMBER OF CHROMOSOMES

Additional Chromosomes. The commonest example of this abnormality is when there is one extra chromosome. This condition is called *trisomy,* and the best known example is trisomy 21. The individual has 47 chromosomes and may be either male or female. The condition is *Down's syndrome,* otherwise known as mongolism (Fig. 3–7). This is always accompanied by mental defect, and the condition is quite common since such affected children are produced with an

FIGURE 3–7. *Down's syndrome.*

This patient exhibits the typical facial appearance of persons having the syndrome. Note the large tongue protruding from the mouth. Particularly characteristic is the presence of an epicanthal fold, which is best seen on the right side (arrow). This is a fold of skin that covers the medial angle of the palpebral fissure and gives the eyes an appearance that superficially resembles that of an Oriental. Down's syndrome can generally be recognized at birth with the diagnosis being confirmed by chromosomal analysis. The mortality is high during the first few years of life, death being related to respiratory infection, congenital heart disease, or leukemia. Dwarfism is common and mental deficiency invariable. Mothers over the age of 35 years are more likely to give birth to an affected child than younger women. (Photograph courtesy of the Department of Clinical Illustration, Birmingham Dental School, Birmingham, England; supplied by Margaret C. Grundy.)

incidence of approximately 1 in every 600 live births. Trisomy of other autosomes is known but is much less common.

The presence of additional sex chromosomes is not uncommon. Certain individuals are found to have an extra "X." Some are apparent males, have the genetic constitution 47,XXY, and have chromatin-positive cells. They have small testes that fail to develop at puberty; there is little facial hair; they may have a female type of breast development (gynecomastia); and they are sterile. These features become evident at puberty; the condition is known as *Klinefelter's syndrome*. Another group of patients have the karyotype 47,XXX and are females, usually with normal secondary sex characteristics and sometimes with mental defect.

In the 47,XYY syndrome, the patients appear as normal males, but in some instances the subject is abnormally tall and exhibits a criminally aggressive temperament. Nevertheless, other individuals with this anomaly appear normal.

Reduction in the Number of Chromosomes. The loss of an autosome is incompatible with postuterine life. In those cases where such a state has been described, a small chromosome is involved and it seems likely that the chromosome is in fact present but has become attached to some other chromosome, *i.e.*, it has been translocated.

The sex chromosomes are less vital for survival and deletion of one is quite compatible with life. In about one in every 3000 births, a female is produced with the karyotype 45,XO. The condition, which is known as *ovarian dysgenesis*, becomes obvious at adolescence when the ovaries fail to function normally, ovulation does not occur, and menstruation is absent (primary amenorrhea). Such individuals tend to be short because of stunted growth and are sterile. Often they have a number of other abnormalities such as webbing of the neck and shieldlike chest with widely spaced nipples. Abnormalities of the cardiovascular system are common—in particular, coarctation of the aorta—and the eponym *Turner's syndrome* is applied. These unfortunate females are chromatin-negative, since only one X chromosome is present.

ABNORMALITIES OF CHROMOSOME STRUCTURE

The recent developments of chromosomal staining have revealed that some individuals have chromosomes differing somewhat from those of the average person. In many instances, these abnormalities are either individual or racial variations and are of no known significance. Any gross abnormality of an entire autosome appears to be incompatible with postuterine life. A number of syndromes have been described in which part of an autosome is missing. For instance, the short arm of chromosome 5 is missing in a syndrome in which the infant exhibits mental defect and cries with a whimpering noise resembling that of a cat in distress (cri du chat syndrome).

So far only one acquired disease has been found to have any consistent chromosomal abnormality. This is chronic myelocytic leukemia, in which the abnormal white cells lack one arm of chromosome 22, usually called the *Philadelphia chromosome*.

AVOIDANCE OF GENETIC DEFECTS

Genetic counseling will dissuade some high-risk couples from procreation, but once conception has occurred, the only course open may be the induction of abortion. Removal (by *amniocentesis*) and testing amniotic fluid can be employed for the prenatal detection of fetal abnormality. The supernatant of the fluid can be examined biochemically and checked for the presence of virus. The amniotic cells (of fetal origin) can be examined for the presence of the X and Y chromatin. They can also be cultured for biochemical investigation and chromosomal analysis. These investigations can usually be completed between the sixteenth and twentieth week of gestation. If a defect is found, an abortion can be performed safely at this time. Whether or not to adopt this course also depends on moral and legal factors.

ACQUIRED DISEASE

Many human diseases are acquired in postnatal life as a result of the action of external factors. The effects of physical and chemical agents, living organisms, and dietary deficiencies are the common causes of these *acquired diseases*. It should be remembered that the developing fetus is also sensitive to environmental factors, and the tragedies that followed administration of thalidomide to pregnant women bear witness to the extreme sensitivity of the fetus under some circumstances. Intrauterine events may produce defects that are present at birth *(congenital)* but are not inherited, since no genetic mechanism is involved. Inherited diseases may be congenital, *e.g.*, achondroplasia, but they may also appear later on in life, *e.g.*, polyposis coli (see Chapter 32). The time of onset of a disease gives no indication as to whether the cause is environmental or genetic.

Review Questions

1. A mother and her child both have the blood group AB. What are the possible genotypes of the father?
2. A patient with galactosemia mates with a heterozygous carrier of this disease. What are the chances that they will have a clinically unaffected child? Will all such children be carriers?
3. Deaf-mutism is inherited as an autosomal recessive trait. Two deaf-mutes marry and have ten children, all of whom have normal hearing. This is not an isolated example of this occurrence. Account for the birth of the children with normal hearing.
4. A man with hemophilia and glucose 6-phosphate dehydrogenase deficiency (inherited as an X-linked dominant trait) has a son. What are the chances that he will have:
    (a) hemophilia only
    (b) glucose 6-phosphate dehydrogenase deficiency only
    (c) both of the above defects
    (d) neither of the above defects.

5. Two phenotypically normal parents have a child with phenylketonuria.
    (a) What is the genotype of each of the parents?
    (b) What is the probability of the next child also having phenylketonuria?
    (c) What is the probability of a normal child of these parents being a carrier of phenylketonuria?

Selected Readings

Emery, A. E. H.: Elements of Medical Genetics. 4th ed. Berkeley, University of California Press, 1975. A short, up-to-date account of the subject.
Hamerton, J. L.: Human Cytogenetics. Vol. 2. New York, Academic Press, Inc., 1971. A reference book.
Leading Article: HL-A antigens and rheumatic diseases. British Medical Journal, 1:238, 1975.
Levine, H.: Clinical Cytogenetics. Boston, Little, Brown and Company, 1971. A reference book.
Thompson, J. S., and Thompson, M. W.: Genetics in Medicine. 2nd ed. Philadelphia, W. B. Saunders Company, 1973. Written for medical students, this book emphasizes the statistical aspects of inheritance.
Valentine, G. H.: The Chromosome Disorders. 3rd ed. London, William Heinemann Ltd., 1975. An excellent, easy-to-read, short account of chromosomal disorders.

Chapter 4

After studying this chapter the student should be able to:

- Describe the concept of a biochemical lesion as a cause of cell damage, and give three examples of such lesions.
- Differentiate between cell death, autolysis, and necrosis.
- List the events that can lead to cellular degeneration, and describe the changes found in damaged cells.
- Give examples of the value of serum enzyme determinations in the diagnosis of
  - (a) liver disease
  - (b) heart disease.
- Define the term "gangrene."
- Describe the pathogenesis of gangrene in the
  - (a) intestine
  - (b) mouth
  - (c) limbs.
- Describe hyaline degeneration and elastosis as applied to collagen.
- Contrast necrobiosis with hyaline degeneration.
- List the conditions in which excess ground substance accumulates in a tissue.

    The importance of the cell as the basic unit of the body has been recognized since the microscope was first applied to the analysis of biological material. This is scarcely surprising, because simple forms of life like the ameba consist entirely of one cell. Just over 100 years ago Virchow published his text-

CELL AND TISSUE DAMAGE

book on cellular pathology; since then our concept of many diseases has centered on abnormalities in cellular behavior or appearance. The cells of any particular organ or tissue usually closely resemble each other, and it is not surprising that a sick cell such as one from the liver is the essential component of a sick liver; likewise, this "sickness" at the cellular level produces a particular clinical syndrome called liver failure. The advent of electron microscopy has greatly increased our knowledge of cellular changes in disease and has further strengthened the concept that abnormalities in cellular appearance and behavior are the building blocks from which disease entities are built. Nevertheless, a morphological view of cellular behavior has its limitations. The application of chemical techniques has considerably widened our views. At a cellular level the techniques of histochemistry allow us to identify particular chemicals within cells. Furthermore, chemists have exerted a quite different influence on the study of disease by adopting another approach. Instead of concentrating on the individual cell or its organelles, they have turned their attention to specific chemical reactions. Thus, with respect to the metabolism of galactose, most cells can be regarded as behaving in a standard way. The disease galactosemia is characterized by a defect in an enzyme that converts galactose to glucose. Deficiency of this enzyme produces a disease leading to microscopic changes in cells that are particularly dependent on this chemical reaction during development. As described previously, the brain, the lens of the eye, and the liver are most severely affected. This second approach to the study of a pathologic condition has been of immense value both in the delineation of disease processes and in the treatment of individual patients. Ultimately, the broad concept of "biochemical disorder" must be reduced to a cellular level. In some instances this has already occurred, and it is convenient therefore to consider some examples of cellular damage caused by lesions of known chemical mechanism.

Biochemical Lesions

The concept of a biochemical lesion was first advanced by Sir Rudolph Peters and was based on the observation that pigeons subjected to a thiamine-deficient diet developed severe neurological symptoms, such as convulsions, and ultimately died. In spite of the severity of the disease, no abnormality could be detected by histological examination of the brain. The cells looked normal, but they were not functioning properly. Thiamine was found to be one of the factors necessary for the conversion of pyruvate to acetyl coenzyme A. This is an important mechanism in the feeding of the Krebs cycle (see Chapter 2). Hence, thiamine deficiency impairs energy production, and this affects the nerve cells, which have a high metabolic requirement. Biochemical lesions can be deliberately induced in cells by feeding them with agents that closely resemble metabolites. Thus, cells fed with 5-fluorouracil respond to the agent as if it were uracil, but the abnormal end-product blocks other essential processes. This deliberate sabotage of cellular metabolism has been called *lethal synthesis* by Peters and has been used with some success in the treatment of malignant disease. Another example of lethal synthesis is the action of chemotherapeutic agents on bacteria. Thus, sulfonamides are treated as para-aminobenzoic acid by some bacteria. This ultimately blocks cellular metabolism. Likewise, penicillin blocks cell-wall synthesis, thus rendering the bacteria extremely fragile and easily destroyed by osmotic effects.

Most agents affect the cell by upsetting some important chemical reaction. The biochemical lesion thus produced is the first change, and this in turn produces secondary results. The structural changes that take place within the cell have been recognized microscopically for many years and are grouped together as the *cell degenerations*. If the adverse influence persists, the cells may die. This in turn leads to the liberation of destructive lysosomal enzymes within the cell, which is thereby lysed by a process of self-digestion, or *autolysis*. When this process occurs after the death of the whole individual, the term *postmortem change* is used. When, however, a group of cells dies in a living person, similar changes occur. It is by recognizing these changes that cell death itself can be determined; to this process the term *necrosis* is applied.

Cellular Degenerations

The various morphological types of cellular degeneration may result from the cell being submitted to a wide variety of adverse circumstances that may be either internal or external events. These may be summarized in the following way:

Internal events
  Genetic error—enzyme defects
  Deprivation of essential chemicals such as hormones, vitamins, and oxygen
  Loss of blood supply
  Hypersensitivity
External events
  Physical: heat, cold, trauma, and radiation
  Chemical: poisons and lack of oxygen
  Microbial: microbial invasion and effects of toxins

Two main types of cellular degeneration were recognized before the advent of electron microscopy (Fig. 4–1).

CHANGES ASSOCIATED WITH THE ACCUMULATION OF WATER

In the first group there is an accumulation of water within the cell. Initially, this gives the cytoplasm a granular appearance *(cloudy swelling)*, sometimes vacuoles become obvious, and finally the cell swells up tremendously and perhaps ruptures *(hydropic degeneration)*. The electron microscopic changes seen in the cells showing these changes are complex. Sometimes there are degenerative changes in the mitochondria, and it is postulated that reduced ATP production leads to impairment of the sodium pump so that the cell becomes water-logged. At other times, the changes appear to be more related to dilatation of the sacs of the endoplasmic reticulum. It has often been assumed in the past that the cellular changes of cloudy swelling or hydropic degeneration are the same, regardless of the organ affected — be it liver, kidney, or heart muscle. Such is clearly not the case. Using the electron microscope, one may probe more deeply into the nature of these changes. Whereas the light microscope can give only a vague impression of intracellular events and can detect the changes only when they are severe enough to affect the cell as a whole, electron microscopy can reveal which parts of the cell are affected and can indicate the sequence of events and metabolic changes occurring. The structure of the cell now appears more complex than did the anatomy of the body as a whole 100 years ago. Just as "coma" ceased to be an intellectually satisfying final diagnosis when specific conditions affecting the brain were recognized, so cloudy swelling is equally unsatisfactory now that organelles are known to exist.

CHANGES ASSOCIATED WITH THE ACCUMULATION OF FAT

The second type of degenerative change that occurs in cells consists of the accumulation of neutral fat. Normally no stainable neutral fat can be seen in cells except in adult fat cells. Under adverse circumstances small droplets of fat appear in the cytoplasm, and ultimately these fuse together to form one large globule that pushes the nucleus to the side (see Fig. 4–1). This fatty change is particularly common in the liver, which plays an essential role in the metabolism of fat (Fig. 4–2). The mechanism for the accumulation of fat is believed to be the following: When liver cells are damaged, as by the action of a poison, they are unable to synthesize protein. Free fatty acids brought to the liver from the fat depots then can no longer be conjugated with protein and liberated as lipoproteins. Instead, they appear within the cytoplasm of the sick liver cell as neutral triglyceride fat. The common cause of this fatty accumulation is alcoholism, and, as noted in Chapter 33, long-term alcoholism can ultimately lead to fibrosis and cirrhosis.

HYALINE DEGENERATION OF CELLS

The appearance of eosinophilic homogeneous material (called *hyaline*) is sometimes a feature of cellular degeneration. The best known example is the hyaline material ("alcoholic hyaline") seen in liver cells following a period of alcoholic debauchery (Fig. 4–3).

ADAPTIVE CHANGES IN DAMAGED CELLS

Although some of the changes seen in damaged cells appear to be degenerative, others are clearly adaptive. A good example of this is the change seen

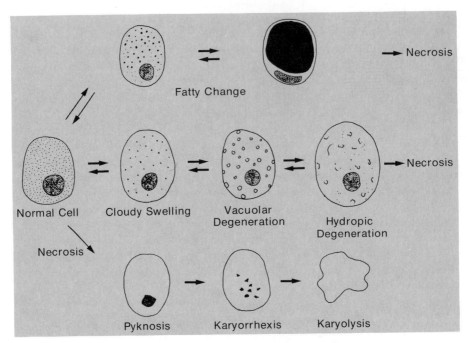

FIGURE 4–1. *Changes that may follow cell injury.*

Mild injury can either cause fatty change or water-logging. These changes are reversible, but if the injury continues, the cell may die. Necrosis follows.

Severe injury may kill the cell rapidly; the nuclear changes of pyknosis, karyorrhexis, and karyolysis indicate necrosis. These changes become evident about 12 hours after cell death and are not reversible. (Drawing by Margot Mackay, Department of Art as Applied to Medicine, University of Toronto.)

in liver cells after the administration of phenobarbital. This hypnotic drug is normally metabolized in the liver. Under the stress of excessive phenobarbital administration, the liver cell shows a tremendous increase in the amount of smooth endoplasmic reticulum, thereby suggesting increased activity in this region (Fig. 4–4). It is believed that the smooth endoplasmic reticulum is responsible for metabolism of many substances, including phenobarbital.

Sometimes localized areas of a cell appear to become degenerate, and the term "focal cytoplasmic degeneration" has been applied. These degenerate areas may be cast off from a surface or sometimes included in membrane-bound structures into which lysosomal enzymes are poured. The membrane-enclosed structures are called *autophagosomes,* or *cytolysosomes,* and an increase in their number is an indication of cell injury.

It is evident that not all the changes described occur under any single circumstance. Cells subjected to adverse conditions show a complex reaction: some changes are degenerative, while others are adaptive. The liver cell showing cloudy swelling due to carbon tetrachloride poisoning would therefore not be expected to show the same changes as one infected with a virus or as a kidney cell damaged by lack of oxygen (hypoxia).

FIGURE 4–2. *Alcoholic liver disease.*

The liver is severely damaged. Some cells show fatty change, the lipid in each cell appearing as a clear intracellular globule (Fat). Other cells are necrotic, and the structure of the liver lobule has collapsed. In the area of necrosis the reticulin fibers will be replaced by collagen fibers. Such a change to fibrous tissue (Ft) has already occurred in another area as a result of a previous episode of necrosis. The amount of fibrous tissue around a bile duct (Bd) is increased (× 250).

Cell Death and Necrosis

Cell death is difficult to define in precise terms, but in practice it may be regarded as having occurred whenever a cell is incapable of further division or of continuing its normal synthetic functions.

The appearance of the dead cells varies according to the cause of the injury. If the cells are killed suddenly as a result of physical or chemical trauma, they show no changes initially other than those directly attributable to the agent concerned, *e.g.*, disruption in electrical injuries and the effects of freezing or burning.

Cells less severely damaged—for instance, by poisons—may develop biochemical lesions that first progress to changes associated with water-logging and fatty change. As noted previously, these changes as detected by light microscopy are cytoplasmic and in themselves do not indicate cell death.

In a dead cell respiration ceases, but glycolysis proceeds for a while; as a result, there is the production of lactic acid and a drop in the pH. The synthetic activities of the cell stop, but the lytic destructive processes resulting from

FIGURE 4–3.   *Alcoholic liver damage.*
The liver cells (hepatocytes) are separated from each other so that the normal arrangement in plates is lost. Some cells contain eosinophilic material termed alcoholic hyaline (Alc H); others are necrotic (Nec). There is a diffuse infiltration by polymorphs (Poly) as evidence of an inflammatory reaction to the necrosis. The patient died of hepatic failure after a long history of excessive drinking (×600).

released lysosomal enzymes continue. As a result of this, the cell undergoes a process of self-digestion *(autolysis)* and within a few hours shows morphological changes by which cell death can be recognized. This process is called *necrosis,* which may be defined as the *circumscribed death of cells or tissues with structural evidence of their death. Necrosis and cell death are therefore not synonymous.*

The microscopic changes of necrosis affect the whole cell. The cytoplasm generally becomes homogeneous — often brightly eosinophilic. At the same time the nucleus shows changes that are pathognomonic of necrosis. Sometimes the nucleus becomes intensely dense-staining, and this is known as *pyknosis.* The pyknotic nucleus either breaks up into fragments *(karyorrhexis)* or becomes indistinct as the nuclear material is digested *(karyolysis).*

The importance of these nuclear changes cannot be overemphasized, because it is by their recognition that the pathologist can diagnose necrosis.

DIAGNOSIS OF NECROSIS BY BIOCHEMICAL MEANS

A diagnosis of the occurrence of necrosis is frequently of great clinical importance. When areas of heart muscle, pancreas, liver, or brain are dying, the

FIGURE 4–4.

Proliferation of the smooth endoplasmic reticulum (ser) in the periphery of a rat liver cell following the administration of ethionine. Phenobarbital can produce a similar change. The proliferated vesicles of the agranular reticulum are tightly packed and well demarcated from the rough endoplasmic reticulum (rer), which can be identified by the ribosomes studded on the membranes. Mitochondria (m) are elongated. (Other abbreviations: cm, cell membrane; lip, lipid droplet.) Tissue was stained by lead hydroxide (× 15,750). (Photograph courtesy of Dr. Katsumi Miyai.)

patient's life is often in jeopardy. As necrosis occurs, various soluble substances such as enzymes diffuse out of the cells and are absorbed into the blood stream where their detection is an aid to clinical diagnosis. Some important examples of this response may be listed. The serum glutamic oxaloacetic transaminase (SGOT), hydroxybutyrate dehydrogenase (HBD), and lactate dehydrogenase (LDH) are all raised after myocardial infarction, since these enzymes are found in high concentrations in heart muscle. An elevation of serum glutamic pyruvate transaminase (SGPT) and LDH is found after liver cell necrosis, such as in viral hepatitis. Some enzymes can be separated into separate fractions by electrophoresis. These separate fractions, each having a similar biochemical activity, are termed *isoenzymes;* specific isoenzymes occur in particular organs. In the case of the LDH, LDH_1 and LDH_2 are released from the heart muscle, whereas LDH_5 is of hepatic origin (Fig. 4–5).

TYPES OF NECROSIS

Coagulative Necrosis. In most tissues the process of necrosis entails the denaturation of cytoplasmic proteins, causing the tissue to become firm and somewhat opaque. The process resembles the change seen in the white of an egg on boiling.

FIGURE 4–5.

The lactate dehydrogenase (LDH) activity of serum is shown as five component isoenzymes separated by electrophoresis. LDH 1 is the fastest component and has traveled farthest in the direction of the arrow toward the anode. In the lower part of the diagram each molecule is depicted as a tetramer made up of varying combinations of either H polypeptides (closed circles) or M polypeptides (open circles). The H and M chains are determined by separate genes. (After Latner, A. L.: Journal of Clinical Pathology, 24, suppl. (Association of Clinical Pathology), 4:8–13, 1970.)

Denaturation often releases active side-chains of the molecules, which are then available for binding to dyes such as eosin. As noted previously, eosinophilia is a useful sign of cell death, and this is particularly helpful when one is looking for early signs of tissue necrosis. Thus, the patient who dies of a heart attack may show increased eosinophilia of the heart muscle fibers, indicating the early changes of an infarct (see below). Likewise, in patients suffering a cardiac arrest, the detection of eosinophilia in brain cells is a useful, reliable indication of permanent cerebral damage. In practice, of course, these changes are seen only at necropsy.

The increased binding capacity of necrotic tissue is also a factor in causing calcification. Necrotic tissue sometimes takes up calcium salts and becomes calcified. This response, which is termed *dystrophic calcification,* is quite frequently seen in necrotic tumor tissue. Since calcium can be detected so early by radiography, its presence has been utilized in diagnosis. In some cancers of the breast, characteristic flecks of calcium deposition can be seen even before the tumor can be palpated. The degenerate tissue of tuberculous lesions also commonly calcifies, as does the material found in atheroma.

A common cause of necrosis is sudden deprivation of the blood supply to the part. The process is called *infarction* and is common in the heart, kidneys, and spleen. These infarcts show the typical changes of coagulative necrosis. Microscopically, in addition to nuclear changes of pyknosis, karyorrhexis, or karyolysis another feature is noteworthy. The general architecture of the tissue may still be recognizable, even though its constituent cells are dead and their nuclei have disappeared. This is called *structured necrosis,* and the appearance has been likened to that of a city of the dead. In other examples of coagulative necrosis, in which there may be no residual structure at all, the effect is called *structureless necrosis;* it is the characteristic change seen in tuberculosis (see "Caseation," Chapter 10).

Colliquative Necrosis.   In the central nervous system, necrotic tissue undergoes softening and liquefaction, so that either the tissue collapses or a cyst is formed. Liquefaction is seen as a secondary event in other tissues when there is suppurative infection (see "Suppuration," Chapter 5) and following caseation in tuberculosis.

FURTHER CHANGES IN NECROTIC TISSUE

Acute Inflammation. Necrotic tissue excites an inflammatory response, which is followed by a phase of demolition and healing. The appearance of the acute inflammatory response, including an infiltration of polymorphs, is an important feature of most necrotic tissues and is a useful microscopic change that helps to distinguish necrosis from postmortem change. Thus, if an area of apparently necrotic cardiac muscle is surrounded by a zone of acute inflammation, the lesion may be safely diagnosed as an infarct. Likewise, the appearance of degenerate renal tubules associated with much edema and separation of tubules indicates premortem tubular necrosis, not a postmortem change. The acute inflammatory reaction is followed by a phase of demolition, as evidenced by the presence of many macrophages. If much lipid is present in the tissue, or if adipose tissue becomes necrotic, these macrophages contain multiple fine fat droplets and are called *foam cells.* This is a striking feature when necrosis affects brain or fatty tissue, such as in the breast. Sometimes macrophages fuse to form giant cells; these are described later in the section on granulomas (see Chapter 8).

Gangrene. Sometimes the dead tissue is invaded by saprophytic protein-splitting anaerobic bacteria, which cause its decomposition with the production of hydrogen sulfide and other foul-smelling substances. There is blackening of the area because of the formation of iron sulfide from the iron of decomposed hemoglobin. This *necrosis with superadded putrefaction is called "gangrene,"* which is an old clinical term that was applied to any black, foul-smelling area in continuity with the living.

CLOSTRIDIAL GANGRENE. The putrefactive bacteria are usually the clostridia of intestinal origin. Therefore, necrosis of the bowel, particularly of the large intestine, is often followed by gangrene. These putrefactive bacteria are of little importance in themselves, because they live on dead tissue and do not invade or harm the living tissues. Nevertheless, gangrenous lesions always contain pathogenic bacteria that invade tissues and cause further destruction. It follows that gangrene is a very serious condition and is fatal unless treated expeditiously.

GANGRENE DUE TO OTHER ORGANISMS. Some putrefactive bacteria are also pathogenic, *e.g.,* certain strains of anaerobic streptococci and members of the family *Bacteroidaceae.* The latter includes the well-known member *Fusobacterium fusiforme,* which is often found in company with a spirochete *(Borrelia vincentii).*

These putrefactive organisms are frequently found in the mouth and are the cause of ulcerative gingivitis, which is often seen following neglect; it is known as "Vincent's infection" or "trench mouth." A more serious gangrenous lesion occasionally affects the soft parts of the face and leads to great tissue destruction. It used to be described in debilitated children, particularly following measles, but it is now extremely rare in civilized countries.

This same group of anaerobic putrefactive organisms is also found in the vagina and is occasionally responsible for gangrene of the uterus following badly conducted labor or ill-performed abortion.

GANGRENE OF THE LIMBS. All the examples of gangrene so far mentioned are "wet." There is progressive tissue destruction, and unless effective treatment is instituted without delay, death results. A similar type of wet gangrene occurs in the limbs. It is usually due to blockage of the main arterial supply and is not infrequently a complication of diabetes mellitus. Generally the legs are affected, rather than the arms.

DRY GANGRENE.   If the blood supply to a limb is slowly occluded, the tips of the digits become black and necrotic and at the same time undergo desiccation. This drying of the part greatly impedes bacterial growth, and infection with pathogenic organisms is minimal. The condition therefore slowly extends until a point is reached where the blood supply to the limb is adequate. A line of demarcation develops, and the dead tissue is discarded by a process of spontaneous amputation. This condition is called *dry gangrene,* but since the amount of putrefaction is minimal, the term is somewhat of a misnomer. The process is, in fact, mummification of an infarcted portion of a limb.

GAS GANGRENE.   This condition is due to invasion by pathogenic clostridia and is described in more detail in Chapter 10.

Damage to Connective Tissue

Degenerations in the fibrovascular connective tissues are common and form as heterogeneous a group as do those affecting cellular parenchymal tissues.

CHANGES IN COLLAGEN

In those organs in which collagen formation stops at the reticulin stage, damage seems to stimulate the maturation of the fibers to ordinary fibrous tissue. The term *fibrosis* is used to describe this response. Good examples are the fibrosis seen in cirrhosis of the liver (see Chapter 33) and the fibrosis of lymph nodes draining areas of chronic infection.

Hyalinization. "Hyaline" is a descriptive term used to describe any glassy, eosinophilic, acellular tissue. Intracellular hyaline has been described previously. Amyloid may be described as hyaline until its true nature is recognized. As generally used, however, the term hyalinization is applied to a change in collagenous tissue when it becomes acellular and homogeneous. The changes are seen in the collagen of old scars, in the fibrous tissue of chronic inflammatory lesions, in the walls of small blood vessels in hypertension, in atheroma, and in "fibroid" tumors of the uterus. Hyalinized collagen has the normal staining properties of collagen, and it appears very inert and stable.

Elastosis of Collagen. Following prolonged exposure to ultraviolet light, the dermal collagen changes in such a way that it takes on some of the staining properties of elastic tissue. This gives the skin the familiar wrinkled, aged look in those fair-skinned individuals whose occupation or pleasures have resulted in excessive sun exposure.

Necrobiosis. Sometimes collagen becomes eosinophilic, weak, and breaks up. This is a characteristic feature of rheumatoid arthritis, and the degenerate collagen excites a chronic inflammatory reaction (see Chapter 40). Necrobiosis in collagen is sometimes described as "fibrinoid necrosis," but this term is also used in other contexts. Thus, the blood vessel walls in malignant hypertension show necrosis and marked eosinophilia. This latter change is probably different from the necrobiosis of rheumatoid arthritis and represents degeneration of the vessel wall as well as infiltration with fibrin.

CHANGES IN THE GROUND SUBSTANCE

Sometimes the connective tissues show an excessive accumulation of ground substance, which appears as a basophilic pool of structureless material. This overhydration of ground substance is sometimes a physiological event and appears to be under hormonal control. Thus, the colorful swelling of the sexual skin of the baboon and the enlargement of the cockscomb of the rooster are in large part due to this change. A similar change occurs in myxedema (see Chapter 39).

Sometimes the accumulation of excessive ground substance is associated with degeneration of the connective tissue fibers. Such a condition is called *myxomatous degeneration.* A good example of this is seen in the aorta when weakness in the vessel wall may cause rupture with consequent dramatic effects.

There is a group of genetically determined diseases involving an abnormality in the metabolism of mucopolysaccharide (the *mucopolysaccharidoses*). These diseases are usually accompanied by skeletal deformities and sometimes by corneal opacity. The best known member of this uncommon group of diseases is *Hurler's syndrome,* which because of the grotesque appearance of the head of its sufferers, is also known as "gargoylism."

Review Questions

1. How would you prove that a patient, under the situations listed below, had had a myocardial infarct:
   (a) during life; use biochemical tests
   (b) at necropsy; use microscopic examination of the heart.
2. Describe the changes caused by an excessive intake of alcohol (ethanol) that can be seen in liver cells. What happens to the reticulin framework of the organ, and what are the possible end results?
3. Compare and contrast the causes and end results of dry gangrene of a limb with those of wet gangrene.

Selected Readings

Peters, R. A.: Biochemical Lesions and Lethal Synthesis, Oxford, Pergamon Press, 1963.
Robbins, S. L.: Pathologic Basis of Disease. Philadelphia, W. B. Saunders Company, 1974. See in particular Chapter 2, "Cell Injury and Cell Death," as a source of further information.
Walter, J. B., and Israel, M. S.: General Pathology. 4th ed. Edinburgh, Churchill Livingstone, 1974. Chapter 4 gives greater details of the topics covered in this chapter.

Chapter 5

After studying this chapter the student should be able to:

- Define the following terms: hyperemia, vasodilatation, opsonization, chemotaxis, surface phagocytosis, macrophage, ulcer, and slough.
- Describe the vascular changes of acute inflammation and relate these to the formation and composition of inflammatory edema.
- Describe the cellular components of the inflammatory exudate and outline the mechanisms involved in their accumulation.
- List the types of acute inflammation and give examples of each.
- List the possible local sequelae of an acute inflammation.
- Describe the process of suppuration.
- Describe the triple response.
- List the important chemical mediators of acute inflammation and indicate their probable role.

    The body's reaction to injury is complex, for it involves not only a generalized response, which is described in Chapter 21, but also a localized response,

ACUTE INFLAMMATION

which has several components. The initial local reaction is concerned mainly with changes in the connective tissues. The blood vessels dilate, and by becoming more permeable, allow white cells and plasma to leak into the affected area. This reaction is termed "acute inflammation" and is familiar to anyone who has ever experienced a boil. It is characterized by four cardinal signs, which were originally described by Celsus in the first century A.D. These signs are *rubor, tumor, calor,* and *dolor,* which indicate that the area is red, swollen, warmer than the surrounding tissues, and painful. Since an inflamed part is often held still, loss of function has been added as a fifth sign of acute inflammation.

Inflammation is extremely common in clinical practice, and it is convenient to use the suffix *-itis* to denote its presence. Thus, tonsill*itis* is inflammation of the tonsils. In itself, this is not a complete diagnosis, for it does not indicate the cause. There can be tonsillitis due to streptococcal infection or tonsillitis due to infectious mononucleosis or to other viral infections.

Causes of Acute Inflammation

The causes are the same as those of tissue injury:

Physical Agents. Traumatic injury, such as cutting and crushing, may cause inflammation. Cuts of the skin become inflamed after several hours and are then more painful than at the time of their infliction. *Thermal* and *freezing injuries* cause typical acute inflammation, and the blisters that form in the skin in both conditions bear witness to the leakage or exudation of plasma from the blood vessels. *Ultraviolet light* and *ionizing radiations* (sunburn and radiation burns) are other physical causes.

Chemical Agents. When introduced into the tissues most chemicals cause inflammation. This may be severe, as with a wasp sting, or minimal as with the introduction of a stainless steel prosthesis, such as in total hip replacement surgery. Consequently, the problem in reconstructive surgery has been to find substances that cause no reaction at all.

Deprivation of Blood Supply. Infarction, which results from obstruction of circulation to an area, is described separately in Chapter 20.

Living Organisms. Inflammation is a feature of many infections, such as when a staphylococcal infection causes a boil. Note that the inflammation is a response to tissue damage rather than to the organism itself. In some infections, such as syphilis and typhoid fever, the invading organisms cause little immediate damage and therefore little immediate inflammation.

Antigen-Antibody Reactions. The IgE antibodies render tissues susceptible to the action of antigen, so that damage is done. Another method by which
immunoglobulins can cause damage is by the formation of immune complexes.
Sensitized lymphocytes can release damaging cytotoxic lymphokines. These
topics are described in Chapter 9.

Changes in Acute Inflammation

Inflammation can be studied in the living animal by observations of thin
tissues. The mesentery of the rat, the stretched-thin tongue of the frog, and the
rabbit ear-chamber (see Chapter 7) have all been used to observe the changing
events of inflammation.

THE VASCULAR RESPONSE

Although most tissues are liberally provided with capillaries, the limited
supply of blood that normally reaches the part is carefully distributed, so that at
any one time only some vessels contain a stream of blood. Indeed, there is a
central or thoroughfare channel, and during inactivity much blood passes
through it directly from the arterioles to the venules (Fig. 5–1). During activity
the thoroughfare channel closes, and blood is diverted to perfuse the tissues in
response to their increased metabolism. In addition, there is arteriolar dilatation, which increases the total volume of blood available. In acute inflammation the response is similar. There is arteriolar dilatation so that more blood
passes into the part. The precapillary sphincters open, so that the capillaries
become distended and blood ceases to flow through the preferential channel
(Fig. 5–1 B). This increased content of blood is termed *hyperemia* and is the
reason why the inflamed part appears red. The skin, being normally cooler than
the arterial blood, becomes warmer because of the increased flow. Dilatation of
blood vessels *(vasodilatation)* is thus a characteristic feature of acute inflammation.

Changes in Blood Flow. In a normal tissue, blood in the arterioles travels
so fast that one cannot discern individual cells. In the large tortuous venules,
on the other hand, the cells can be seen to occupy the central or axial part of
the stream and are separated from the endothelial lining by a clear zone of
plasma *(plasmatic zone)*. This arrangement is dictated by physical laws and has
the advantage of reducing the viscosity of blood. In acute inflammation, plasma
leaks from the vessels, and the blood consequently becomes more viscid; the
lubricating action of the plasmatic zone is impaired, and the stream slows
down. This process is termed *stasis*. Meanwhile, two other important changes
occur. The endothelial cells become swollen, and electron microscopy shows
that the spaces between adjacent cells become widened, thereby permitting
plasma and cells to pass between them. At the same time, white cells move
into the plasmatic zone and stick to the altered vessel wall. This adhesion is
highly characteristic of acute inflammation and is best seen in the venules. At
first, the cells adhere for a short time, and then they either roll gently along the
endothelial lining or get swept back into the blood stream. Later, however, the

FIGURE 5–1. *Diagrammatic representation of the vascular bed in normal tissue (A) and in acutely inflamed tissue (B).*

In the normal resting tissue much of the blood passes from the arteriole to the venule directly through the thoroughfare channel (T.C.). One capillary is closed (Cap. 1), while some blood passes through the other capillary (Cap. 2). The hydrostatic pressure at the arteriolar end of the capillary is 32 mm Hg and at the venous end is 12 mm Hg. These forces tend to drive fluid out of the vessel and are countered by the osmotic pressure of the plasma proteins—about 25 mm Hg. The interstitial extravascular fluid normally contains very little protein. Hence, fluid tends to leave the vessel at the arteriolar end and to be reabsorbed at the venous end.

In an inflamed tissue (B) the arteriole is dilated, the thoroughfare channel is closed, and both capillaries are dilated by the increased blood flow. The hydrostatic pressure at each end of the capillary is increased as shown. Plasma proteins have leaked from the vessels so that their concentration in the interstitial tissue fluid approximates that in the plasma. The osmotic effect of the plasma proteins tending to drive fluid into the vessels is thereby neutralized. Fluid is exuded along the entire length of the capillary, therefore, and is ultimately halted by a rise in tissue tension. (Drawing by Margot Mackay, Department of Art as Applied to Medicine, University of Toronto.)

cells become more firmly adherent and line the endothelium, forming masses that may even block the lumen. This phenomenon is known as *pavementation of the endothelium* and is the prelude to the emigration of the white cells from the blood stream into the interstitial tissue spaces.

FORMATION OF THE EXUDATE

The most characteristic feature of acute inflammation is the formation of an exudate that has both a fluid and a cellular component.

The Fluid Exudate. Under normal conditions the vascular endothelium is virtually impermeable to the plasma proteins, and the fluid that escapes from the vessels has a low protein content; on reaching the interstitial tissues, it either returns to the venules or is gathered by the lymphatics and returned to the circulation. In acute inflammation the increased vascular permeability allows the plasma proteins to leak through the vessel wall, causing the osmotic pressure effect of the plasma proteins to be lost. An increased volume of fluid therefore leaves the vessels, and this forms the inflammatory exudate (Fig. 5–1 *B*). A useful method of investigating this phenomenon is to tag the blood albumin either with a dye such as trypan blue or with a radioactive isotope of iodine. The accumulation of tagged albumin in the interstitial tissues of an area of inflammation then becomes an index of the change in vascular permeability. This type of investigation indicates that increased permeability occurs in two phases (Fig. 5–2). The initial phase of exudation appears to occur from the venules, whereas the later and more prolonged phase occurs from the capillaries.

There is another factor that plays an important part in the formation of the inflammatory exudate: one of the first detectable changes in experimental lesions is an alteration in the ground substance, causing it to become more fluid. The effect of this increased fluidity is to allow the exudate to diffuse into surrounding tissues more readily and thereby to prevent an immediate rise in tissue tension. Nevertheless, the tissue tension eventually increases, thereby limiting the amount of exudate formed, because it tends to drive fluid back into the venules. The increased tissue tension is one important factor in the causation of pain. It follows that inflammation in a densely compact tissue or in an enclosed space causes severe pain. This is well shown by the pain that is experienced in infections of the pulp of a finger and in acute osteomyelitis where the marrow is encased in unyielding bone.

The fluid leaving the blood vessels in acute inflammation has almost the same composition as plasma, and it contains antibacterial substances (such as complement) as well as specific antibodies. If present in the plasma drugs and antibiotics also appear in the exudate. The importance of the early administration of therapeutic agents is obvious when one recalls that these agents are merely carried to the inflamed area in the exudate and are in no way concentrated there. Furthermore, the fluid in the exudate is in a state of flux, since it is in equilibrium with the circulating plasma. Therapeutic agents must therefore be administered continuously if their concentration is to remain at a therapeutic level in the area of inflammation.

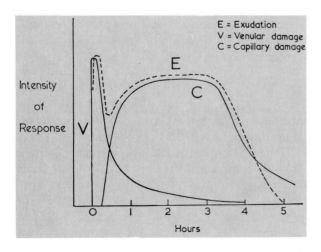

FIGURE 5–2. *Multiphase vascular response to mild thermal injury (54° C for 40 min.) in the rat cremaster muscle.*

(From A. A. Miles: Current notions about acute inflammation. *In* C. Illingworth (Ed.): Wound Healing. London, J & A Churchill Ltd., 1966.)

The fluid of the exudate has additional effects. It dilutes any irritating chemicals and bacterial toxins that might be present. The fibrinogen in it is converted into fibrin by the action of tissue thromboplastins (see Chapter 26), and a fibrin clot forms. This fibrin forms a fine network of fibers and has three main functions:

1. It forms a *union* between severed tissues.
2. It forms a *barrier* against bacterial invasion (see Chapter 6).
3. It aids *phagocytosis* (see later in this chapter).

The Cellular Exudate.   The white cells adhering to the endothelium of blood vessels soon push pseudopodia between adjacent endothelial cells, penetrate the basement membrane, and emerge on the external surface of the vessel. This remarkable process is called *emigration of the white cells;* for the most part, neutrophil polymorphonuclear leukocytes* predominate during the early phases of an acute inflammatory response. The gap that is left by the emigrating white cell soon closes behind it, although sometimes a few red cells escape at the same time. A variable number of lymphocytes and monocytes also leave the blood vessels. Figure 5–3 shows the typical appearance of an acutely inflamed tissue. The fixed tissue cells are separated by edema, and fibrin threads can be seen bathed in the edema fluid. Numerous white cells—for the most part polymorphs—are seen lying within the fluid exudate.

The movement of white cells into the interstitial tissues of an inflamed part appears to be a purposeful event, but it is obvious that the cells are not capable of independent, thoughtful action and that there must be some mechanism by which they are enticed from the vessels into the area of damage. It is generally believed that the attraction is of a chemical nature. Directional movement of cells in response to a chemical gradient is well known in biology and is called *chemotaxis*. An example of this movement is seen in the reproduction of the fern. The spermatozoids of the male are attracted by malic acid produced by the female germ cells.

A great deal of research has gone into the identification of the chemicals responsible for chemotaxis in acute inflammation in humans. Both polymorphs and monocytes have been shown to be attracted *in vitro* to a number of agents (Fig. 5–4) such as starch and certain bacteria. Other chemotactic agents are antigen-antibody complexes and dead tissue. These function only if complement is present and activated (see Chapter 9). The activated trimolecular complex C567 and the anaphylatoxins C3a and C5a are the chemotactic agents. The kinins, discussed later in the chapter, and nucleic acid derivatives also appear to be chemotactic.

One of the characteristic features of the inflammatory exudate is that in the initial stages polymorphs predominate, but as time goes by, these are replaced by monocytes. One explanation of this phenomenon is that polymorphs, having a very limited life span (probably a few hours), soon die off, leaving the long-lived mononuclear cells to replace them. Until recently it was thought that all agents attracting polymorphs also attract monocytes, and that the change in population of the inflammatory exudate could be explained on the basis of a

---

*These cells are commonly called "PMNs," "polys," or "polymorphs." The abbreviation *polymorph* is used frequently in this book.

FIGURE 5–3. *Acute appendicitis.*

This section was taken through the wall of an acutely inflamed appendix. The smooth muscle cells (Musc) are separated by inflammatory edema, and the whole area is heavily infiltrated by inflammatory cells, mostly polymorphs (Poly). Macrophages (Mac) and red cells (RBC) are also present in the exudate (× 600).

slow, steady recruitment of monocytes in the face of rapid destruction of polymorphs. It is now known that this is an oversimplification of the process and that the immune response plays a part (see Chapter 9). Thus, the reaction of antigen with IgE appears to release a chemotactic factor that specifically acts on eosinophils: cells that are prominent in certain allergic inflammations and in parasitic infections. Another important source of chemotactic agents is derived from sensitized lymphocytes. When these cells are acted upon by specific an-

FIGURE 5–4. *The Boyden chamber for detecting chemotactic activity.*

The Boyden chamber consists of two tissue culture chambers placed one on top of the other and separated by a membrane of 3 μm pore size (A). A suspension of polymorphs is placed in the upper chamber, and the test substance is placed in the lower. The number of cells that migrate to the lower surface of the filter is a measure of the chemotactic effect (B).

tigens, they release a number of factors called *lymphokines.* These have not been clearly defined, but some appear to have a specific chemotactic effect on polymorphs, eosinophils, or monocytes.

Lymphocytes are found in areas of inflammation, particularly during the healing process. In certain instances they are the predominant cell in the early phase of acute inflammation; viral infections and acute dermatitis are good examples in which this occurs. The mechanism of their accumulation is not known, because no definite chemotactic agents have been found that affect these cells. As noted above, lymphocytes can release lymphokines; they may therefore play several roles in acute inflammation.

FUNCTIONS OF CELLULAR EXUDATE: PHAGOCYTOSIS

Polymorphonuclear Leukocytes. The main function of these cells is *phagocytosis.* They ingest bacteria and other foreign particles (Fig. 5–5). Phagocytosis is aided by two mechanisms:

1. OPSONIZATION. Opsonins are proteins present in the plasma that coat organisms and cause them to be more easily phagocytosed. Some opsonins appear to be quite nonspecific and are present in all normal individuals, whereas others are immune antibodies and are therefore specific for the particular organisms that excited their formation. It follows that phagocytosis is more marked in the inflammation of an individual who has been immunized against the particular infecting organism.

2. SURFACE PHAGOCYTOSIS. The fibrin clot of the inflammatory exudate provides a network on which polymorphs can trap organisms. This method of phagocytosis can occur in the absence of opsonins and is presumably of value to the individual who is not immune.

Polymorphs show loss of their granules following phagocytosis. The granules are, in fact, lysosomes; they fuse with phagocytic vesicles and their lytic enzymes enter the common sac where digestion proceeds (Fig. 5–5).

Polymorphs release various chemicals following phagocytosis. These include *lysosomal enzymes*, which play a part in the digestion of dead tissue during the phase of healing as well as endogenous *pyrogen*, which is a major factor in the pathogenesis of the fever that accompanies any acute inflammation other than the most trivial.

The way in which organisms are killed by polymorphs and macrophages is complex and incompletely understood. The energy for phagocytosis is derived

FIGURE 5–5. *Phagocytosis.*

   A human peripheral blood polymorphonuclear leukocyte that has been exposed to zymosan particles (Z). At the right is a particle that has been bound to the cell but has not yet been ingested. In the lower portion of this picture are zymosan particles in phagocytic vacuoles. Lysosomes surround the particles and have degranulated into the vacuoles (arrows). Bacteria are treated in a similar manner and may later be destroyed (× 21,500). (Courtesy of Dr. Sylvia Hoffstein and Dr. Gerald Weissmann, New York University Medical Center.)

from glycolysis, and the lactic acid produced by this anaerobic process is bactericidal. Nevertheless, bactericidal activity is dependent mainly on oxidative reactions, with glucose being oxidized via the hexose monophosphate shunt (see Fig. 2–11). Hydrogen peroxide appears to be one of the vital bactericidal agents produced as a result of this.

Macrophages. The monocytes that accumulate in the area of acute inflammation are highly phagocytic; as with the polymorphs, their ingestion of virulent organisms is aided by opsonins. A pyrogen is also released. The monocytes are termed *macrophages* when they show morphological evidence of having phagocytosed material within them. Thus, the monocyte may be regarded as a resting cell that circulates in the blood. Once it enters an area of inflammation, it enlarges, becomes highly phagocytic, and is then termed "a macrophage." Another important function of the macrophage is that it appears to play a part in the initiation of the immune response (see Chapter 9).

Types of Acute Inflammation

Although all types of acute inflammation have many features in common, some types have been categorized on the basis of some particular gross or microscopic feature. The categories are useful for descriptive purposes and are commonly used, but the differences are of no fundamental importance.

Serous Inflammation. In inflammation of serous sacs and loose tissues such as the subcutaneous tissues around the vulva, scrotum, and eyes, the fluid component of an inflammatory exudate exceeds the cellular one, because the limiting factor of increased tissue tension is absent. There results a large accumulation of inflammatory edema, which is termed *serous inflammation.*

Fibrinous Inflammation. Fibrin formation is an obvious feature of inflammation in the lungs and on the surface of the serous membranes. Thus, it forms a well-marked feature of pericarditis and peritonitis (Figs. 5–6 and 5–7). Fibrinous inflammation of this type is often accompanied by an accumulation of serous fluid; thus, the term "sero-fibrinous inflammation" is an apt one.

Hemorrhagic Inflammation. The blood-stained exudate indicates severe vascular damage and bleeding. It is therefore a feature of vasculitis due to either organisms or chemical irritants. When blood-stained exudates are found in the pleural cavity or peritoneum, the two causes that first come to mind are tuberculosis and cancer. In both diseases, bleeding is common because of involvement of blood vessel walls.

Catarrhal Inflammation. This is seen when a mucus-secreting mucous membrane is involved in an acute inflammatory reaction. There is some destruction of the epithelial cells and a profuse mucus secretion from those cells that remain as well as from the underlying glands. The common cold provides an excellent example of this type of inflammation.

Pseudomembranous Inflammation. In diphtheria inflammatory exudate combines with necrotic epithelium to produce a gray membrane that is adherent to the affected part—usually the tonsils or the pharynx. This response is termed a pseudomembranous inflammation and can be contrasted with a *membranous inflammation* in which the membrane consists of an inflammatory

FIGURE 5–6. *Acute pericarditis.*

Two hearts have each been opened in the routine way at necropsy. *A*, Heart from 24-year-old female who had been diagnosed as having systemic lupus erythematosus. In spite of treatment, the patient developed the nephrotic syndrome and died of renal failure. At necropsy the pericardial sac contained 60 ml of straw-colored clear fluid; in some areas overlying the left ventricle, the pericardium was covered by a thin layer of fibrinous exudate (arrow). Elsewhere the pericardium is thin, shiny, and normal-appearing. This is an example of a serofibrinous inflammation. *B*, Heart from patient who had been operated on for cancer of the stomach but in whom the area of surgery had become infected. At necropsy pus was present in the left pleural space (thoracic empyema or pyothorax). Infection has spread to the pericardial sac, which also contained thick pus. The pericardial surface of the heart is seen to be covered by a thick, shaggy inflammatory exudate. Compare with *A*.

exudate and mucus. This latter type of inflammation is, in fact, extremely uncommon and is seen only rarely in the respiratory tract and colon.

 Gangrenous Inflammation.   Gangrene occurs in inflammation when the dead tissue is invaded by putrefactive organisms (see Chapters 4 and 10).

 Suppurative Inflammation.   Inflammation resulting in the formation of pus is described later in this chapter.

VARIABILITY OF THE CELLULAR EXUDATE

 Certain inflammations do not show the usual neutrophil polymorph response. Sometimes eosinophils are plentiful—particularly with inflammations produced by parasitic worms and with some allergic conditions, such as hay fever. Lymphocytic infiltration is frequent in inflammatory lesions produced by viruses, even in the early stages. It is also a feature of acute inflammation in many skin diseases. Occasionally macrophages are the predominant cell in the inflammatory response (see typhoid fever). The reason for this variation in cellular response is not known, but recent work indicates that many chemotactic factors are involved in the cellular exudation in acute inflammation.

FIGURE 5–7. *Acute pericarditis.*

This section is from the heart illustrated in Figure 5–6B. The pericardial surface is covered by a thick, inflammatory exudate consisting of a network of fibrin (Fib) in which many polymorphs are trapped. The epicardium, with its fat cells (Fat), overlies the cardiac muscle (Musc). It is inflamed and shows a heavy infiltration by acute inflammatory cells, mostly polymorphs (× 250).

Local Sequelae of Acute Inflammation

The changes following acute inflammation are shown in Figure 5–8 and depend upon two major factors: (1) the amount of tissue damage sustained; and (2) whether or not the causative agent remains in the body.

FIGURE 5–8. *The local sequelae of acute inflammation.*

RESOLUTION

In acutely inflamed tissues in which cellular damage has been relatively slight and reversible, necrosis does not occur. If the causative agent is eliminated by the inflammatory reaction—for instance, the pneumococcus in lobar pneumonia—or if the agent itself acts only once, such as in an acute sunburn, the acute inflammatory reaction terminates by resolution (Fig. 5–9). The polymorph cellular infiltrate is replaced by macrophages that engulf degenerate fibrin, red cells, polymorphs, and any other dead tissue that remains. Some of the fluid exudate returns to the blood in the venules, but most of it is carried away by the lymphatics to the regional lymph nodes. The reticuloendothelial cells remove cellular debris, and the fluid is returned to the circulation. With the removal of the inflammatory exudate and subsequent return of the macrophages to the lymphatics, the tissue is restored to its normal, previous state. *Resolution is the term applied to the process by which the tissue returns to normal following acute inflammation.*

ORGANIZATION OF EXUDATE

Occasionally the inflammatory exudate is not removed expeditiously enough, and it becomes invaded by granulation tissue and converted into scar tissue. It is a very common event to find fibrous adhesions between the visceral and parietal layers of the pleura. These are the organized remnants of some previous pleurisy. Likewise, fibrous adhesions are very common in the abdomen. They may occur around a site of previous inflammation such as an inflamed appendix, or they can follow previous surgery. Such adhesions make subsequent surgery more difficult; they can render it impossible to undertake sterilization by ligating the Fallopian tubes through a peritoneoscope.

SUPPURATION

When the noxious agent produces much necrosis of the tissue involved, resolution is impossible. If the exudate contains many polymorphs, the center of the inflammatory lesion becomes a cavity filled with a liquid containing dead tissue and numerous polymorphs, which are now called *pus cells*. The fluid is referred to as *pus*, and an inflammation with this type of response is termed *pyogenic*. A typical pyogenic infection is a boil; the hair follicle and adjacent dermis undergo necrosis, and a small sac of pus is formed. The necrotic tissue in an area of suppuration softens by virtue of the proteolytic lysosomal enzymes of the polymorphs as well as by autolysis mediated by the tissue's own enzymes. The creamy fluid is contained in a cavity called an *abscess* (see Fig. 44–4), and surrounding this there is a *pyogenic membrane*, which at this stage consists of inflamed and necrotic tissue with much fibrinous exudate and polymorph infiltration. The pus itself is composed of (a) leukocytes, some of which are dead; (b) other components of the inflammatory exudate, such as edema fluid with fibrin; (c) organisms, many of which are alive and can be cultured; and (d) tissue debris, such as nucleic acids and lipids. The pus tends not to remain at the site of its formation but rather to track in the line of least resistance until a free surface is reached. Then the abscess bursts and discharges its

FIGURE 5–9. *Bronchopneumonia.*

A, Instead of containing air, the alveoli are filled with inflammatory exudate, the cellular component of which is the most obvious. An inflamed lung such as this is airless (*consolidated*); the condition is called pneumonia (× 250). B, Higher magnification of one alveolus from the same case as A. The cellular exudate contains many macrophages (Mac) in addition to the polymorphs (Poly). The pneumonia is beginning to resolve (× 600).

contents spontaneously. In clinical practice this is usually anticipated by surgical drainage, because until the pus has been evacuated, healing is much delayed. If drained, an abscess heals by granulation tissue, but if the causative agent persists, chronic inflammation ensues. This response is considered in later chapters.

If, as occasionally happens, the abscess is not drained and remains localized or sequestered in the tissues, its walls become organized into dense fibrous tissue, and the pus undergoes thickening, or *inspissation.* It develops a porridgelike consistency and eventually calcifies.

When an acute suppurative inflammation involves an epithelial surface, the covering is destroyed and an ulcer is formed (Fig. 5–10). An *ulcer* is a term used to describe a localized defect of a covering or a lining epithelium. In the first instance the floor of the ulcer is covered by necrotic tissue and acute inflammatory exudate; this layer is called a *slough* and is at first adherent, because the dead tissue has not yet become liquefied. Eventually, however, the slough becomes detached, and the ulcer heals by the processes of repair and regeneration as described in Chapter 7.

CHRONIC INFLAMMATION

The other sequela of acute inflammation is progression to a state of chronicity. This occurs whenever the cause of tissue damage persists. In essence, chronic inflammation is a condition in which the causative agent persists, and the persisting acute inflammation is combined with healing and repair proceeding side by side.

Conclusion: Definition of Inflammation

Inflammation may be defined as *the reaction of the vascular and supporting elements of a tissue to injury, provided the injury has not been severe enough to destroy the area, and results in the formation of a protein-rich exudate.* Acute inflammation is mainly a vascular phenomenon and cannot occur in an avascular tissue like the cornea. The reaction is usually beneficial but may not be so under all conditions. The inflammatory cells, particularly macrophages, can themselves spread infection; this is a feature of tuberculosis. Furthermore, inflammatory edema may in some situations endanger life. Thus, in acute laryngitis the patient, particularly if it is a young child, may asphyxiate. Inflammation must be regarded as a mechanism that has evolved to protect the individual from a wide range of hazards. On the whole, it is a beneficial reaction; under certain circumstances the reaction itself becomes a hazard.

The Chemical Mediators of Acute Inflammation

The apparent uniformity of the acute inflammatory response — regardless of its cause — has led many investigators to presume that the changes are mediated by chemical agents that are formed when the tissue is damaged, rather than

FIGURE 5–10. *Suppurative appendicitis with mucosal ulceration*

The wall of the appendix shows the changes of acute inflammation. Edema separates the muscle fibers, and there is a heavy infiltration by polymorphs, which cannot be identified at this magnification. On the right there is necrosis. The overlying epithelium has been cast off, thereby leaving an area of ulceration. This is an example of suppurative inflammation with ulceration of a mucous membrane ($\times$ 60).

being caused directly by the injury itself. The search for these mediators has a practical as well as a theoretical objective. If these chemical substances could be identified, antagonistic drugs might be designed and administered to prevent or modify the acute inflammatory response.

HISTAMINE

At first, it appeared that the major mediator in acute inflammation was histamine. This is a simple amine of the amino acid histidine; if it is injected into the skin, it produces a reaction that is very similar to that produced by injuring the skin mechanically.

The Triple Response. Shortly after a firm stroking of the skin, a *red line* appears that is due to capillary dilatation. Soon after this, a more diffuse and widespread *flare* appears surrounding the red line. This results from arteriolar dilatation. Finally, a swelling or a *weal* appears at the site of the red line, and this is due to exudation of fluid through the altered vascular wall (Fig. 5–11). This triple response of the red line, flare, and weal was first noted by Sir Thomas Lewis to be very similar to the local changes that follow an injection of histamine. Indeed, there is little doubt that injury to the skin releases histamine from mast cells and that histamine is responsible for the phenomenon

FIGURE 5–11. *The triple response*

This game of tick-tack-toe was started on the skin of the back about three minutes before the photograph was taken. Red lines developed and were soon replaced by well-marked weals. The response is more marked in this subject than in the average person, but the ability to write on the skin in this way is not uncommon and is termed *dermatographism*. It is generally asymptomatic as in this 21-year-old female.

of the triple response. It now appears that histamine is the important mediator of the early phase of acute inflammation. Antihistaminic drugs have been developed, and their administration, while blocking the early phase of exudation, is without effect on the second phase (see Fig. 5–2). Histamine is especially important in inflammation having a type I allergic basis (see Chapter 9), and antihistaminic drugs are of some value in the treatment of hay fever. Nevertheless, in the acute response to most infections, particularly in the important and prolonged second phase of increased vascular permeability, histamine appears to play no part. Antihistamines are therefore of limited value in practice.

THE KININS

The blood contains an enzyme called *kallikrein,* which exists as a precursor and can be activated under certain circumstances. The kallikrein acts on a plasma protein and produces a polypeptide called *bradykinin.* This was so named because it causes a slow contraction of guinea pig small intestine *in vitro.* Bradykinin is an extremely potent chemical that causes an increase in vascular permeability and is chemotactic to white cells. It causes pain and clearly is a good candidate for being a mediator of acute inflammation. There is good evidence that bradykinin is formed following injury; as with histamine, however, it seems that its role is limited strictly to the early phase of acute inflammation. Tissues become refractory to the prolonged action both of bradykinin and histamine; therefore, neither can be mediators of the prolonged second phase.

BIOLOGICALLY ACTIVE CLEAVAGE PRODUCTS OF COMPLEMENT

Complement can be activated not only by antigen-antibody interaction but also by tissue damage. A number of fragments of complement, *e.g.*, C5a and C3a, can release histamine from mast cells. Likewise, there is a chemotactic component C567 (see Chapter 9).

BIOLOGICALLY ACTIVE COMPONENTS OF POLYMORPHS

Although inflammation can occur in the absence of polymorphs, these cells can release vasoactive compounds that may play a part in the inflammatory reaction. Among these are lysosomal enzymes that can activate kallikrein and indirectly can lead to the formation of bradykinin. In addition, they can lead to local tissue destruction. This is an important mechanism in the pathogenesis of immune-complex reactions.

PROSTAGLANDINS

The prostaglandins are a group of long-chain fatty acids that were first identified in human semen. They are highly active pharmacologically and cause vasodilatation and smooth muscle contraction. When injected into the skin, they cause a well-marked vasodilatation that lasts for some hours. Together with polymorph lysosomal enzymes, they are the present contenders for the role of mediators of the prolonged phase of acute inflammation. Prostaglandins can be synthesized in human platelets — an action that is inhibited by aspirin. Here then may be a clue to the action of this well-used but poorly understood anti-inflammatory agent.

CONCLUSION

Many other agents have been suggested as chemical mediators of acute inflammation but their relative importance is not known. There has been a tendency to stress the uniformity of the inflammatory reaction regardless of its cause, but this uniformity may be more apparent than real. Recent observations of the details of the vascular response to injury have revealed that it is a multiphased response with both early and delayed components affecting capillaries and venules. The precise changes vary according to the type of injury and the species of animal involved. It is therefore hardly surprising that no single common chemical mediator is involved. So far, much research has been directed to the vasodilatation and increased vascular permeability of acute inflammation caused by trauma and chemical agents. The much more complex cellular changes and the intricacies of infection have been largely neglected.

Review Questions

1. Describe the four cardinal signs of acute inflammation; explain how they occur.
2. An irritant solution is accidentally injected into one pleural cavity. Predict the possible results of this injection.

3. Describe the origin and functions of the macrophage in acute inflammation and its sequelae.
4. Describe the morphological types of acute inflammation that might be encountered in the peritoneal cavity. Name some likely causes of the inflammation.
5. Describe the possible role of complement in the pathogenesis of acute inflammation.

Selected Readings

Leading article: Mechanisms of eosinophilia. Lancet, 2:1187–1188, 1971.
Stossel, T. P.: Phagocytosis: The department of defense. New England Journal of Medicine, 286:776–777, 1972.
Weissmann, G. (Ed.): Mediators of Inflammation. New York, Plenum Press, 1974, 205 pp.
Ward, P. A.: The inflammatory mediators. Annals of the New York Academy of Sciences, 221:290, 1974.
Zweifach, B. W., Grant, L., and McCluskey, R. T. (Eds.): The Inflammatory Process. 2nd ed. New York, Academic Press Inc., 1974. This reference book, now in three volumes, covers many facets of the inflammatory response in considerable depth.

INFECTION

Chapter 6

After studying this chapter the student should be able to:

- Define the difference between intoxication and infection and give two examples of each.
- Describe how organisms are transmitted to the body.

- Discuss the importance of hospital infections.
- Describe the body's defenses against infection by using the skin, the intestine, and one other mucosal surface as examples.
- Discuss the three major patterns of infection, using as examples infection by:
    - (a) *Staphylococcus aureus*
    - (b) *Corynebacterium diphtheriae*
    - (c) *Salmonella typhi*
- Describe the various avenues through which infection can spread.
- List the factors that are of importance in predicting whether a particular infection will spread.
- List five examples of opportunistic infection.

From the moment of conception, the human body is exposed to microorganisms, some of which can produce lethal effects. Intrauterine development is rarely complicated by infection; the main microbial assault occurs after birth. Organisms can cause disease in two ways: either they gain access to the tissues of the host, multiply, and cause *infection,* or they manufacture powerful toxins that are subsequently introduced into the body and cause an *intoxication.*

Intoxication

Staphylococcal food poisoning provides an important example of an intoxication. If staphylococci of a suitable strain are allowed to grow for a few hours in a sample of food, the unfortunate victim who eats it will subsequently develop an acute attack of enteritis with accompanying diarrhea and vomiting. This reaction occurs even if the food is cooked, because even though heat kills staphylococci, it does not inactivate the toxin. It is obvious that anyone with a staphylococcal skin lesion, such as a boil, should not be allowed to handle food. Another example of intoxication is *botulism,* which fortunately is very rare. It occurs when food is contaminated with *Clostridium botulinum,* and when sufficient time has elapsed for the organism to grow and produce its toxin. Most outbreaks have been due to the ingestion of home-canned food in which the sterilizing process has been inadequate to destroy the highly resistant spores of the organism. When food containing toxin is ingested, the toxin is absorbed into the blood stream and affects the nervous system—apparently by interfering with acetylcholine release at nerve endings. Paralysis results, and in many instances it is progressive and fatal.

Infection

The most important method whereby microorganisms cause disease is by their *invasion of and multiplication in the living tissues of the host.* This is the definition of *infection,* and organisms capable of producing it are termed pathogens. With the exception of some rare congenital conditions, all infection is derived from the external environment. The organisms may be injected directly into the host by the bite of an insect or through an injury, but more often they are first deposited on a surface of the body which is thereby contaminated. Contamination may or may not be followed by infection.

TRANSMISSION OF ORGANISMS TO THE BODY

The following modes of transmission are important:

DIRECT CONTACT.   The causative agents of syphilis, gonorrhea, and other venereal diseases pass from one individual to another by direct contact. So also do staphylococci when they are transferred from the hands of one person to the skin surface or wound of another.

INHALATION.   Droplets or particles of dust containing pathogenic organisms cause contamination of the respiratory tract when they are inhaled. It is in this manner that some viral diseases such as influenza, measles, and chickenpox are contracted. So also are diphtheria, streptococcal sore throat, and meningococcal meningitis.

Droplets are formed during talking, coughing, and sneezing when air passes rapidly over a mucous membrane covered by saliva, or over tracheal or nasal secretions. Droplets soon dry and float in the air for long periods as particles of dust. Some organisms, such as the tubercle bacillus, are capable of surviving prolonged desiccation and are readily transmitted in this form.

INGESTION.   Food may be contaminated directly by the dirty hands of a human carrier or indirectly by flies. These insects carry pathogens from feces on which they feed to food on which they alight so readily. It is in this way that typhoid fever, bacillary dysentery, amebiasis, poliomyelitis, and infectious hepatitis are transmitted. Milk may contain bacteria because the animal itself is diseased, *e.g.,* brucellosis in goats and bovine tuberculosis in cows may be transmitted to man via the milk from these animals. Salmonella infections of fowls are passed on in their eggs.

HOSPITAL INFECTION

Whenever human beings live together in confined quarters, there is always the danger that there will be carriers of pathogenic organisms. Although not suffering from clinical illness themselves, they may pass on the organisms to others who succumb to the infection because of their reduced resistance. In turn, they further transmit the disease. This process is called *cross-infection;* in the past there have been many examples of epidemics of meningococcal meningitis and dysentery occurring in nurses' homes, army camps, and other places housing large numbers of people.

In hospitals it is not uncommon for patients to acquire severe infections from their environment; this is hardly surprising, because many patients are debilitated and their resistance to infection is lowered. Furthermore, surgical incisions provide a ready avenue for the invading bacteria. Extensive burns are particularly liable to become infected, and such patients should be isolated from possible sources of infection. This is termed *reverse isolation.*

A particularly unfortunate feature in hospitals is that the staff acquire pathogenic organisms from their patients, become carriers, and further disseminate the organism. Often, the strain is one that is resistant to the antibiotics in common use in that particular hospital. The infection is therefore all the more serious.

In the past, streptococcal infections have been serious, particularly in maternity wards. Identification of the strain of organism involved and a subsequent search for the source of infection has usually incriminated microbes in the throats of a few members of staff. The exclusion and treatment of such carriers and general measures designed to improve aseptic techniques have usually brought such an epidemic to a halt. Penicillin therapy is very effective in streptococcal infections, since resistant organisms do not occur. It follows that outbreaks of streptococcal hospital infection are not a problem at the present time.

The staphylococcus has, on the other hand, attained a much more prominent position. Outbreaks of postoperative wound infection are not uncommon, and the methods of control that proved effective with streptococcal outbreaks are quite inadequate. Often the majority of the staff are found to be carriers, and in addition the hospital itself—the floors, air-conditioning plant, and patients' bedclothes—is also contaminated with a virulent strain of staphylococcus. Although human carriers provide the reservoir, the hardy staphylococcus often infects patients by indirect means: for instance, in airborne dust particles. The problem of control is not easy; indeed, there is no simple answer to an outbreak of staphylococcal wound infection.

Other organisms that sometimes cause hospital infection are the coliform group, particularly the *Proteus* species, and *Pseudomonas pyocyanea.* As with the staphylococcus, the transfer of these organisms is usually indirect—via dust, contaminated articles, and fomites.* The source of organisms is often a patient with urinary-tract infection who contaminates his immediate environment—bedclothing, urine bottle, and other articles with which he has contact.

The Body's Defenses Against Infection

It is evident that the body surfaces are commonly contaminated by pathogenic organisms. Whether infection follows depends upon two factors: (1) the mechanical integrity of the body surface; and (2) its powers of removing organisms, *i.e.,* its powers of *decontamination.*

The protective mechanisms vary greatly from one tissue to another. Some examples will be considered below, others will be described under individual organs.

---

*Fomites are articles such as bedding or clothing that are capable of acting as a medium for the transmission of organisms that may give rise to infection.

MECHANICAL INTEGRITY OF BODY SURFACES

The mechanical strength of the epidermis with its tough outer layer of keratin is an important defense mechanism. Intact skin appears to be completely impervious to invasion by organisms, and it is only after injury that infection is established. Excessive sweating may macerate the keratin layer and render it incapable of repelling organisms. For this reason, skin infections are very common in the tropics, and boils are frequently seen in moist areas like the axillae (armpits). Boils are also common on the buttocks, a condition presumably related to the trauma of continual pressure in the sitting posture.

In other areas, the integrity of the covering epithelium is of less importance in repelling infection. Thus, in the mouth, esophagus, and stomach minor trauma causing superficial ulceration is common, and yet infection rarely occurs. In these situations the underlying connective tissue seems to have some special ability to prevent infection. The nature of this local immunity is not understood, but without it, every dental extraction would present a severe hazard, for not only is the underlying fibrous tissue exposed, but also the socket penetrates deeply into the bone of the jaw. In other situations, exposed bone is readily infected, and yet in the jaw following dental extraction, osteomyelitis is very uncommon.

DECONTAMINATION

Pathogenic organisms that are deposited on a body surface are generally removed expeditiously. Contamination is followed by decontamination. In the case of the skin, this can be readily demonstrated by deliberately contaminating the hands with hemolytic streptococci and subsequently estimating their rate of disappearance by taking swabs at regular intervals. The organisms are often removed or destroyed within two or three hours.

The mechanisms of decontamination vary with each individual surface and can be considered under three headings: *mechanical, biological,* and *chemical.*

Mechanical.   The surface keratin flakes of the skin are continually being rubbed off. This shedding carries away any surface organisms. Mucous membranes have a covering of fluid, and its movement has a washing effect that tends to remove organisms. The flow of tears over the conjunctiva, the upward moving sheet of mucus of the respiratory tract, the flow of saliva in the salivary ducts, and the flow of urine in the urinary tract are all mechanical methods that serve to wash away any organisms that have alighted on the surface.

Biological.   Most body surfaces are not sterile but are contaminated by organisms constituting the resident flora. This flora is characteristic of each particular surface. In the case of the skin, it includes *Staphylococcus albus* and diphtheroids. In the mouth, alpha hemolytic streptococci (*Streptococcus viridans*) predominate. In the large intestine on the other hand, bacteroides, coliforms, and enterococci abound. These organisms, constituting the resident flora, are so adapted to their environment that they do not normally cause infection. In fact, they provide protection to the host by producing antibiotic substances and by competing with other organisms for essential foodstuffs. If the resident flora is upset by antibiotic therapy, subsequent contamination by pathogenic organisms can lead to infection. This is sometimes seen when potent broad-spectrum antibiotics are administered by mouth. The flora of the intestine is so altered that an acute, fulminating — sometimes lethal — gastroenteritis can result from infection with *Staphylococcus pyogenes. Candida albicans* can likewise cause a troublesome stomatitis and pruritus ani.

Chemical. The various secretions that are found on each body surface often contain chemicals that destroy unwanted pathogens. The chemicals vary from one tissue to another. In the stomach, the hydrochloric acid is of great importance and destroys many pathogens. This is a very important method by which ingested food is broken down and common pathogens such as pneumococci and streptococci are destroyed. The stomach also forms an important defense mechanism for the respiratory tract, since pathogens present in the expectorated mucus are destroyed when this is swallowed.

Two other antibacterial substances are noteworthy in body secretions. *Lysozyme* is an enzyme present in many secretions and is capable of removing the cell wall of some bacteria. This was first described by Fleming, who is better known for his discovery of penicillin. The other important chemical agent is immunoglobulin, particularly IgA (see Chapter 9).

PATTERNS OF INFECTION

The relationship between a host and its invading pathogens is a complex one. Three main patterns will be described: (1) *Invasive organisms producing local damage;* (2) *toxic organisms;* (3) *invasive organisms producing little local damage.*

Invasive Organisms Producing Local Damage. Some infecting organisms produce toxins which, by causing local tissue destruction, excite an acute inflammatory reaction. *Staphylococcus aureus* is an example of an organism that produces such an infection; in the skin, this response can vary from a mild *folliculitis* involving the superficial part of a pilosebaceous follicle to a *boil* involving the whole hair follicle apparatus and leading to abscess formation. Local spread of infection leads to involvement of the subcutaneous tissues so that a *carbuncle* is formed (see Fig. 10–1). Spread into the lymphatic vessels leads to inflammation of the tissues around these vessels *(lymphangitis).* When these vessels are superficial, the inflammation appears as red streaks under the skin. When organisms reach the regional lymphatic nodes, there is swelling and tenderness of the nodes as evidence of *lymphadenitis.* Finally, the organisms may penetrate the barrier of the lymph nodes and enter the blood stream via the thoracic duct. The local tissues and the inflammatory reaction form the *first defense against infection,* and the *lymph nodes form the second,* but it is in the blood stream that the third and most effective defense mechanism is encountered. This is the *reticuloendothelial system.* The cells of this system have the property of being able to phagocytose circulating organisms, and frequently they destroy them. If the cells of the reticuloendothelial system are capable of destroying such organisms, the presence of organisms in the blood is both of short duration and little consequence. It sometimes happens that during the course of an infection blood is taken for culture and organisms are grown. The presence of these organisms in the blood is termed *bacteremia,* and it signifies the presence of a positive blood culture in the absence of any marked symptoms.

Sometimes organisms engulfed by the reticuloendothelial system are not destroyed but are allowed to proliferate in the cytoplasm of the cells. This situation occurs when immunity is low and results in vast numbers of organisms being produced in the cytoplasm of the reticuloendothelial cells. When these cells undergo necrosis, the organisms and their toxic products are released into the blood stream. The blood culture is again positive, but on this occasion the patient is gravely ill. Such a condition is known as *septicemia*. It indicates a positive blood culture and a complete overwhelming of the defenses of the body. It is therefore a grave condition, which frequently proves fatal.

Toxic Organisms.   Some organisms manufacture extremely potent exotoxins that produce local tissue damage. In addition, these toxins can enter the blood stream and cause damage at distant sites. An excellent example of this type of infection is diphtheria. When the causative organism, *Corynebacterium diphtheriae,* alights on a tonsil, it proliferates and produces diphtheria toxin. This leads to local tissue necrosis and a local acute inflammation, recognized clinically as a sore throat. The tonsils are covered by a layer of necrotic epithelium and exudate, which is called a *pseudomembrane.* Surrounding edema can be so severe that life is threatened by involvement of the larynx. However, the serious effects of diphtheria are related to the effects of disseminated toxin. Damage to nerves can cause paralysis, *e.g.,* of the palate, and damage to the heart leads to a toxic myocarditis and heart failure. It should be noted that the manifestations of diphtheria are entirely due to the exotoxin. The organisms themselves are not invasive, but remain on the surface of the tonsils or on the pharyngeal wall.

In tetanus there is a similar pattern of disease. Spores of the organism are introduced into a wound, germinate if circumstances are favorable, and produce tetanus exotoxin. This agent is absorbed both via perineural spaces and directly into the blood stream. When the toxin reaches the central nervous system, its actions lead to violent spasms of skeletal muscles and ultimately to paralysis and death. Once again the organisms remain localized, but the disease is attributable to the effects of exotoxin. Gas gangrene is another example of an infection with a toxic organism (see Chapter 10).

Invasive Organisms Producing Little Local Damage.   Some organisms appear to produce little or no local tissue damage and therefore no inflammatory response at the site of entry. Such organisms can proliferate rapidly and spread throughout the body via the lymphatics and ultimately via the blood stream. Infection with this type of organism is common, and the manner by which lesions are produced can be understood by a study of the disease typhoid fever.

PATHOGENESIS OF TYPHOID FEVER.   The pathogenesis of mouse typhoid (infection with *Salmonella typhimurium)* has been studied in considerable detail. By analogy, the sequence of events in man is as follows:

Typhoid fever is contracted by the ingestion of food contaminated with *Salmonella typhi.* The organisms reach the lumen of the intestine and are taken up by phagocytes on its mucosal surface. In the cytoplasm of these cells the organisms are carried into the mucosa itself and then to the local lymphoid tissue (Peyer's patches). Scarcely any local tissue damage occurs, and little or no inflammation ensues. The organisms multiply, and some pass on through lymph vessels to the mesenteric nodes and finally reach the blood stream via the thoracic duct. In this way a bacteremia develops and the phagocytic cells of the reticuloendothelial (RE) system engulf them. However, since the bacteria are pathogens they are able to live and multiply in the RE cells; by about the tenth day the parasitized cells undergo necrosis and cause the blood stream to be flooded with large numbers of bacilli. This is the end of the *incubation period* (usually 10 to 14 days), and the patient becomes seriously ill with septicemia (Fig. 6–1).

The *septicemic phase* lasts about a week and is characterized clinically by a progressive rise in temperature, by constipation, and by severe constitutional symptoms. The mind becomes clouded, coma ensues, and death may occur. Diagnosis rests on one's obtaining a positive blood culture.

The next phase of the disease is marked by the onset of diarrhea associated with ulceration of the small intestine and by the appearance of organisms in the feces. The bacilli reach the gut via the bile, which is heavily contaminated as a result of passage of bacteria from the RE cells of the liver. The ulceration occurs over the inflamed Peyer's patches and is accompanied by enlarged mesenteric lymph nodes. In both the ulcers and the lymph nodes there is an accumulation of macrophages; polymorphs are conspicuously absent. The most likely explanation of these events is that following the initial infection the local lymphoid tissue of the gut becomes sensitized to the organisms or their products, and that subsequent contact with the organisms produces damage. The sensitizing antibodies are presumably produced locally, because the blood

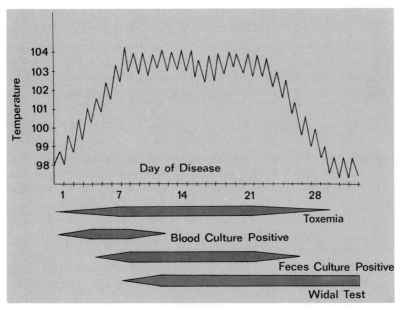

FIGURE 6–1.

Chart correlating the clinical course of a typical case of untreated typhoid fever with the principal methods of bacteriological diagnosis. Note the step-ladder rise in temperature during the first week. (Drawing by Anthony J. Walter.)

level of antibodies detectable as agglutinins does not rise until later in the course of the disease. During the second week of typhoid fever, diagnosis depends upon the finding of the organism in the feces.

Typhoid fever therefore represents an infection by a highly invasive organism in which tissue damage appears to be produced by some type of antigen-antibody interaction. Since antibody production takes 10 to 14 days to begin, it follows that symptoms do not occur until after the organism has spread widely. The incubation period is therefore long and contrasts with the short incubation period of diseases caused by invasive organisms that produce direct local tissue damage, e.g., staphylococci and streptococci.

Toward the end of the second week of typhoid fever, antityphoid antibodies appear in the blood, and their titer subsequently rises. These antibodies are usually detected as agglutinins; the test employed is referred to as the *Widal reaction* (see Fig. 9–6). Since a rising titer of agglutinins is particularly significant in the diagnosis, a specimen of blood should be taken early in the course of a suspected case of typhoid fever so that its titer of antibodies can be compared with that of later samples. This method of confirming the diagnosis of an infective illness is particularly valuable if the causative organism has not been isolated. It is particularly useful in viral disease, since the infective agent is often difficult to isolate once the disease is clinically apparent. The method is also of use if the virus laboratory is not immediately at hand.

Other invasive organisms produce a disease similar in overall pattern to that of typhoid fever. In syphilis there is widespread dissemination of organisms, and a local ulcer does not appear for three to four weeks (see Chapter 10). In many viral infections (e.g., smallpox and measles), widespread dissemination of the disease organisms occurs before the onset of the characteristic disease. Once again, the incubation period tends to be about two weeks. It is interesting that in many instances the ability of the organisms to spread is inversely proportional to their ability to produce immediate local tissue damage. Thus, staphylococci produce local inflammatory lesions but tend to remain localized, whereas the organism of syphilis produces no immediate damage yet is highly invasive.

Other Patterns of Infection. Many other patterns of infection can be recognized. Some organisms can produce a local lesion with minimal inflammation such that the incident goes unnoted. This is a *subclinical* infection. Some organisms can enter into a symbiotic state with their hosts — either permanently or between phases — when they cause damage. An example of the latter type of infection is the common coldsore due to the herpes simplex virus. The virus causes the characteristic blisters of the skin; between attacks, however, it resides in the ganglion of a sensory nerve supplying the part. A special group of virus infections (oncogenic viruses) is known that will produce tumors; these are described in Chapter 17. It is evident that infection proceeds according to many different patterns, and the situation is further complicated by the fact that one particular strain of organism can, under different circumstances, produce different types of infective illness. Thus, *Streptococcus pyogenes* can on the one hand produce a relatively minor local infection in the form of a sore throat, but under other circumstances (e.g., when it is introduced into a cut sustained while a necropsy examination is performed) can lead to a fulminating septicemia. Likewise, the herpes simplex virus can remain as a latent infection in some individuals, while in others it causes coldsores, pneumonitis, or encephalitis. It may even be a major factor in the etiology of cancer of the uterus.

Spread of Infection

Following is a summary of the ways in which infection can spread (Fig. 6–2):

SPREAD BY CONTINUITY: DIRECT SPREAD

The natural cohesion of tissues tends to prevent the spread of organisms. Nevertheless, the tissue fluids are in constant motion because of movement of the part, and organisms are carried in any stream of fluid that may be present. Since muscular activity causes considerable fluid movement, the time-honored treatment of inflammation is to rest the part. Two features should be noted. First, the actual motility of the organism appears to play no part in the spread of infection. Thus, *Clostridium tetani* is a motile organism but the infection (tetanus) is a localized affair. Second, the degree of local spread is inversely proportional to the amount of damage produced by the organism. Damage leads to an inflammatory reaction, and this is often an efficient local defense mechanism. Thus the deposition of fibrin sometimes appears to be important in walling off an infection; for example, fibrinous adhesions prevent the spread of infection from an acutely inflamed appendix (see Chapter 32).

Local spread can occur in an entirely different way. Some organisms are ingested by phagocytes and are transported by these cells. This is an important means of spread in tuberculosis and almost certainly occurs in other infections.

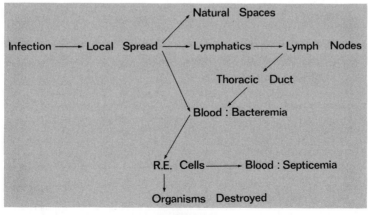

FIGURE 6–2.

Diagram illustrating the sequence of events that can follow the spread of infection.

SPREAD BY NATURAL CHANNELS

If local spread implicates a natural passage, infection may extend by this route. The following examples are important:

Peritoneum. Infection may spread rapidly throughout the peritoneal space from a localized lesion. Acute appendicitis is therefore serious, because following perforation of the organ, the entire peritoneal cavity can become infected. A large surface is involved, and there is rapid absorption of toxic substances, causing the patient to become severely ill. Likewise, infection can spread throughout the pleural cavity, the subarachnoid space, the pericardium, and joint spaces.

Infection can also spread along tubes, like the bronchi (with bronchopneumonia and tuberculosis), the ureter, and the gut.

Lymphatics. In acute inflammation the lymphatic vessels are held open widely by the increased tissue tension. The permeability of the vessel walls is increased and so also is the flow of lymph. Invading organisms that gain access to the lymphatics are carried to the nearest lymph node where, for a time at least, they are held up by the local reticuloendothelial cells. Lymphangitis and lymphadenitis are characteristic of certain types of infection, *e.g.*, streptococcal and tubercular infections.

Blood Stream. There are several ways by which organisms enter the blood stream. These will be elaborated on in the following sections.

DIRECT INVASION OF BLOOD VESSELS. A few organisms may invade the blood vessels during the course of any local infection. The infection may itself be quite trivial, but the adjacent blood vessels can be ruptured by trauma, thereby allowing organisms to enter. Gingival infection or abscesses related to the apices of the roots of teeth are common lesions in which this invasion occurs. Such spread of infection often follows dental extraction, scaling of teeth, or even chewing hard food. When small numbers of organisms enter the blood stream in this way, they are rapidly removed by the reticuloendothelial system, and the bacteremia that occurs causes no symptoms. An exception to this is when the bacteremia is due to one of the gram-negative bacilli of the coliform group. In this instance, the patient sometimes has rigors and develops a fever. This is occasionally seen in the bacteremia that follows passage of a catheter up the urethra.

Bacteremia cannot be dismissed as a completely inconsequential event. Under certain circumstances, it can lead to serious sequelae.

Metastatic Lesions. Experimentally it can be shown that when an animal has a bacteremia, histamine injected at any site will precipitate a local infection by the organism concerned. Trauma has a similar effect. It is believed that this is the origin of acute osteomyelitis. A child who happens to have a staphylococcal bacteremia and traumatizes a limb then develops an acute infection of the bone (see Chapter 40). Another danger of a bacteremia is that the organisms can be filtered off by the kidneys, and if there is a simultaneous obstruction of the outflow of urine, a kidney infection *(pyelonephritis)* results. A further hazard of bacteremia is that the organisms may colonize a damaged heart valve and cause endocarditis (see Chapter 28).

SEPTIC THROMBOPHLEBITIS. When infection spreads to a vein, its walls become inflamed and thrombosis occurs. The condition is called *thrombophle-*

bitis. If the thrombus is invaded by a pyogenic organism, it may soften and parts of it become detached, leading to the condition of pyemia (see Chapter 20).

SPREAD FROM THE LYMPHATIC SYSTEM. Organisms that are not held up in the tissues at the site of entry or in the lymph nodes reach the venous circulation via lymphatic ducts. This has already been described in the instance of typhoid fever.

Along Nerves. This is not a common route of infection and in fact is restricted to some viruses, such as the virus of rabies.

Factors Determining Localization or Spread of Infection

The following sections include a summary of the factors that determine whether a particular organism is likely to spread from the site of infection or to remain localized.

FACTORS INVOLVING THE ORGANISMS

VIRULENCE. Within each species of organism there are many different strains, each with differing virulence. For example, there are many strains of staphylococci, and some of these are associated with particularly severe infection. Likewise, some strains of diphtheria bacilli produce more exotoxin than do others.

DOSE. A large dose of organisms tend to produce a more severe infection than a small dose.

PORTAL OF ENTRY. This is a most important factor, because some organisms will cause infection only if administered by a particular route. For example, *Vibrio cholerae* can be injected subcutaneously without harm, but if it is swallowed, it causes cholera. Likewise, many of the coliform organisms produce no damage in the intestine, but cause infection if introduced into the urinary tract.

SYNERGISM. The combined effect of two organisms may be more severe than the effect of either acting alone. Staphylococcal infection of a wound, for example, can precipitate the onset of gas gangrene (see Chapter 10).

PRODUCTS OF THE ORGANISM. The toxic products of organisms can presumably aid their infection. They act in many ways; some destroy tissue locally. Leukocidins damage white cells, hyaluronidase depolymerizes the ground substance, whereas streptokinase aids in the lysis of fibrin by activating plasmin (see Chapter 20).

FACTORS INVOLVING THE HOST

General Factors. The *general state of health* of the host is important. Patients who are starved or who suffer from chronic debilitating diseases like chronic nephritis and diabetes mellitus are less capable of resisting infection. The factors involved are complex and probably involve both humoral factors (*e.g.,* a low complement level) and an impaired activity of phagocytes.

THE IMMUNE STATE. This involves both nonspecific factors like complement and the presence of specific antibodies of acquired immunity.

LOW WHITE CELL COUNT. Whenever the neutrophil polymorph count is low (agranulocytosis), there is a tendency for infection to occur.

ABNORMAL WHITE CELLS. Occasionally patients are encountered in whom there is an inherent defect in white cell function. These patients tend to suffer from repeated bacterial infections that commence in childhood. Specialized techniques are now available for investigating the phagocytic and bactericidal activity of polymorphs.

Local Factors. The presence of necrotic tissue is an important predisposing cause of local infection. Foreign bodies and chemicals that cause necrosis are therefore harmful. Another important factor is the local blood supply. Ischemia of any origin, by impairing the local inflammatory reaction, is detrimental to the body's efforts at repelling infection. Infection and ulceration can follow quite trivial injuries to the legs of patients who have varicose veins or suffer from arteriosclerosis. Likewise, tetanus can sometimes follow the local injection of epinephrine if a dirty needle is used.

OPPORTUNISTIC INFECTIONS

It is now apparent that some organisms that in the past have been considered to be avirulent can cause infection under certain circumstances. This is called *opportunistic infection* and may occur when either local or general factors operate in favor of the organism.

Abnormal Local Conditions. Prosthetic heart valves provide an admirable site for infection with a wide range of organisms, including rickettsiae and fungi, which normally do not produce endocarditis. Another example is related to the use of broad-spectrum antibiotics. As noted previously, these drugs can so alter the flora of the gut that fulminating gastroenteritis can be caused by *Staphylococcus aureus.* Secondary infections stemming from alteration of the microbial flora by antibiotic therapy are usually called *superinfections.*

Immunologically Suppressed Patient. The administration of glucocorticoids and anticancer drugs, particularly to patients with malignant disease of the reticuloendothelial system (*e.g.,* Hodgkin's disease), can create conditions favorable to opportunistic infections. Thus, it is not uncommon for such patients to die of infections by fungi that in normal people rarely cause infection. Furthermore, organisms (*e.g., Candida*) that commonly produce a local infection can become widely disseminated in the immunologically suppressed patient (see Chapter 13).

Conclusion

The traditional division of organisms into pathogens and nonpathogens, while serving a useful purpose under most circumstances, is an artificial separation. Before deciding whether an organism is causing a particular infection one must consider the organism in relation to the circumstances of a particular patient. In the ongoing battle between man and microbe there are no simple rules for distinguishing friend from foe.

Review Questions

1. Explain the following complications of untreated or inadequately treated typhoid fever: (a) suppurative parotitis; (b) bronchopneumonia; (c) boils; (d) pyelonephritis; and (e) typhoid osteitis and periosteitis.
2. The incubation period of diphtheria is 2 to 7 days, whereas that of typhoid fever is about 10 days. Based on your knowledge of the pathogenesis of the two diseases, account for this difference.
3. Why is a wound infection with *Staphylococcus aureus* of greater importance than one due to *Streptococcus pyogenes*?
4. When placed in reverse isolation, a patient is protected from organisms that are carried by visitors, including the attending medical and nursing staff. Give some examples of patients who should be placed in reverse isolation and indicate the reason for doing this.

Selected Readings

Leading article: What makes bacteria pathogenic? Lancet, 2:266, 1972.

Youmans, G. P., Paterson, P. Y., and Sommers, H. M.: The Biologic and Clinical Basis of Infectious Diseases. Philadelphia, W. B. Saunders Company, 1975.
Chapter 2, "Characteristics of Host-Bacteria Interaction: External Defense Mechanisms," elaborates on many of the topics covered in this chapter.

Chapter 7

After studying this chapter the student should be able to:

- Describe the differences between repair, regeneration, and reconstitution of tissue.
- Compare wound contraction with cicatrization.
- Describe how wound contraction can be measured experimentally.
- Describe the mode of formation and the components of granulation tissue.
- Describe how an incised skin wound heals and compare it with the healing of a skin wound with separated edges.
- List the important causes of slow wound healing.
- List the important complications of wound healing.
- Describe the main features of healing in liver, kidney, tendon, and muscle.
- Compare and contrast healing in the peripheral nervous system with healing in the central nervous system.

Introduction; Definition of Terms

Sustaining injury is one of the inevitable tribulations of life. It follows that the individual's ability to heal wounds is one of the fundamental processes in pathology. The term "wound healing" is taken to include all those processes that follow the inflammation secondary to the infliction of tissue damage. The types of injury include not only obvious traumatic damage such as those caused by a surgical incision or stab wound but also those examples of tissue damage produced by heat, freezing, radiation, infection, chemical toxins, ischemia, and the results of damaging antigen-antibody interaction. The process of healing has obvious survival value for the individual, and has therefore been highly developed in all forms of life. Nevertheless, it differs from one species to another as well as from one tissue to another within the same individual.

Wound healing has two important aspects: (1) *contraction*—a process by which the size of a wound decreases during the first few days following the infliction of the wound; and (2) *replacement of lost tissue*—a process by which migration of cells as well as division of adjacent cells provides extra tissue to fill the defect. This can be accomplished in two ways:

Repair. This is a process by which the lost specialized tissue is replaced by granulation tissue, which later matures to form scar tissue. It is an inevitable end-result when the surviving specialized cells do not possess the ability to proliferate.

Regeneration. This term is applied to the process by which the lost tissue is replaced by a tissue similar in type. Thus, when liver cells have been damaged, more liver tissue is produced by a proliferation of the surrounding undamaged specialized cells.

Reconstitution. This term describes the coordinated regeneration of several types of lost tissue, and it results in the re-formation of whole organs or limbs. The process is well seen in lower forms of life. For example, if the limb of a newt is amputated, a new mass of cells develop that proceeds to differentiate into the skeletal and other structures of a new limb. Among the crustaceans, new limbs, claws, and eyes can be re-formed in a similar manner. It is obvious that the processes concerned in reconstitution are complex and resemble the embryonic development of the limb or asexual reproduction, such as occurs in lower forms of life. One would have thought that the ability to reconstitute a lost limb or organ was so useful to survival that it would have been retained during evolution. Such has not been the case. The higher animals—including humans—do not have the ability to replace limbs following their amputation. In humans, the nearest approach to this process is the re-formation of new liver tissue following partial hepatectomy.

Before the coordinated process that occurs during simple skin wound healing is described, it is convenient to describe wound contraction and granulation tissue formation. These are two components of the process that can be studied experimentally and can be quantitated.

WOUND CONTRACTION

This is a dynamic process that can be studied in the experimental animal by excising a small, circular, full-thickness disk of skin from the back or flank. Figures 7–1 and 7–2 show the result of such an experiment. The size of the wound is measured at regular intervals; after an initial period of two to three days, there follows a phase of rapid contraction, which is largely completed by the fourteenth day. New tissue formation is not included, since the measurements are made from the original wound edges. The importance of wound contraction is illustrated in Figure 7–3. It can be seen that with good contraction a small scar is produced, while with inadequate contraction, a large scar results, with all the cosmetic and functional complications that follow.

Much experimental work has been carried out with a view to understanding the process of wound contraction so that it may be brought under control when necessary. It is generally agreed that the contractile force resides in the new granulation tissue that forms around the circumference of a healing wound. This has been called the *picture frame area.* Although the mechanism is not fully understood, it appears that the tissues become remodeled. Perhaps contraction of the fibromyoblasts of granulation tissue plays a role in this process.

Wound contraction can be inhibited by the systemic administration of glucocorticoids and by the local application of ionizing radiations. Mechanical factors, such as tethering of the wound edges, are also effective in preventing contraction. This is well illustrated by the large chronic ulcers that occur around the ankle in patients with venous stasis (Fig. 7–4). Dense, fibrous tissue fixes the wound edges to the periostium of the tibia, and healing results in very extensive scar tissue formation. The scar is covered by thin (atrophic) epidermis and is liable to ulcerate with subsequent injury—even quite trivial injury.

GRANULATION TISSUE FORMATION

Granulation tissue is formed by the proliferation and migration of surrounding connective tissue elements. In the first instance, it is composed of *capillary loops* and *fibroblasts,* together with a variable number of inflammatory cells. Initially, granulation tissue is highly vascular, but with the passage of time it becomes avascular scar tissue. The manner of its formation can be studied experimentally in various ways. A convenient method is by observations of the rabbit ear–chamber, which is illustrated in Figures 7–5 to 7–8.

Buds of endothelial cells grow out from existing blood vessels at the wound margin, undergo canalization, and form a series of vascular arcades by joining with their neighbors. At first the new-formed vessels all appear similar and have a thin wall consisting of only endothelium. These vessels leak protein readily, so that the fluid bathing the area consists virtually of plasma and forms an admirable nutrient medium. Very soon differentiation occurs: some vessels acquire a muscular coat and become arterioles, while others form thin-walled large venules. Some persist as part of the capillary bed, while the remainder disappear as the granulation tissue steadily becomes modified.

At the same time that the vessels grow into the clot, fibroblast-like cells around the wound margin multiply and accompany the vascular invasion.

Text continued on page 112

Control   Days   1,650 r

1.

8.

10.

17.

FIGURE 7–1. *Wound contraction in the rat and the effect of x-radiation.*

The edges of the skin wounds have been tattooed with carbon to render them easily visible. Note how the delivery of 1650r to the wound on the right has delayed the contraction process. (From G. H. Blair, D. Slome, and J. B. Walter: Review of experimental investigations on wound healing. *In* J. Patterson Ross (Ed.): British Surgical Practice: Surgical Progress. London, Butterworth & Co. (Publisher) Ltd., 1961.)

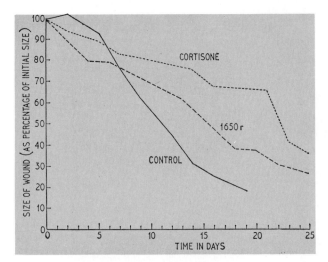

FIGURE 7–2. *Graphic representation of wound contraction in the rat.*

Three groups of animals were used; a standard 1-cm excised wound was made on the back of each animal. One group of animals was given a daily injection of cortisone acetate. Another received one dose of a 1650r x-ray immediately after infliction of the wound; the third group acted as the control. Each wound was measured daily, and the average wound area within each group was calculated. The graphs show that both irradiation and cortisone administration caused considerable delay in wound contraction.

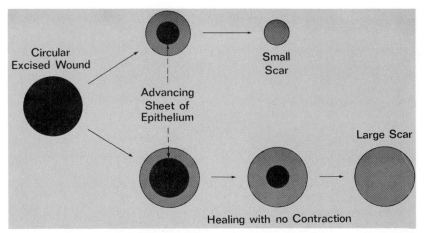

FIGURE 7–3. *Diagram showing how contraction accelerates the healing of a wound and produces a small scar.*

Note that in actual practice a circular wound invariably shows considerable distortion in shape by the time healing is complete. (Compare this diagram with Figure 7–1.) (Drawing by Anthony J. Walter.)

FIGURE 7–4. *Chronic leg ulcer in patient with varicose veins.*

The ulcer is almost circular and is covered by a dark blood-stained slough. A thin layer of regenerating epidermis is beginning to grow across the ulcer bed. The surrounding skin is thickened as a result of edema and fibrosis of the dermis. It is firmly tethered to the underlying muscle sheaths and bone. Hence, there can be no contraction in such an ulcer. The discoloration of the skin is due to the deposition of blood and hemoglobin-derived pigment (hemosiderin). There is also increased melanin pigmentation of the epidermis.

FIGURE 7–5. *Diagrammatic representation of one type of rabbit ear-chamber with wedge cut out to show its construction.*

The chamber is composed of a Perspex base plate which has a raised central table and three peripherally arranged pillars. The coverslip consists of a disc of mica supported at the edge by a ring of Perspex. The coverslip is placed upon the three pillars and is held in position by screws that are inserted into threaded holes in the pillars. The height of the pillars is such that the gap between the top of the table and the mica is 50 to 100 μm. (Drawing by S. P. Steward.)

FIGURE 7–6. *Two rabbit ear–chambers in position.*

The one in the left ear shows the clear central area in which observations are made. In the chamber on the right, the area of the central table is still filled with blood clot. (From G. H. Blair, H. A. S. van den Brenk, J. B. Walter, and D. Slome: Experimental study of effects of radiation on wound healing. In D. Slome (Ed.): Wound Healing. New York, Pergamon Press, 1961, pp. 46–53.)

Thus, the clot is converted into a living vascular granulation tissue, and the process is called *organization.* The cells are generally termed "fibroblasts," but they differ from the fibroblasts seen in other situations. The cells have contractile elements in their cytoplasm and have therefore been termed "fibromyoblasts." Some authorities believe that these cells can contract and that this is the mechanism of wound contraction. At first, the cells are large and plump and have in their cytoplasm the endoplasmic reticulum necessary for the formation of collagen. Hence, collagen fibrils steadily form around cells that become thin and elongated and finally resemble the inert fibrocytes of adult tissue (Fig. 7–9). The fibromyoblasts are also responsible for the formation of ground substance.

Lymphatic vessels grow into the maturing granulation tissue in much the same way the blood vessels do. The two sets of vessels do not anastomose, and the lymphatics form blind-ended channels. At the same time, there is an ingrowth of nerve fibers so that not only do blood vessels acquire an autonomic nerve supply but also the tissue regains sensation.

As maturation proceeds, there is a general remodeling of granulation tissue. Some vessels undergo atrophy and disappear, whereas others exhibit thickening of their coats and eventual obliteration of the lumen. This process of devascularization and collagen formation eventually results in the formation of an avascular scar.

Healing of Skin Wounds

Skin wounds are so common that one takes it for granted that they will heal. Nevertheless, the process by which this occurs is by no means well understood. Following is a description of the healing of two separate types of wound.

FIGURE 7–7. *Granulation tissue formation in the rabbit ear–chamber.*

Photographs taken at the following times after the insertion of the chamber: *A,* 9 days. *B,* 12 days. *C,* 17 days. *D,* 21 days. *E,* 24 days. *F,* 44 days. At 9 days vessels are seen to be invading the dark clot in the center, and by 24 days organization is complete. The large tortuous vessels are venules; the arterioles are more difficult to see at this magnification. The arrow in F indicates an arteriole that divides almost immediately. Note how by 44 days changes have occurred in the course of many blood vessels, although the original pattern of certain venules can still be recognized on the left-hand side of the picture. A lymphatic vessel is now visible at the top of the chamber (×8.5).

FIGURE 7–8. *The growing edge of granulation tissue in a rabbit ear–chamber.*

The rapidly moving stream of blood in the capillary loops at the top produces a streaked effect, and individual red cells cannot be distinguished; in the right-hand vessel, white cells are adherent to the endothelium and appear as transparent globules. In the lower half of the picture, the capillary buds, which contain plasma with few cells, show no flow. Rouleaux formation is seen in one of the capillary buds.

HEALING OF A CLEAN, INCISED WOUND WITH APPOSED EDGES

This process is sometimes described as *healing by primary intention,* and it is the desired result in all healing surgical incisions. Little tissue is lost, and the separated skin edges are brought together by the use of sutures, clips, or tape.

Bleeding occurs immediately after injury and a small amount of blood clot forms in the wound area. An acute inflammatory reaction follows, and the fibrinous exudate helps to join the cut margins of the wound together.

Epithelial Changes.   Within 24 hours of injury, the epithelial cells from the adjacent epidermis migrate into the wound and slide in between the inert dermis and the overlying clot (Fig. 7–10). A continuous layer of epidermal cells soon covers the surface, and overlying this is a crust or scab of dried clot. During the next 24 hours these epidermal cells invade the space where connective tissue will eventually develop. In this way, spurs of epidermal cells are formed not only in the area of incision but also along the tracts of any sutures that have been inserted. These epidermal cells are derived from the cut epidermis and from any severed hair follicle or sweat-gland cells.

FIGURE 7–9. *Maturing granulation tissue from the base of a healing ulcer.*

The fibroblasts and their associated collagen fibers tend to be aligned parallel to the plane of the ulcer surface. The blood vessels (bv), on the other hand, tend to run at a right angle to the surface (×250).

FIGURE 7–10. *Diagrammatic representation of the healing of an incised wound held together by a suture of which the track alone is shown.*

A, The wound rapidly fills with clot. *B,* Shortly afterward, the epithelium migrates into the wound and down the suture tracks. *C,* Epithelial spurs are formed, and granulation-tissue (Gran.) formulation proceeds. *D,* The suture has been removed, and scar tissue remains to mark the site of the incision and the suture tracks. The epithelial ingrowths have degenerated.

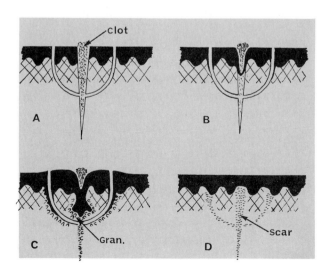

Connective-Tissue Changes.   Following the initial acute inflammatory reaction, the edema subsides and the polymorphs are replaced by monocytes.
These cells, which become phagocytic and perform a scavenger function, are
then called *macrophages*. This *demolition phase* is an essential prelude to the
organization that follows.

ORGANIZATION.   By about the third day, the area of the wound is invaded
by granulation tissue from the adjacent subepithelial layers. The major part of
this ingrowth occurs from the subcutaneous tissues, since there is little or no
contribution from the dense, inert reticular dermis.

Soon after the granulation tissue appears, collagen formation commences.
At first this appears as reticulin fibers, but these later mature into collagenous
bundles. This collagen is of vital importance to the wound, because it forms the
main connecting tissue between the originally divided skin. The amount of
collagen can be assessed subjectively by examining sections of wounds. A
more accurate method is to measure the amount of hydroxyproline in hydrolysates of wound tissues. By this technique it can be shown that the *tensile
strength* of a wound during the first month is proportional to the amount of
collagen formed. The tensile strength can be measured experimentally by excising the entire wound area and applying a disrupting force across the wound.
The force needed to cause separation of the wound edges is measured, and from
this information it is possible to calculate the amount of energy necessary to disrupt the wound. Such measurements are not of purely academic interest, because the strength of a wound is of prime importance when one considers the
way in which surgical incisions heal. Were it not for the tensile strength of a
laparotomy wound, this common surgical incision could burst open and the abdominal contents would spill out to the exterior. This is an occasional
catastrophe following surgery; it is often fatal. A remarkable experimental finding is the fact that the tensile strength of a wound continues to increase for
many months, long after the total amount of collagen has ceased to increase. It
is thought that the formation of new bonds between adjacent collagen bundles
accounts for this phenomenon (see Chapter 2).

The granulation tissue that is formed in a healing wound appears to
prevent excessive epithelial migration into the wound. The epithelial spurs
noted previously soon undergo degeneration and are replaced by granulation
tissue. Only the surface epithelial cells persist, and these divide and differentiate so that a multilayered covering of epidermis is re-formed. It first covers a
vascular granulation tissue, so that the wound has a pink color. Gradually,
devascularization occurs; the scar shrinks in size and changes in color from red
to white.

In the healing of a simple incised wound, it therefore appears that the
epithelial cells are first stimulated to divide, and they then migrate into the
wound. The stimulus for the epithelial growth and migration is not known. Experimentally it has been noted that cells in tissue culture continue to divide
until they have established contact with similar cells, at which point mitosis
stops. This process is termed *contact inhibition*. The epithelial cells appear to
excite a connective tissue response; this results in the formation of granulation
tissue, which in its turn prevents excessive epithelial migration into the
wound. The presence of epithelial ingrowths along a suture tract explains why

granulation tissue is formed in this situation. It is a common finding that if stitches remain *in situ* for three days or more, their site is marked subsequently by small punctate areas of scarring that remain permanently. It is to avoid these ugly punctate marks that surgeons often use tapes to hold skin edges together. A subcuticular stitch is used to hold the wound together while healing proceeds. It should be noted that puncture wounds due to injections do not form such scars, because the wound is not held open, and therefore no epithelial invasion occurs.

HEALING OF A WOUND WITH SEPARATED EDGES (HEALING BY SECONDARY INTENTION)

When the edges of a wound are not approximated or when there is extensive tissue loss, either by direct trauma or following infection, a large defect is present that has to be corrected. Since the main bulk of tissue to perform this service is granulation tissue, this type of healing is sometimes known as healing by granulation. The term, however, is a poor one, since it wrongly implies that granulations are not formed in a simple incised wound. The difference between primary and secondary intention healing is quantitative, not qualitative.

In healing by secondary intention the wound edges are widely separated so that healing has to proceed from the base outward as well as from the edges inward. From a practical point of view, healing of a well-approximated incised wound is fast and leaves a small, neat, linear scar. Healing of a wound with separated edges is slow and results in a large distorted scar. The difference lies in the type of wound and not in the type of healing. The following account of the healing of a large uninfected wound is illustrated in Figure 7–11.

1. There is an initial inflammatory reaction affecting the surrounding tissues, and the wound area is filled with a coagulum consisting in part of inflammatory exudate and in part of blood clot. This coagulum dries on its surface and forms a scab or crust.

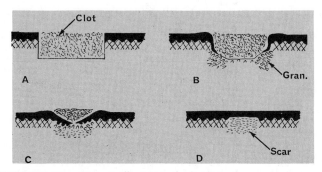

FIGURE 7–11. *Diagram illustrating the healing of an excised wound.*

The wound is rapidly filled with clot. A. Epithelium soon migrates in from the margins to undermine the clot, which dries to form a crust. B, Granulation tissue (Gran.) grows into the wounded area and is most profuse around the circumference where it is derived from the subcutaneous fat. C, Epithelial ingrowth continues, and spurs are produced; these, however, do not persist. D, The end-result is a scar covered by epidermis that lacks rete ridges. During the healing process, contraction has taken place so that the final scar is considerably smaller than the original wound.

2. The wound contracts, as has already been fully described. This process is important, because it reduces the size of the wound and the amount of tissue that has to be produced to fill in the gap.

3. The epidermis adjacent to the wound shows mitotic activity, and the epithelial cells migrate into the wound as a thin tongue that grows between the pre-existing viable connective tissue and the central area of coagulum, which includes some necrotic epithelium and connective tissue. The epithelial cells secrete a fibrinolytic enzyme that aids their penetration between the fibrinous crust and the viable connective tissue.

4. Demolition follows acute inflammation, and the clot in the center of the wound is invaded and replaced by granulation tissue. This grows from the sub-cutaneous tissues at the edge of the wound; it is believed that this zone is responsible for wound contraction. Granulation tissue is also formed in the base of the wound, the amount depending upon the nature of the area and its vascularity.

When the wound is viewed with a magnifying glass, the surface (under the scab, if one is present) is deep-red and granular, the capillary loops forming elevated mounds. It is very fragile, the slightest injury causing bleeding. It is this granularity that is responsible for the name "granulation tissue." The covering of a wound by granulation tissue serves an important protective role, because it has the ability to withstand bacterial infection. Under experimental conditions, organisms introduced into a recent wound are likely to cause infection. However, if the wound is first allowed to granulate, infection does not occur. Thus granulation tissue forms a temporary protective layer until the surface is finally covered by epithelium.

5. The migrating epidermis covers the granulation tissue. A mushroom-shaped scab is thus formed with a central attachment that finally becomes nipped off.

6. The regenerating epidermis becomes thicker and re-forms the multicellular layer of epidermis. This epidermis tends to be abnormally thin and lacks the normal rete ridges. Although cells from hair follicles and sweat glands can contribute to the re-formation of epidermis, these structures themselves are not re-formed. The healing of epidermis falls into the category of regeneration, but the regeneration is imperfect, because in man none of the appendages are replaced.

A scar differs from normal skin in many respects. The epidermis is thin and lacks hair follicles and sweat glands. Melanocytes are not re-formed in normal numbers, and the area therefore appears hypopigmented. The underlying scar tissue consists mainly of collagen, but its arrangement is quite different from that of the structured dermis.

Factors Influencing Wound Healing

The ability of wounds to heal is of fundamental interest in the practice of surgery. Surgeons must pay great attention to anything that could influence the healing process. It would be desirable to analyze the factors that influence repair according to whether they affect granulation tissue formation, collagen production, contraction, or some other process. Unfortunately, this is rarely possible, since we are ignorant about many of these fundamental processes. In practice, the factors affecting wound healing may be divided into two groups: those that act locally, and those whose influence is general.

LOCAL FACTORS

Blood Supply. The normal blood supply varies greatly from one part of the body to another. The scalp and face have an excellent blood supply and wounds there heal quickly. It is possible to remove stitches on the third day without having the wound gape, provided undue traction is not applied. The skin of the leg has a poor blood supply and wounds heal much more slowly.

Pathological changes affecting the blood vessels have an enormous effect on wound healing. Patients who have varicose veins or atheroma in the leg vessels show very slow healing: trivial injuries can lead to ulceration, which takes many months to heal. Other causes of poor blood supply are local pressure and chronic inflammation. *Bed sores* are caused by local pressure, which is also a factor in their poor healing. Likewise, *chronic inflammation* is liable to be accompanied by endarteritis obliterans, ischemia, and slow healing. An excellent example of this is x-ray dermatitis, in which ulceration is notoriously slow to heal. Finally, the slow wound healing of old age is in part related to a poor circulation.

Continued Tissue Breakdown and Inflammation. Any condition causing continued tissue breakdown leads to persistent inflammation, and this delays the completion of the healing process. The most important examples are infection, the presence of a foreign body or irritant chemical, and excessive movement.

INFECTION. If a simple incised wound becomes infected, the two edges do not become adherent, and the wound tends to gape. Furthermore, the infection may cause tissue destruction, causing healing to proceed, in effect, by secondary intention.

FOREIGN BODIES AND OTHER IRRITANTS. The presence of a foreign body in a wound may delay healing, either as a result of its direct irritant properties or by encouraging infection. The overenthusiastic use of irritating antiseptics may cause considerable damage and may delay healing. The use of potent antiseptic and antibiotic agents was once popular in the local treatment of wounds, but it is now appreciated that they frequently do more harm than good. Sometimes hypersensitivity develops and leads to extensive inflammation. A good example of this is the acute allergic contact dermatitis that can follow the use of ointments containing neomycin.

MOVEMENT. It is a time-honored dictum that injured parts should be kept at rest. Movement delays healing because the edges of the wound are continually disrupted and this damages the delicate granulation tissue, leading to repeated injury, and consequently to inflammation.

Adhesion to an Underlying Bony Surface. By anchoring the wound edges, this adhesion prevents contraction.

Direction of the Wound.   Skin wounds made in a direction parallel to the crease lines of the skin heal faster than those made at right angles to them. Skin incisions made across the lines tend to gape, and their healing is delayed. Therefore, when one plans a surgical incision, these lines should be taken into consideration. Incisions parallel to or in the crease lines heal more readily than those in other directions and the scars are less visible.

The Presence of a Large Hematoma.   Some blood clot is always present in a wound, but a large hematoma should be avoided. Its presence favors infection, and in any case the space caused by its presence leads to delayed healing and to the formation of a large scar.

GENERAL FACTORS

Age.   Wound healing is fast in the young and is generally of normal rate in old age unless there is some associated debilitating disease or ischemia.

Nutrition.   Animals starved of protein show poor wound healing and defective collagen formation. This abnormality can be corrected by the administration of proteins containing methionine and cystine.

Vitamin C Deficiency.   Vitamin C is essential for the formation of collagen (see Chapter 2). Animals deficient in this vitamin therefore show poor wound healing. Wound contraction is normal and so are epithelial regeneration and granulation tissue formation. The abnormality is in the absence of normal collagen formation, and the wound is therefore very weak. Capillaries are unduly fragile and bleeding occurs. Although overt scurvy is uncommon in civilized countries, minor degrees of vitamin C deficiency are not infrequent in patients on a marginal intake of the substance, and in those who are stressed.

The Role of Zinc.   The addition of zinc salts to the diet of rats has been shown to promote wound healing. The mechanism of this is not known, but the oral administration of zinc sulfate has been tried in man and claimed to accelerate wound healing. These claims have not been substantiated by all workers, and the role of zinc in healing of human wounds remains problematic.

Glucocorticoids.   The administration of excessive amounts of these steroids delays wound contraction and the formation of granulation tissue.

Temperature.   It is the general experience that wounds of the exposed parts heal more slowly in cold weather. Experiments on animals that hibernate have lent some support to this observation.

Complications of Wound Healing

Infection.   Wounds form a ready avenue for the invasion of pathogenic bacteria. All the techniques of aseptic surgery are devoted to preventing infection of surgical wounds.

Delayed Healing.   Any of the factors mentioned above—either local or general—may produce delayed healing.

Wound Dehiscence.   The bursting open of a wound is described as *dehiscence.* It occurs when stress is applied before the wound has healed sufficiently. It is a particularly serious complication of an abdominal incision, because it results in the exposure of the abdominal contents to the outside atmosphere. Quite apart from delayed healing due to infection and the other factors just considered, another important contributing element is increased intra-abdominal pressure, such as is caused by heavy coughing.

Cicatrization. Scar tissue tends to contract in an erratic way such that the wound becomes greatly distorted. This process is quite different from contraction, because it occurs as a late event and appears to be due to some change in the dense avascular collagenous scar tissue. The mechanism is not understood. Cicatrization is a frequent complication in the healing of skin following extensive burning. It produces great deformity and can immobilize joints in the affected area. Cicatrization involving hollow viscera such as intestine, esophagus, or urethra is an important cause of stenosis.

Keloid Formation. Occasionally, an excessive amount of collagen results in the appearance of a raised nodule of scar tissue called a *keloid*. The precise cause of this is not known, but keloid formation is particularly common in young women (particularly if they are pregnant) and in Blacks. Keloids are found most frequently in the region of the neck and shoulders. They are especially frequent after burns. One should be particularly wary of performing nonessential surgery on patients who are prone to develop keloids. Thus, the removal of a small nevus for cosmetic purposes can result in the formation of a large ugly keloid, far more disfiguring than was the original lesion. The treatment is quite unsatisfactory, because removal is followed by even more keloid formation. Postoperative radiotherapy can be given in an effort to prevent this.

Weak Scars. If the scar tissue is subjected to continuous strain, it may stretch. Incisional wounds may therefore bulge and, in the abdomen, produce incisional hernias.

Healing in Specialized Tissues

It is generally stated that the greater the degree of specialization of a tissue, the less well developed are its powers of regeneration. Certainly, nerve cells are highly specialized and are incapable of division, but degrees of specialization in the cells are as difficult to define as are degrees of specialization among human beings. Is a liver cell more or less specialized than a simple unstriped muscle fiber? Liver cells show remarkable powers of proliferation and yet perform functions of which they alone are capable. Similarly, it is impossible to compare the degree of specialization of the different types of epithelium, each of which has its own particular characteristics. It seems likely that the power of regeneration is best developed in those organs and tissues that are most liable to injury and the replacement of which has survival value for the individual and for the species.

REGENERATION IN EPITHELIAL TISSUES

All covering epithelia show good regenerative power. They are repeatedly subjected to trauma, and the integrity of the surface therefore depends upon the ability of the cells to regenerate. The re-formation of the squamous epithelium of epidermis has already been described in the healing of skin wounds, and a similar regeneration is seen in the mucosa of the mouth, the intestine, the respiratory tract, and the urinary tract.

The solid epithelial organs show varying regenerative capacity. In the liver it is quite remarkable; if three quarters of the liver of a rat is resected, there is such active division of the remaining cells that within a few weeks the organ is restored to its original weight. Its anatomical shape is different, but normal liver lobules are formed in relationship to new blood vessels and bile ducts. As noted previously, this is a simple type of reconstitution. In man, regeneration of liver cells is seen following any type of necrosis, provided the patient survives. The end-result of this regeneration varies widely, depending on the type of necrosis (see Chapter 33 for a consideration of this important subject). Kidney tubules show excellent regenerative capacity, and in patients with extensive tubular necrosis (as occurs in shock) it is common for regeneration to result in complete recovery, provided the patient does not die in the acute phase. This type of renal disease is therefore most eligible for treatment by dialysis (artificial kidney), since the ultimate prognosis is good. If entire nephrons or glomeruli are destroyed, there is no replacement.

REGENERATION IN CONNECTIVE TISSUES

As a general rule, specialized connective tissues show good regeneration if circumstances are favorable. The *mesothelial lining* of the peritoneum and other serous cavities is readily re-formed from exposed underlying connective tissue cells, which take on the form and function of flattened mesothelium. Were it not for this, abdominal surgery would be hazardous. One can leave extensive areas of tissue exposed in the abdominal cavity, and they will be rapidly covered by newly formed mesothelium: adhesions do not form, unless healing is complicated by infection or by the presence of chemical irritants such as the talc or starch in glove powder. Likewise, synovial cells are readily re-formed. With cut *tendons* regeneration is good, provided the severed ends are carefully proximated and are held in good position. It is important that the ends be meticulously sewn together; otherwise, the space between them becomes organized and ultimately union is by scar tissue. Since scar tissue is relatively weak, it will stretch. *Unstriated muscle* shows little regenerative capacity, and destroyed muscle tissue is replaced by scar tissue. Thus, if the patient has a deep penetrating gastric ulcer, even though it may heal, scar tissue remains for life to indicate the site of the previous ulceration. *Heart muscle*, unfortunately, shows no regenerative capacity either, and patients who suffer extensive myocardial necrosis are forever destined to have a scar replacing the pre-existing muscle. With *striated voluntary muscle*, the situation is somewhat more variable, and under good conditions striated muscle can regenerate, so that a clean surgical incision through a voluntary muscle will ultimately unite and no scar tissue will remain to indicate the site of previous surgery.

HEALING IN NERVOUS TISSUE

Adult nerve cells are unable to divide, and therefore when part of the brain or spinal cord is destroyed, no new neurons are produced. The common "stroke" therefore inevitably results in the formation of scar tissue (see Chapter 44). When the axons of the nerve cells are damaged, the situation is quite different, because the body of the cell itself is not directly affected. The effects vary according to whether the axon is in the peripheral or central nervous system.

Peripheral Nervous System. Following the section of a nerve fiber, the corresponding nerve cell shows degenerative changes. Sometimes the cell dies, but more usually it recovers. The severed axis cylinder itself becomes irregular in shape, and by 48 hours has broken up. With myelinated nerves the surrounding myelin shows fragmentation, and the Schwann cells enlarge, proliferate, and become phagocytic. These changes are known as *Wallerian degeneration*, and they affect the nerve fiber distally to the point of section and proximally up to the first node of Ranvier. The original nerve becomes replaced by a mass of Schwann cells. From the proximal portion of the cut axon numerous neurofibrils sprout out and are seen to invaginate into the cytoplasm of the Schwann cells. They push their way distally through the Schwann cells at a rate of about 1 mm per day. Many of the fibrils lose their way and degenerate, but one may reach an appropriate end organ and persist to form the definitive replacement axon. It is evident that accurate apposition of the cut ends of the nerve is of vital importance in facilitating this process. The final process involves the re-formation of the myelin sheath by the Schwann cells as the regenerating nerve axon matures and increases in diameter.

The functional end-result of nerve damage depends on various factors. If the axons are damaged but the nerve trunk itself is not severed, an excellent result may be expected. When the nerve is severed, careful suturing and avoidance of infection are important. Functional recovery is more complete when a pure motor or a pure sensory nerve is cut. Recovery from section of a mixed nerve—like the median nerve—is often poor, and this is presumably because motor nerves often find themselves arriving at sensory nerve endings and vice versa.

Central Nervous System. In the central nervous system the oligodendroglia takes on the functional and anatomical function of the Schwann cells in relation to the axons. For reasons that are not clear, regeneration of long axon tracts does not occur. In some experiments on mammals a limited degree of regeneration has been reported, but with humans, when long tracts such as the corticospinal and spinothalamic tracts have been destroyed, no effective regeneration occurs. Degenerating tissue is phagocytosed by macrophages, and the area becomes replaced by a type of granulation tissue. Unlike the granulation tissue of ordinary connective tissue, the proliferating cells are astrocytes rather than fibroblasts. The end-result is a glial scar containing astrocytes with their matted processes but with relatively little collagen and few fibrocytes.

Mechanism of Repair and Regeneration

When one considers that in a healing wound there is cell and tissue proliferation proceeding at a rate exceeding that seen in most malignant tumors, it is humiliating to admit how little we know of the mechanisms involved. We understand neither the signal that starts the process nor the mechanisms that control and maintain it. Many workers have claimed that local wound hormones, or *trephones*, are responsible for healing; none of these substances, however, has been isolated from animal tissue. In the plant world, growth hormones have certainly been isolated and have found considerable use as weed killers.

An alternative hypothesis is that tissues normally produce inhibiting substances *(chalones)* that are responsible for inhibiting mitotic activity. Following injury, there is destruction of tissue and removal of this inhibiting substance, so that cell division is stimulated. The remarkable regenerative capacity of liver has stimulated much research, but no definite answer has been discovered as to why the liver regenerates following partial hepatectomy, or what stops liver growth when the mass of tissue has been restored to normal. Metabolic factors and hormones have been postulated, but none has been isolated. A failure to identify the mechanism by which normal tissue homeostasis is maintained is particularly disappointing, since any understanding of the major disorder of cell division (cancer) must surely be related to a knowledge of the normal controlling mechanisms of cell growth.

Review Questions

1. A surgeon opens the abdominal cavity and removes a portion of small intestine that is 3 feet long. The cut ends of the gut are sutured together by an end-to-end anastomosis. Describe the healing processes that take place in the intestinal wall.
2. It is claimed that a new compound, when given by a daily injection, has a beneficial effect on the healing of a skin wound. Describe how you would attempt to prove this in a group of experimental animals.
3. A patient receives a severe burn over one shoulder. It involves an area approximately 8 inches in diameter. What are the possible local complications?

Selected Readings

Bucher, N. L. R.: Experimental aspects of hepatic regeneration. New England Journal of Medicine, *277*:686–696; 738–746, 1967.
Editorial: To heal the wound. Lancet, *1*:84, 1973.
Editorial: Zinc in human medicine. Lancet, *2*:351–352, 1975.
Forrester, J. D.: Mechanical, biochemical, and architectural features of surgical repair. Advances in Biological and Medical Physics, *14*:1–34, 1973.
Gabbiani, G., Hirschel, B. J., Ryan, G. B., Statkov, P. R., and Majno, G.: Granulation tissue as a contractile organ. Journal of Experimental Medicine, *135*:719–734, 1972.
Gillman, T.: Healing of cutaneous wounds. Glaxo Volume, *31*:5–31, 1968.
King, G. D., and Salzman, F. A.: Keloid scars. Surgical Clinics of North America, *50*:595–598, 1970.
Ordman, L. J., and Gillman, T.: Studies in the healing of cutaneous wounds. Parts I and II. Archives of Surgery, *93*:857–882; 883–928, 1966.
Peacock, E. E.: Biologic frontier in the control of healing. American Journal of Surgery, *126*:708–713, 1973.
Walter, J. B.: Wound healing. Journal of Otolaryngology, *5*:171–176, 1976.
Weinbren, K.: Problems in restoration of the liver. *In* Illingworth, C. (Ed.): Wound Healing. London, Churchill Livingstone, 1966, pp. 69–77.

CHRONIC INFLAMMATION

Chapter 8

After studying this chapter the student should be able to:

- Define chronic inflammation.
- Enumerate the causes of chronic inflammation.
- Give examples of chronic suppurative inflammation and describe the microscopic appearance of a pyogenic membrane.
- Define the term *granuloma* and describe the three types of the tuberculoid variety.
- Discuss the role of healing in relation to the tissue reaction seen in chronic inflammation.
- Discuss the role of the immune response in relation to the cause of chronic inflammation and in terms of the tissue response seen.
- Discuss the general effects of chronic inflammation and relate these to the reticuloendothelial system.

DEFINITION

When an irritant substance that has caused acute inflammation persists locally, it leads to *chronic inflammation,* which may be defined as *a prolonged process in which destruction and inflammation are proceeding at the same time as attempts at healing.*

The tissue response to injury has been divided into three phases: (1) *acute inflammation,* which is characterized by vascular and exudative phenomena; (2) *demolition,* which is accomplished by macrophage activity; and (3) *healing,*

126

CHRONIC INFLAMMATION

the final phase, by which lost tissue is replaced by the combined processes of repair and regeneration. Pathologically, chronic inflammation is a mixture of the effects of tissue damage, acute inflammation, demolition, and healing.

CAUSES OF CHRONIC INFLAMMATION

Any cause of tissue damage can, if it persists, lead to chronic inflammation. Three main groups can be recognized:

1. *Infections.* The body has a limited ability to destroy certain organisms, *e.g.*, the tubercle bacillus and *Treponema pallidum*. Infection with these agents therefore commonly leads to chronic inflammation (Fig. 8–1). Moreover, if local or general conditions impair the body's defenses, an organism that usually produces a self-limiting acute inflammation may persist to cause a chronic one. Thus, *Staphylococcus aureus*, which can produce a boil that generally heals rapidly, can also produce chronic inflammation in some situations, such as in the bone marrow (see *chronic osteomyelitis*, Chapter 40). Any of the causes of delayed healing may so turn the scales against the host that there develops the "frustrated healing" that chronic inflammation has so aptly been called.

2. *Insoluble Particulate Irritants.* Silica and asbestos are examples of irritant particles that the body cannot easily remove. Inhalation of such substances leads to persistent chronic inflammation of the lungs (see *pneumoconiosis*, Chapter 30).

3. *Hypersensitivity.* The development of hypersensitivity is an important factor in chronic infective diseases, of which tuberculosis is the prototype. Much of the chronic damage produced by persisting tubercle bacilli is mediated by damaging antigen-antibody interactions. There is also a group of diseases in which damaging antibodies are produced against the body's own tissues. This group of autoimmune diseases is typified by rheumatoid arthritis.

TYPES OF CHRONIC INFLAMMATION

Chronic inflammation is encountered in all organs of the body; many examples will be described later. Pathologically, these inflammations share certain features. All consist of varying mixtures of the basic pathological reactions previously described as acute inflammation, demolition, and healing (Table 8–1). The reaction encountered under any particular circumstance consists of varying mixtures of these three basic ingredients. Cells involved in an immune response are often added to this mixture and add to the variety of the tissue response to chronic irritation.

FIGURE 8–1. *Tuberculous pericarditis.*

The patient was a 22-year-old man who had had pulmonary tuberculosis for 5 years. The specimen shows the opened pericardial sac, in which the heart is seen to be covered by a thick fibrinous exudate. Over the apex there is a layer of blood clot due to recent hemorrhage. The parietal pericardium is greatly thickened and is also covered by fibrinous exudate and blood clot. (EC 12.1, Reproduced by permission of the President and Council of the R.C.S. Eng.)

Chronic Suppurative Inflammation. Suppuration is frequently followed by chronic inflammation if the causative agent is not removed or if the pus is not adequately drained. A chronic abscess consists of a central cavity filled with pus and lined by a pyogenic membrane. The latter consists of acutely inflamed granulation tissue. Examples of this type of lesion are seen in the lung following bronchopneumonia, in chronic osteomyelitis, and in a chronic brain abscess (Fig. 44–4). The term *empyema* denotes a collection of pus in a cavity. Thus, in *empyema thoracis* there is pus in the pleural cavity. This condition often becomes chronic, especially if the pus is badly drained. Empyema thoracis follows the rupture of a lung abscess into the pleural cavity, and in preantibiotic days it was high on the list of the complications of pneumonia.

Granulomatous Inflammation. In some types of chronic inflammation the predominant cell is the macrophage. By tradition, an inflammation showing a heavy macrophage infiltration is called *proliferative*, in contrast to the exudative lesions of suppuration. This concept was based on the supposition that the macrophages were derived from local histiocytes by mitosis. In fact, most of them are derived from blood monocytes, but the term "proliferative" is still re-

Table 8-1 COMPONENTS OF CHRONIC INFLAMMATION

COMPONENT	TISSUE RESPONSE
Acute Inflammation	Polymorph Infiltration
	Edema
	Fibrin
Demolition	Macrophage Formation
	Epithelioid Cell Formation
	Giant Cell Formation
Healing	
Repair	Granulation Tissue
	Blood vessels
	Fibroblasts
	Collagen
	Neuroglia in CNS
Regeneration	Epithelial Overgrowth
	Specialized Connective Tissue
	Overgrowth
Immune Response	Lymphocytes
	Plasma Cells
	Eosinophils

tained. Since the accumulation of macrophages can produce a tumorlike swelling, and since there is an underlying mass of granulation tissue, the term "granuloma" is in common use.

DIFFUSE TYPE OF GRANULOMATOUS INFLAMMATION. Under some circumstances, the macrophage infiltration is diffuse, causing a nearly uniform enlargement of the tissue, perhaps with some areas of nodularity. This type of reaction is uncommon, but it is seen typically in lepromatous leprosy.

TUBERCULOID TYPE OF GRANULOMATOUS INFLAMMATION. Under certain circumstances, macrophages enlarge, and the pale eosinophilic cytoplasm becomes poorly defined. These cells then lose their phagocytic ability and are termed "epithelioid" cells because of their resemblance in appearance to the epithelial cells of the epidermis. Epithelioid-cell formation is accompanied by a tendency for the cells to be arranged in groups rather than in diffuse sheets. The formation of groups of epithelioid cells is characteristic of the reaction to the tubercle bacillus. An inflammation characterized by the formation of groups of epithelioid cells is traditionally called a *tuberculoid reaction* (see Fig. 10-3).

When macrophages encounter insoluble material, they frequently coalesce to form giant cells (Fig. 8-2). This response is seen around exogenous foreign bodies, *e.g.*, catgut, silk, talc, and plastic sponges. Coalescing macrophages are also seen around endogenous debris such as dead bone, cholesterol crystals, and uric acid crystals (in gout). They are formed in response to the tubercle bacillus, to fungi, and to many other organisms that cause chronic inflammation. It frequently happens therefore that in a tuberculoid reaction, in addition to epithelioid cells, a considerable number of giant cells are also present.

The reason for the macrophage predominance in certain chronic inflammations and for their change to epithelioid cells is not well understood. The development of hypersensitivity is thought to play an important role in this type of

FIGURE 8–2. *Foreign-body reaction.*

This is a section of an Etheron sponge that had been implanted for 40 days subcutaneously in a rat. The clear areas were occupied by fragments of sponge that have been dislodged during processing. They were surrounded by exuberant giant cells. Many of these have peripherally disposed nuclei and are of the Langhans type. Only a few have the nuclear arrangement of foreign-body giant cells. A similar type of chronic inflammatory reaction with giant-cell formation is seen around other foreign material, e.g., nylon or silk sutures (×150).

reaction. Certainly, the hypersensitivity can lead to necrosis, which is often a feature of tuberculoid granulomatous inflammation. Indeed, three variants of this are recognized: (1) *noncaseating tuberculoid granuloma,* as seen in sarcoidosis, tuberculoid leprosy, and early lesions of tuberculosis (Fig. 10–3); (2) *caseating tuberculoid reaction,* as commonly seen in tuberculosis and also in some lesions produced by deep-seated fungi (Fig. 10–4); and (3) *suppurative tuberculoid reaction,* in which small abscesses filled with polymorphs are found and surrounded by a mantle of epithelioid cells. The commonest example of this is cat-scratch disease.*

Chronic Inflammation with Features of Healing.   The formation of granulation tissue is a feature of many types of chronic inflammation. The tissue consists of endothelial cells forming blood vessels and lymphatics, fibroblasts forming collagen, and an infiltration by numerous lymphocytes and plasma

---

*This curious disease is thought to be caused by a virus, although the agent has never been isolated. The appearance of an ulcerated nodule at the site of a cat scratch is followed by enlargement of the regional lymph nodes. These nodules suppurate, and the overlying skin may ulcerate so that the pus drains spontaneously. The pattern of infection and tissue response in the nodes closely resembles the changes seen in lymphogranuloma venereum (see Chapter 11).

cells. In hematoxylin and eosin sections it is often difficult to identify each cell as either lymphocyte or plasma cell; therefore, the term *small round cell* is often used to encompass both groups. A heavy infiltration by such cells is a common finding in chronic inflammation.

Inflammatory granulation tissue is seen in the pyogenic membrane surrounding a chronic abscess and in the chronic inflammatory tissue in the base of an ulcer. Since the vascularity of the tissue can result in easy bleeding, chronic peptic ulcers are associated with intestinal bleeding. Likewise, chronic inflammation of the bronchial tubes leads to hemoptysis (coughing up of blood).

Fibroblasts are prominent in most chronic inflammation; since they lay down collagen, the end-result is fibrosis. This scar formation is characteristic of many chronic inflammatory lesions. It is seen in fibroid tuberculosis, in the base of a chronic peptic ulcer, and in the wall of an abscess. If fibrin is the hallmark of acute inflammation, fibrosis can be considered the salient feature of chronic inflammation. As scarring proceeds, the lumina of small arteries and arterioles are gradually obliterated by the thickening of the tunica intima; this process is called *endarteritis obliterans*. The end-result is a mass of dense avascular scar tissue. *Contracture* or *cicatrization* follows, and this leads to many important complications of chronic inflammation. Thus, chronic inflammation of the heart valves leads to stenosis and distortion of the valves; chronic gastric ulcers proceed to pyloric stenosis; and a chronic arthritis, such as rheumatoid arthritis, results in fibrous adhesions in the synovium and around joints.

EVIDENCE OF REGENERATION. In chronic inflammatory lesions involving specialized tissue, there is sometimes evidence of regeneration. This is usually seen in covering or lining epithelia; at times, the regeneration is followed by definite hyperplasia and even tumor formation. One of the best examples of this event is found in ulcerative colitis, which can proceed to polypoid overgrowth of epithelium and ultimately to cancer formation. In general, however, chronic inflammation in most organs is an infrequent precursor of cancer.

Chronic Inflammation with Evidence of an Immune Reaction. Although a few lymphocytes and plasma cells are found in uninflamed granulation tissue, many examples of chronic inflammation are characterized by a heavy infiltration of these cells (Fig. 8–3). Together with macrophages they are engaged in the processing of antigen and in the manufacture of antibodies—either sensitized T cells or immunoglobulins. An infiltration by eosinophils is found in some examples of chronic inflammation in which hypersensitivity plays a part, *e.g.,* some parasitic infections.

GENERAL EFFECTS OF CHRONIC INFLAMMATION

The general effects of chronic inflammation depend on the nature and extent of the responsible agent. In a localized foreign body reaction, or in a chronic ulcer of the leg, there is no noteworthy general response at all. On the other hand, in chronic infective diseases like tuberculosis there may be widespread changes in the reticuloendothelial system and in the blood stream.

FIGURE 8–3. *Plasma cells.*

The section is of a chronically inflamed gum and shows numerous plasma cells. Note that the nuclei are placed eccentrically in the cells and that a clear zone is visible in the cytoplasm (arrows). This is the Golgi apparatus (×600).

Changes in the Reticuloendothelial System. Most chronic inflammatory reactions lead to hyperplasia of the reticuloendothelial (RE) system. The local accumulation of macrophages in some types has already been described; in addition, the lymph nodes draining a chronic inflammatory lesion generally show hyperplasia of the RE cells and sometimes of the germinal centers and medullary cords.

If organisms gain access to the blood stream, they are taken up by the other members of the RE system. These cells may destroy the organism or may themselves become parasitized. Overgrowth of the RE cells can lead to enlargement of the RE organs: of clinical importance is the enlargement of the spleen, since it can be detected readily. This RE hyperplasia is, in part, due to the immune response.

The Immune Response. Antibody production is a feature of most chronic inflammatory diseases, and the demonstration of specific antibodies is often a useful diagnostic procedure. Likewise, the detection of cell-mediated hypersensitivity is available as a diagnostic test.

The immune response is sometimes reflected in generalized enlargement of the reticuloendothelial system. Enlargement of lymph nodes, the spleen, and—at times—the liver is a manifestation of this response.

Finally, the long-continued stress on the antibody-producing mechanism may be associated with amyloid disease (see Chapter 25).

Review Questions

1. Describe the role of the macrophage in chronic inflammation. Discuss its origin, functions, appearance, and the cells to which it may give rise.
2. It is sometimes stated that an infiltration by lymphocytes and plasma cells is typical of a chronic inflammatory reaction, and that a polymorph response is typical of acute inflammation. Elaborate on this statement.

Selected Readings

Walter, J. B., and Israel, M. S.: General Pathology. 4th ed. Edinburgh, Churchill Livingstone, 1974. Note, in particular, Chapter 11, which gives a detailed account of chronic inflammation as well as references to specific examples.

Chapter 9

After studying this chapter the student should be able to:

- Define the terms antigen, epitope, hapten, active immunity, and passive immunity.
- Describe the development of the lymphoid tissues of the body and distinguish the B-cell system from the T-cell system.

134

THE IMMUNE RESPONSE

- Describe the chemical nature of the immunoglobulins.
- Discuss how Ig produces (a) immunity to a toxic organism such as *Corynebacterium diphtheriae;* (b) immunity to an invasive organism such as the pneumococcus; and (c) hypersensitivity.
- Distinguish between type I, type II, and type III hypersensitivity reactions.
- Describe the symptoms, pathogenesis, and treatment of acute anaphylaxis in man.
- Give four examples of a type III reaction.
- List the lymphokines and relate their *in vitro* activity to (a) cell-mediated immunity; and (b) type IV hypersensitivity.
- Describe (a) transfer factor; (b) blast transformation of lymphocytes; (c) specific immunological tolerance; and (d) the Koch phenomenon.
- Define the following terms: autograft, homograft, allograft, syngeneic graft, and xenograft.
- Discuss the types of allograft rejection, the mechanisms involved, and the steps that can be taken to combat rejection.
- Classify the immunological deficiency diseases.
- Contrast the instructive theory of antibody formation with the selective theory.
- List the circumstances under which autoantibodies can be formed, and discuss the role of these antibodies in disease processes.

INTRODUCTION

A remarkable feature of the adult mammal is its ability to distinguish between its own constituents ("self") and those of external, or foreign origin ("nonself"). Foreign material excites a reaction now called the *immune response,* and this results in the elimination of the alien matter. Since many of the foreign substances encountered are living organisms or their toxins, it follows that their elimination results in immunity to infection or limitation of its spread. In the first description of antibody formation in the last century, it was shown that animals injected with tetanus toxin produced substances that were capable of neutralizing the toxin. The antibodies, termed *antitoxins,* gave protection against the disease; the subject naturally grew around this central theme of immunity to infection. The immune response has presumably been evolved by animals during evolution as a means of self-preservation in a world teeming with microorganisms. Nevertheless, the immune response is not selective, and antibodies are formed against foreign substances regardless of whether they are bacterial products or not. Under certain circumstances these antibodies can react with foreign material, if it is reintroduced, and can produce

135

severe damage to tissue components. The term *hypersensitivity* is applied to such a reaction. It is evident that the immune response is not concerned solely with immunity to infection, but that it plays a part in many disease processes and under some circumstances causes hypersensitivity.

Substances that are capable of eliciting an immune response are termed *antigens;* the antibodies that are formed are highly specific for the antigen evoking their formation. Antigens are high-molecular-weight substances, nearly always protein, and are recognized as foreign by special features of their chemical structure—probably by particular configurations of their external shape. The areas of the molecular surface that are involved are called *epitopes* or *determinant sites;* one protein may have several such sites. Hence, antibodies with separate specificities can be produced even with the injection of a single pure protein substance. Furthermore, it is possible to add a new epitope to a protein by the addition of a simple chemical substance called a *hapten.* The antigenic properties of a protein are altered by this procedure to such an extent that if the hapten-antigen combination is injected into a suitable animal, some antibodies that are produced are specific for the hapten. Thus, *haptens are substances that are not antigenic in themselves but behave as antigens when combined with a suitable carrier protein.* They are of great importance in human pathology as a simple example will illustrate: Iodine and nickel are not antigenic but if applied to the skin of some individuals act as haptens. They combine with body proteins so that a new antigenic complex is formed. This stimulates the production of antibodies that are specific for iodine or nickel. The next occasion on which the agent is applied to the skin a damaging antigen-antibody reaction occurs, and this produces an inflammatory response that manifests itself as allergic contact dermatitis (see Chapter 41).

The immune response results in the formation of antibodies, and these may be either *immunoglobulins* or *cell-bound.* It is believed that there are two distinct immune systems involved. To understand this, one must first appreciate the formation and structure of the antibody-forming tissues.

THE ANTIBODY-FORMING TISSUES

The cell most intimately concerned in the immune response is the small lymphocyte. This cell resides in the bone marrow, the thymus, the spleen, in lymphoid aggregates such as the tonsils and the Peyer's patches of the small intestine, and in the circulating blood. The development and functions of the lymphocyte have been subjected to intense investigation.

The lymphocytes first formed in the fetus appear in the bone marrow. From there, they migrate either to the *thymus* or to a structure that in birds is termed the *bursa of Fabricius* (Fig. 9–1), an organ that is situated near the cloaca. Although no such structure is present in mammals, it is believed that there is an equivalent tissue that is more widely distributed and forms the lymphoid tissues of the appendix, colon, and Peyer's patches (bursal equivalent lymphoid tissue). The bursa and the thymus are believed to play an essential part in the subsequent development of the lymphoid tissues. Lymphocytes from these two organs migrate into the blood stream and settle in various sites to populate the peripheral lymphoid tissue of lymph nodes, spleen, and other

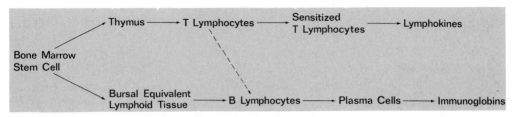

FIGURE 9-1. *Diagram showing the postulated development of the peripheral lymphoid tissue.*

When stimulated by antigen, the T lymphocytes become sensitized, or committed, and on further contact with the same antigen, release lymphokines. B lymphocytes, on the other hand, develop into plasma cells and manufacture immunoglobulins. T cells act as helpers in the stimulation of B lymphocytes.

such structures. The lymphocytes that developed in the bursa (or the bursal equivalent in mammals) are termed *B lymphocytes* (also called "B cells") and are found in the medulla and in the cortex of lymph nodes where they tend to be aggregated in groups called *follicles* (Fig. 9–2). B cells tend to remain sessile in the lymphoid tissues. When stimulated in an immune response, the B lymphocytes develop an endoplasmic reticulum that leads to the formation of immunoglobulin. The fully developed cell is then known as a *plasma cell*, and in the lymph node it is found mainly in the medulla.

The cells that migrated from the thymus are termed *T lymphocytes*. They settle in the peripheral lymphoid tissue, predominantly in the paracortical zone of the lymph nodes. T cells are mobile and long-lived. They enter the lymphatics, pass via the thoracic duct into the blood, and soon reach the lymphoid tissues again. T cells circulate in this way several times each day (Fig. 9–2).

When stimulated by an antigen T cells develop into *sensitized lymphocytes* that are capable of reacting specifically with the antigen that elicited their formation. Thus, the immune response can be regarded as having two distinct components: (1) *the B system of lymphocytes, which leads to the formation of immunoglobulins,* and (2) *the T system of lymphocytes, which produces immune or sensitized lymphocytes.* The immune response takes place in the peripheral lymphoid tissue. The thymus and bursal equivalent tissues play no direct part in this but are essential for the proper development of the immune system. This can be shown quite easily experimentally: If the thymus is removed from a developing embryo, the animal subsequently lacks T lymphocytes and never exhibits the cell-mediated component of the immune response.

THE B-CELL SYSTEM—IMMUNOGLOBULIN PRODUCTION

When an antigen such as diphtheria toxin is introduced into an animal for the first time, there is an interval of about two weeks before any immunoglobulin can be detected in the serum. Then follows a rise in antibody titer that reaches a plateau and subsequently declines (Fig. 9–3). This is termed a *primary response.*

When the same antigen is injected on a second occasion, there is a rapid rise in antibody titer that reaches a high level and subsequently falls again.

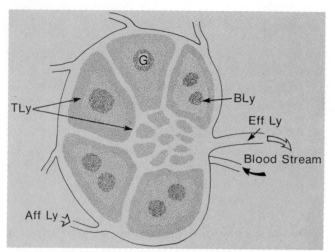

FIGURE 9–2 *Diagram of a lymph node.*

Lymph enters the node through several afferent lymphatic vessels (Aff Ly) and percolates through a meshwork formed by reticulum cells and their reticulin fibers. In the medulla the fluid is collected into sinuses that are lined by phagocytic sinus-lining cells, which—like the reticulum cells—are members of the reticuloendothelial system. The cortex contains collections of B lymphocytes (B Ly), some of which have one or more germinal centers (G). Surrounding these areas, there is a mantle of T lymphocytes (T Ly); this is designated the *paracortical zone*. In the medulla there are groups, or cords, of B cells—both lymphocytes and cells that have differentiated into plasma cells. The B cells tend to remain in the node and are therefore described as being sessile. T cells, on the other hand, leave the node via the solitary efferent lymphatic vessel (Eff Ly), enter the blood via the thoracic duct, and finally return to a lymph node. They leave the blood stream by passing through the walls of the postcapillary venules in the paracortical zone. Lymph containing lymphocytes from tissues or other lymph nodes also enters the lymph node through one of the afferent lymphatics (Aff Ly). (Drawn by Margot Mackay, Department of Art as Applied to Medicine, University of Toronto.)

This is a *secondary response.* Note that the time lag is shorter and there is a greater production of antibodies than at the first introduction of antigen. Evidently, the introduction of antigen in the first instance leads not only to the formation of antibodies but also to the formation of cells that have a "memory." On subsequent contact with the same antigen, consequently, there is rapid proliferation and formation of immunoglobulin. This *immunological memory* is an important component of the immune mechanism (see *Blast Transformation,* discussed later in this chapter).

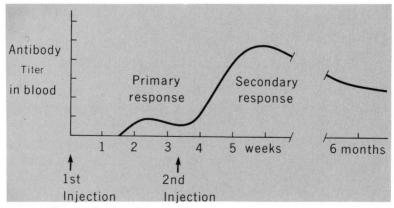

FIGURE 9–3. *Diagram showing differences between a primary and a secondary response to an antigenic stimulus.*

(Drawn by Margot Mackay, Department of Art as Applied to Medicine, University of Toronto.)

THE NATURE OF IMMUNOGLOBULINS

Immunoglobulins are composed of four polypeptide chains joined together, as shown in Figure 9–4. Two of the chains are termed *long* and are identical chemically, whereas two are termed *short* and also resemble each other. Five classes of immunoglobulin are recognized and differ from each other in having different long chains. The antigenic specificity of each is the same. With a primary response, the first formed immunoglobulin is IgM. With the secondary response, the major component is IgG, an immunoglobulin that forms about 70 per cent of the plasma immunoglobulins. IgA is important in that it appears predominantly in secretions and is probably manufactured by local cells. Thus, it is present in the tears and mucus of the mouth, respiratory tract, and gastrointestinal tract. IgE is important because it has affinity for certain cells and renders them highly sensitive (see *Type I Hypersensitivity*, discussed later in this chapter).

THE DETECTION OF IMMUNOGLOBULINS

Although the chemical nature of immunoglobulins is known in some detail, chemical analysis of plasma can determine only the total immunoglobulin content. Antibodies are highly specific, and a variety of techniques have been developed for measuring the amount of a particular antibody. If the antibodies produced after injection of a simple soluble protein, *e.g.*, egg albumin, are mixed with the appropriate antigen, a precipitate is formed when the antibody and antigen meet in approximately equivalent concentrations. An antibody that behaves in this way is termed a *precipitin* (Fig. 9–5). When the antigen is a particle, *e.g.*, a red cell or bacterium, antibodies produced to it can lead to the aggregation of the particles thereby forming visible clumps. This reaction is termed *agglutination* and antibodies that produce it are termed *agglutinins* (Fig. 9–6).

FIGURE 9–4. *Structure of the immunoglobulins.*

Each immunoglobulin has two identical long, or heavy, chains and two identical short, or light, chains. There are five classes — IgG, IgA, IgM, IgD, and IgE — each differing in their heavy chains, which are γ, α, μ, δ, or ϵ, respectively. Of each class there are two types — type K and L — the type depending on whether the light chain is κ (kappa) or λ (lambda). The specificity of each molecule is related to the two binding sites, which are indicated by the two arrows on the IgG type κ. Antibodies are therefore divalent. Note that following immunization by a single antigen, ten distinct types of immunoglobulin can be formed. They each have the same antibody specificity but differ in other respects, such as in chemical structure, physical properties, and in ability to sensitize, to fix complement, and to cross the placenta.

FIGURE 9–5. *A precipitin reaction used to identify an antigen.*

A young child developed signs of meningitis and was admitted to a hospital after having received an antibiotic. A sample of cerebrospinal fluid (CSF) was obtained by lumbar puncture; although it contained many polymorphs, no bacteria could be cultured. Nevertheless, bacterial antigen was demonstrated by the technique of *countercurrent immunoelectrophoresis*, which is shown in the figure. The test is carried out in a sheet of agarose gel. CSF is placed in the four wells on the right, and specific antisera are placed in separate wells on the left. The meaning of each abbreviation is as follows: Pn, antipneumococcal serum. H.i.'b', antihaemophilus influenzae B serum; M'I', antimeningococcal-type I serum, M'II', antimeningococcal type II serum. A current is passed through the gel, and bacterial antigen, which has a strong negative charge, is driven toward the anode (+). Under the conditions of the test, antibody moves toward the cathode (−). Hence, antigen and antibody move toward each other, and a precipitate is formed where specific antibody meets antigen in optimum proportions. The well-marked precipitin line that is shown indicates that the CSF contains *Haemophilus influenzae* antigen. This test is useful in demonstrating antigen when bacteria cannot be cultured because of previous antibiotic therapy. The test is also used in identifying bacterial antigens in sputum and blood.

Precipitin reactions can be performed by allowing antigen and antibody to diffuse toward each other from separate wells in an agar sheet. However, the test is less sensitive, since diffusion occurs all around the periphery of the wells and the reagents are thereby diluted. Application of an electric field drives the two agents toward each other and thereby makes the test more sensitive. (Courtesy of Dr. C. Krishnan.)

Antibody-antigen combinations can also produce another important effect. The combined molecule can combine with a protein in blood that was originally called *complement,* but is now known to consist of a group of at least nine separate proteins. Union of antigen-antibody complex with the first component of the complement system can lead to the subsequent activation of the other components in a cascade manner as shown in Figure 9–7. The importance of this complement activation is that many agents are produced that can have a potent effect on blood vessels and white cells. Furthermore, complete activation of complement can damage cell membranes and lead to cell destruction. Thus, if red cells are mixed with anti–red-cell antibodies in the presence of complement, the red-cell envelopes are damaged and the cells lyse. The antibody is called a *hemolysin.* Similarly, antibodies that lyse bacteria are termed *bacteriolysins.* Such antibodies which are capable of activating complement are termed *complement-fixing antibodies.* If the antigen is a protein, no visible

| 1 in 2 | 1 in 4 | 1 in 8 | 1 in 16 | 1 in 32 | 1 in 64 | 1 in 128 | 1 in 256 |

FIGURE 9–6. *Agglutination test.*

A series of tubes is prepared, the first containing neat serum (left-hand tube), with each subsequent tube containing serum diluted with saline in proportions of $\frac{1}{2}$, $\frac{1}{4}$, $\frac{1}{8}$, etc. (i.e., doubling the dilution). To each tube is added an equal volume of suspension of particles—bacteria, red cells, or latex particles coated with antigen. The tubes are incubated at 37°C for a suitable time. The final dilution of the serum in the last tube to show definite agglutination is described as the *titer of the antibody*. In this illustration the titer is 1 in 128. Sometimes the left-hand tube, which contains the highest concentration of antibody, fails to show agglutination. Such a situation is described as the *prozone phenomenon*. Examples of this type of agglutination test are the Widal (for typhoid fever), the Weil-Felix (for typhus fever), and the Paul-Bunnell (for infectious mononucleosis).

FIGURE 9–7. *Pathway of the activation of complement.*

The complement system consists of at least nine proteins, labeled C1 to C9. The classic pathway of activation is shown. When attached to a receptor site (E) on a red cell a specific antibody (A) initiates the process. Each component is depicted as adding on to the complex, and in turn, as activating the next component. The end-result is damage to the cell membrane and lysis of the cell. During activation, cleavage products of the complement components (e.g., C3a and C5a) are formed as well as activated components in a soluble phase (C567). These agents have important properties, since they are chemotactic to white cells or lead to the release of histamine from mast cells (anaphylatoxins). When attached to a particle the component C3b aids phagocytosis (opsonic activity).

In the *alternate pathway* of complement activation, C3 is activated by other agents such as bacterial endotoxins and aggregated antibodies, which do not activate complement by the classical route. C1, C2, and C4 are not involved. Activation of the terminal components of complement by the alternate pathway can explain how complement can play a part in the pathogenesis of lesions (e.g., in inflammation) that are not immunologically mediated.

FIRST REACTION	SECOND, OR DETECTOR, REACTION (HEMOLYTIC SYSTEM)
Patient's Serum	*Sheep Red Cells*
Previously heated to 56° C for 30 min to inactivate complement; may or may not contain syphilitic antibody.	
+	+
Antigen	*Hemolysin*
A standard quantity	Serum of a rabbit immunized against sheep red cells
+	+
Complement ──────────────────→ *Complement*	
A carefully measured amount	If unused in the first reaction

FIGURE 9–8. *The Wasserman reaction for syphilitic antibody.*

The test is carried out in two stages. In the first reaction, patient's serum (depleted of complement) is mixed with antigen and complement. If the patient's serum contains antibody, it combines with antigen and activates the complement, which is consumed or "fixed." Hence, no complement is available for the second reaction and hemolysis does not occur. Conversely, if the patient's serum does not contain antibody, complement is available for the detector reaction (hemolytic system), and hemolysis occurs.

The antigen used in this test is an extract of heart muscle, which by chance has antigenic properties in common with *Treponema pallidum*. By the use of treponemal antigen the test can be made more specific. In practice, other tests are also employed (see Chapter 10).

reaction may be detected when it reacts with its specific complement-fixing antibody, but the fixation of complement can nevertheless be detected (Fig. 9–8). This is an important phenomenon and is used to detect antibodies in syphilis, gonorrhea, and many viral infections.

Some antibodies are capable of coating organisms (*e.g.*, pneumococci) and rendering them more readily susceptible to phagocytosis by polymorphs and macrophages. Such antibodies are termed *opsonins,* and their presence can be detected *in vitro* by incubating a suspension of organisms with polymorphs in a suitable medium. Opsonins are important *in vivo* in providing immunity to infection.

Effects of Immunoglobulin in the Body

IMMUNITY

The exotoxins of the causative agents of diphtheria, tetanus, gas gangrene, and botulism are potent antigens, and their introduction into the body leads to the formation of antitoxins. These antibodies provide immunity to these diseases, since their presence in the blood leads to neutralization of toxin and to its subsequent elimination. An individual who has had diphtheria or even a subclinical attack is invariably immune for life, since immunological memory will lead to the rapid formation of antibody (secondary response) if the organism is ever encountered again. This immune state can be produced artificially by injecting *toxoid.* Toxoids are toxins that have been rendered less toxic by addition of formaldehyde but which, nevertheless, are still highly antigenic. It is now a common practice to give a series of injections of tetanus toxoid and diphtheria toxoid so that active immunity is produced. *Active immunity* means that subjects are producing their own antibodies because of antigenic stimulations. In the case of patients suffering from these diseases, immunity can be provided by injecting specific immunoglobulin derived from an immune animal or another human being. This is *passive immunity.* It is a useful emergency procedure, because it provides immediate immunity. It is of a temporary nature, however, and as the antibodies are broken down (catabolized), immunity is lost.

In the case of most infective agents, the antibodies that are produced in response to infection are directed against antigenic components of the organism itself. These antibodies are therefore called *antibacterial, antiviral,* or *antifungal,* and because the organisms have many antigenic determinants, antibodies are produced that have different specificities. Some of these antibodies can lead to protection against subsequent infection, but others appear to have no protective activity; their detection in the blood, however, is useful in diagnosis. Examples of the latter are the detection of agglutinins during the second and third week of typhoid fever (Chapter 6) and the VDRL test (from Venereal *Disease Research Laboratory*) in secondary syphilis (see Chapter 10). With invasive organisms, active immunization is carried out by injecting a suspension of the organism itself. Such a preparation, which is termed a *vaccine,* may contain either living or dead organisms. The precise preparation that is used is the one found in practice to produce the most effective immunity. Production of vaccines is very much a matter of trial and error. In the case of the staphylococcus, an effective vaccine has yet to be produced. Injecting a dead suspension of *Hemophilus pertussis,* on the other hand, has been found to be an effective means of preventing whooping cough. With tuberculosis, vaccines containing dead organisms are of no value, but those with living organisms are effective. The organism commonly used is a tubercle bacillus (used in the *bacille Calmette-Guérin* vaccine, BCG), which has been grown in artificial media for so long that it has lost its virulence. A vaccine of this *attenuated* organism produces a very local infection, which leads to a reasonable (but not absolute) degree of immunity. Attenuated smallpox virus is used for "vaccination" against that disease. Vaccines should not be confused with toxoids. A vaccine is a suspension of microorganisms, either alive or dead. A toxoid is a chemically altered preparation of bacterial toxin.

Passive antibacterial immunity can be provided by injecting human or animal sera containing specific antibodies. This has been used in the past (*e.g.,* antipneumococcal sera), but the discovery of potent antibiotics has made their use unnecessary. Passive immunization against viral infections still has a useful role; for example, antimeasles serum is used to prevent very young children from contracting this infection.

Antibacterial antibodies provide immunity to infection in a variety of ways. Some act as opsonins and aid phagocytosis. Other activate complement and lead to lysis of the organisms. The activation of complement also releases important factors. For example, C3b (Fig. 9–7) acts as an opsonin. The anaphylatoxins and chemotactic factors augment the inflammatory response, which itself limits the spread of infection. Agglutinins may also limit the spread of infection, but their role in immunity is probably a minor one.

It should be noted that the globulin antibodies have been named according to the nature of the test used to detect them. It was at one time thought that each type of antibody was a distinct entity, but it is now known that in many cases a single antibody can perform several functions, depending upon the conditions under which it is examined. Thus, a substance may be capable of neutralizing toxin, *e.g.*, diphtheria toxin, in an *in vivo* experiment; it is therefore rightly called an "antitoxin." However, *in vitro* it can produce a precipitate with its antigen and may then be labeled a "precipitin." Some agglutinins, such as to red cells, produce agglutination only in the absence of complement. When this is present, there is lysis and complement is fixed.

Nevertheless, not all antibodies are the same. It is known that a single antigen can lead to the formation of a heterogeneous group of immunoglobulins, each with the same specificity but differing in chemical composition (IgG, IgA, etc). This is reflected in their properties, such as their ability to fix complement, cross the placenta, and sensitize.

HYPERSENSITIVITY

Immunoglobulins can produce hypersensitivity in three distinct ways:

Type I Hypersensitivity or Anaphylaxis. This is best illustrated by a simple experiment. If a guinea pig is given an injection of a simple protein, such as egg albumin, it shows no obvious discomfort. About two weeks later, specific immunoglobulins (precipitins) appear in the plasma. A second injection of egg albumin is then given intravenously. Antigen reacts with a sensitizing antibody, and the animal rapidly develops difficulty in breathing. It becomes unconscious, convulses, and dies within a few minutes. The reaction, termed *generalized anaphylaxis* or *anaphylactic shock*, is highly specific; it is due to a damaging antigen-antibody reaction occurring on the surface of certain cells, which causes *histamine* to be liberated. The histamine produces vasodilatation (dilatation of blood vessels), lowering of the blood pressure, and spasm of the bronchial muscle. In the guinea pig the second injection must be large and given intravenously. It first neutralizes the circulating plasma antibodies, and enough then remain to combine with sensitizing antibody that is fixed to cells. When anaphylaxis occurs in humans, the manifestations are the following:

1. *Bronchospasm,* which causes great difficulty in expiration. The sudden onset of wheezing dyspnea is characteristic.

2. *Edema* due to a generalized increase in vascular permeability. Sometimes edema of the larynx adds to the respiratory difficulty.

3. *Pallor.*

4. *Low blood pressure.*

In humans, the reaction is due to the formation of sensitizing IgE, which has a great affinity for certain cells (particularly mast cells) to which it becomes firmly attached. Very little need be present in the blood. Hence, unlike the situation of the guinea pig, very small doses of antigen can cause acute anaphylactic shock. Although rare, it is encountered under three circumstances:

(1) When horse gamma globulin is given to patients who are sensitized to horse protein, *e.g.*, in passive immunization against diphtheria and tetanus, whether prophylactic or therapeutic.

(2) When a drug that is capable of acting as a hapten is injected into a patient who is sensitive to it. Penicillin is such a drug; each year a number of people die of anaphylaxis from this therapy.

(3) Following the sting of a bee or wasp in highly sensitive individuals.

The danger of anaphylaxis should always be kept in mind by anyone administering animal sera or drugs by injection. At the first sign of anaphylaxis, 1.0 ml of a 1/1000 solution of epinephrine should be given intramuscularly and 0.5 ml repeated as necessary. Edema of the larynx may necessitate emergency tracheostomy.

DUST AND FOOD HYPERSENSITIVITY. This group of hypersensitivity reactions occurs after the ingestion of certain foods and the inhalation of pollen or dust. The symptoms differ according to the route of absorption. The offending agent may be a complete antigen or a hapten.

Types. *Inhalation* of antigens like pollen, horse dander, and dust usually produces watering of the eyes or symptoms involving the respiratory tract: congestion of the nasal mucosa (allergic rhinitis or hay fever) and bronchial asthma.

Ingestion of certain foods produces either gastrointestinal symptoms or urticarial skin rashes. Some people are particularly sensitive to such foods as shellfish, mushrooms, strawberries and milk. The lesions of this group of hypersensitivities are mostly exudative in type and are mediated by histamine. The antihistaminic drugs therefore have an ameliorative effect. Sensitive people can be detected by injecting into or pricking the skin with a minute dose of the offending antigen. Redness and a wheal appear *within a few minutes.* It will be noted that the phenomena of type I hypersensitivity appear within a minute or two of contact with antigen. For this reason the term *immediate hypersensitivity* is often applied to the group.

Patients with this type of hypersensitivity frequently give a family history of similar complaints. One member may have hay fever, another asthma, and a third, atopic dermatitis. It seems that the capacity to react to certain antigens with the production of sensitizing IgE antibodies is related to genetic make-up. Individuals who have such a family background are termed *atopic* and are liable to suffer from *eczema in childhood.* They may later develop *allergic rhinitis* (hay fever), or *bronchial asthma* and are particularly liable to become susceptible to anaphylactic shock. It therefore follows that before any injection is given to a patient, any personal or familial liability to hypersensitivity should be determined.

DESENSITIZATION. Attempts to desensitize atopic patients are sometimes made by injecting small doses of the antigen (*e.g.*, pollen extract) at weekly intervals. The dose is steadily increased, with an aim to produce an excess of antibody in the blood so that antigen is intercepted before it reaches cells sensitized by IgE. Specific blocking IgG antibodies may be produced. Unfortunately, the procedure of desensitization is not uniformly successful.

FIGURE 9–9. *The Arthus reaction in a rabbit.*

This section is from the subcutaneous tissues and includes striated muscle (Musc). The blood vessel in the center is sectioned obliquely and shows occlusion of its lumen by thrombus. Its walls are heavily infiltrated by polymorphs (Poly), many of which are degenerating. Free red cells (RBC) in the tissues bear witness to the severity of the vascular damage ($\times$ 550).

Type II Hypersensitivity — Cytotoxic.   This is an uncommon type of hypersensitivity and is manifested by the production of antibodies capable of destroying cells. An example of this is occasionally seen with penicillin therapy. The drug, acting as a hapten, becomes attached to the red-cell membrane. Antibodies are formed, react with penicillin, and lead to red-cell damage by activating complement on the red-cell surface. A hemolytic anemia therefore follows.

Type III Hypersensitivity — Immune-Complex Reactions.   As noted previously, some types of antibodies have the property of combining with their respective antigen to form complexes that can activate complement. Chemotactic factors are liberated (Fig. 9–7), and polymorphs, which are attracted to the complexes, release damaging lysosomal enzymes. Four examples in which damaging immune-complexes produce disease will be described below.

THE ARTHUS PHENOMENON.   Repeated weekly subcutaneous injections of antigen given to an animal lead to progressively more severe local reactions. Swelling and redness appear within one hour, and over the next few hours hemorrhage and necrosis develop. The pathogenesis is as follows: The injected antigen diffuses into vessel walls and encounters the specific IgG that is present in the blood. Antigen-antibody complexes activate complement in the vessel wall. Polymorphs accumulate and release their lysosomal enzymes. The vessel wall is damaged and thrombosis follows (Fig. 9–9). The Arthus reaction is thought to be the explanation of some types of vasculitis in man, such as that seen in gonococcal septicemia (see Chapter 10).

SERUM SICKNESS.   Serum sickness is a condition characterized by fever, joint pains, and urticarial eruptions that occur about 14 days after the administration of a large dose of foreign serum, such as horse immunoglobulin. The pathogenesis is explained in Figure 9–10.

DRUG HYPERSENSITIVITY.   Hypersensitivity to drugs is a common clinical event and is due to the drug or one of its degradation products acting as a hapten and stimulating the formation of sensitizing antibodies. Virtually any drug can produce a reaction, but common offenders are penicillin, sulfonamides, aspirin, barbiturates, and quinine. *Anaphylactic reactions* (Type I reaction) can range from urticaria to severe anaphylactic shock. Sensitizing IgE antibodies are responsible. *Later drug reactions* begin several days after the administration of the drug and are much more common. Some of these have the features of immune-complex reactions. They are characterized by skin rashes that may be urticarial, papular, or petechial and are usually widespread, brightly erythe-

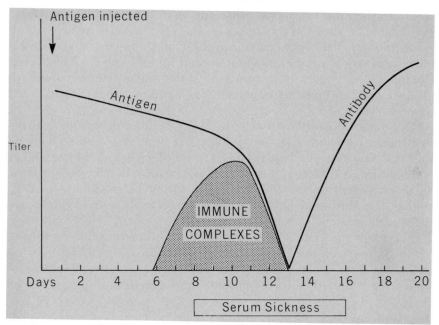

FIGURE 9–10.   *Graph indicating changes in antigen and antibody titer during serum sickness.*

Following a single injection of a large dose of antigen, free antigen is present in the blood in higher titer. The titer drops rapidly with the onset of the immune response. As antibody enters the blood, antigen-antibody complexes form and are rapidly eliminated from the circulation by the activity of the reticuloendothelial system. It is during the period of circulating immune complexes that the illness of serum sickness occurs. The complexes are deposited in the kidney, skin, and joints. Complement is activated, polymorphs accumulate, lysosomal enzymes are released, and damage is done. It is not known why the lesions tend to be restricted to those three sites. As the immune complexes are catabolized, the symptoms of the illness subside, and free antibody appears in the blood. This illustrates how the immune response results in elimination of foreign protein from the body. (Drawn by Margot Mackay, Department of Art as Applied to Medicine, University of Toronto.)

matous, and intensely itchy. The rash is accompanied by fever and sometimes by pain in the joints, thereby showing some similarity to serum sickness. The antibodies concerned are IgG or IgM. Note that some later drug effects such as thrombocytopenia, hemolytic anemia, erythema multiforme, jaundice, and a syndrome resembling systemic lupus erythematosus are not clearly understood. Sometimes cytotoxic antibodies are produced (*e.g.*, as with penicillin), and sometimes immune complexes may be incriminated, but often the pathogenesis is quite obscure.

CHRONIC IMMUNE-COMPLEX DISEASE. If daily injections of antigen are given to an animal in such quantity that antigen-antibody complexes are formed in the blood, a chronic glomerulonephritis develops. It is believed that some types of human glomerulonephritis have a similar pathogenesis (see Chapter 35). Likewise, the acute rheumatic fever that follows streptococcal sore throat is probably of similar nature.

THE T-CELL SYSTEM

CELL-BOUND ANTIBODY

Following the injection of antigen, particularly if combined with Freund's adjuvant or in the form of a living organism, an animal produces cell-bound antibodies. These are sensitized lymphocytes or *effector cells,* which morphologically resemble the small lymphocytes of the blood. They react specifically with antigen and release a number of agents called *lymphokines,* which have a variety of actions. These agents are at present ill-defined chemically but have been named according to specific demonstrable activity. They may be listed as follows:

1. MIGRATION-INHIBITION FACTOR (MIF). This acts on macrophages and prevents their migration in a tissue culture system (Fig. 9–11). This agent is probably the same as the *macrophage-activating factor,* which makes cells more phagocytic and better able to kill organisms. It may be supposed that MIF is an important agent, which leads to the accumulation of macrophages during the demolition phase of acute inflammation and in many types of chronic inflammation.

2. TRANSFER FACTOR. This substance specifically transfers sensitization to previously uncommitted lymphocytes. Therefore, it probably recruits new cells to the site involved, *e.g.*, the site of infection, and is therefore important in multiplying the effect of cellular immunity and also in multiplying the effect of cellular hypersensitivity.

3. LYMPHOTOXIN. This agent has the property of destroying cells, an effect that can be demonstrated in fibroblast tissue cultures. Presumably, lymphotoxins can also destroy cells *in vivo.*

4. SKIN REACTIVE FACTOR. This is presumed to be responsible for some of the phenomena of the Mantoux test, which is described later in this chapter.

5. CHEMOTACTIC FACTOR. Several types are produced and can attract neutrophils, monocytes, or eosinophils.

6. MITOGENIC FACTOR. This agent causes blast transformation of lymphocytes and stimulates mitosis.

NO ANTIGEN   OVALBUMIN   TOXOID

NORMAL
CELLS

OVALBUMIN
SENSITIVE
CELLS

TOXOID
SENSITIVE
CELLS

FIGURE 9–11. *Specific inhibition by antigen of the migration of cells from sensitized animals.*

The cells, mostly macrophages and lymphocytes from a peritoneal exudate, are placed in capillary tubes and incubated in a microchamber. Normally, the macrophages migrate from the open end and produce a tufted appearance. The cells derived from animals with delayed hypersensitivity show no migration in the presence of specific antibody. (From J. R. David, S. al-Askari, H. S. Lawrence, and L. Thomas: Delayed hypersensitivity in vitro. Journal of Immunology, 93:264–273, 1964.)

7. INTERFERON. This agent prevents intracellular viral replication and is described in detail in Chapter 12.

8. IMMUNOGLOBULIN.

As with the humoral immune response, the presence of cell-bound antibody can be associated with either immunity to infection or hypersensitivity. Immunoglobulins are not concerned, and neither cellular immunity nor hypersensitivity can be transferred to another animal by transferring serum. Transfer can be effected only by lymphocytes. With animals the cells must be alive, but with humans extracts of lymphocytes are effective. The agent responsible is called *transfer factor*, and it acts on the recipient's lymphocytes to render them sensitized.

CELL-MEDIATED IMMUNITY

Although it is relatively easy to assess humoral immunity by measuring the titer of specific immunoglobulins, there is no simple way of assessing cell-mediated immunity. Only the response to a challenging infection can reveal its presence; in animals, this is difficult, while in humans it is virtually impossible.

Cell-mediated immunity is probably a factor in immunity to all infections, but it is particularly important in relationship to infections with viruses, fungi, and acid-fast bacillary infections, such as tuberculosis and leprosy (see Immunological Deficiency Diseases, discussed later in this chapter).

Cell-mediated immunity is thought to be mediated by the lymphokines; lymphocytes are recruited and divide; chemotactic factors attract phagocytes, and the monocytes are prevented from leaving the site of infection as well as being more actively phagocytic.

CELL-MEDIATED HYPERSENSITIVITY

This is also known as *type IV* or *delayed hypersensitivity* and is exemplified by the Koch phenomenon.

The Koch Phenomenon. If tubercle bacilli are injected into a normal guinea pig, there is an incubation period of 10 to 14 days before the appearance of a nodule at the site of injection. Ulceration follows, bacilli spread to local lymph nodes, and finally they reach the blood stream. The animal dies of a generalized infection within 6 to 12 weeks. The injection of more tubercle bacilli into a different site in the same animal infected 4 to 6 weeks previously evokes a completely different type of response. A nodule appears within 1 to 2 days, ulcerates, and then heals. There is little tendency to spread to the local lymph nodes. This second type of response was first described by Robert Koch. It should be noted that the reaction of a tuberculous animal to the tubercle bacilli differs from that of a healthy one in three important respects: (1) the incubation is greatly shortened (this may be described as *hypersensitivity*); (2) the lesion heals quickly; and (3) there is little spread. *These are the features of immunity.*

The heightened tissue response of the tuberculous animal can be demonstrated not only with the living tubercle bacillus but also with a protein extract of the organism. Koch originally used a crude extract called *old tuberculin;* more recently, a purified protein derivative (PPD) has been introduced.

The injection of a small quantity of PPD into a normal animal results in a negligible inflammatory response. In the tuberculous animal, however, an indurated red lesion develops that appears within 12 to 24 hours and reaches a maximum by 48 to 72 hours. This is the *tuberculin,* or *Mantoux, test;* a positive result indicates the existence of hypersensitivity to tuberculoprotein.

This type of hypersensitivity differs in many important respects from the type I reactions described previously. Characteristics of the Koch phenomenon are as follows:

1. The reaction is delayed: *It takes at least 12 hours* to develop, as compared with only *a few minutes* in other types of hypersensitivity reactions.

2. Although there is a mild acute inflammatory reaction, the phenomenon is characterized by an accumulation of lymphocytes and macrophages rather than polymorphs.

3. The reaction is not mediated by histamine or by any of the other known mediators of acute inflammation. It is not blocked by antihistaminic drugs.

4. Immunoglobulins are not involved in the reaction. If plasma from a Mantoux-positive individual is injected into a Mantoux-negative person, there is no transfer of sensitivity.

5. Delayed hypersensitivity can be transferred to a normal animal by the

transfer of T lymphocytes. Passive hypersensitivity persists for as long as the injected cells live in the new host. In some way, the transplanted cells alter the host's own lymphocytes so that these also take part in the delayed type of skin reaction that is subsequently elicited. In man, delayed hypersensitivity can be transferred not only by living cells but also by extracts of lymphocytes. First described by Lawrence in 1955, the action of the *transfer factor,* which is one of the lymphokines, is not known. However, it is evidently very potent, because a single injection of lymphocyte extract can render the recipient hypersensitive for many months.

Examples of Cell-Mediated Hypersensitivity

1. FOLLOWING INFECTION.   A positive Mantoux reaction indicates past or present infection with the tubercle bacillus. The hypersensitivity reaction probably plays a major part in the production and persistence of tuberculous lesions. Delayed hypersensitivity is a feature of many other chronic infections — leprosy and histoplasmosis, for example. Much of the damage in these infections is produced not by the organism itself but by the host's own reaction.

2. ALLERGIC CONTACT DERMATITIS.   This follows the application of a sensitizing chemical to the skin. The reaction has been described previously.

3. THE GRAFT REACTION.   See below.

4. EXPERIMENTAL.   Delayed hypersensitivity also follows the injection of antigen mixed with Freund's adjuvant. The latter consists of an oil-and-water emulsion mixed with killed tubercle bacilli or other mycobacteria. It is not known how this curious concoction can potentiate the sensitizing effect of an antigen, but the injection of antigen with Freund's adjuvant mimics the natural events that follow infection by organisms such as the tubercle bacillus.

Blast Transformation.

One of the most remarkable observations of recent times is that the small lymphocytes of the blood can be stimulated *in vitro* to enlarge, develop basophilic cytoplasm, and undergo mitosis. Such cells are termed *immunoblasts* and are thought to be able to develop into plasma cells or lymphocytes. Agents that cause lymphocytic transformation are:

1. PHYTOHEMAGGLUTININ.   This is an extract of the broad bean; the reason for its causing blast transformation is not understood.

2. ANTIGEN IF ADDED TO THE LYMPHOCYTES OF A SENSITIZED INDIVIDUAL.   This occurs regardless of whether the sensitization is of the immediate or delayed type.

3. CONTACT WITH FOREIGN CELLS.

4. ANTIGEN-ANTIBODY COMPLEXES.

The precise role of blast transformation phenomenon in the intact animal is not known, but various suggestions have been made, as follows:

1. The proliferating cells form the germinal centers of lymph nodes, and in fact represent clones that produce antibody. The cells can develop endoplasmic reticulum and differentiate into plasma cells.

2. The blast cells can revert to a type of small lymphocyte, which could have several possible functions. It could act as a *memory cell,* so that when next simulated by antigen it could be transformed and produce antibody. It could also contain cell-bound antibody and act as an *effector cell* in cell-mediated responses.

TISSUE GRAFTS*

In addition to its practical value in surgery, the transplantation of tissue has done much to extend our knowledge of the body's response to foreign tissue. To a considerable extent the fate of a graft depends upon its origin. The three types — autograft, homograft, and heterograft — will therefore be described separately.

AUTOGRAFTS

An autograft is a graft of tissue made from one site to another site in the same individual. Provided the graft obtains an adequate blood supply, it usually lives and functions normally.

Autografts have been used extensively in plastic surgery. Free grafts of skin may be applied to raw surfaces, *e.g.*, following a burn or wide excision of a tumor such as carcinoma of the breast. Whole-thickness flaps of skin may be used as pedicle grafts and swung from one part of the body to another area. With such a procedure, part of the original blood supply is maintained until the portion that has been moved acquires a new blood supply. When the latter is thought to be adequate, the original connection with the donor site is divided.

HOMOGRAFTS

A homograft is a transplant made from one individual to another of the same species. If the two individuals are of identical genetic structure, the graft is termed *syngeneic* or *isogeneic*. Such a graft is accepted as self, does not provoke an immune response, and behaves like an autograft.

An *allogeneic graft,* or *allograft,* is a graft made between individuals of the same species but of different genetic constitution. This is the common type of graft that is used in clinical practice.

As a general rule, allogeneic homografts are rejected. Three patterns of rejection are encountered:

Hyperacute. The graft never becomes vascularized and is rapidly destroyed. This hyperacute rejection is mediated by immunoglobulins that have been preformed against the graft antigens. In clinical practice it is therefore important to test a person who is about to receive a graft for immunoglobulins that are specifically directed against the graft, particularly its major blood group antigens.

Acute Rejection. Provided preformed immunoglobulins are not present, most allogeneic grafts become vascularized. About two weeks later, however, the graft undergoes necrosis and is rejected. It can be shown that this rejection is due to the development of specific sensitized lymphocytes that infiltrate the graft and destroy it.

The application of a second graft from the same donor, or from an animal that is syngeneic, results in an *accelerated graft rejection phenomenon.* The graft no longer becomes vascularized but is rejected within a few days. This reaction is also mediated by sensitized lymphocytes.

---

*The terms *transplant* and *graft* are used interchangeably.

Chronic Rejection. This type of response occurs after about one year; its mechanism is not clearly understood. Both immunoglobulins and cellular antibodies are probably involved. The rejection is particularly important in the case of renal transplantation. Histologically, the reaction is characterized by gradual reduction in the size of the lumen of the vessels supplying the graft.

The vigor with which a graft is rejected is related to the type and amount of transplantation antigens present in the graft but not represented in the host. Some tissues contain much antigen; these are rejected rapidly. Thus, in humans, skin and heart transplants have met with little success. Renal grafts, on the other hand, are of great value. A beginning has been made in identifying the transplantation antigens in man, and it is now possible to match the host and the graft more closely. The antigens are determined by genes that are part of a single complex and are called the *HL-A system.*

Various attempts have been made to prolong the life of allografts. In general, these involve the suppression of the immune response either by ionizing radiation, or by the administration of drugs. Ionizing radiation is dangerous, and its effects are difficult to control. Glucocorticoids such as prednisone and cytotoxic drugs, particularly azathioprine (Imuran), are the mainstay of therapy. Their careful use has led to the success of kidney transplantation. In many patients these grafts endure for many years—some, perhaps, indefinitely.

The function of the graft is dependent on the continued survival of its cells and is an example of a *homovital graft.* This contrasts with a *homostatic graft,* in which the cells die, but the matrix persists and performs a useful function. The best example of this is a bone graft. The bone cells die, but the matrix remains and is gradually replaced by living bone tissue. In the meantime, the bone provides valuable support. The cornea and heart valves have also been used as homostatic grafts.

HETEROGRAFTS (XENOGRAFTS)

These are grafts from one individual to another of a different species. In general, vital grafts of this nature are invariably rejected. Xenografts are not used in clinical practice.

Immunological Deficiency Diseases

Primary immunological deficiency diseases are rare, but their existence has strengthened the view that the immune response has two separate components. In one group, the most common of which is congenital sex-linked agammaglobulinemia, there is a failure in the development of the B lymphocytes, and the subjects possess few plasma cells and manufacture little immunoglobulin. They are susceptible to repeated bacterial infections, which usually results in early death. In another group, there is failure of thymic development and T lymphocytes are absent. These individuals suffer from viral, fungal, and acid-fast bacterial infections. They also fail to develop delayed hypersensitivity. In the most severe type of immunological-deficiency disease there is complete failure of both T and B lymphocytes, and life is limited to a year or two.

Acquired immunological deficiency is of much greater practical importance and occurs in generalized lymphoma (particularly Hodgkin's disease), leukemia, and other related conditions. It is also a feature of therapy with cytotoxic drugs and glucocorticoids.

FUNCTIONAL STEPS IN THE IMMUNE RESPONSE

The following steps may be postulated as occurring after the introduction of an antigen: (1) *recognition* of antigen; (2) *processing* of antigen; and (3) *production* of antibody.

Recognition. A mechanism must exist for recognizing an antigen as foreign. In addition, the system must have a memory so that the same antigen can be recognized again. A cell that is capable of recognizing antigen and initiating an immune response—although not necessarily producing antibody itself—is termed an *immunologically competent cell.* Morphologically, such a cell is a small lymphocyte.

Processing.   Once having been recognized, an antigen must have its determinants processed in such a way that a specific antibody can be produced. It is probable that macrophages perform this function, since they ingest antigen and appear to release factors that act on the antibody-producing cells.

Production.   The final outcome of the immune response is the manufacture of antibody. This involves the synthesis of a range of specific proteins as well as the formation of immune lymphocytes. The production system must be *regulated* in some way so that the immune response can be turned off when the antigenic stimulation is withdrawn.

Immunoglobulin is formed in the cytoplasm of plasma cells. These are the end-product of differentiation of B lymphocytes. It also seems that T cells are required at some stage of immunoglobulin manufacture. Precisely how these T cells act as "helper cells" is not clear. They may act as recognition cells; certainly, since they are more mobile, they are better adapted for this function than are the sessile B lymphocytes.

Theories of Antibody Production

The Instructive Theory.   It has been postulated that antigens play an instructive role and that the extraordinary specificity of antibodies is related to the antigens acting as molds, or templates, during antibody synthesis. The theory, although superficially satisfying, has many drawbacks. It assumes that the antigen remains in the body throughout the period of antibody production—a period that extends for months or even years. There is little direct evidence that antigens can persist for such long periods, for indeed the immune response is responsible for their rapid elimination. It is difficult to envisage how a protein molecule or its determinants could modify the synthesis of a specific globulin in a cell. An alternative explanation is that contact with antigen produces a permanent modification of the antibody-producing cell. According to this theory there must be a change of a self-replicating nature, because it is handed down to the progeny of the cells for many generations. The nature of this hypothetical change is quite unknown.

The Selective Theory. This postulates that in the adult there are cells capable of mounting an immune response against any nonself antigen that the individual is likely to meet. The antigen *selects* these cells and stimulates them to grow and produce antibody. Hence, the antigen determines the *quantity* of antibody produced but not its specificity.

This theory, formulated by Jerne and elaborated upon by Burnet, provides one explanation of the phenomenon of specific immunological tolerance (see below). It is postulated that during the early stages of embryonic development many somatic mutations occur in the immunologically competent cells. These mutations result in the formation of a whole range of cells that between them are capable of mounting an immune response specific for any antigen that the body may subsequently meet. In the adult, contact with antigen stimulates growth of these cells and in this way forms a body of cells, or clone.*As the clone increases in size, antibody production increases in intensity.

It is obvious that if somatic mutation occurs so frequently, cells are produced which can produce antibodies against all possible antigens and inevitably some mutations will result in cells capable of forming antibodies against the host's own developing tissues. As liver cells with liver antigens are produced, antiliver antibodies also should appear. Since this does not occur, there must be some mechanism, activated *during embryonic life,* for the destruction of these harmful, or *forbidden clones.* Any antigen present in the developing embryo is recognized as self, and at birth there are no cells present that could make antibodies against it.

SPECIFIC IMMUNOLOGICAL TOLERANCE

The administration of an antigen to an embryo results not in the formation of antibodies but in the acceptance of the foreign substance as "self." This phenomenon of specific immunological tolerance was first noticed by Medawar when embryo mice were injected with donor allogeneic cells, *i.e.,* from a mouse of a different genetic constitution. When the injected embryonic mice were born and reared, it was found that they would accept skin grafts from the same strain as the original donor but not from those of any other strain (Fig. 9–12). The tolerance was therefore specific and was not due to a generalized depression of the immune response.

Specific immunological tolerance to nonliving antigens can also be induced, but it persists only for as long as the antigen remains. Therefore, repeated injections are usually required. Tolerance can be induced in adult animals, but with difficulty. Usually large doses of antigen must be given, and the lymphoreticular system must first be damaged either by the administration of cytotoxic drugs or by ionizing radiation. When antibody formation is temporarily in abeyance, it seems that the regeneration of the immunologically competent cells in the presence of antigen can lead to tolerance.

The precise explanation of tolerance is not known. It is possible that, in the presence of a large quantity of antigen, the immunologically competent cells become tolerant. An alternative explanation, which is more favored, is

---

*A clone is a group of cells of like hereditary constitution that has been produced asexually from a single cell. The word is derived from the Greek *klon,* meaning a cutting used for propagation.

that tolerance results in the elimination of potentially reactive cells. This explanation is in keeping with Burnet's theory, since the presence of antigen will result in destruction of any potentially harmful or forbidden clone.

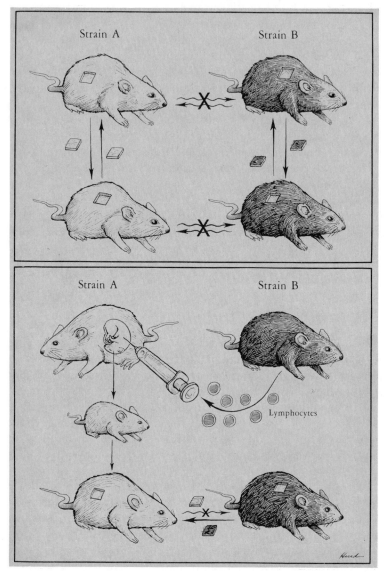

FIGURE 9–12.   *Representation of Medawar's experiment illustrating the fetal induction of tolerance in the mouse.*

Note that skin grafts can be exchanged between any two untreated mice of strain A or strain B but cannot be exchanged between mice of strain A and strain B. Injection of strain B cells into fetal strain A mice induces tolerance. If the cells consist of adult lymphocytes (immunologically competent cells), they may react against the host. This is called a *graft versus host* (GVH) reaction. If it is severe enough the baby mice are stunted and may die. Such a condition is called *runt disease.* The severity of the GVH reaction depends on the number and strength of tissue antigens present in the host (*i.e.*, strain A) and not present in the donor lymphocytes. (From J. A. Bellanti: Immunology. Philadelphia, W. B. Saunders Company, 1971.)

AUTOIMMUNITY

Although it is evident that under normal conditions the body does not make antibodies against its own tissues, the mechanisms that prevent their formation may occasionally break down.

MECHANISM OF AUTOANTIBODY FORMATION

In theory, antibodies could be made against the individual's own tissues (*autoantibodies*) under three circumstances:

1. *Alteration in Antigenicity of Tissue Proteins.* This may be due to either of the following:

(1) DEGENERATIVE LESIONS. Following necrosis of tissue, such as in skin burns, antibodies may be produced to a slightly altered skin protein. These antibodies are an effect of the disease and not its cause.

(2) ATTACHMENT OF HAPTEN. With a condition such as allergic contact dermatitis, the antibodies are directed more specifically against the hapten than against the normal skin.

2. *Release of a Previously Isolated Antigen.* It is possible that some tissue antigens are anatomically isolated from the immunologically competent cells, and are therefore not recognized as "self." When antigens are released into the tissues following injury or disease autoantibodies are formed. It has been postulated that thyroglobulin in the thyroid acini is one such substance, and that antibodies to it could damage the thyroid cells and lead to Hashimoto's disease (see Chapter 39). The evidence is not convincing.

3. *Altered Reactivity of the Immune Mechanism.* In this case "self" protein would no longer be recognized. There is little doubt that this does occur in lymphocytic leukemia. Autohemolysins are sometimes produced, causing a hemolytic anemia—a good example of a condition caused by an autoantibody.

EXPERIMENTAL AUTOIMMUNE DISEASE

The injection into an animal of normal syngeneic or allogeneic tissue mixed with Freund's adjuvant may result in a disease of the respective organ, which is presumed to be due to autoantibody production. If thyroid tissue is used, a condition resembling Hashimoto's disease is produced. If brain tissue is used, a cell-mediated allergic encephalomyelitis results. This bears considerable resemblance to the human disease that may follow administration of rabies vaccine, which itself contains rabbit spinal-cord tissue (see Chapter 12).

TYPES OF ANTIBODY

It may be postulated that the autoantibodies will either be immunoglobulins or cellular. The immunoglobulins might be of any class and of one of two types: (1) *Organ-specific immunoglobulins*, whose specificity is directed against a determinant present in one organ, *e.g.*, hemolysins and antithyroid antibodies; or (2) *Nonorgan–specific antibodies*, which are exemplified by those directed against DNA (in systemic lupus erythematosus), mitochondria, and immunoglobulin determinants (rheumatoid factor) (Fig. 9–13).

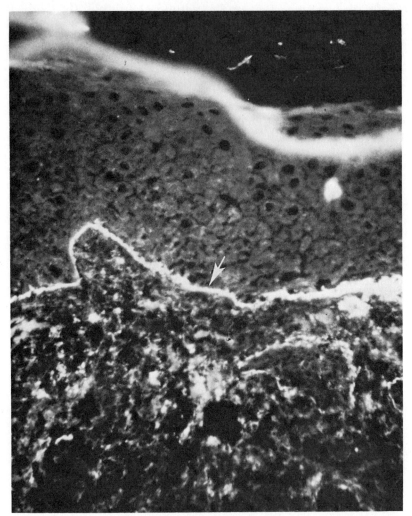

FIGURE 9–13. *Deposition of IgG antibody in the basement membrane zone of skin in bullous pemphigoid.*

Bullous pemphigoid is a skin disease characterized by the formation of blisters, either vesicles or bullae (see Chapter 41). IgG anti–basement membrane antibodies are present in the blood and are deposited in the basement membrane zone of skin and mucous membranes. A frozen section of skin from a patient with this disease was treated with fluorescein-labeled antihuman IgG and examined microscopically under ultraviolet light. The fluorescein fluoresces brightly and acts as a stain for IgG. The linear staining of the basement membrane, indicated by the arrow, is characteristic of this disease and is useful as a diagnostic test. It is not known whether the skin lesions are caused by the deposition of antibody. Possibly, the skin is damaged by some other mechanism and the IgG deposition is a secondary incidental event.

The labeled antihuman IgG used in this test is obtained by immunizing an animal with human IgG. The animal is bled and the antibody is purified. Attachment of fluorescein to the molecule is performed chemically.

ROLE OF ANTIBODIES IN DISEASE PROCESSES

Antibodies may directly attack a tissue and cause damage. The immuno-globulins acquire destructive properties by activating complement, *e.g.*, hemolysins damage red cells, which results in acute hemolytic anemia. Cell-bound antibodies can also destroy cells, such as in allergic encephalomyelitis. Autoantibodies can also combine with antigen and form damaging antigen-antibody complexes. The lesions of this immune-complex disease can resemble serum sickness if acute, but if the process is chronic the kidney is the organ most often affected. Diseases in which the major lesions are caused by an immune mechanism may justifiably be called autoimmune diseases. However, it must be stressed that the autoimmunity merely provides a mechanism in the pathogenesis of a disease. It does not explain the cause, which as noted below, may be inherited or acquired.

ETIOLOGY OF IMMUNOLOGICALLY MEDIATED DISEASES

1. **Genetic Factors.** There is a definite tendency for some autoimmune diseases (*e.g.*, systemic lupus erythematosus and rheumatoid arthritis) to be familial.

2. **Acquired Factors.** Some extrinsic factors are known to precipitate an autoimmune process. Certain drugs and sunlight can precipitate the onset of lupus erythematosus. Mycoplasmal pneumonia is sometimes complicated by an autoimmune hemolytic anemia. When the cause of a disease is clearly established—as in smallpox—the immunologically mediated manifestations of the disease, such as the skin eruption, are readily accepted as part of the entire condition. It is when the cause of a disease is not known, such as with rheumatoid arthritis, that emphasis is given to the autoimmune component of the illness. The label "autoimmune disease" should not delude one into thinking that one knows the cause of the disease; only part of the pathogenesis has been described.

Summary

When antigen gains access to the tissues of the body, a complex series of events occurs. It is taken up by the phagocytic cells of the reticuloendothelial system, and this uptake is followed by some permanent change in the immunologically competent cells. In this way the macrophages, lymphocytes, and plasma cells are altered; under some circumstances, specific immunoglobulins and sensitized lymphocytes pass into the blood stream. The appearance of these antibodies is therefore the final event in a sequence of changes, the whole of which constitutes the immune response.

The relationship of this immune response to hypersensitivity and of immunity to infection is complex.

With simple protein antigens, or with haptens that combine with body proteins, it is the immunoglobulin type of antibody that is produced. If the antigen is a bacterial toxin or a component of a bacterium, the antibody can afford immunity to infection. Sometimes the immunoglobulin antibodies are of such a type (IgE in humans) that they sensitize the cells of the body to the action of antigens, which in turn mediates hypersensitivity of the anaphylactic type. Sometimes antibodies form damaging complexes with antigen, leading to a nonspecific injury to various parts of the body, commonly the kidney and blood vessels. This is immune-complex disease or type III hypersensitivity. Occasionally antibodies are specific for a particular tissue, as when hemolysins are formed. This is the type II reaction.

When the body is invaded by foreign living cells, cell-bound antibodies are formed and reside in the lymphocytes. Such lymphocytes, when confronted with the appropriate antigen, release a variety of lymphokines. These may attack the target cells directly, or they may recruit macrophages and enhance the inflammatory response. The cell-mediated immune response can lead to the rejection of grafts and cause damage to the skin in acute allergic contact dermatitis. Similarly, it can mediate immunity to microbial infection. The role of type IV hypersensitivity is more difficult to understand, since it is a factor in prolonging the effect of some infections that thereby become chronic. It must be admitted that the precise relationship between immunity and hypersensitivity in relation to infection is not clearly understood.

The value of a response that eliminates foreign grafts is of no obvious evolutionary advantage. It has been suggested that the immune response, particularly the cell-mediated type, has evolved as a mechanism for eliminating abnormal cells that have been produced in the body as a result either of damage or genetic change. This scrutinizing or surveillance action of the lymphocytes may therefore be an important homeostatic mechanism by which damaged and neoplastic cells are destroyed and eliminated (see Chapter 17). It is of interest in this connection that malignant disease, especially lymphoma, is more common in the immunological deficiency diseases, particularly the primary group. Another role suggested for cellular immunity is that in mammals it has evolved to prevent the invasion of the mother by fetal cells during gestation.

Review Questions

1. Describe what is meant by atopy. Under what circumstances is an atopic person liable to react adversely to medical treatment?
2. Describe the possible functions of a cell that morphologically resembles a small lymphocyte.
3. Compare type I hypersensitivity with type IV hypersensitivity with respect to the following:
    (a) antibodies involved
    (b) means of passive transfer to another individual
    (c) detection by skin testing.
4. Describe the pathogenesis of the various hypersensitivity reactions that can follow the injection of penicillin.
5. A newborn infant is found to have no thymus. Predict what might happen if
    (a) he is given no treatment
    (b) he is injected with live syngeneic small lymphocytes from his identical twin
    (c) he is injected with live allogeneic small lymphocytes from a parent.

6. Compare and contrast antitoxins with antibacterial antibodies with respect to their:
- (a) chemical properties
- (b) *in vitro* reactions with antigen
- (c) ability to prevent infection
- (d) ability to provide immunity to disease.

Selected Readings

Bigley, N. J.: Immunological Fundamentals. Chicago, Year Book Medical Publishers. 1975. A recent elementary introduction to the subject in 225 pages.

Bloom, B. R.: In vitro methods in cell-mediated immunity in man. New England Journal of Medicine, 284:1212–1213, 1971.

Cooper, M. D., Faulk, W. P., Fudenberg, H. H., et al.: Classification of primary immunodeficiencies. New England Journal of Medicine, 288:966–967, 1973.

Craddock, C. G., Longmire, R., and McMillan, R.: Lymphocytes and the immune response. New England Journal of Medicine, 285:324–331; 378; 1971.

David, J. R.: Lymphocyte mediators and cellular hypersensitivity. New England Journal of Medicine, 288:143–149, 1973.

Good, R. A., and Fisher, D. W. (Eds.): Immunobiology. Stamford, Conn., Sinauer Associates, 1971. A multi-author textbook in 305 pages in which the fundamentals of immunology are presented in graphic style by many of the best-known immunologists.

Haurowitz, F.: The evolution of selective and instructive theories of antibody formation. Cold Spring Harbor Symposia on Quantitative Biology, 32:559–567, 1967.

Humphrey, J. H., and White, R. G.: Immunology for Students of Medicine. 3rd ed. Oxford, Blackwell Scientific Publications Ltd. 1970, 757 pp.

Leading Article: Immunosuppression and malignancy. British Medical Journal, 3:713–714, 1972.

Leading Article: Transfer factor. Lancet, 2:79–81, 1973.

Leading Article: Lymphokines. Lancet, 1:1490–1491, 1973.

Leading Article: Immunological tolerance. Lancet, 1:555–556, 1975.

Lepow, I. H., and Rosen, F. S.: Pathways to the complement system. New England Journal of Medicine, 286:942–943, 1972.

Mackaness, G. B.: Cell-mediated immunity to infection. Hospital Practice, 5(9):73–86, 1970.

Ogra, P. L., and Karzon, D. T.: The role of immunoglobulins in the mechanism of mucosal immunity to virus infections. Pediatric Clinics of North America, 17:385–400, 1970.

Orange, R. P., and Austen, K. F.: Chemical mediators of immediate hypersensitivity. Hospital Practice, 6(1): 79–89, 1971.

Roitt, I. M.: Essential Immunology. Oxford, Blackwell, 1971, 220 pp.

Ruddy, S., Gigli, I., and Austen, K. F.: The complement system in man. New England Journal of Medicine, 287:489–495; 545–549; 592–596; 642–646, 1972.

Tomasi, T. B.: Secretory immunoglobulins. New England Journal of Medicine, 287:500, 1972.

Waldman, R. H.: Immune mechanisms on secretory surfaces. Postgraduate Medicine, 50:78–82, 1971.

Chapter 10

SOME BACTERIAL INFECTIONS—PYOGENIC, ANAEROBIC, MYCOBACTERIAL, AND SPIROCHETAL

After studying this chapter the student should be able to:

- Describe the characteristics of the following organisms and the common diseases caused by them: staphylococci, streptococci, pneumococci, gonococci, and meningococci.
- Classify the gram-negative intestinal bacilli and list the types of infection they produce.
- Compare and contrast gas gangrene with tetanus.
- Discuss the prophylaxis of tetanus in relation to the immune state of the patient.
- Describe the properties of *Mycobacterium tuberculosis* and the tissue reaction to the organism.
- Differentiate between the following types of tuberculosis: (a) infection caused by the bovine and the human strains; (b) childhood and adult types of infection.
- Describe the Koch phenomenon.
- List the factors that predispose to tuberculosis.
- Differentiate between lepromatous and tuberculoid leprosy with respect to: (a) tissue reaction, (b) the immune state, (c) the number of bacilli present in the lesions, and (d) clinical features.
- Describe three diseases caused by organisms of the genus *Borrelia*.
- Outline the sources of infection and the clinical features of human leptospirosis.
- Describe the three stages of syphilis and relate the gross findings to: (a) the pathogenesis of the disease, (b) the number of organisms present in the lesions, and (c) the diagnosis of the disease.

PYOGENIC INFECTIONS

Organisms that cause infection leading to suppurative inflammation are termed *pyogenic*. Important examples of such organisms are staphylococci, streptococci, pneumococci, gonococci, meningococci, and the coliform group of bacteria. The pathological effects of these bacteria are all similar. There is an acute inflammatory response culminating in a massive infiltration of polymorphs. If the inflammation succeeds in destroying the organism, the lesion abates. If the organisms gain the upper hand, the condition proceeds to tis-

163

sue destruction and suppuration. The abscess so formed may burst spontaneously onto a free surface or may be drained surgically. The destroyed tissue is ultimately replaced by regeneration or repair. Sometimes, if the body's resistance is poor or if the organism is extremely virulent, there may be rapid local spread of infection and generalized dissemination. Fatal septicemia or pyemia is the result. Not infrequently, infection with pyogenic organisms results in chronic suppurative inflammation. Indeed, these organisms are responsible for much of the chronic bacterial inflammation that plays such an important role in everyday clinical practice.

Staphylococcal Infections

Staphylococci are gram-positive cocci that tend to grow in clusters. They are common inhabitants of the skin and can be divided into two groups:

Staphylococcus albus. This organism, which is so named because of the white appearance of its colonies, is almost nonpathogenic and a normal member of the skin's flora. It occasionally produces infection under unusual circumstances, such as with mainline drug abusers in whom it causes endocarditis (see Chapter 28).

Staphylococcus aureus. This organism is found on the skin of some normal people, particularly those who live in crowded communities such as those of hospitals. The reservoir of pathogenic staphylococci is in the anterior part of the nose. About 40 per cent of healthy adults are nasal carriers, but the figure may rise to over 70 per cent in a hospital population. From the nose, the organisms are readily transferred to the skin, particularly the hands. Here the organisms can multiply and spread to other objects and to other people.

LESIONS PRODUCED BY STAPHYLOCOCCUS AUREUS

The typical staphylococcal lesion is a circumscribed area of inflammation with suppuration. Skin lesions are frequent and include boils, carbuncles, paronychia (inflammation of the nail fold), and impetigo (Fig. 10–1).

In *impetigo* the organisms invade the superficial layers of the skin and produce characteristic subcorneal bullae and pustules. This is common on the face in children. The blisters soon rupture and become covered by a honey-colored crust.

Infection of the hair follicles is common; the type of lesion produced depends upon how deeply the organisms penetrate. Since pus is produced, the term *pyoderma* is employed to describe this whole group of skin diseases. In *superficial folliculitis* numerous small pustules are seen at the openings of adjacent hair follicles. The face is a common site for this eruption to occur.

A more destructive and severe infection of the hair follicle is the *boil*, or *furuncle;* when pus is produced, it is discharged from a single opening. A *stye* is a particular type of boil in which an eyelash is implicated. Boils are particularly common in the axillae and on the back of the neck (see Chapter 6).

In a *carbuncle* the staphylococcal infection extends to the underlying fatty subcutaneous tissue and spreads laterally. The subcutaneous tissue is divided

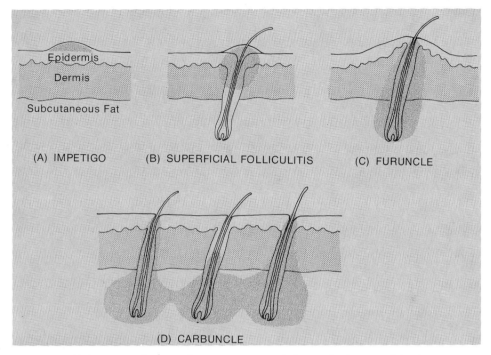

FIGURE 10–1. *Diagram illustrating some staphylococcal infections of the skin.*

A, Impetigo. The infection is very superficial, and a pustule forms beneath the stratum corneum of the epidermis. *B, Superficial folliculitis.* The suppurative inflammation involves the superficial part of a hair follicle. Clinically this appears as a small pustule; the condition is called impetigo of Bockhart. *C, Furuncle, or Boil.* The infection involves an entire hair follicle, and the inflammatory edema produces a considerable swelling, which can be 1 cm or more in diameter. Nevertheless, a boil has one head only. *D, Carbuncle.* The infection involves the subcutaneous tissues and loculated pockets of pus are present. These pockets are formed between fibrous septae, which are not shown in the diagram. Note the multiple heads through which pus can be discharged. (Drawing by Margot Mackay, Department of Art as Applied to Medicine, University of Toronto.)

into compartments by fibrous septa, which extend from the deep fascia to the dermis. It therefore follows that subcutaneous infections tend to be loculated, with each individual abscess bursting to the surface through its own hair follicle orifice. Thus, a carbuncle has multiple heads, and extensive areas of skin become undermined and are eventually sloughed off.

Staphylococci are the commonest cause of wound infection, usually the result of hospital cross-infection. Other important staphylococcal infections are bronchopneumonia, enterocolitis, and osteomyelitis, all of which are discussed elsewhere in this text. Staphylococcal infections sometimes involve veins (a condition called *phlebitis*), and this leads to thrombosis. If the thrombus is invaded by the organisms, it tends to soften and break off, forming septic emboli. This condition is called *pyemia* and is characterized by multiple pyemic abscesses and septic infarcts (see Chapter 20).

Streptococcal Infections

Streptococci are gram-positive organisms that tend to grow in chains, particularly in a fluid culture.

TYPES OF STREPTOCOCCI

The four major groups are recognized by the type of colony produced on blood agar:

1. *Alpha-hemolytic streptococci,* also called *Streptococcus viridans,* grow on a blood-agar plate as small colonies that produce an ill-defined surrounding zone of partial hemolysis. Two important infections produced by this group of organisms are on the one hand the relatively trivial apical infections of teeth and on the other its lethal complication, subacute bacterial endocarditis (see Chapter 28).

2. *Beta-hemolytic streptococci* produce a sharply demarcated zone of complete hemolysis on the agar plate. The strain of beta-hemolytic streptococcus that produces disease in man is termed *Streptococcus pyogenes.* Other strains produce disease in animals, such as bovine mastitis, in which the udder is infected.

3. *Nonhemolytic streptococci* are also called *enterococci,* since they commonly occur in the gut.

4. *Anaerobic streptococci* are a separate group that is considered later.

LESIONS PRODUCED BY STREPTOCOCCUS PYOGENES

The typical streptococcal lesion is a spreading infection of the connective tissues—a condition called *cellulitis.* Abscesses occur later than in staphylococcal infections, and the pus tends to be watery and often blood-stained. Streptococci are occasional causes of wound infection and are also responsible for a number of cases of *impetigo. Erysipelas* is a classic streptococcal lesion and consists of a spreading infection in the dermis. It affects the face and is seen as a raised, bright red plaque with a sharply defined edge that steadily advances.

Streptococci are important causes of *tonsillitis* and *pharyngitis.* Infection can spread to the middle ear to produce *otitis media* and down the tracheo-bronchial tree to lead to *bronchopneumonia.*

In days gone by, streptococcal infections of the uterus following labor were common *(puerperal sepsis).* This was one of the major causes of death following childbirth before the introduction of aseptic techniques and chemotherapy.

Some streptococci produce an *erythrogenic toxin,* which is absorbed into the blood and produces a punctate erythematous rash termed *scarlet fever.* The skin lesions are sterile, since they are produced entirely by this exotoxin. The usual streptococcal infection leading to scarlet fever is a sore throat.

Two other important diseases associated with streptococcal infections are *acute rheumatic fever* and *acute glomerulonephritis.* Both are thought to be related to the development of hypersensitivity and to be manifestations of immune-complex reactions (see Chapter 9).

Pneumococcal Infections

Pneumococci closely resemble streptococci but have a well-defined capsule and tend to occur in pairs. The organism is a common commensal of the throat; about 80 different serotypes are known. A few of these types are highly virulent and can cause infection in healthy individuals. The organisms penetrate the defenses of the respiratory tract, invade the lung, and cause *lobar pneumonia*. This is accompanied by a septicemia that at times is complicated by metastatic lesions such as meningitis. The other category of pneumococci tends to be relatively avirulent but can act as secondary invaders causing *bronchopneumonia* either in elderly debilitated patients or in persons who have had a previous virus infection (see Chapter 30).

Gonorrhea

Gonorrhea is caused by the gonococcus, a gram-negative diplococcus whose only known host is man. The disease is generally transmitted by sexual intercourse. In the male, an acute urethritis appears two to eight days after infection. A purulent penile discharge is the main symptom and is combined with difficulty and pain on passing urine. If treated correctly—usually with penicillin—the disease clears up rapidly. Untreated, the infection can spread to involve the seminal vesicles and epididymis. Chronic infection and its attendant fibrosis is a well-known cause of urethral stricture.

In the female, gonorrhea causes acute urethritis and cervicitis, but symptoms are frequently ignored or absent, and the infection goes unnoticed. These asymptomatic females are the main reservoir of gonorrhea in our society. Spread to involve the Fallopian tubes leads to *acute salpingitis* and associated peritonitis. This event can present as an acute surgical abdominal emergency; the patient presents with abdominal pain and fever. Chronic gonococcal infection is a very common cause of pelvic inflammatory disease (PID) and may follow an acute attack or appear *de novo*. Salpingitis leads to fibrosis of the Fallopian tube, which is an important cause of sterility in the female.

Two nonvenereal infections with the gonococcus are worthy of note:

ACUTE VULVOVAGINITIS. This can occur in epidemic form in girls' schools and is transmitted by towels and communally used clothing. This infection does not occur after puberty, because the hormonal activity associated with menstruation leads to an acid pH in the vagina, and this acts as an efficient bactericidal chemical barrier.

GONOCOCCAL CONJUNCTIVITIS AND OPHTHALMITIS. Infection of the baby's conjunctiva during delivery results in an acute purulent conjunctivitis. Corneal involvement with ulceration and even perforation is a dreaded complication, since it leads to blindness. This disease was said to be responsible for about 50 per cent of blindness in children before effective prophylaxis abolished it. As a routine, a drop of 1 per cent silver nitrate is placed in each conjunctival sac of a newborn child.

Gonococcal conjunctivitis is occasionally seen in adults when pus from a urethral discharge is transmitted to the eyes, generally by the patient's own hands.

The introduction of the gonococci usually leads to a local infection, but the invasive potential of the organisms should not be forgotten. Bacteremia can result in metastatic lesions of which acute septic arthritis is the most common. Gonococcal septicemia has recently become an important complication. It usually affects young women, and its onset is triggered by a menstrual period.

FIGURE 10–2. *Gonococcal septicemia.*

    The patient was a 24-year-old woman who complained of pain that flitted from one joint to another (polyarthralgia) and had been present for about five days. The pain dated from the onset of her last menstrual period. Pain and discomfort were particularly marked in the right knee; on examination, this joint was shown to be swollen and somewhat tender. A day or two after the onset of her arthralgia, she noted a rash that consisted of scattered lesions on the distal part of her arms and legs. Some of these lesions were small erythematous papules, but others were enlarged and developed hemorrhagic pustules in their centers. The figure shows one of these lesions on a finger. During the course of the disease the patient felt unwell, lost her appetite, and developed a mild fever every evening. A biopsy of one of the skin lesions showed an acute vasculitis. This finding, together with the history and clinical features, strongly suggested a diagnosis of gonococcal septicemia. A slight vaginal discharge was noted. A swab of the cervix subsequently grew gonococci. Penicillin therapy was started, and an uninterrupted recovery ensued.

    The patient had been on a holiday two weeks before the onset of the illness. During that time she had had intercourse with a new acquaintance. Prior to that she was not aware of having had intercourse with anyone who had any discharge.

The fever, arthralgia (pain in the joints), and the development of skin lesions due to vasculitis are the outstanding symptoms of the condition (Fig. 10–2).

Meningococcal Infections

    The meningococcus closely resembles the gonococcus morphologically and is a normal commensal of the nasopharynx. The first encounter with the organism causes an inconsequential infection in most individuals, but occasionally the organism spreads to produce a septicemia; finally, it settles in the subarachnoid space to cause *meningitis.* Septicemia is usually accompanied by a petechial skin rash, which gives the disease its alternative name of "spotted fever." Meningitis usually occurs in those individuals who lack immunity (usually children), but it also may appear in susceptible adults. The disease occasionally becomes epidemic when large numbers of adults are crowded together in confined quarters, such as in army barracks.

Gram-Negative Intestinal Bacilli*

This is a large group of rod-shaped bacteria; the pus-producing members include *Escherichia coli, Proteus* species, and *Pseudomonas pyocyanea* (also called *Pseudomonas aeruginosa).* The organisms, commonly grouped as the "coliforms," are normal commensals of the lower small intestine and the colon where they cause no damage; indeed, their presence is beneficial. Once outside the confines of the gut, they cause infection with suppuration. They are always predominant in infective lesions derived from the bowel contents, *e.g.,* appendicitis and generalized peritonitis following perforation of the gut.

°Salmonella and *Shigella* also belong to this group and cause typhoid fever, food poisoning, and bacillary dysentery. These organisms are considered briefly elsewhere.

Table 10–1 COMMON PYOGENIC INFECTIONS

ORGANISM	SOURCE OF INFECTION	COMMON INFECTIONS
Staphylococcus		
Staphylococcus aureus	Skin of carrier or patient	Wound and skin infections; pyemia; pneumonia; osteomyelitis
Staphylococcus albus	Normal flora of skin	Mild wound infections; endocarditis
Streptococcus		
Streptococcus pyogenes	Throat of carrier or patient	Throat infections; wound infections; pneumonia
Streptococcus viridans	Normal flora of mouth	Apical tooth infection; endocarditis
Nonhemolytic streptococci (enterococci)	Normal flora of intestine	Wound infections; urinary tract infections; peritonitis
Pneumococcus	Normal flora of nose and throat; carriers	Pneumonia; meningitis
Gonococcus	Patients with chronic genital infection	Genital tract infections; gonococcal conjunctivitis; and ophthalmitis
Meningococcus	Normal flora of nose and throat; carriers	Meningitis
Gram-negative intestinal bacillus		
Escherichia coli *Proteus* species *Pseudomonas pyocyanea*	Normal flora of intestine; fomites	Wound infections; urinary tract infections; peritonitis; pneumonia

Furthermore, the coliforms are the commonest agent in *urinary-tract infec-tions*, reaching the kidney as part of a normal bacteremia from the colon, or else being introduced into the bladder by catheterization. The coliform orga-nisms are sometimes troublesome causes of *wound infection* in hospitals. Not infrequently they cause *bronchopneumonia* and *middle-ear infection*. Septice-mia may complicate any of these infections and is a potent factor in inducing shock (see Chapter 21).

The common pyogenic infections are summarized in Table 10–1.

ANAEROBIC INFECTIONS

Clostridial Infections

The Clostridia comprise a group of organisms that are normal commensals of the intestine, form spores that are extremely resistant to destruction, and grow only in the absence of oxygen. The strict anaerobic requirement for growth makes laboratory isolation difficult and explains the curious circum-stances under which these bacilli cause human disease. *Clostridium botulinum* has already been described in Chapter 6. This section deals with the clostridia that cause gas gangrene as well as *Clostridium tetani*, which causes tetanus.

GAS GANGRENE

Gas gangrene follows the contamination of a wound with spores of the pathogenic clostridia. Considering the ubiquitous presence of these spores and the rarity of gas gangrene, it is evident that a healthy wound that is contami-nated does not develop infection. The essential factor necessary for spore ger-mination is a reduced oxygen tension. This is present in a severely lacerated wound that contains dead tissue — particularly dead muscle that has lost its blood supply. The presence of soil in a wound is particularly dangerous, because the calcium salts in it may lead to considerable tissue necrosis. Any co-incidental infection by one of the aerobic pyogenic organisms, such as staphy-lococci or streptococci, serves to augment the anaerobic conditions. Most ex-amples of gas gangrene are exogeneous in origin, and are due to the gross contamination of a severely lacerated dirty wound. Gas gangrene is frequent in battle casualties and in agricultural accidents. Indeed, it was during the First World War that this group of organisms was studied intensively and finally classified — so important was this type of infection in causing deaths. Occa-sionally, gas gangrene is endogenous and occurs when a wound is contamin-ated with the patient's own feces.

Pathogenesis and Lesions of Gas Gangrene.   Gas gangrene is never due to infection by a single type of clostridium; it is the result of a combined assault by several organisms working together. The true pathogens, best known of which is *Clostridium welchii* (also called *Clostridium perfringens),* produce powerful exotoxins that are liberated locally and produce tissue necrosis. Since muscle is usually involved, an extensive and progressive local muscle necrosis around the area of the original wound follows. At this stage the muscle appears red and is obviously dead, since it does not contract. The dead muscle excites an acute inflammatory response characterized by a tremendous outpouring of fluid with remarkably few polymorphs. The extensive inflammatory edema impairs the blood supply of the muscle, so that further growth and invasion of the organism is favored. As noted above, many organisms are involved in the clinical condition of gas gangrene. The saphrophytic group of clostridia, typified by *Clostridium sporogenes*, produces no potent toxins, but has the property of splitting protein. They attack the dead muscle and liberate hydrogen sulfide and other foul-smelling gases. The hydrogen sulfide combines with iron from hemoglobin, and the iron sulfide so formed gives the whole area a black color. The wound that is complicated by gas gangrene rapidly becomes black and discharges foul-smelling fluid in which there are bubbles of gas. Absorption of toxic substances, particularly the exotoxins of the pathogenic clostridia, leads to shock, and the patient dies unless the limb is expeditiously amputated.

Treatment of Gas Gangrene. In the treatment of gas gangrene it is usual to give an antiserum prepared against the exotoxins of the main pathogens. Penicillin or other antibiotics are also useful, because they destroy the growing bacteria. For prophylaxis it is important that wounds be adequately treated surgically so that all dead tissue is removed and adequate drainage assured. This is as important as the administration of appropriate antibiotic therapy.

TETANUS

The spores of *Clostridium tetani* infrequently contaminate wounds, but as with gas gangrene organisms, a reduced oxygen tension is essential for their germination. The conditions conducive to tetanus infection are therefore similar to those described above. Nevertheless, quite often the degree of trauma appears to be mild, because an insignificant puncture wound, such as the prick of a thorn contaminated with manure, has quite commonly been the site of origin of a fatal tetanus infection.

Clinical Features. The incubation period varies from a few days to several weeks; the shorter it is, the worse is the prognosis. Tetanus is clinically a disease of the central nervous system. The local lesion may be so mild that only a very careful search will reveal it, yet the exotoxin produced by the local infection may be sufficient to cause death.

After peripheral absorption, the toxin reaches the central nervous system — probably by passing along the motor nerve trunks to the spinal cord or medulla oblongata. At first, the toxin acts locally, which explains the phenomenon of local tetanus. Early symptoms include spasm of those muscles controlled by the same spinal segment as that supplying the area infected. Stiffness of the muscles appears, and this is soon followed by an increase in muscular tone and painful spasms. After a while, the spasms become generalized; particularly striking is contraction of the jaw muscles, resulting in closure of the lower jaw or trismus (inability to open the mouth, or "lockjaw"). Finally, generalized convulsions occur, and death from asphyxia follows involvement of the respiratory muscles.

Prophylaxis of Tetanus. Since tetanus may complicate quite trivial wounds, by far the best method of prophylaxis is active immunization. This is carried out by giving a course of three injections of tetanus toxoid, thereby inducing a high blood level of specific antitoxin immunoglobulin.

In a patient who has sustained a deep wound — particularly if there is much ragged laceration of tissue, or if it has been contaminated with animal fecal material — the procedure used depends upon whether the patient has had previous active immunization or not. If previous injections of tetanus toxoid have been given, all that needs to be done is to give a further dose of toxoid. A rapid secondary type of response leads to a high level of antitoxin within one or two days. If, on the other hand, there has been no previous immunization, passive immunization with antitoxin must be considered. In the past, the administration of horse antitetanic serum (ATS) has been advised, but the danger of inducing anaphylactic shock or serum sickness is considerable. Furthermore, the duration of passive immunity is short, particularly if the subject has had previous injections of horse serum (see Fig. 9–10). Since the use of human antitetanic serum obviates these difficulties, it should be given whenever it is available. At the same time it is also advisable to give the first injection of tetanus toxoid. The patient should be instructed to return for further toxoid administrations. Tetanus is now an uncommon disease in the Western World, but the situation in the poorer countries is quite different. It has been estimated that over one million people die of tetanus each year, and that it is the leading cause of death in hospitals in many developing countries. Injecting quinine (for malaria), ear piercing, circumcising, and applying soil or even dung to the umbilicus of the newborn are all common modes of contamination that lead to infection in the unprotected population.

Gram-Negative Anaerobic Intestinal Bacilli

The gram-negative intestinal bacilli of the genus *Bacteroides* form the bulk of organisms in the feces, and they are present also as part of the normal flora of the mouth and vagina. These organisms do not produce spores and are strictly anaerobic. They cause wound infection, pelvic abscesses, puerperal sepsis, and occasionally oral infection. But in these instances their role is probably secondary to infection with more pathogenic organisms. Their presence

Table 10–2 COMMON ANAEROBIC WOUND INFECTIONS

ORGANISM	SOURCE OF INFECTION	COMMON INFECTIONS
Clostridium welchii and others	Animal feces; normal flora of human intestine	Wound infection; myositis (gas gangrene); gangrenous lesion of intestinal tract
Clostridium tetani	Animal feces; occasional member of flora of human intestine	Mild wound infection with severe toxic effects (tetanus)
Anaerobic streptococci *Bacteroides* species	Normal flora of intestine, vagina, and the mouth, to a lesser extent	Wound infections; gangrenous lesions of intestinal tract: peritonitis; postpartum uterine infection (puerperal sepsis)

should be suspected in any infection associated with a foul odor. The organisms may on occasion invade the blood stream and cause septicemia with shock.

Anaerobic Streptococci

Anaerobic streptococci are normal inhabitants of the bowel and vagina. They were important causes of puerperal infection in the past and occasionally are associated with wound infection and gangrenous lesions.

The important anaerobic infections are summarized in Table 10–2.

MYCOBACTERIAL INFECTIONS

The mycobacteria or acid-fast bacilli have features that distinguish them from other bacteria. They are difficult to stain (see *ZN stain*, below), and the two important human pathogens *Mycobacterium tuberculosis* and *Mycobacterium leprae* grow slowly *in vivo*. They have some affinity with fungi and were so named on this account (*mykes* is Greek for "fungus").

Tuberculosis

The importance of tuberculosis cannot be judged by its present incidence in the Western World. In the past it was a common and dreaded disease, but the sanitoria and hospitals for "consumption" (as the disease was once called) either have shut down or have changed their names and directed their attention to other diseases. In part, this has been effected by early diagnosis and better treatment; in the main, however, improvement in social conditions, removal of slums, and the pasteurization of milk have played the major role. In parts of the world where poverty and overcrowding are rife, so also is tuberculosis.

The Causative Organism. Tuberculosis is caused by *Mycobacterium tuberculosis* of which there are several strains, the most important being the *human* and the *bovine* varieties. The organisms contain a waxy material in their cell walls that is responsible for their special properties. Since stains cannot easily penetrate the organism, a smear receiving the ordinary Gram stain will show no bacteria. A special stain must be employed: heating a smear with strong carbolfuchsin. Once this stain has penetrated the organism, it cannot easily be removed by acid or alcohol. This forms the basis of the Ziehl-Neelsen stain. Mycobacterium tuberculosis is therefore spoken of as being "acid-alcohol-fast." The organism is demanding in its cultural requirements and takes several weeks to produce visible colonies. It follows that tuberculous specimens treated in a routine way will be reported as sterile. Special methods must be employed, and the laboratory technicians must be aware of the necessity for this. The organisms also grow slowly *in vivo*, and tuberculous infections tend to develop slowly and to be chronic.

The Tissue Reaction to Tuberculous Infection. When tubercle bacilli are introduced into a tissue, there is a rapid acute inflammatory response with a

FIGURE 10–3.   *Tuberculosis of lymph node; early lesion.*

In the center of the picture there is a circumscribed collection of epithelioid cells forming a follicle that stands out clearly against the dark background provided by the closely packed small lymphocytes. On the right-hand side several follicles have fused together.

polymorph infiltration. This tends to be quite mild and fleeting. It is soon followed by massive accumulation of macrophages, which ingest the bacilli and then become modified to form *epithelioid cells*. These have more cytoplasm than the typical macrophage, and lose their ability to ingest material. The accumulation of epithelioid cells tends to be focal, and small nodules or tubercles are formed (Fig. 10–3). These are about 0.5 to 1.0 mm in diameter and are just visible to the naked eye. Some macrophages, instead of becoming epithelioid cells, form giant cells that are of the Langhans type. Surrounding the mass of epithelioid cells, there is a diffuse zone of lymphocytes with a few plasma cells and fibrocytes. Within two weeks necrosis begins in the mass of tissue containing not only the epithelioid cells but also those cells peculiar to the part involved. The necrosis is called *caseation,* and the dead tissue forms a dry, firm, coagulated mass, which has fancifully been likened to cheese. Caseation is probably caused by the development of hypersensitivity to the products of the bacilli, as explained in Chapter 9.

The end-result is a fully formed tubercle follicle (Fig. 10–4). It consists of a central mass of caseation surrounded by epithelioid cells and occasional giant cells. This, in turn, is surrounded by a wide zone of small round cells. The appearance is highly characteristic of tuberculosis, but a similar reaction can be seen in other infections, particularly those caused by fungi. Adjacent tubercles tend to fuse, and as the caseous process extends, wide areas of tissue are destroyed. The lesion can now be seen with the naked eye, and the caseation can extend for many centimeters. Progressive caseation is the hallmark of spread of tuberculosis. In some instances, the firm caseous tissue undergoes liquefaction. The precise reason for this is not known, but increased hypersensitivity is generally incriminated. A cavity is then formed containing liquefied caseous material that is teeming with bacilli. Conventionally, this is called pus, although technically this term is inaccurate, since few polymorphs are present. The tuberculous pus tends to track in the line of least resistance, providing for one means by which a tuberculous lesion can extend.

Tubercle bacilli are typically intracellular parasites and can be spread locally in the tissues by the migration of macrophages. Satellite lesions are therefore formed, and their eventual fusion with the original focus is the means by which the lesion enlarges. Tubercle bacilli also spread via the lymphatic vessels, causing the regional lymph nodes to contain typical tubercles. In susceptible individuals this spread continues to the blood stream, and widespread dissemination occurs. The subject becomes severely ill, having numerous tubercles, particularly in those organs with a high reticuloendothelial content such as the spleen, bone marrow, and liver. The meninges are also affected, and *meningitis* frequently accompanies this condition, which is called *general-*

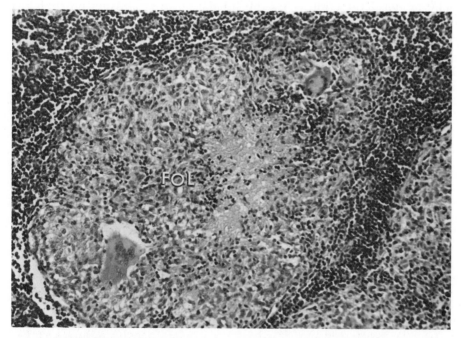

FIGURE 10–4. *Tuberculosis of lymph node; follicle with caseation.*

Compared with the lesion shown in Figure 10–3, this tuberculous follicle (Fol) has enlarged, and its center has become caseous. Two giant cells are shown. The one with many nuclei arranged around its periphery has the characteristic features of a Langhans giant cell. Although this is an active tuberculous lesion, bacilli are scanty and would be very difficult to find in a section stained with Ziehl-Neelsen's carbol-fuchsin. Culture in a suitable medium or guinea-pig inoculation is used to isolate the organism.

ized miliary tuberculosis. The name is derived from the numerous small tubercles that at one time were likened to millet seeds.

TUBERCULOSIS DUE TO THE BOVINE STRAIN OF TUBERCLE BACILLUS

Tuberculosis causes mastitis in cows, and the organism is therefore present in milk. On ingestion of the milk by man, a local infection occurs either in the tonsils or in the small intestine. This local lesion is small and clinically silent, but the organism spreads to involve regional lymph nodes in a massive way. The situation is similar to that of tuberculosis in the guinea pig. Bovine tuberculosis was once common in children in whom large masses of caseous cervical or mesenteric lymph nodes were characteristic. Human beings have considerable innate immunity to tuberculosis, and the disease usually stopped its spread at this point. Occasionally, continued spread resulted in miliary tuberculosis and death.

The eradication of tuberculosis from our herds and the almost universal pasteurization of milk have made bovine tuberculosis so rare that this form of the disease virtually ceased to exist in the Western World.

TUBERCULOSIS DUE TO THE HUMAN TUBERCLE BACILLUS

The mode of infection is by the inhalation of organisms present in fresh droplets or in the dust of dried sputum expectorated by a person having an open case of pulmonary tuberculosis.

It has been recognized for a long time that tuberculous infection manifests itself differently in children and adults. At all ages the lung is the principal organ involved.

Childhood Tuberculosis.   In childhood the primary focus (the Ghon focus)

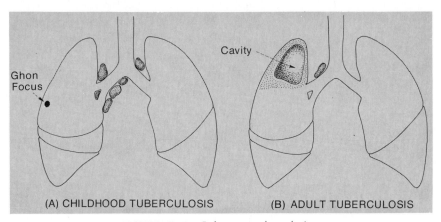

FIGURE 10–5. *Pulmonary tuberculosis.*

In childhood tuberculosis, the lung lesion is small, but the spread to hilar and mediastinal lymph nodes is extensive. In adult tuberculosis, there is a destructive lung lesion (often apical and with cavitation), and the lymphatic spread to the hilum is minimal. (Drawing by Margot Mackay, Department of Art as Applied to Medicine, University of Toronto.)

FIGURE 10–6. *Tuberculosis of lung.*

This section of lung shows a circumscribed, partly calcified lesion called a *Ghon focus* (see also Fig. 10–5A), which is indicated by the upper right arrow. This is thought to be the primary focus of a previous tuberculous infection. The adjacent pleura is thickened, and the overlying pleural space is obliterated by fibrous adhesions. In Europe this type of lesion is usually due to a previous tuberculous infection; however, it is often difficult to prove this by finding organisms in the focus itself. In North America histoplasmosis can produce a lesion that has an identical appearance.

The specimen was from a patient who had died of miliary tuberculosis. The Ghon focus had evidently become reactivated, and bacilli had spread throughout the body via the blood stream. Two miliary tubercles are indicated by arrows. (Specimen courtesy of the Boyd Museum, University of Toronto.)

is a small lesion situated at the periphery of the lung field. This subpleural focus may heal and produce no clinical illness, while the infection may spread to the hilar lymph nodes, which become greatly enlarged and caseous and eventually form a conspicuous primary complex (Fig. 10–5 A). It either heals and calcifies (Fig. 10–6), or the infection spreads and the child dies of miliary tuberculosis with meningitis.

Adult Tuberculosis. In adult life a pulmonary focus is almost always either apical or subapical. The lesion either heals or progresses slowly with softening and liquefaction. In this way a cavity is formed (Figs. 10–5 B and 10–7). The destruction of lung tissue leads to bleeding, which often leads to hemoptysis. This is accompanied by a chronic cough, low-grade fever, and a raised erythrocyte sedimentation rate (ESR). Depending upon the resistance of the patient, there is a tendency for either healing with fibrosis, or extension of the cavitating process. In severe cases there can be great destruction of lung tissue.

FIGURE 10-7. *Chronic pulmonary tuberculosis in an adult.*

This radiograph shows a typical chronic destructive tuberculous infection in the right upper lobe. Two areas of cavitation are evident. The large one is indicated by the two arrows; below and slightly to the right there is a smaller cavity. The infection has now spread to the lower lobe where extensive areas of tuberculous bronchopneumonia are evident. (Photograph courtesy of Dr. D. E. Sanders.)

At any time, caseous debris may be inhaled into other bronchi to produce areas of tuberculous bronchopneumonia. This may occur on a small scale and result in extension of the disease, but if it is widespread in a highly sensitized person, it can lead to massive consolidation of lung tissue. This is quite uncommon nowadays.

In summary, adult tuberculosis is a chronic disease in which phases of spread alternate with phases of healing and fibrosis.

Precisely why the morphology of adult tuberculosis of the lung is so different from that seen in childhood is not known. One explanation is that the adult type is a reinfection. The previous infection induces immunity, so that with a reinfection the disease does not spread but remains localized to the lung. Unfortunately, hypersensitivity leads to extensive destruction of lung tissue. Undoubtedly, there is some truth in this explanation, but although the situation is similar to that seen in the Koch phenomenon, it is not exactly the same. In the Koch phenomenon the lesion of reinfection heals because immunity develops (see Chapter 9), whereas in human pulmonary adult tuberculosis, the lesion tends to heal slowly, and the disease remains chronic and progressive.

Metastatic Tuberculosis. At any stage in the development of a tuberculous lesion, a transient bacteremia can occur. This can result in small metastatic tuberculous lesions being produced in virtually any organ of the body. These usually remain quiescent, but years later they may become active and produce active tuberculous lesions at that site. Bone, kidney, brain, epididymis, Fallopian tube, and joints are areas where this response is particularly frequent. The lesions are typically those of a chronic inflammation with progressive destruction of parenchyma and its replacement by fibrous tissue. Caseation is usually an obvious feature; if there is liquefaction, the pus can spread in the line of least resistance. With renal tuberculosis, the pus ruptures into the pelvis of the kidney and is passed in the urine. Large cavitated areas extend from the pelvis of such a kidney. When tuberculous pus is formed adjacent to tuberculosis of the spinal column, the pus enters the psoas sheath, tracks down to below the inguinal ligament, and finally opens onto the skin surface.

Factors Determining the Response of Tissues to Tuberculous Infection. It is evident that a tuberculous infection may be followed by a minimal reaction that heals rapidly or may lead to a progressive disease with rapid spread culminating with a fatal disease. The factors determining tissue response are the following:

1. THE DOSE AND VIRULENCE OF THE ORGANISM.

2. INNATE IMMUNITY. For the most part, human beings have considerable immunity to tuberculosis, but it does seem that certain races (*e.g.,* the Eskimos and the Irish) are especially susceptible. Nevertheless, it is difficult to separate the effects of environment from those of innate immunity, because poverty, starvation, and ignorance are the forerunners of tuberculosis in any race.

3. AGE AND SEX. In days gone by, tuberculosis was particularly common in early adulthood, particularly in females. With the improvement in social conditions and the great decline in the incidence of tuberculosis, this trend is no longer apparent. In old age, immunity to tuberculosis diminishes, and the disease even now is not infrequent in our senior citizens.

4. GENERAL HEALTH OF THE INDIVIDUAL. Malnutrition and chronic debilitating disease, particularly diabetes mellitus, are notorious predisposing factors to tuberculosis. For example, an attack of measles can activate a previously quiescent tuberculous focus.

5. OCCUPATIONAL FACTORS. Those whose work carries the hazard of atmospheric pollution by particles of silica (*e.g.,* tunnelers, miners, and quarrymen) are liable to develop pulmonary tuberculosis. To a lesser extent the same hazard applies to those who manufacture asbestos products.

6. ACQUIRED IMMUNITY AND SENSITIVITY. This has been described previously (see Chapter 9). It is generally held that the immunity to tuberculosis is T cell–dependent. It follows that in diseases where T cell function is impaired, tuberculosis is particularly liable to occur; if infection has already been acquired, it is likely to spread. Patients with Hodgkin's disease and other lymphomas treated with immunosuppressant drugs are extremely susceptible to terminal fulminating tuberculosis infection.

Leprosy

INTRODUCTION

Leprosy is caused by *Mycobacterium leprae,* which was one of the first bacteria to be incriminated as a cause of human disease and will probably be the last to be cultured in an artificial medium. Investigation of the disease, in particular the sensitivity of the organism to antibiotics, has been greatly hindered by our inability to grow the organism and the great difficulty encountered in infecting laboratory animals. So far, the organism has only been grown in the foot pads of mice and in the armadillo. In practice, pathological diagnosis depends on demonstrating the organism by ZN staining of smears or sections.

Although the disease is of great antiquity, it is uncertain whether the accounts in the Old Testament in fact describe leprosy. There seems little doubt that the disease was present in the Middle East before the birth of Christ, and during the Middle Ages it was common in Europe, having been introduced there by the returning Crusaders. The disease has now retreated from Europe and is endemic in the Far East, India, the Middle East, Africa, and Central and South America. The disease was probably introduced into the United States by the Negro slaves, and is still endemic in some southern states and Hawaii.

MODE OF INFECTION

The mode of infection is unknown, but the disease is probably spread by contaminated nasal secretions. The disease is generally acquired in childhood, and the first lesion is an insignificant scaly skin patch. This *indeterminate lesion* may heal spontaneously or progress to one of the two major forms of the disease.

TYPES OF LEPROSY

Tuberculoid Leprosy. This type of leprosy occurs in individuals with a high state of immunity. The skin lesions consist of one or several *well-demarcated* papules or plaques, which are associated with local nerves, causing the skin of the area to become anesthetic. Microscopically the skin and involved nerves show a noncaseating tuberculoid reaction similar to that seen in early tuberculosis. Lepra bacilli are extremely sparse. The lepromin reaction, which is similar to the Mantoux, is positive and indicates a high state of cell-mediated immunity.

Lepromatous Leprosy. In lepromatous leprosy the lesions consist of multiple macules, papules, and plaques, which are of *widespread distribution* and tend to be *symmetrical.* The lesions are *poorly delineated,* and often there is a diffuse infiltration of the skin. Microscopically the dermis is diffusely packed with macrophages, which are themselves stuffed with lepra bacilli. Since the lesions tend to occur in the cold parts of the body, the hands and face are particularly affected. The diffuse thickening of the skin of the face leads to a lionlike appearance (leonine facies). There is diffuse involvement of nerves, so that a symmetrical peripheral neuritis is characteristic.

FIGURE 10–8. *Leprosy.*

This patient is a voluntary resident of a leper colony in the Caribbean. Years before this picture was taken she was found to be suffering from lepromatous leprosy, and has been taking a sulfone or other antileprous drug ever since. Her condition is not now infectious; indeed, she may be completely free of the lepra bacillus, although this is difficult to prove. Nevertheless, she exhibits some of the devastating effects of the disease. Inflammation of the nasal mucosa (rhinitis) accompanied by destruction of the nasal bones has resulted in collapse of the bridge of the nose. Repeated attacks of iritis have led to glaucoma and cataract so that the sight of both eyes has been gravely affected. The left eye is completely blind, but the right is able to detect movement and the difference between light and dark. Because the patient has a left-sided facial nerve paralysis, the muscles of the left side of the face do not move. This can be detected by the drooping of the left eyelid, and the failure of the left side of the mouth to move backwards when the patient smiles or talks.

In lepromatous leprosy, the nasal mucosa is also infiltrated by bacteria–laden macrophages, and the destruction of the nasal bones leads to the characteristic appearance (Fig. 10–8). Because the nasal secretions contain a large number of bacilli, it is probable that this is the manner by which the disease is disseminated.

In lepromatous leprosy there is defective T-cell immunity, causing the lepromin reaction to be negative. As if to compensate for this, there is an overproduction of immunoglobulins, and the hyperimmunoglobulinemia is associated with *acute reactional phases* that are a great hazard in leprosy. Exacerbation of the skin lesions, iridocyclitis, orchitis, nerve damage, fever, prostration, and death can occur during these acure phases, which may either develop spontaneously or be precipitated by ill-advised vigorous treatment. The damage is probably mediated by the deposition of immune complexes with antigen excess (see Chapter 9). The large number of bacilli present in the lesions provides the antigen for the formation of these complexes.

Leprosy provides a fascinating example of the effects that an immune response has on the pattern of an infection. In the tuberculoid type, T-cell immunity is well developed, the lepromin test is positive, few bacilli are present in the lesions, and the inflammatory response is characterized by a tuberculoid reaction with plentiful Langhans giant cells. The pattern of reaction is similar to that encountered in the common type of tuberculous infection. In lepromatous leprosy on the other hand, T-cell function is in abeyance, the lepromin test is negative, and vast numbers of bacilli are present in the lesions, which are characterized by a diffuse infiltration by macrophages ("lepra cells"). Occasionally an analogous situation is encountered in tuberculosis. In the terminal stages of miliary tuberculosis, the tuberculin test becomes negative, and the lesions teem with bacilli.

Borderline or Dimorphous Leprosy. Cases occur in which the clinical and pathological features are between the two polar types of tuberculoid and lepromatous leprosy. In these borderline cases, acute reactional states are particularly common, and the disease tends to terminate in one of the two major forms, often the lepromatous type.

Leprosy is a chronic disease that is now amenable to treatment with a number of chemotherapeutic drugs. The sulfones are the mainstay of these drugs, because they are not only effective but also readily available and cheap.

SPIROCHETAL DISEASES

Spirochetes are long, slender, spiral filamentous organisms. The human pathogens are classified according to three genera: *Borrelia, Leptospira,* and *Treponema.*

Borrelia

Two species of *Borrelia* cause relapsing fever. The European type is spread by lice, whereas the African variety is tickborne. Relapsing fever has an incubation period of three to four days and is characterized by a high fever and the appearance of spirochetes in the blood stream. After three to five days, circulating immunoglobulin antibodies appear, the blood is cleared of organisms, and the fever abates. Some days later, organisms return to the blood, and another attack of fever ensues. Up to ten similar attacks may occur, thereby giving the disease its descriptive name.

The pathogenesis of this remarkable relapsing disease is that the organisms are able to mutate with extreme rapidity. No sooner does the immune response develop and kill off the organism than a new immunological variant emerges, followed by a relapse of fever until the host has had time to develop new specific antibodies. A similar type of relapsing fever is also seen in trypanosomiasis; this, too, is due to the high mutability of the organism.

Borrelia vincentii is another large spirochete; it is a naturally occurring contaminant of the mouth. When local resistance is impaired, *e.g.,* in agranulocytosis and leukemia, the organism in association with *Bacteroides* causes ulcerative oral lesions. It is also an important member of the bacteria that are incriminated in gingivitis. During the First World War the condition of acute ulcerative gingivitis was so common in soldiers that it was known as "trench mouth." This was due to poor nutrition and poor dental hygiene.

Leptospirosis

Many strains of leptospira are known, and are normally carried in the kidneys of many species of animals such as rodents, dogs, cattle, birds, and amphibians. The organisms rarely cause harm in their usual host, but if transmitted accidentally to another animal species or to human beings they give rise to a clinical infection called leptospirosis. Leptospirosis is transmitted to man in water contaminated by the urine of carrier animals, usually rats or dogs. It is therefore an occupational hazard of such persons as sewer workers, military personnel, and veterinarians.

Leptospirosis can vary from a mild influenzalike disease to a severe illness with renal and hepatic damage. The latter type is known as Weil's disease. Occasionally meningitis is a dominant feature of the clinical presentation.

Syphilis

The causative organism of syphilis, *Treponema pallidum,* is a delicate spiral filament or spirochete, which is difficult to stain and has never been cultivated in a synthetic medium. It is difficult to infect animals with this organism; rabbits, however, develop an acute orchitis after intratesticular inoculation. This method is used to obtain a supply of spirochetes for use in some diagnostic tests.

During the course of infection, the patient develops immunoglobulins that are of great diagnostic importance. The best known is the Wassermann antibody, which fixes complement in the presence of a phosphatide extract of heart muscle (cardiolipin), or produces a precipitate in the presence of a similar type of antigen (Kahn reaction, the Venereal Disease Research Laboratory [VDRL] test, and other modifications). Since the antigen used can hardly be regarded as a specific component of the spirochete, it is not surprising that these standard tests for syphilis (STS) are also sometimes positive in nonspirochetal diseases — for example, leprosy, malaria, and systemic lupus erythematosus. Pregnancy, too, is occasionally associated with a false positive reaction.

In recent years it has been found that syphilitics also develop a more specific treponemal antibody in their sera. When mixed with a suspension of live organisms it leads to their immobilization, and this forms the basis for the treponemal immobilization (TPI) test. Specific treponemal antibody will adhere to the organism, and this can also be detected by a fluorescent technique (fluorescent treponemal antibody test, FTA). These tests are not performed routinely but are of great value in verifying ambiguous results and eliminating false positive reactions. It is unfortunate that even the specific tests cannot distinguish between syphilis and yaws.*

---

*Yaws is a disease that has much in common with syphilis and is caused by *Treponema pertenue.* It is frequent in some tropical countries and is not of venereal origin. The primary lesion is extragenital; secondary and tertiary stages follow. Significant cardiovascular and nervous system involvement is rare as compared with syphilis. It is possible that *Treponema pallidum* developed as a variant of *Treponema pertenue,* which became adapted to venereal transmission.

FIGURE 10–9. *Primary chancre of syphilis.*

For a more complete description, see Case History I.

The Disease. Apart from congenital syphilis, the infection is nearly always acquired venereally. Unlike the tubercle bacillus, *Treponema pallidum* is very rapidly destroyed both in water and by drying. Intimate direct contact is therefore necessary for infection to occur. The spirochete is one of the most invasive organisms known, for once having penetrated the surface, it spreads along the lymphatics to the regional nodes and reaches the blood stream in a matter of hours. Therefore, systemic dissemination occurs long before any local manifestations appear.

The disease is divisible into three stages, described below, each of which is followed by a latent period.

PRIMARY SYPHILIS

The primary lesion of syphilis is the *chancre,* which usually appears on the genital area two to four weeks after infection. It commences as an indurated nodule, which breaks down to form an ulcer that characteristically is painless and is accompanied by enlargement of the regional lymph nodes (Fig. 10–9). Extragenital chancres are not uncommon (*e.g.,* around the anus, and on the lips, tip of tongue, tonsil, or other part of the oral cavity). The chancre heals even without treatment and leaves little scarring. Its occurrence can easily be missed, particularly in women, in whom the lesion can be on the cervix or vaginal vault.

Case History I. (See Figure 10–9.)   The patient, who had been consorting with a number of sexual partners, had noticed a small ulcer on the penis about a week before this picture was taken. This ulcer had steadily enlarged. Although it was not painful, he was persuaded to seek medical advice when he noticed swelling of his left inguinal region. On examination an oval ulcer with a firm base on the penis was noted, and this was associated with large inguinal lymph nodes on the left side. Characteristically, the ulcer was not painful. The ulcer was firmly squeezed, and its base gently rubbed with a bacteriological loop. The drop of fluid that was obtained was examined by dark-field illumination and showed numerous active spirochetes. A blood sample taken at this time showed a negative VDRL. Following the administration of penicillin, the ulcer healed and the lymphadenopathy subsided. The patient's sexual partners were traced, and only two were found to have had intercourse with him during the last three months. Both were found to have a positive VDRL and were treated for syphilis. This case illustrates three important points: (1) A VDRL can be negative during the early stages of primary syphilis. (2) The response to penicillin is dramatic. (3) Contacts must be traced in an effort to prevent the further spread of the disease. Tracing the contacts is an important public health function.

The fact that the spirochetes become disseminated long before there is any local lesion suggests that hypersensitivity plays an important part in the pathogenesis of the lesion. The chancre is not comparable with a boil, for it is not a local inflammatory reaction tending to limit the infection. A possible explanation is that sensitizing antibodies are first formed at the site of infection and in the regional lymph nodes. During the incubation period, the organisms multiply; as sensitizing antibodies are produced, a damaging antigen-antibody reaction occurs to produce the primary lesion and its associated lymphadenitis.

A definite diagnosis of primary syphilis rests entirely upon finding the organisms in the lesion by direct microscopic examination using the dark field method (see Chapter 1). Soon after the appearance of the chancre, antibodies appear in the blood and the serological tests for syphilis become positive.

SECONDARY SYPHILIS

Within two to three months of exposure, the disease becomes clinically generalized. Tradition has it that syphilis was introduced into Europe by the

FIGURE 10–10. *Lesions of secondary syphilis.*
For a more complete description, see Case History II.

returning sailors of Columbus in 1492, and that the disease was than sufficiently severe to warrant naming it the "Great Pox." Nowadays, secondary syphilis is much milder and is characterized by the appearance of a generalized macular or papulosquamous erythematous rash. Characteristically, this does not itch and affects the whole body, including the palms and soles (Fig. 10–10).

Case History II.   (See Figure 10–10.) The patient had developed a generalized nonitching rash composed of red palpable lesions (0.2 to 1.0 cm in diameter) covered by loose, keratin scales (this constitutes a generalized, nonpruritic, erythematous, papulosquamous eruption; see Chapter 41). Lesions were most obvious on the trunk, but they were also present on the limbs, including the palms and soles. (Because the patient was in the habit of taking a barbiturate sleeping pill each night, the possibility of the rash's being due to an adverse drug reaction was also considered.) However, drug rashes generally itch, and the presence of a nonitching rash, particularly if it affects the palms and soles, is very suggestive of secondary syphilis. The patient denied ever having had an ulcer on his penis but admitted to having had homosexual encounters. Blood was taken for a VDRL test. The patient was treated with penicillin. Within eight hours he had developed a fever, and the rash had become more obvious before it faded. The VDRL was subsequently reported as being strongly positive.

This case illustrates the following points:
1. Any generalized nonpruritic papulosquamous rash, particularly one affecting the palms and soles, should be diagnosed as syphilis until proved otherwise.
2. The VDRL test is always positive in secondary syphilis.
3. No history of a primary lesion is obtainable in some patients — particularly in females and in male homosexuals.
4. Successful treatment with penicillin often causes an immediate accentuation of of the lesions. This response is known as the Herxheimer reaction and is presumed to be due to the massive release of bacterial antigen as the organisms are killed.
5. The patients should be treated before laboratory confirmation is obtained. This helps to prevent the spread of the infection.

A low-grade fever, headaches, joint pains, iritis, and many other symptoms may be noted at this stage. Shallow ulcers may occur on the mucous membranes; these, like other secondary lesions, are teeming with organisms and are highly infectious. Diagnosis at this stage depends either on identification of the organism by microscopy or on confirmation by serological means. The serological tests are always positive in secondary syphilis. If a negative result is reported, the prozone phenomenon should be suspected (see Chapter 9).

TERTIARY SYPHILIS

Local destructive lesions may appear two to three years after infection and continue to erupt sporadically for many years. The lesions are presumably due to marked hypersensitivity, since spirochetes are few and the reaction to them is excessive. Two types of lesions can be recognized: localized gummas and diffuse inflammatory lesions characterized by parenchymatous destruction.

LOCALIZED GUMMAS.   The gumma is the classic lesion of tertiary syphilis. It is usually a solitary tumorlike mass and consists of a central large area of coagulative necrosis surrounded by a granulomatous inflammatory reaction. Gummas are described as being most frequent in the liver, testes, subcutaneous tissues, and bones — including the nasal and palatal bones. In the latter situations the destruction produced by the gummas leads to perforation of the hard palate and depression of the nose, causing a saddle-shaped deformity. With the introduction of penicillin and other antibiotic treatment of syphilis, *gummas are now extremely uncommon.*

DIFFUSE LESIONS. The really severe effects of tertiary syphilis fall on the cardiovascular and the nervous systems.

In *syphilitic aortitis* the elastic aortic wall is steadily destroyed by a chronic inflammatory reaction and is replaced by fibrous tissue. The weakening of the aorta results in aneurysmal dilatation; ultimately, the vessel may rupture. The disease tends to affect the thoracic aorta, causing widening of the aortic ring, which can lead to incompetence of the aortic valve.

Cerebral syphilis may be meningovascular or parenchymatous. In the former type there is focal meningitis and vascular occlusion of small vessels. Isolated cranial nerve paralyses are produced.

Parenchymatous neurosyphilis includes the two well-known conditions of general paralysis of the insane and tabes dorsalis. *General paralysis of the insane* (GPI) is a chronic syphilitic meningoencephalitis in which the frontal lobes are particularly affected. This results in progressive dementia and paralysis. *Tabes dorsalis* is a degenerative condition of the posterior columns of the spinal cord and the posterior roots of the spinal nerves. The loss in sensation leads to loss of postural sense and a typical staggering gait.

The diagnosis of tertiary syphilis is primarily clinical, but it may often be substantiated by serological examination of the blood and cerebrospinal fluid. In most cases of overt syphilis the serological reactions are positive. Gummas are usually diagnosed by biopsy or following excision. It has frequently been stressed that syphilis is the great mimic in medicine and that virtually any lesion or disease can be faithfully copied by syphilis. Hence, a routine VDRL test is a common clinical procedure. Note, however, that the serological tests for syphilis frequently remain positive during the latent periods and that a syphilitic patient can suffer from other diseases. Thus, a mass present in the lung in a patient with a positive VDRL is more likely to be a carcinoma, which is common, than a gumma, which is rare.

CONGENITAL SYPHILIS

During the first two years of infection, an untreated syphilitic mother is very liable to transmit the disease to her fetus, particularly in the later months of pregnancy. Abortion may result, or a severely affected infant may be born alive but die soon after birth.

More frequently, the child survives and may then exhibit early stigmata of the infection: skin eruptions, nasal infection (snuffles), and involvement of bones. Sometimes stigmata appear only in later childhood. The notched, deformed incisor teeth, inflammation of the cornea, periostitis, and nerve deafness are all well-known features. In effect, the early lesions of congenital syphilis are comparable to those of the secondary stage, whereas the later manifestations have the destructive features of tertiary syphilis as encountered in the adults.

Table 10–3 SPIROCHETAL DISEASES

ORGANISM	SOURCE OF INFECTION	DISEASE PRODUCED
Borrelia		
Borrelia recurrentis	Body louse	European relapsing fever
Borrelia duttonii	Ticks	African relapsing fever
Borrelia vincentii	Normal flora of mouth	Gingivitis, gangrenous lesions of mouth
Leptospira		
Leptospira icterohaemor-rhagiae and others	Urine of rodents, dogs, and many other species	Leptospirosis (Weil's disease)
Treponema		
Treponema pallidum	Human case of syphilis	Syphilis
Treponema pertenue	Human case of yaws	Yaws

The spirochetal diseases described in this section are summarized in Table 10–3.

Review Questions

1. Compare and contrast infections with *Staphylococcus aureus* with those produced by *Streptococcus pyogenes* in terms of the following:
    - (a) site of infection
    - (b) type of local lesion produced
    - (c) spread of infection
    - (d) lesions produced by exotoxin
    - (e) sterile lesions produced by immune mechanisms.
2. List the lesions produced by the gonococcus. Indicate how the organism reaches each of the sites mentioned.
3. A patient has driven a fork through his foot while digging in the garden. What measures should be taken to prevent the development of tetanus under these conditions:
    - (a) if he has had tetanus toxoid injections previously
    - (b) if he has never had tetanus toxoid or does not know whether he was ever given toxoid.
4. A soldier sustains a gunshot wound of the thigh. The lacerated wound is contaminated by soil, and he is unable to receive medical attention for 24 hours. Describe the signs and symptoms that indicate the development of:
    - (a) infection with a pyogenic organism, such as a gram-negative intestinal bacillus
    - (b) tetanus
    - (c) gas gangrene.
5. Compare a chronic staphylococcal lung abscess with a cavitated tuberculous lesion with respect to:
    - (a) the tissue reaction
    - (b) the contents of the cavity
    - (c) the methods of demonstrating the causative organism.

6. Compare and contrast leprosy with tuberculosis in terms of the following areas:
   - (a) properties of the organisms
   - (b) methods of diagnosis
   - (c) tissue response to infection
   - (d) immune response to infection
   - (e) organs or tissues affected.
7. Syphilis is an excellent example of a disease in which the lesions are produced, not by the organism acting alone, but by an interplay between the organism and the host reacting to it. Discuss this response in relation to the three stages of the disease.

Selected Readings

Christie, A. B.: Infectious Diseases. 2nd ed. Edinburgh, Churchill Livingstone, 1974. See, in particular, Chapter 22, "Tetanus" and Chapter 28, "Leptospiral Infections."

Cruickshank, R., Duguid, J. P., Marmion, B. P., and Swain, R. H. A.: Medical Microbiology. 12th ed. Vol. 1. Edinburgh, Churchill Livingstone, 1973. An excellent account of medical microbiology, with the accent on laboratory findings and the properties of bacteria and viruses.

Browne, S. G., and Bullock, W. E.: Mycobacterial diseases: leprosy. In: Fitzpatrick, T. B. et al. (Eds.): Dermatology in General Medicine. New York, McGraw-Hill Book Company, 1971.

Moschella, S. L., Pillsbury, D. M., and Hurley, H. J., Dermatology. Philadelphia, W. B. Saunders Company, 1975. See pp. 808–825 for a well-illustrated, detailed account of leprosy.

Robbins, S. L.: Pathologic Basis of Disease. Philadelphia, W. B. Saunders Company, 1974. See Chapter 10, "Infectious Diseases" which provides a useful reference to the pyogenic infections and tuberculosis.

Scofield, C. B. S.: Sexually Transmitted Diseases. 2nd ed. Edinburgh, Churchill Livingstone, 1975.

Woodruff, A. W. (Ed.): Medicine in the Tropics. Edinburgh, Churchill Livingstone, 1974. See Chapter 24, "Leptospirosis."

Youmans, G. P., Paterson, P. Y., and Sommers, H. M.: The Biological and Clinical Basis of Infectious Diseases. Philadelphia, W. B. Saunders Company, 1975. An excellent account of medical microbiology and infectious disease, with particular emphasis on the clinical features.

Chapter 11

After studying this chapter the student should be able to:

- Outline the main features of mycoplasmal pneumonia and the organism that causes it.
- Compare chlamydia with mycoplasma and describe the important human diseases caused by members of the chlamydial group of organisms.
- List the four types of typhus fever and describe the main features of one of them.
- Name two diseases other than typhus that are caused by a rickettsial infection.

This chapter describes infection with members of three groups of organisms. The microorganisms are all much smaller than the true bacteria; many of them are obligatory intracellular parasites, and some of them in the past have been confused with viruses. Nevertheless, unlike viruses they are capable of simple division and do not exhibit the complex intracellular mode of reproduction that is so characteristic of viruses.

Mycoplasmal Infections

Mycoplasma are the smallest organisms (150 to 250 nm) that are capable of growth in a cell-free medium. They lack a cell wall and therefore tend to be very pleomorphic; coccobacillary, filamentous, and branching forms are com-

190

MYCOPLASMAL, CHLAMYDIAL, AND RICKETTSIAL INFECTIONS

mon. The only known human pathogen is *Mycoplasma pneumoniae,* an organism causing a type of pneumonia that tends to occur in small epidemics. The onset is insidious, and the x-ray changes of patchy consolidation are often more extensive than the clinical picture would suggest. Recovery is invariable and can be hastened by tetracycline therapy (Fig. 11–1). Before the nature of the causative organism was understood, the disease was labeled "primary atypical pneumonia" or "viral pneumonia" (see legend of Fig. 13–1). A curious feature of the disease is the development of cold autohemagglutinins (see Chapter 26) and a positive standard test for syphilis.

Case History I. (See Figure 11–1.)   The patient was a 36-year-old female who had developed an upper respiratory infection that persisted for two weeks and was accompanied by a dry, hacking cough. Although she was treated with penicillin, she showed no improvement. At the end of the third week the patient still felt ill and was troubled by a persistent cough, shortness of breath, and an evening fever. She was diagnosed to have mycoplasmal pneumonia.

Since the patient was found to be three months pregnant, she was not administered tetracycline, the usual drug of choice. Tetracycline is contraindicated in pregnancy, particularly during the last three months, because it impairs fetal tooth development. The patient was given erythromycin and made a slow recovery.

Chlamydial Infections

The chlamydia, previously called *Bedsonia* after Samuel Bedson who was a pioneer in the field, are small, obligatory intracellular parasites about 300 nm in diameter. Several are pathogenic to human beings. Since growth in tissue cultures is difficult, the organisms are generally isolated by injecting a suitable laboratory animal.

Psittacosis (Ornithosis).   This is a disease of birds of the parrot family (psittacine birds) as well as of other related birds. Infection in humans is caused by inhalation of dust containing contaminated bird excreta, and it usually presents as a type of pneumonia. The regulations relating to the importation of psittacine birds have made this an uncommon disease. Occasional outbreaks still occur, however, because native birds, such as poultry and pigeons, can harbor the organism.

Trachoma.   This is an infection of the conjunctiva that becomes chronic, tends to spread to the cornea, and causes scarring. The disease is uncommon in

191

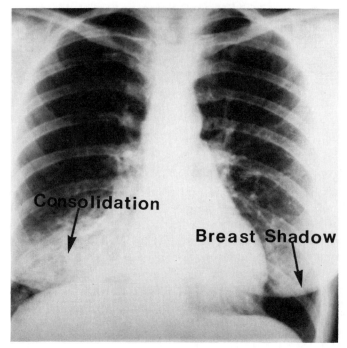

FIGURE 11–1.   *Chest radiograph of patient with mycoplasmal pneumonia.*

Note bilateral, patchy consolidation, most marked in the lower lung fields, particularly on the right side. A diagnosis of mycoplasmal pneumonia was confirmed by the finding of specific antibodies of a titer of 1 in 3000. (Photograph courtesy of Dr. D. E. Sanders.) For a more complete description, see Case History I.

the Western World but is a very important cause of *blindness* in the Middle East and other areas of poverty and overcrowding.

Inclusion Conjunctivitis.   This disease is so named because inclusion bodies can be seen in infected cells. It affects newborn babies (in whom it forms a type of ophthalmia neonatorum) as well as adults (causing "swimming pool conjunctivitis"). The organism is transmitted venereally and causes urethritis in the male ("nongonococcal urethritis") and cervicitis in the female. Indeed, the genital area is the reservoir of infection. Transfer to the eyes of babies occurs during labor; transfer in adults occurs via the hands or imperfectly chlorinated pool water. The TRachoma–Inclusion Conjunctivitis chlamydia are often grouped as the TRIC organisms.

Lymphogranuloma Venereum.   This is an uncommon venereal disease, which is characterized by the appearances of a local genital ulcer and regional lymph node enlargement.

Rickettsial Infections

The rickettsial organisms are obligatory intracellular parasites that are widely distributed in nature, infecting many species of mammals that form their natural reservoir. Infection is transferred by lice, fleas, ticks, and mites.

Humans are infected when they accidentally intercept the life cycle of infection from insect vector to animal reservoir. The only exception to this mode of transfer is with epidemic typhus, in which humans, themselves, are the only known reservoir.

TYPHUS

The typhus group of fevers is currently of little day-to-day importance; in the past, however, it has been responsible for epidemics of ferocious intensity. These have occurred in times of war when rats, fleas, humans, and lice have shared a common habitation. No doubt, future catastrophes will once again highlight the virulence of the rickettsiae, and it is for this reason that some knowledge of this group of diseases is important.

Mode of Infection.   Some rickettsiae are injected by the bite of an infected tick or mite. On the other hand, lice and fleas pass contaminated feces as they feed on their animal host, causing rickettsial organisms to be introduced when the site of the bite is scratched.

Types.   The typhus fevers have an incubation period of 7 to 10 days, and their onset is of dramatic suddenness with rigors, fever, and severe headaches accompanied by prostration. The organisms multiply in the endothelial cells of blood vessels and the far-reaching vascular damage accounts for the widespread nature of the lesions seen in the disease. A skin rash appears in most cases about the fourth day of clinical illness. The following types of typhus are important:

1.   EPIDEMIC, LOUSE-BORNE TYPHUS.*   Caused by *Rickettsia prowazeki*, this disease is associated with a high mortality and was responsible for the typhus epidemics of the two World Wars. DDT, with its lousicidal activity, proved to be an effective weapon in controlling this disease. Unlike the case in all other forms of typhus, with this disease man is the only mammal host. Since infected lice soon die, one would expect the disease to die out. A parasite that often kills its only hosts should not be successful. The explanation of the paradox is that following an attack of the disease humans can harbor the organism for many years. A recrudescence of the disease (Brill-Zinsser disease) can occur; the illness is mild but of great importance, because the victim constitutes a potential source of infection. If he happens to harbor lice, and lives in overcrowded squalor, he can initiate the next epidemic.

2.   ENDEMIC, FLEA-BORNE TYPHUS.   This disease is endemic in many parts of the world, including the U.S.A. It is caused by *Rickettsia mooseri* and is transmitted by the *rat flea*.

3.   ROCKY MOUNTAIN SPOTTED FEVER.   This disease, endemic throughout North America, is caused by *Rickettsia rickettsii* and is a severe form of typhus transmitted by the bite of a tick. A widespread hemorrhagic rash is an outstanding feature. Similar types of tick-borne diseases occur in other parts of the world.

---

*In addition to rickettsiae, the body louse also transmits one type of relapsing fever (see Chapter 10). Infestation can generally be recognized by the presence of itchy papules and numerous scratch marks ("vagabond's disease"). It is important to note that the parasite lives in clothing and not on the skin. Hence, when infestation is suspected, the underclothing—particularly its seams—should be carefully examined.

4. SCRUB TYPHUS.   This was the type of typhus that constituted a problem in the Pacific area in World War II.

Laboratory Diagnosis.   Patients with typhus develop antibodies that by chance agglutinate certain strains of proteus organisms. This reaction has been utilized in a diagnostic test, which is called the Weil-Felix reaction and is analogous to the Widal reaction for typhoid. A rising titer during the course of a febrile illness helps to confirm the diagnosis. Specific antirickettsial antibodies can also be demonstrated. Isolation of the organism is performed by inoculating a suitable laboratory animal.

Treatment.   Treatment of typhus has been revolutionized by the introduction of chloramphenicol and tetracycline. Typhus now has a low mortality, unless the patient is already the victim of other disease or starvation.

Two other forms of rickettsial disease are of interest:

TRENCH FEVER.   This disease, which is spread by lice, was a problem in World War I and on Germany's eastern front in World War II. As with other rickettsial diseases, the onset is sudden and is soon followed by fever and very severe pains in muscles and bones. Although symptoms sometimes persist for three weeks, no fatal cases have been recorded.

Q FEVER.   Q (for *query*) fever, caused by *Coxiella burneti,** is transmitted from animal to animal by the bite of a tick. Sheep, goats, and cows are naturally infected, and human disease is caused either by drinking contaminated milk or by inhaling dust contaminated by animal material. Q fever in humans is characterized by a long incubation period (about 19 days), and the disease resembles other forms of typhus, except that although a rash is very uncommon, evidence of pneumonia or hepatitis is frequently found.

Review Questions

1. Describe the antibodies that are formed during the course of an infection with mycoplasmal or rickettsial organisms. How may these aid in diagnosis? How may their presence cause confusion with other diseases?
2. How does infection with *Rickettsia prowazeki* in humans differ from infection with other rickettsial organisms?
3. Write brief notes on the infections caused by the TRIC group of organisms.
4. List the diseases that are spread by the body louse. Where would one expect to find this parasite in a verminous person?

Selected Readings

Castleman, B. (Ed.): Case records of the Massachusetts General Hospital. A case of Rocky Mountain spotted Fever. New England Journal of Medicine, *288*:1400–1404, 1973.
Cruickshank, R., Duguid, J. P., Marmion, B. P., and Swain, R. H. A.: Medical Microbiology. 12th ed. Edinburgh, Churchill Livingstone, 1973, Chapters 50–52.

*Named after Burnet, the Australian virologist, who is better known for his concepts in immunology (see Chapter 9). The genus *Coxiella* is closely related to the genus *Rickettsia*.

VIRAL INFECTIONS

Chapter 12

After studying this chapter the student should be able to:

- Compare and contrast viruses with higher organisms with respect to the following:

    (a) size
    (b) structure
    (c) chemical composition.

VIRAL INFECTIONS

- Describe how viruses enter a cell, how new viral material is produced, and how new particles are released.
- Describe the range of effects that a viral infection can have on a cell.
- Describe the immunity that a viral infection can evoke, particularly in relation to the following:
     - (a) immunoglobulin formation
     - (b) T-cell immunity
     - (c) interferon production.
- List the nine groups of viruses described in this chapter and give examples of the common members within each group.
- Distinguish among the following: the incubation period, the prodromal stage, enanthem, and exanthem. Use measles and smallpox as examples.
- Describe the pathogenesis of poliomyelitis as well as the means available for preventing this disease.
- Describe the hazards of vaccination against smallpox.
- Discuss the relationship between varicella and zoster. Outline the clinical features of each.
- Compare infective hepatitis with serum hepatitis in regard to these factors:
     - (a) incubation period
     - (b) mode of transmission
     - (c) clinical features and complications
     - (d) etiology.
- Describe the three particles that have been found in the blood of patients with serum hepatitis. Indicate their antigenic inter-relationship.

INTRODUCTION

Viral infections are common and are of many types. At times, some have reached epidemic proportions and have been so severe that through the ages man has made strenuous attempts at preventing them; by chance, some attempts have been successful. Thus, Jenner, who knew nothing of virology, found a way to prevent smallpox. Pasteur postulated that the cause of rabies was an infinitesimally small microorganism, and without ever isolating it, he devised a means of protecting against rabies. Pasteur's theory was finally confirmed by Iwanowsky in 1892, when he showed that tobacco mosaic disease was due to an agent so small that it could pass through the pores of a filter that would retain all known bacteria. It was at the turn of the century that the first human disease, yellow fever, was proved to be caused by a similar ultramicroscopic, filterable virus. Until the advent of electron microscopy, the structure of viruses was poorly understood. We now have a wealth of knowledge concerning their structure and chemical composition, and this can best be understood in relation to the properties of bacteria.

GENERAL PROPERTIES OF VIRUSES

Bacteria are all within the range of the light microscope and are complete cells surrounded by a cell membrane and often by a cell wall.* They contain both DNA and RNA together with many chemicals, such as enzymes, for their own maintenance and reproduction. They multiply by simple division. Since bacteria are complete cells, the majority of them can be grown by the bacteriologist on an artificial medium; the causative organisms of leprosy and syphilis are the two notable exceptions. Viruses, on the other hand, are much smaller, although the large poxviruses are just within the range of the conventional light microscope. Viruses contain either RNA or DNA, but never both. They have no mitochondria and cannot produce high-energy adenosine triphosphate (ATP). They possess no ribosomes. Indeed, viruses consist of little more than structural protein and nucleic acid. They can multiply only in the protoplasm of another cell, and they do this by utilizing the structures and chemicals of the infected cell and perverting them for their own purposes. Indeed, the essential differences between viruses and all other organisms is that the synthetic processes that attend multiplication take place within the protoplasm of the infected cell in viruses but in the body of the organism itself in all other infective agents.

STRUCTURE OF VIRUSES

A complete infective virus particle that can exist outside a cell is called a *virion,* and it consists of a core of either DNA or RNA, which is surrounded by a protein sheath, or *capsid.* Electron microscopy has shown the coat to consist of subunits, or *capsomeres,* each of which is made of protein and consists of a hollow tube pointing outwards. The capsomeres are closely packed and so arranged with their neighbors that the virion has a definite geometric shape. Two major types of viruses can be recognized as follows: (a) *viruses with cubical symmetry,* which have the form of an icosahedron, a solid, roughly spherical structure having 20 facets, each consisting of an equilateral triangle and meeting at 12 corners (Fig. 12–1); and (b) *viruses with helical symmetry,* which consist of a filament with capsomeres arranged around the nucleic acid as a *helix* (Fig. 12–2). Other viruses are known, which have a more complex structure (Fig. 12–9). Thus, bacteriophage, a virus that infects bacteria and is commonly called "phage" for short, has a head attached to a central core from which arise six tail filaments (Fig. 12–3).

GROWTH OF VIRUSES

Viruses will grow only in living cells. In the early days of virology, whole live animals were used for growth of these structures, but the animal's immune response was a complicating factor and the method was ethically undesirable as well as expensive. Also, the animals often harbored their own viruses, and

---

*Animal cells do not possess a cell wall. Penicillin acts by inhibiting the formation of cell-wall material. After division, penicillin-treated bacteria have a defective cell wall, are fragile, and are easily killed.

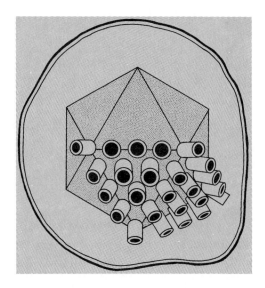

FIGURE 12–1. *Diagrammatic representation of a typical virus showing cubical symmetry.*

The core of the virus has the form of an icosahedron having 20 facets. It is covered by symmetrically arranged capsomeres, each consisting of a hollow tube. The covering of capsomeres constitutes the viral capsid. The virion (consisting of the genetic material and the capsid) has an outer membrane that is derived from the altered host plasma or nuclear membrane. (Drawing by Frederick Lammerich, Department of Art as Applied to Medicine, University of Toronto.)

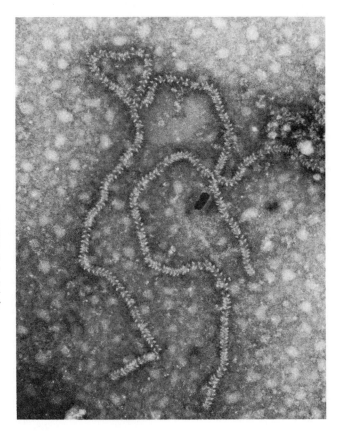

FIGURE 12–2. *Helical arrangement of capsomeres.*

The covering membrane of a paramyxovirus has been ruptured; its RNA content has been released. The photograph shows the long thread of nuclear protein surrounded by the capsomeres arranged in a helical fashion (× 117,450). (Photograph courtesy of Micheline Fauvel, Department of Medical Microbiology, Faculty of Medicine, University of Toronto.)

FIGURE 12–3. *Diagrammatic representation of the entry of bacteriophage into a bacterial cell.*

The bacteriophage consists of a head containing DNA, a rigid core surrounded by a sheath to which is attached a tail piece, and tail fibers. *A,* The first event in the entry of the phage is the attachment of the tail fibers to the receptors of the bacterial cell wall. *B,* Contraction of the sheath results in the injection of viral DNA into the bacterial cell substance. *C,* The protein component of the phage shown attached to the cell wall is subsequently lost, leaving the viral DNA within the substance of the bacterium. Here, it can replicate and lead to lysis of the bacterial cell, or it can remain latent as prophage. (Drawn by Sue Reynolds.)

these sometimes served as contaminants. Embryonated hen's eggs were next used, but apart from the absence of an immune response they had similar disadvantages. Cell culture has now largely replaced these methods (Fig. 12–4).

Animal cells (*e.g.,* kidney cells or fibroblasts) will grow as a single mono-layer on a glass surface if this is covered by a suitable culture medium. Subcul-

FIGURE 12–4. *Normal HeLa cells in tissue culture.*

The confluent sheet is composed of plump polygonal cells derived from a malignant epithelial cell line that originated from a carcinoma in a patient named *Helen Lane*—hence, the name "HeLa." A giant cell form is conspicuous in this field. This photograph was obtained by using phase contrast microscopy (× 200).

tures can be obtained from such a growth; unfortunately, after repeated subculture, however, the cells cease to multiply and die off. Apparently normal animal cells cannot live forever. Occasionally, the cells undergo an alteration and continued subculture is possible. The process is called *transformation,* and the cells do not show contact inhibition (see Chapter 7). Established cell lines of this type can be kept growing indefinitely and are used for virus culture. Unfortunately these cells are malignant, and they cannot be used to prepare vaccines for human use. The best known cell line is the HeLa cell, originally derived from the cells of a cancer of the cervix of a patient, *Helen Lane.*

Mechanism of Viral Growth. The first stage of virus-cell interaction is *attachment* of the virion to the cell surface. This is believed to be the result of an affinity of the virus for some specific cell receptors. With the relatively simple bacteriophage, the protein capsid of the organism remains on the outside of the cell, but the phage acts as a type of microsyringe, its DNA content being squirted into the cell substance (Fig. 12–3). With animal viruses the process is less simple, because the stage following attachment is *penetration* of the virus particle into the cell by a process of *endocytosis.* To begin with, the virus is contained within a phagosome; then, by means that are not clearly understood, it escapes from the phagosome and enters the cytoplasm proper. The next stage is one of *uncoating* of the virus so that the free nucleic acid is released. The virus now ceases to exist as a particle and may not even be infective. Nevertheless, its component parts can still be detected. This stage in viral multiplication is known as the *eclipse phase* and is a feature of the reproductive cycle of all true viruses.

The information in the viral nucleic acid is transcribed and diverts the host's cell activity into synthesizing viral coded enzymes, regulating protein synthesis, and ultimately leading to the production of more viral nucleic acid and viral structural proteins. The precise way in which this occurs varies considerably from one virus to another. Thus, with the DNA viruses, the DNA encodes for a specific mRNA, and this is translated on host ribosomes. With the RNA viruses, the RNA serves as a source of genetic information and acts directly as a type of mRNA. The site of nucleic acid replication varies. Often the

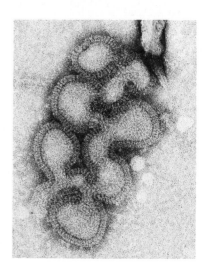

FIGURE 12–5. *A myxovirus.*

An electron micrograph of influenza A/2, England 4272, which is demonstrated by negative staining. The irregular shape of the virus is clearly seen, and the well-marked covering membrane from which numerous prickles project is also observable. These projections contain hemagglutinin; it is to these structures that red cells become adherent. The RNA within the virion is not apparent in this photograph (× 120,000). (Photograph courtesy of Micheline Fauvel, Department of Medical Microbiology, Faculty of Medicine, University of Toronto.)

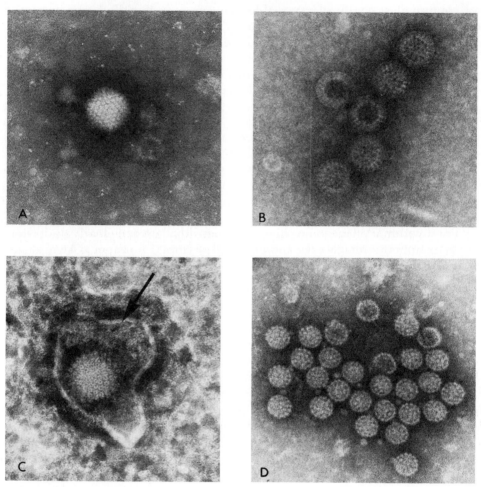

FIGURE 12–6.

A, Adenovirus. This virus, which is demonstrated by negative staining, has the typical icosahedral form and has no outer envelope (× 167,760). *B, Rotavirus.* This virus, also called an "orbivirus," has not yet been grown in tissue cultures. It can be found by electron microscopy in the stools of some infants with acute gastroenteritis. This disease is a major cause of illness during childhood and is particularly common in infants under the age of two years; it often occurs in winter. Some cases are due to bacterial infection (e.g., *Salmonella, E. coli*), but most cases appear to be due to viruses (× 136,300). *C, Herpes simplex virus.* The envelope, which is clearly shown (arrow), is derived from the modified nuclear membrane of an infected cell. The hollow capsomeres of the virion are clearly visible (× 139,800). (Compare this with Figure 12–1.) *D, Papovavirus, S.V. 40.* This organism was found as a contaminant in a culture of African Green Monkey kidney cells. Another important member of this group of viruses is the polyoma virus. In tissue culture, the cells show characteristic vacuolation. The name "papova" is derived from *PA*pilloma, *PO*lyoma, *VA*cuolating agent (× 136,300). (Photographs courtesy of Micheline Fauvel, Department of Medical Microbiology, Faculty of Medicine, University of Toronto.)

FIGURE 12–7. *HeLa cells in culture infected with adenovirus.*

The sheet of cells is broken up, and the swollen, refractile cells have fused to form irregular masses. This response is called the *cytopathic effect of the virus.* Specific antisera will inhibit this effect. Using known antisera, one can identify a particular virus. Likewise, if cultures of a known virus are used, the ability of a serum to inhibit the cytopathic effect can be used to estimate the titer and specificity of antibody (× 200).

DNA replicates in the nucleus of cells, whereas the protein of the capsomeres is formed in the cytoplasm. The end-result of viral activity is the reformation of mature virus particles by assembling nucleic acid with protein.

Release of Virus Particles. The virus-infected cell may be so damaged that it disintegrates, and mature virus particles are released in a burstlike fashion. Under other circumstances, the cell is not destroyed, and virus particles are released slowly. In the latter type of infection, the virus frequently receives an additional coat, termed an *envelope,* from a cell membrane. Thus, the orthomyxoviruses receive an envelope of cell membrane (Fig. 12–5). This membrane is not completely normal cell membrane, but one that has been modified by the effect of virus and contains viral type antigens. Herpesvirus, a DNA virus that is assembled in the nucleus, acquires an envelope of modified nuclear membrane from the host cell (Fig. 12–6).

EFFECT OF VIRUSES ON CELLS

As noted above, viruses sometimes kill the cells that they infect. In tissue culture this is termed a *cytopathic effect* and is useful in diagnostic virology. If known specific antiserum is added to a culture, inhibition of the cytopathic effect helps to identify an unknown virus (Figs. 12–7 and 12–8).

Sometimes an infecting virus alters the cell, but it does not kill it. A common effect is the formation of a mass of homogeneous material, called an *inclusion body,* either in the nucleus or in the cytoplasm of the infected cell. Inclusion bodies consist of maturing viral material and can be used as markers in the identification of a viral disease. Thus, the finding of characteristic inclusion bodies (Negri bodies) in the neurons of a dog is diagnostic of rabies.

FIGURE 12–8. *HeLa cells infected with poliovirus.*

The cells have undergone profound disintegration, so that only a few shrunken survivors are still present. The polioviruses are much more destructive than the adenoviruses to the cell cultures (× 200).

Viral nucleic acid can sometimes enter the nucleic acid pool of the host cell and become incorporated into the host's genetic material. The viral nucleic acid then replicates when the cell divides; in fact, it behaves like a gene. This symbiotic relationship can result in the cell showing no evidence of infection. The virus is *latent*.

Under certain circumstances the nucleic acid of a latent virus can replicate and behave once more as an infective agent. The cell may then be damaged. Some examples illustrating the implications of this remarkable relationship are as follows:

1. Some bacteria contain a latent bacteriophage. This can suddenly lead to lysis of a whole culture. Such a strain of bacteria is termed *lysogenic.*

2. Herpes simplex virus can remain latent for many months or years in human beings. The development of fever from any cause, exposure to sunlight, or the onset of menstruation can upset the balance between the person and the virus, and then herpes blisters, or *cold sores*, appear on the skin.

3. The cell containing a latent infection may show altered function. Thus, production of toxin by the diphtheria bacillus is determined by the presence of a phage.

4. Some viruses can cause normal animal cells to be transformed into cancer cells. Since such cells are stimulated to grow, this response has very important implications when one considers the possible causes of cancer (see Chapter 17).

CLASSIFICATION OF VIRUSES

It was once fashionable to classify viruses according to the tissue they affected. Thus, a *derma*totropic virus affects the skin, whereas a *neuro*tropic one involves the nervous system. This classification is quite unsatisfactory, because many viruses can affect different tissues. Thus, the dermatotropic virus, herpes simplex, which causes cold sores, in fact lies latent in the nerve cells of the ganglion that is related to the sensory nerve supply of the part affected. Herpes simplex virus can cause pneumonia and encephalitis. It is therefore quite unreasonable to classify it as a dermatotropic virus. The modern classification of viruses is under constant review, but major groups are now being separated with reference to the following criteria:

1. The type of nucleic acid present; that is, whether it is DNA or RNA.
2. The shape of the virus; that is, whether it is icosahedral, filamentous, or some other shape.
3. The antigenic structure of the virus. Some viruses share common antigens with others, and these are then included in one group; for example, the adenoviruses all possess a common group antigen.

MECHANISM OF IMMUNITY TO VIRAL INFECTIONS

The mechanism of immunity to viral infection is complex and has several components.

Immunoglobulin Antibodies. Plasma antibodies play an important part, especially in the disseminated infections. Most viruses possess several antigens, some associated with the protein envelope and others with the nucleoprotein. The antibodies reacting with the protein coat are those that are of importance in immunity; they prevent the virus from attaching itself to the cell receptor. The virus is invulnerable to antibody when it is intracellular. These plasma, virus-neutralizing immunoglobulins belong to the IgG class.

Note that after recovery from an attack of poliomyelitis, or following immunization with living attenuated virus administered orally, a subsequent dose of poliovirus does not flourish in the cells of the small bowel. This is due to the action of IgA antibodies produced locally in the intestine and present in the secretions. People who have been immunized with a killed suspension of poliovirus administered parenterally (Salk vaccine) usually exhibit unhindered multiplication of viruses in the small bowel despite a considerable antibody response in the blood.

Cellular Immunity. There is also a T-cell–mediated immunity independent of circulating antibodies. Children with congenital immunoglobulin deficiency can resist viral infections, but if they have a T-cell defect, death is often due to widespread viral disease. The lymphokines liberated by sensitized lymphocytes (see Chapter 9) include interferon. Cellular immunity is particularly important in herpesvirus and poxvirus infections.

Viral Interference. The infection of a cell with one virus sometimes prevents a second infection by another virus. This phenomenon is termed "viral interference," and an important mechanism is the production of a protein called *interferon* by the cell. Interferon is a protein of low molecular weight, which readily diffuses from the cell and causes other cells to produce agents called *translation-inhibiting proteins* (TIP), which are thought to prevent translation of viral mRNA. Interferon has no effect on the cell's protein synthesis, but by being able to distinguish between viral and cellular mRNA can prevent viral replication in the cell. The production of interferon does not save an infected cell, but by affecting neighboring cells, the interferon can conceivably prevent the spread of a viral infection within the body. Various attempts have been made to use interferon as a prophylactic agent; unfortunately, interferon is species specific. To be effective in humans, it must be produced in human cell cultures, and this has posed some technical difficulties.

VIRAL CHEMOTHERAPY

The very close relationship between the virus and its host cell at one time made it appear unlikely that specific chemotherapeutic agents could be developed for viral diseases. If a virus utilized cell ribosomes and other enzymes, then it seemed unlikely that a specific blocking agent could be found. This initial pessimism was not justified. Viruses have very specific actions, starting with their attachment to the cell, their penetration, their uncoating, their production of viral material, and their assembly and release. These are highly specific events, each of which is a point of attack. Already a number of compounds are known which will act as chemotherapeutic agents, but they have not yet come into general use. Some are toxic, whereas others have to be given at an early stage of the disease, often before diagnosis is usually possible. However, the hopes are that in the future better agents will be available and capable of use for mass prophylaxis in the face of a serious epidemic such as smallpox or influenza.

EXAMPLES OF VIRAL INFECTIONS

These will be described under nine headings: (1) The Enteroviruses; (2) The Poxviruses; (3) Viruses Affecting the Respiratory Tract; (4) The Arboviruses; (5) The Herpesviruses; (6) The Papovaviruses; (7) Viral Hepatitis; (8) Rabies; and (9) The Slow Viruses.

The Enteroviruses

Three main groups are recognized.
1. THE COXSACKIE VIRUSES. This group was so named because they were first isolated in the town of Coxsackie in New York State. There are a large number of viruses in this group, and they cause a variety of illnesses ranging from an upper respiratory infection resembling a cold to meningitis and myocarditis.
2. THE ECHO VIRUSES.* There are many types, causing a variety of infections, as do the Coxsackie viruses.

---

*ECHO = Enteric, cytopathic, human, orphan viruses. These viruses were first noted in children's feces and could not at first be linked with any disease.

3. POLIOVIRUS. Poliomyelitis is an important disease and will be discussed in some detail.

Poliomyelitis. Poliomyelitis (infantile paralysis) is the most important of the enterovirus infections. There are three separate strains of the organism, and the disease is acquired by ingesting material that has been contaminated by virus-containing feces. The virus proliferates in the cells of the bowel, and if the infection is not arrested at this stage, the virus enters the blood stream via the lymphatics. It multiplies in various extraneuronal sites, and after 7 to 14 days (the incubation period of the disease) virus particles re-enter the blood stream and fever commences. Even at this stage of viremia, the disease may be arrested without severe effect.

If the condition proceeds, the virus finally settles in the central nervous system and localizes in the motor nerve cells of the medulla and spinal cord. Some of the infected cells are destroyed, and paralysis ensues. It should be stressed that although many people are infected with poliomyelitis, only a few develop a clinical disease, and of these only some develop paralysis. A number of factors are known which appear to precipitate paralytic poliomyelitis. One of these is local trauma. If a patient who is already infected with poliomyelitis has his tonsils removed, paralysis of the pharynx can occur. This is known as the bulbar type of disease. Likewise, an injection at any site can precipitate paralysis. It is therefore important that during an epidemic of poliomyelitis, no one should be subjected to unnecessary surgical trauma nor should injections for immunization against other disease, such as diphtheria, be given.

ACTIVE IMMUNIZATION. The first effective vaccine was devised by Salk, who used poliovirus grown in monkey kidney cells and subsequently inactivated by formaldehyde. The Salk vaccine is administered by intramuscular injection, and three or four doses are given to ensure adequate antigenic stimulation. The vaccine stimulates the production of immunoglobulins. This does not prevent infection of the intestine with poliovirus, but it does prevent subsequent spread of the virus to involve the central nervous system. The vaccine can advantageously be combined with other vaccines and toxoids.

The vaccine developed by Sabin is a live attenuated virus and is given by mouth. The attenuated virus causes an intestinal infection that, like the Salk vaccine, stimulates the formation of immunoglobulin antibodies. However, there is one important difference between the vaccines: the Sabin vaccine also produces intestinal immunity because of the local formation of IgA. Thus, the Sabin vaccine prevents the subsequent infection with poliovirus, and it may be presumed that if large populations are immunized with Sabin vaccine, virulent strains of the virus will eventually die out. Because the Sabin vaccine is easier to administer and more effective, it has become the more popular of the two methods of immunization. It is usual to give the three separate strains of poliovirus. As noted previously, the infection of a cell with one virus sometimes prevents infection with other viruses. To overcome this interference, three separate doses of the trivalent vaccine are administered.

The Poxviruses

The poxviruses are a group of large, brick-shaped DNA-containing viruses, which produce vesicular and pustular lesions of the skin. Many animals have

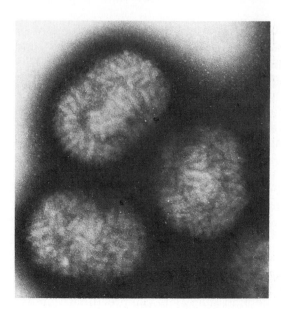

FIGURE 12–9. *Poxvirus from molluscum contagiosum.*

Molluscum contagiosum is a viral disease of the skin that is characterized by the formation of small umbilicated papules. It is common in children and is a self-limiting disease. A suspension of material from a human lesion was mixed with a solution of 2 per cent phosphotungstic acid and allowed to dry on a suitably prepared copper grid coated with a film of carbon. Under the electron microscope, the electron-dense background produced by the phosphotungstic acid allows the viral particles to stand out quite clearly. This technique, which is known as "negative staining," is frequently used to demonstrate viral particles. Poxviruses are large, square, and structurally complex. The outer protein layer consisting of strands is shown here. Because vaccinia and smallpox viruses have a similar morphology, the identification of particles of this type in a case of suspected smallpox would lead to a provisional diagnosis of this disease. Confirmation by culture and serological means would be required (× 105,850). (Photograph courtesy of Micheline Fauvel, Department of Medical Microbiology, Faculty of Medicine, University of Toronto.)

their own variety of pox disease, *e.g.*, cowpox and mousepox. The human disease is *smallpox*, or *variola* (Fig. 12–9).

SMALLPOX

The disease is acquired by inhalation of virus either directly from a patient or indirectly from fomites. The bedding is particularly dangerous as a fomite, and there are many instances on record where laundry workers have acquired the disease. It is believed that the primary site of infection is in the nasopharynx and that following local multiplication of virus, the organism spreads via the lymphatics; following a transient primary viremia, it spreads to involve the reticuloendothelial system. Viral multiplication is followed by a second phase of viremia about 10 days later, and this coincides with the onset of symptoms. The initial illness, before the development of the rash, is called the *prodromal stage* and lasts for about four days. The rash starts first on the mucous membranes (the *enanthem*) and then on the skin (the *exanthem*). Skin lesions are at first erythematous but rapidly become vesicular and pustular. Characteristically all the lesions are at the same stage of development, and they tend to be more frequent on the face and distal parts of the body. The trunk, particularly the front of the chest and abdomen, is relatively spared. Smallpox is highly infectious, and in the past has been responsible for devastating epidemics having a mortality of up to 50 per cent. In those who survive, the skin lesions heal with scarring, which leaves the typical "pockmarks" on the face.

Active Immunization. The first really effective attempt at smallpox immunization was performed by Edward Jenner, who discovered that the natural pox infection of bovine animals, cowpox, could produce a similar but localized lesion in human beings and that this would lead to protection against subsequent smallpox infection.

Since then a third virus has emerged: vaccinia virus. Its origin is obscure. It is believed to be a mutant of either variola or cowpox viruses; probably most strains used at the present time originated from cowpox.

Until recently, vaccination has been a recommended procedure for protection against infection with smallpox. However, it has certain dangers:

1. ECZEMA VACCINATUM. Patients with pre-existing skin disease, particularly atopic dermatitis, can develop a generalized rash which somewhat resembles smallpox itself. This is known as *Kaposi's varicelliform eruption* (Fig. 12–10). It appears to be due to generalized spread of the vaccinia virus in those patients who are particularly susceptible. Occasionally a similar type of generalized eruption is seen from herpes simplex virus infection.

2. GENERALIZED VACCINIA. This condition occurs as a blood-borne spread from the local vaccination site. It is a self-limiting, relatively benign condition.

FIGURE 12–10. *Kaposi's varicelliform eruption.*

The patient is a young man who was eager to travel; he was vaccinated at his own request by his physician. As a child he had suffered from infantile eczema and periodically had developed areas of atopic dermatitis. At the time of vaccination he appeared normal; nevertheless, shortly afterward he developed a widespread eruption that was particularly severe on the chest, neck, and back. Each lesion consisted of a pustule, the center of which was somewhat depressed and umbilicated in appearance. (Note: Any patient with a widespread skin eruption—particularly atopic dermatitis—should not be vaccinated against smallpox.) Accidental inoculation of the lesions with the virus produces Kaposi's varicelliform eruption; if widespread, this can be fatal. A similar widespread infection can occur in patients with burns. Herpes simplex can also produce a similar clinical picture. Electron microscopy of the fluid from one of the pustules is an easy means of distinguishing between the two types of infection.

3. PROGRESSIVE VACCINIA.   In this condition the local lesion continues to spread and the outcome is generally fatal. This disease occurs in patients who have T-lymphocyte deficiency.

4. POSTVACCINAL ENCEPHALOMYELITIS.   About two weeks after vaccination an encephalitis occurs that has a 50 per cent mortality. It appears to be due to some type of autoimmune reaction, but its precise pathogenesis is not understood.

In view of these unpleasant, though admittedly rare, complications of vaccination, the wholesale use of vaccination is less widely practiced today. This is particularly relevant as antiviral antibiotics are becoming available.

Viruses Affecting the Respiratory Tract

ORTHOMYXOVIRUSES

This is a group of filamentous RNA-containing viruses having a helical symmetry and a characteristic envelope that has the property of adhering to red cells (Figs. 12–2 and 12–5). The orthomyxoviruses cause influenza—an illness characterized by an acute tracheobronchitis of abrupt onset. The severity of the illness varies from a mild upper respiratory infection with fever and chest pains (the 'flu) to a rapidly fatal illness with extensive pneumonia. The pneumonia may be due to the virus itself or to a coexistent bacterial infection—generally streptococcal or staphylococcal. Three types of influenza virus are known. *Influenza virus type A* is the most important and causes epidemics or pandemics of varying severity. In some, such as the pandemic of 1918, tens of millions of people died. Influenza virus type A readily mutates so that new strains are continually appearing. Occasionally a virulent strain emerges, and an epidemic ensues because the population has no immunity to it. *Influenza virus type B* causes endemic cases and occasional epidemics, although these tend to affect a localized area. Type B virus shows less antigenic variation than type A. *Influenza virus type C* appears to exist as one single type and causes a subclinical or very mild upper respiratory infection.

PARAMYXOVIRUSES

These viruses resemble the orthoviruses in morphology but are larger and more pleomorphic. The group includes the viruses described below:

PARAINFLUENZA VIRUSES.   These cause respiratory infections similar to influenza.

MUMPS VIRUS.   Mumps is a disease that has a long incubation period (18 to 21 days) and is characterized by fever and enlargement of one or both parotid glands (acute parotitis). In adult males this may be complicated by involvement of one or both testes (acute orchitis). Infection of the ovaries may also occur, and in both sexes meningoencephalitis and pancreatitis are well recognized complications.

MEASLES (MORBILLI).   This is the most infectious of the common fevers. A 10-day incubation period is followed by a 4-day illness with fever, tracheobronchitis, and conjunctivitis. The characteristic enanthem appears on the buccal mucosa as grains of salt on a red background; these "Koplik's spots" are diagnostic of the disease during this early catarrhal infectious phase. On the fourteenth day after exposure, the characteristic maculopapular exanthem appears. *German measles* (rubella) resembles measles clinically but has a longer incubation period (16 to 18 days), and the prodromal stage is mild or absent. This otherwise trivial disease is of importance because it causes malformations and other abnormalities in the unborn child of pregnant women who contract the disease (see Chapter 16). The virus of German measles is probably not a paramyxovirus, and as yet it remains unclassified. It is included here for convenience.

ADENOVIRUSES

The adenoviruses are DNA-containing viruses that are common commensals of the upper respiratory tract. They cause a variety of mild upper respiratory infections and conjunctivitis (Fig. 12–6A).

RHINOVIRUSES

These are small RNA-containing viruses, which cause the common cold. They are now grouped with the enteroviruses and are classified as *picornaviruses.**

Arboviruses

The arboviruses are so named because they are arthropod-borne. They are RNA viruses and usually spread by mosquitoes, but ticks and sand flies are implicated in some varieties. The most severe disease of this group is yellow fever, which is spread by a mosquito. The disease is endemic in West Africa and Central America. It causes a severe illness with hepatic necrosis and renal failure and has a high mortality.

ARBOVIRUS ENCEPHALITIS

Many types are known and tend to be restricted to particular parts of the world. Some (*e.g.*, Western equine encephalitis of North America and Venezuelan equine encephalitis) are mild, while others (*e.g.*, Eastern equine encephalitis of North America and Japanese B encephalitis) are severe.

ROTAVIRUSES. The rotaviruses, or orbiviruses, are closely related to the arboviruses and have recently attained importance as a possible cause of infantile diarrhea (Fig 12–6B).

The Herpesviruses

VARICELLA AND ZOSTER

Although the well-known clinical features of varicella (chickenpox) and zoster are poles apart, there is good evidence that they are both caused by the same virus.

---

*Pico, meaning small (they measure 27 nm in diameter), and *RNA*-containing viruses.

FIGURE 12–11. *Shingles (zoster).*

A, The photograph shows the right thigh of a patient with early zoster. Skin lesions consist of grouped, tender water blisters (vesicles), each surrounded by a zone of redness (erythema). The lesions are distributed along the second lumbar nerve. As the disease progresses, the lesions dry up and become encrusted. *B,* This print shows a typical case of zoster at the stage of crusting. Note how the lesions follow the line of the cutaneous nerves that parallel the ribs. The lesions do not cross the midline; this is an important sign that helps to distinguish zoster from other localized blistering diseases, such as a contact dermatitis. The lesions of zoster heal with scarring and are often painful, particularly in elderly patients.

Chickenpox. This disease has a pathogenesis similar to that of smallpox. It exhibits an enanthem with vesicles on the oral mucosa followed by an exanthem of vesicles on the skin, which subsequently become pustular. Clinically, the disease bears some resemblance to smallpox, but the prodromal stage is much less severe; the skin eruption tends to occur in crops, so that lesions at a different stage of development are present at the same time, and the distribution of the rash is different. In chickenpox the lesions are not clustered in areas of pressure and tend to be most profuse on the trunk. In smallpox the limbs, face, and back are most severely affected.

Zoster. Following an attack of chickenpox the virus may lie latent in the posterior root ganglia of the spinal, trigeminal, or facial nerves. In later life the virus can be reactivated, and can spread down the nerve fibers to the skin, producing the lesions of herpes zoster (Fig. 12–11). Children exposed to a patient with zoster can develop chickenpox if they are susceptible.

HERPES SIMPLEX

The virus of herpes simplex is one of the most widely distributed viruses in human beings (Fig. 12–6C). It has been estimated that about 60 per cent of the population is affected. Of these, only 10 per cent exhibit primary childhood lesions, such as gingivostomatitis, keratoconjunctivitis, and vulvovaginitis.

Abrasions of the skin sometimes lead to primary herpetic infection (traumatic, or inoculation, herpes simplex). A good example of this is the painful *herpetic whitlow*, which is seen in nursing attendants working in neurosurgical wards. These people acquire their infection while inserting endotracheal tubes into the mouths of unconscious patients.

Usually, however, the primary infection remains subclinical, and the virus remains latent in the cells of the host. This symbiosis tends to be disturbed by intercurrent infections, such as the common cold, pneumonia, and malaria, and in very susceptible victims even by menstruation, emotional strain, and exposure to sunlight. There then develop typical *herpetic blisters*, especially around the mucocutaneous junction of the lips. Occasionally lesions recur in the conjunctiva and cornea. The remarkable feature of herpes simplex is the tendency for lesions to recur at the same site. Thus, one patient complained of developing lesions on the left knee every spring for six consecutive years.

Herpes simplex can also affect the genitalia, particularly in the female. The virus concerned is of a different strain from the one that causes oral lesions.

The tendency for herpes simplex to recur at the same site as well as its continued chronicity has led to the belief that the virus resides in the sensory root ganglia and that the pathogenesis is therefore similar to that of zoster.

Infectious Warts and Other Papovavirus Infections

The common wart is due to a small DNA-containing virus, which belongs to a group of organisms that also cause papillomas in other animals (Fig. 12–6D). They have been labeled the *papovaviruses*. Included in this group is a passenger virus quite commonly found in monkey kidney cells—the *SV-40* virus, which under some circumstances is capable of inducing tumor formation. It is for this reason that monkey kidney cells are not used for the preparation of vaccines for human use.

Viral Hepatitis

There are two distinct diseases that come into this category. They are traditionally called infective hepatitis and serum hepatitis.

INFECTIVE HEPATITIS

This has an incubation period of about *one month* and tends to occur in epidemics in places where young adults are crowded together, such as in military and academic institutions. Fecal contamination of ingested food appears to be the mode of spread. The onset of the disease is usually insidious and is accompanied by malaise and mild gastrointestinal upset. Aversion to cigarette smoking is a curious early symptom, and sometimes urticaria and joint pains are prominent, suggesting that immune complexes play a part in the pathogenesis of this stage of the disease. After a few days, jaundice and other evidence of liver cell damage appear. Following a prolonged course of several weeks, recovery occurs. The disease has a low mortality.

FIGURE 12–12. *Hepatitis B; negative-stained preparation of Australia-antigen positive serum.*

Three types of particles can be seen: spherical particles 20 nm in diameter (a); elongated tubular filaments up to 230 nm in length, 20 nm in diameter (b); and Dane particles, 42 nm in diameter and having a double shell (c) (× 119,700). (Photograph courtesy of Micheline Fauvel, Department of Medical Microbiology, Faculty of Medicine, University of Toronto.)

SERUM HEPATITIS

This disease has an incubation period of about *three months* and tends to be more severe than infective hepatitis, although an absolute distinction between the two is not possible on clinical grounds. The disease has an appreciable mortality, and there is a tendency for it to be followed by progressive liver damage and cirrhosis. Serum hepatitis is nearly always contracted by the injection of blood or serum from a person carrying the infective agent. Minute quantities are capable of transferring infection. In the past the disease has occurred in venereal disease clinics where patients were lined up and therapeutic agents were injected with a common needle. Likewise, it is a major hazard among drug addicts. The disease is also rife in those who handle human blood or work in hemodialysis units.

In spite of the fact that serum hepatitis is due to an infective agent (termed *virus B*), it has proved to be incredibly difficult to isolate the agent. The virus is clearly no ordinary virus! Indeed, the first clues as to its nature came from a most unlikely source: an abnormal antigen of lipoprotein constitution was noted in the serum of an Australian aborigine, and this was at first believed to be a plasma protein of unusual type determined by an abnormal gene. The antigen was subsequently found in cases of leukemia, lepromatous leprosy, and finally in patients who had a history of having had hepatitis. The antigen was called the Australia antigen, and its presence in the blood was found to be associated with the ability of the blood to transmit serum hepatitis. Electron microscopy of Australian antigen-positive serum revealed two types of particles, marked "a" and "b" and shown in Figure 12–12. At first it seemed that these must be the infective agents of serum hepatitis, but the discovery that neither of them contained nucleic acid proved to be a stumbling block. Surely no infective agent could exist without nucleic acid! The search for Australia antigen-positive individuals was greatly aided by the observation that patients who had received many blood transfusions, (e.g., hemophiliacs) and also those who had recovered from serum hepatitis had a variable titer of antibodies against this particular antigen. Further investigations of patients with serum hepatitis revealed a third type of particle now known as the *Dane particle* (in Fig. 12–12). This consists of a central core that is surrounded by a double-shelled structure. The shell and the other two particles share a common antigen, and this is now termed the HB_SAg. This is the original Australian antigen. It is not infective and cannot be the cause of serum hepatitis. The core of the Dane particle, on the other hand, has another antigen, which is now labeled HB_CAg (Fig. 12–13). The core contains some RNA and also a DNA polymerase. This indeed appears to be the essential agent in serum hepatitis, and the Dane particle is currently regarded as the virion responsible for this disease. Identification of the core antigen is at present difficult, owing to the lack of suitable antisera. For the time being, detection of HB_SAg is used to screen blood for its likely infectivity in transfusion work. It seems that the two particles depicted in Figure 12–12 (*a* and *b*) as well as the outer coat of the Dane particle are protein components of the virus, and that these are produced in excess during an infection of serum hepatitis.

Although serum hepatitis is commonly transmitted by the transference of infected serum, there must be some other means of transmission. Ingestion of contaminated material (*i.e.*, feces) is one possibility, but two other alternatives have recently been investigated. Infection could occur during sexual intercourse when the male acquires infection from the menstrual blood of the female. Secondly, infection could be congenital, since it has been shown that antigen-positive mothers give birth to antigen-positive babies. The investigation has indeed come almost full circle, for in the first instance it was believed that the Australia antigen was a genetically determined factor passed from the parent to the child! This perhaps reiterates again the close similarity between the genetic material contained within viruses and the genetic material contained within chromosomes.

The infective agent of infective hepatitis, tentatively termed *virus A*, has proved to be even more elusive than that of virus B. During the last five years, viruslike particles have been isolated from the stools of patients with infective hepatitis. The investigation of these particles has been hampered by the fact that they appear to be infectious only to certain strains of monkeys and chimpanzees – apart from man. The supply of monkeys and chimpanzees is precarious, and it has to be augmented by "volunteers" from penitentiaries. It is a sad reflection on our current civilization that there are now more human "volunteers" than there are available monkeys!

The subject of hepatitis has been dealt with at some length, partly because the disease is of current interest and tends to affect young healthy adults, and

FIGURE 12–13. *Immune electron microscopy test with Dane core antigen incubated with human serum.*

A concentrated sample of Dane particles was treated with a detergent (polysorbate 80) in order to disrupt the outer coat and to release the internal component. This Dane core measures 27 nm in diameter. The suspension of particles was incubated with serum from a patient who had recovered from an attack of virus B hepatitis. An anticore antibody causes the core particles to adhere to each other and to form immune complexes. This method can be used to detect anti-HB$_c$Ag (see text; *B* and *C* are negative tests; bars represent 100 nm)($\times$ 119,700). (From Fauvel, M., Babiuk, L., Sheaff, E. T., and Spence, L.: Preparation of a Dane core (hepatitis B) antigen from human plasma. Canadian Journal of Microbiology, *21*(6):905–910, 1975.)

partly because it illustrates the fact that the pathogenesis of viral diseases is by no means simple. The relationship is not as straightforward as that between the staphylococcus and a boil.

Prophylaxis of hepatitis is possible. Immune serum administered after infection will largely prevent type A hepatitis. With type B or serum hepatitis, the position is less certain, perhaps because the antibody titer of globulin used has been so low that it is virtually ineffective.

Rabies

Rabies is caused by a bullet-shaped virus belonging to the group of rhabdoviruses, which normally infect certain species of animals. The disease is rare in human beings, but it is of intense interest for two reasons. With one possible exception there has never been recorded a human case of rabies that survived. While many diseases are fatal, the mode of death in rabies is particularly unpleasant. An initial phase of excitement with spasms and convulsions is characteristic. Particularly common are painful contractions of the pharyngeal muscles initiated by attempts to swallow water. Hence the term *hydrophobia*, meaning that the patients fear water. The stage of excitement is followed by one of generalized paralysis, and death usually occurs within a few days of its onset. Treatment is entirely supportive; the only hope is that the diagnosis is wrong. The second reason for considering rabies important is that the infection is always a threat in North America and in continental Europe. Only in England is the disease virtually unknown and likely to remain so, owing to the strict quarantine regulations that are enforced.

Rabies is endemic in the fox population in Europe, whereas in North America it affects many species of animals, particularly the skunk. Following the bite of an infected animal the virus spreads to the nervous system via the nerve fibers. Rabies in dogs is invariably fatal within 10 days, and if a person is bitten by a dog, it is important to keep the dog under surveillance for this period. If the dog dies or is killed, examination of the brain for Negri bodies is an important investigation.

If the person is bitten by a rabid animal, or by an animal that escapes, the question of immunization is of paramount importance. It has been estimated that about 30,000 persons in the U.S.A. are given treatment each year for rabies immunization.

The original method of immunization against rabies was devised by Pasteur. He noted that rabbits infected with rabies developed a virus of fixed virulence. By taking the spinal cords of infected rabbits and drying them for varying periods, it seemed that the virus had lost its pathogenicity. Thus material derived from a rabbit spinal cord that had been dried for some time failed to produce rabies on injection into a human being. A series of 14 injections, each given at daily intervals, was administered—each one being from a rabbit cord preparation dried for a lesser period of time. Unfortunately, the injections are painful and produce ever-increasing local inflammatory reactions. The repeated injection of foreign spinal cord tissue can on occasion lead to an autoimmune encephalomyelitis (see Chapter 9). The problem with rabies prophylaxis is whether the risk of inducing a disabling encephalomyelitis outweighs the risk of developing rabies. Antiserum prepared in horses is now available, and vaccines prepared in duck eggs have been developed. The latter are used for immunizing animals, but whether they are sufficiently potent for human use, or indeed whether they are safe, has yet to be determined.

Slow Viruses

Scrapie is a disease of sheep that is characterized by itching and degeneration of the brain. It can be transmitted to sheep, goats, and mice, but the incubation period is long — rarely less than four months. The infective agent has unusual properties: it can withstand boiling, x-irradiation, and treatment with formalin. It contains little, if any, nucleic acid. Its nature is not understood, but it is grouped with other similar agents as a *slow virus*.

Kuru is a slowly progressive degenerative nervous disease of the Fore people of New Guinea and was originally thought to be inherited. It usually affected women and children of either sex, but not men. A tribal ritual was for women and children to eat the brains of diseased relatives, and it is believed that the disease is caused by a slow virus acquired by this quaint tribute to the dead.

These rare and curious diseases have been mentioned not because they are ever likely to be encountered by a medical practitioner but because they reveal the existence of patterns of infective disease quite different from those previously recognized. Two other human "degenerative" nervous diseases are known to be caused by viruses. One is Creutzfeldt-Jakob disease and the other subacute sclerosing panencephalitis. The latter is caused by the measles virus acting in an obscure way that is quite different from that seen in ordinary measles. The hope is that other diseases will be found to be of similar nature, and ways will be found to combat them.

Review Questions

1. Compare and contrast the methods available for the production of immunity against the following:
    (a) smallpox (variola)
    (b) poliomyelitis (infantile paralysis)
2. It was once fashionable to classify viruses according to the tissues that they affected. Describe why this is now considered an unsatisfactory approach to classification. In particular, use the following viruses to illustrate your answer: the poliovirus, the mumps virus, herpes simplex virus, and the influenza virus.
3. How does the immunity to a virus infection differ from that produced against a bacterial infection? Illustrate your answer with reference to diphtheria, influenza, poliomyelitis, and smallpox.
4. Under what circumstances would you consider it inadvisable to vaccinate a person against smallpox? What are the possible complications of vaccination?
5. List the viruses that cause an upper respiratory infection.

Selected Readings

Cruickshank, R., Duguid, J. P., Marmion, B. P., and Swain, R. H. A.: Medical Microbiology. 12th ed. Vol. 1. Edinburgh, Churchill Livingstone, 1973. Chapters 12, 13, and 14 give a good account of the general properties of viruses. All of Part III is devoted to a detailed account of viral diseases.

Dale, S.: Early events in cell-animal virus interactions. Bacteriological Reviews, 37:13–135, 1973.

Holland, J. J.: Slow, inapparent, and recurrent viruses. Scientific American. 230:32–40, 1974.

Leading Article: Diagnosis and management of human rabies. British Medical Journal, 3:721–722, 1975.

Middleton, P. J., Szymanski, M. T., Abbott, G. D., Bortolussi, R., and Hamilton, J. R.: Orbivirus acute gastroenteritis of infancy. Lancet, 1:1241–1244, 1974.

Temin, H., and Baltimore, D.: RNA-directed DNA synthesis and RNA tumor viruses. Advances in Virus Research, 17:129–186, 1972.

Timbury, M. C.: Notes on Medical Virology. 5th ed. Edinburgh, Churchill Livingstone, 1974. An introduction to elementary virology in 150 pages.

Youmans, G. P., Paterson, P. Y., and Sommers, H. M.: The Biologic and Clinical Basis of Infectious Diseases. Philadelphia, W. B. Saunders Company, 1975. Chapters 4, 5, and 6 describe the general properties of viruses. Individual infections are discussed in other parts of the book in terms of regional or clinical findings.

Chapter 13

After studying this chapter the student should be able to:

● Classify the fungi into four groups on the basis of their morphology.
● List the various regional types of ringworm.
● Describe the forms of *Candida* infection and relate them to the types of people who are liable to be affected.
● Describe cryptococcosis, histoplasmosis, candidiasis, North American blastomycosis, and South American blastomycosis with respect to:
(a) geographic distribution
(b) primary site of infection
(c) organs affected in the disseminated forms.

Classification of Fungi

In the past, fungi have been regarded as plants without roots, stems, and leaves and as being incapable of photosynthesis because they lack chlorophyll. They are now regarded as neither plants nor animals; they are placed in a separate group. Although their classification is complex and unsatisfactory, for practical purposes four varieties can be recognized:

1. *Molds*, which grow as long filaments (*hyphae*), which branch and interlace to form a meshwork or *mycelium*.

2. *Yeasts*, which are unicellular and grow by budding only.

220

FUNGAL INFECTIONS

3. *Yeastlike fungi,* which grow partly as yeasts and partly as long filamentous forms called *pseudohyphae.*

4. *Dimorphic fungi,* which can grow either as hyphae or as yeasts, according to the cultural conditions.

The great majority of fungi are saprophytic and play an important part in nature by breaking down organic material. They have been of great service to man in the production of bread, cheese, and alcoholic beverages. In the last several decades, they have attracted interest because they produce antibiotic agents.

Infection of the skin by fungi is very common and usually is quite trivial. Nevertheless, there are a number of fungi that can produce a generalized infection, and these have come recently to the fore because they complicate illnesses in which there is impairment of the T-cell component of the immune response.

Diseases Caused by Fungi

Ringworm or Tinea. Ringworm is caused by a group of fungi that are termed the *dermatophytes* and have the property of digesting the keratin of skin or hair. The dermatophytes are molds that grow as a mycelium and reproduce by the formation of various types of spores.

Ringworm, which is due to invasion of keratin by one of the dermatophytes, can affect the scalp (causing *tinea capitis* in which involvement of hair shafts causes a bald patch), the body skin (causing *tinea corporis* with its variant *tinea cruris* affecting the inguinal region), the foot (causing athlete's foot, or *tinea pedis*), the hands (causing *tinea manuum*), and sometimes the nails (causing *tinea unguium*). Clinically, each type of ringworm has its own particular characteristics, but in general the lesions are erythematous, scaly, sometimes vesicular, and tend to have a sharp red spreading border that gives the lesions a ringlike shape from which the disease acquires its name. Diagnosis is easy: Scrapings of keratin can be examined by direct microscopy for hyphae, and from the culture one can readily identify the particular strain of mold responsible. Local antifungal treatment is effective, except in the case of ringworm of the nails, for which the only effective treatment is prolonged oral administration of griseofulvin, one of the few antibiotics that is effective against fungi.

Not all ringlike lesions are ringworm. Psoriasis and nummular eczema can mislead the unwary; vigorous, ill-advised treatment can lead to contact dermatitis. Most patients who complain of "ringworm" and "athlete's foot" do not have a fungal infection.

221

Candidiasis (Moniliasis).   Infection with *Candida* species is one of the most frequent fungal infections in man. The organism most commonly involved is *Candida albicans* (previously called *Monilia albicans*), a yeastlike fungus that reproduces by budding but sometimes elongates to form pseudohyphae. The yeast form is characteristic of superficial candidal infections, whereas the pseudomycelial growth is found when the organism invades deeper tissues. *Candida albicans* is a common commensal in the *oral cavity, alimentary tract,* and *vagina.* Infection occurs when general or local conditions become suitable. Superficial infections of the mucous membrane appear as white patches called *thrush.* In the mouth this is very common in infants—especially premature ones—and it may be accompanied by perianal lesions. Oral candidiasis can occur at any age during the course of any debilitating disease. Vaginal thrush is common during pregnancy, in women using the contraceptive pill, and in patients with diabetes mellitus. Cutaneous candidiasis can occur around the corners of the mouth, in moist intertriginous areas, such as under the breasts, and in the nail folds (chronic paronychia) of those whose occupations brings their hands repeatedly into water.

Generalized infection with *Candida albicans* is occurring more frequently and is a serious and often fatal opportunistic infection (see Chapter 6). Steroid therapy, the presence of lymphomas, the administration of cytotoxic drugs, and indeed any disease in which cell-mediated immunity is impaired are predisposing factors for widespread invasion by the organism. Disseminated lesions affect many internal organs.

Less extensive candidal infections are seen under particular circumstances. Endocarditis occurs in addicts who inject themselves intravenously with narcotics. Mouth lesions can spread to produce extensive gastrointestinal infections following the prolonged oral administration of a broad-spectrum antibiotic that upsets the balance of the local bacterial flora. Finally, there is an inherited type of immunological, T-cell deficiency, in which there is a selective susceptibility to *Candida* infection. These patients have persistent widespread skin and mucous-membrane infections with *Candida* that defy all treatment. Nevertheless, despite the distressing skin lesions, dissemination to the internal organs does not occur.

DEEP-SEATED FUNGAL INFECTIONS

In certain parts of the world fungal infections are of considerable importance. In general, the organisms are found as saprophytes in the soil, and infection is acquired by inhalation. A primary lesion may occur in the lungs, but in the majority of people it is asymptomatic and is followed by healing. Occasionally, however, the organisms produce more severe local damage and spread to involve other organs. In their pathogenesis the diseases therefore resemble tuberculosis to a considerable extent. Indeed, the tissue reaction to these organisms sometimes also closely resembles that seen in tuberculosis.

Cryptococcosis.   The causative organism, *Cryptococcus neoformans* (previously called *Torula histolytica*), is a yeast, and of worldwide distribution. The primary lung lesion is usually small, heals by fibrosis, and passes unnoticed. Occasionally, the organism spreads widely and has an affinity for the central nervous system, where it causes *meningitis.* This widespread dissemination is particularly common in patients with T-cell deficiency.

Histoplasmosis. The causative organism, a dimorphic fungus named *Histoplasma capsulatum,* has a worldwide distribution; infection, however, is particularly common in the Mississippi valley of the U.S.A. Once again the primary lesion is in the lung and the disease closely resembles tuberculosis. Healing usually occurs with calcification. Occasionally the lung lesion cavitates, and metastatic lesions occur elsewhere. Even more rarely, the fungi invade the blood stream in a massive way and cause a generalized infection. An extract of the organism is used in the *histoplasmin test* (analogous to the tuberculin reaction) and is positive in infected individuals.

Case History I. In 1953 at the age of 25 years, the patient, an Englishwoman, developed a flulike illness that was accompanied by pain in the chest on taking a deep breath. Pleurisy complicating "virus pneumonia" was diagnosed initially, but markedly enlarged hilar lymph nodes and normal lung fields were revealed by a chest radiograph. The diagnosis was changed to primary tuberculosis, but since the patient produced no sputum, the diagnosis was never proven; nevertheless, her tuberculin test was initially negative and became strongly positive. This Mantoux conversion was taken as good evidence of a tuberculous infection. Three months of rest in a sanatorium was ordered. The patient made a rapid recovery, married, and had two children without recurrence of the lung infection. She emigrated to North America in 1965.

In 1971 at the age of 43, the patient developed another "flulike" illness (see radiograph, Fig. 13–1). A "coin lesion" was noted in the right lung field (*A*), and a tomogram (*B*) revealed the shadow with greater definition. Although the patient was a

FIGURE 13–1.

Chest radiograph of a 43-year-old female patient with histoplasmosis. *A,* Note "coin lesion" in the right lung field. *B,* Tomogram reveals the shadow with greater definition. (Radiographs courtesy of Dr. D. E. Sanders.)

nonsmoker, a diagnosis of lung cancer was considered. However, a radiograph taken two years previously showed a lesion of similar size to be present. A cancerous lesion probably would have enlarged during this period. Nevertheless, it was decided that this was insufficient evidence on which to exclude such a serious disease. A needle biopsy was performed under local anesthesia, and necrotic tissue was obtained. Neither organisms nor tumor cells could be identified in this. A histoplasmin test proved to be strongly positive. Histoplasmosis is much more common in North America than in England, and the presence of a lung lesion with a strongly positive histoplasmin test in a recent immigrant was regarded as presumptive evidence of primary histoplasmosis. No treatment was given and the patient remains well to this day.

This case illustrates four points:

1. Persistent lung infections in young people should always raise the possibility of tuberculous infection.
2. The development of hypersensitivity to an organism or its products during the course of a disease is good evidence of infection by that organism, provided the clinical features are consistent with such a diagnosis.
3. A lung lesion in a person over the age of 40 should be regarded as cancerous until proven otherwise.
4. A knowledge of the geographic incidence of disease can help in the physician's attaining a correct diagnosis.

Coccidioidomycosis. This disease is caused by *Coccidioides immitis,* a dimorphic fungus that is common in the dry desert regions of California, Arizona, and Argentina. In these places the majority of the inhabitants acquire a primary infection of the lung, but as with other diseases of this type, the lesion soon heals and is either asymptomatic or else causes a mild influenza-like illness known locally as "valley fever" or "desert fever." Occasionally, the disease is progressive, and the destructive lung lesions closely resemble tuberculosis. Rarely the organism invades the blood and infection of many organs may subsequently occur.

North American Blastomycosis. This is caused by infection with the yeast *Blastomyces dermatitidis.* The primary lesion is usually in the lung but may be cutaneous. Widespread dissemination occasionally occurs and tends to involve the bones, skin, and lung.

South American Blastomycosis (Paracoccidioidal Granuloma). The causative organism, *Paracoccidioides brasiliensis,* is a yeast that usually produces a primary infection in the region of the nasopharynx. Destructive local lesions and regional lymphadenopathy ensue. Untreated, the disease runs a prolonged course, and ultimately death ensues as a result of spread to lung, skin, and other organs. It is a more serious infection than the other deep-seated mycoses mentioned; unless treated, it is frequently fatal.

TREATMENT OF FUNGAL INFECTIONS

Few drugs are available for the treatment for the deep-seated fungal infections. Amphotericin-B offers some hope in the treatment of systemic fungal infections, but unfortunately the drug causes renal damage. Topical nystatin is effective for superficial candidal infections but cannot be administered systemically.

FIGURE 13-2. *Blastomycosis of the lung.*

The alveolar walls are intact, but the alveoli themselves (ALV) are *consolidated,* being completely air-less and filled with inflammatory exudate (compare with Figs. 5–9A and 30–1). This condition is called *consolidation.* The exudate contains amorphous fibrinous material, disintegrating polymorphs, and large numbers of fungi (× 250). The inset is from the same case, but it shows a section that has been stained by a silver impregnation method. The budding form of the fungus, marked by the arrow, is typical (×·600).

OTHER FUNGAL INFECTIONS

Over 100,000 species of fungi are known, and of these about 100 are pathogens. Apart from those previously described, there are others that occasionally produce infection under particular circumstances. For the most part they act as secondary invaders in the course of other diseases, or they occur as opportunistic infections when immunity is weakened. One of the best known examples of the latter is the *Aspergillus* species, which sometimes affects the lung.

In India, injuries to the feet are sometimes infected with fungi, leading to chronic suppurative lesions involving the skin, subcutaneous tissues, and bone; such a condition is known as *Maduromycosis* or *Madura foot.* Not only is this caused by various species of fungi, but also by certain higher bacteria.

In conclusion, it can be appreciated that although serious infections due to fungi are not common, fungal disease can assume considerable importance under specific conditions. These circumstances include climate and treatment of patients in specialized units with cytotoxic or immunosuppressive drugs.

Review Questions

1. A coin lesion, similar to that shown in Figure 13–1, is found in a radiograph taken as part of a routine health inspection. List the possible causes. Modify this list after reading Chapters 16, 17, and 30.
2. Classify the fungi into four groups and give at least one example of each group.
3. A patient has several red scaly skin lesions, ranging from 1 to 3 cm in diameter, each having a raised border. How would you attempt to arrive at a diagnosis?

Selected Readings

Cruickshank, R., Duguid, J. P., Marmion, B. P., and Swain, R. H. A.: Medical Microbiology. 12th ed. Volume 1. Edinburgh, Churchill Livingstone, 1973. Chapter 53 gives a good review of the pathogenic fungi.

Youmans, G. P., Paterson, P. Y., and Sommers, H. M.: The Biologic and Clinical Basis of Infectious Diseases. Philadelphia, W. B. Saunders Company, 1975. Chapter 26 gives a detailed account of histoplasmosis, coccidioidomycosis, and blastomycosis.

HELMINTHIC INFECTIONS

Chapter 14

After studying this chapter the student should be able to:

● Distinguish between the definitive and the intermediate host of a parasite.
● Describe the major differences between the tapeworms, the flukes, and the roundworms.
● Describe the life cycles of the helminths listed in Table 14–1 and outline the effects on human beings of infection with these parasites.

The worms, or helminths, that plague mankind are classified as belonging within two phyla of the animal kingdom (Table 14–1).

The phylum *Platyhelminthes*, or flatworms, is further subdivided into two classes: (1) *Trematoda*, and (2) *Cestoda*. The *Trematoda*, or *flukes*, are flat, leaf-like creatures that live in the *intestine, liver,* or *lung* (the distomes) or in the *blood stream* (the schistosomes). The *Cestoda*, or *tapeworms*, are segmented and possess a head or scolex, a neck, and a varying number (often hundreds) of proglottides. Both cestodes and trematodes are hermaphroditic.

The phylum *Nemathelminthes* contains the roundworms, which are never segmented, possess an alimentary canal, and in general have separate sexes.

The helminths of medical importance form a very small fraction of the total number known, and their study and recognition is a very specialized field.* Only some common examples will be described in this chapter.

The life cycle of many worms is complex. The *definitive host* is the one in which the parasite reaches maturity and produces gametes. The *intermediate host* is one in which the parasite passes through its larval stage or stages; in some instances, several intermediate hosts are required. Most parasites are extremely exacting in their demands, and knowledge of their host requirements is a valuable weapon in designing methods of eliminating them.

In general, the spread of parasites is encouraged by unsanitary conditions, overcrowding, and a warm climate. The Arctic is less hospitable for harboring

---

*The diagnosis of parasitic infections generally depends on identification of the worm itself or its ova. In some instances, specific antibodies demonstrated by complement fixation or the presence of delayed hypersensitivity is useful in diagnosis.

HELMINTHIC INFECTIONS

Table 14–1   CLASSIFICATION OF WORMS DESCRIBED IN THIS CHAPTER

PHYLUM	CLASS	EXAMPLES
Platyhelminthes (Flatworms)	*Trematoda* (Flukes)	Distomes *Fasciola hepatica* *Clonorchis sinensis* *Fasciolopsis buski* *Paragonimus westermani*
		Schistosomes *Schistosoma hematobium* *Schistosoma mansoni* *Schistosoma japonicum*
	Cestoda (Tapeworms)	*Taenia saginata* *Taenia solium* *Diphyllobothrium latum* *Echinococcus granulosus*
Nemathelminthes (Roundworms)	Nematoda (Roundworms)	*Ascaris lumbricoides* Ancylostomes *Ancylostoma duodenale* *Necator americanus*
		Enterobius vermicularis (pin- or threadworm) *Trichuris trichiura* (whipworm) *Trichinella spiralis*
		Filariae *Wuchereria bancrofti* *Onchocerca volvulus* *Loa loa* *Dracunculus medinensis*

these organisms than the Nile. It follows that helminthic infections are much more common in the tropics. Nevertheless, a worm can travel by air as easily as its host; even in temperate climates, therefore, it is important to be aware of common "tropical diseases."

The Trematodes or Flukes

The life cycle of the flukes involves one or two intermediate hosts (Fig. 14–1). Man is the definitive host and acquires the infection by ingestion of in-

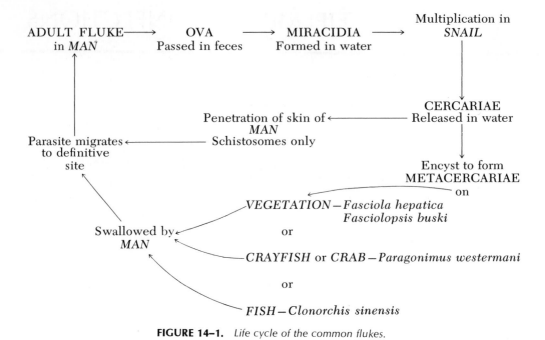

FIGURE 14–1. *Life cycle of the common flukes.*

Note that the schistosomes have only one intermediate host: a snail. The other parasites shown have a second intermediate host: freshwater *vegetation,* a *crab* or other *crustacean,* or a *fish.* The parasites are shown in capital letters, Roman type, whereas the hosts are in capital letters, italic type.

fected fish, crayfish, or vegetation (causing the disease distomiasis) or by penetration of the skin by the parasite (schistosomiasis).

THE DISTOMES

The Liver Flukes. *Fasciola hepatica* is a common parasite of sheep and is occasionally acquired by human beings following the ingestion of watercress containing metacercariae (the resting stage of a trematode parasite). The parasite reaches the intestine, penetrates the wall, crosses the peritoneum, and reaches the liver, where it matures to form an adult fluke.

Clonorchis sinensis, or Chinese liver fluke, has a similar life cycle, but the metacercariae are found beneath the scales of a freshwater fish. Eating raw fish is the mode of infection. The flukes can obstruct the bile ducts, cause inflammation, and ultimately lead to hepatic fibrosis and cirrhosis.

Intestinal Flukes. Infection with *Fasciolopsis buski* is limited to the Far East. Adult worms live in the upper small intestine.

Lung Flukes. *Paragonimus westermani* resides in the lungs, where it causes recurrent hemoptysis and, ultimately, chronic lung inflammation with fibrosis. Infection results from eating raw crayfish in which the metacercariae reside.

THE BLOOD FLUKES OR SCHISTOSOMES

Schistosomiasis (also called bilharziasis after Bilharz [1852], who discovered the worm) is the most important disease caused by flukes, because of its worldwide distribution and the severity of its lesions. It is caused by three closely related flukes described below.

Schistosoma hematobium. The adult flukes live in the portal venous system; after copulation they migrate against the blood flow to the venous plexus around the bladder, where the female lays eggs. As these mature, they secrete a lytic substance that destroys the surrounding tissues. Some ova die and become calcified. A chronic cystitis with hematuria ensues, and the epithelial hyperplasia that is a component of this process sometimes progresses to carcinoma. Viable ova that penetrate the mucosa are passed in the urine. On contact with fresh water, the ova hatch and liberate ciliated forms—the *miracidia*. These have about eight hours in which to search for the intermediate host, a specific snail. If the search is successful, the parasite proliferates in the snail, and one to two months later thousands of infective larvae, called *cercariae*, are liberated into the water. Cercariae are able to penetrate the skin of an unsuspecting bather, then enter venules, and finally pass through the lungs and heart, reaching the portal vein to start their remarkable life cycle once again. This type of schistosomiasis is common in the African continent, particularly in the Nile Valley.

Schistosoma mansoni. This type of schistosome has a life cycle similar to that of *Schistosoma hematobium* and is found in South America, the Caribbean, and Africa. The adult worm resides in the intrahepatic portal veins, from which the ova are distributed to the venules of the colon, rectum, liver, and lung. An

FIGURE 14–2. *Schistosome ova in pancreas.*

The ova are probably dead, since they are calcified and stain deeply with the hematoxylin owing to their calcium content. In spite of their being dead, they can still excite a chronic inflammatory reaction (× 250).

FIGURE 14–3. *Tapeworms.*

A, Part of the tapeworm *Diphyllobothrium latum.* The total length of the worm is over 30 feet. The head is about 1 mm in diameter, and the immature segments are much smaller than the mature segments shown above (× 1.5). *B,* Part of the worm shown in *A.* It is made up of many proglottides or segments, each of which is wider than it is long. *C,* Part of the tapeworm *Taenia saginata.* Each segment is longer than it is wide.

initial phlebitis with surrounding inflammation is eventually followed by fibrosis. Intestinal involvement causes diarrhea, pain, and melena. The liver becomes fibrosed, and portal hypertension leads to esophageal varices and splenomegaly. Pulmonary fibrosis is less common. Ova are passed in the feces, contaminate fresh water, and develop into cercariae. The cycle starts once again.

Schistosoma japonicum. This fluke causes schistosomiasis in the Orient and is similar to the mansoni type but is more severe. The colon, the liver, the lungs, and other organs—including the spinal cord—are involved, and death usually occurs within five years of onset unless effective treatment is given (Fig. 14–2).

The continued existence of schistosomiasis is related to poor sewage disposal as well as to the popular habit of passing urine and feces into water channels that are used for bathing. The reversal of such habits is difficult, and education is all-important.

Villages can be located away from known contaminated streams. Mass treatment of patients and snail control are other methods of checking this disease. Nevertheless, schistosomiasis is a disease of great antiquity, and it gives no evidence of decreasing in frequency. Indeed, estimates suggest that the disease is spreading and is increasing in prevalence. Schistosome eggs have been identified in the Egyptian mummies of the twentieth dynasty (1200 to 1190 B.C.). Present estimates of 180 million infected persons bear witness to the continued success of this parasite.

The Cestodes or Tapeworms

Tapeworms possess a head (scolex) and a neck followed by a chain of segments or proglottides arranged in a ribbon, often many feet long (Fig. 14–3). Two hosts are necessary; man is the definitive host of three common tapeworms and the intermediate host of one other (hydatid disease).

Taenia saginata.   The beef tapeworm grows only in the human intestine. It has up to 2000 segments and can be 30 feet long. The mature terminal segments contain vast numbers of eggs, which are passed in the feces. As mature segments are cast off at one end, new ones are formed in the neck region. The worms are very long-lived—some have reportedly lived over 40 years.

When cattle eat the mature proglottides or isolated eggs, the embryos hatch out, penetrate the intestine, and migrate to the skeletal muscle, where they form the next larval stage, which is cystic (this stage of the tapeworm is called the *cysticercus*). Man becomes infected by eating undercooked infected beef. Symptoms consist of vague abdominal pains or skin eruptions (*e.g.*, urticaria) due to hypersensitivity.

Taenia solium.   This is the pork tapeworm. It has up to 1000 segments

FIGURE 14–4.   *Hydatid cysts.*

The patient had emigrated to North America at 21 years of age after having previously lived and worked on a sheep farm in Yugoslavia. Nine years later he developed a rapidly expanding mass in the upper abdomen. Laparotomy was performed, and multiple hydatid cysts were found in the liver. The largest of these were drained, but unfortunately some of the cysts' contents were spilled into the peritoneal cavity. The parasite was thus disseminated. During the next 10 years, four further operations were necessary for removal or drainage of cysts in the peritoneal cavity, spleen, mediastinum, and pleural cavities.

The figure shows five separate hydatid cysts. These have an epithelial lining from which small cysts or brood capsules develop. These are pinhead sized (see arrow), and within them scoleces of the head of the worm project. The inset shows one scolex with its characteristic hooklets. On being ingested by a dog or wolf this structure will form the head of a new tapeworm.

and can extend to 20 feet in length. The intermediate host is the pig. Humans acquire intestinal infection by eating undercooked pork containing cysticerci.

Occasionally man eats the eggs of *Taenia solium,* and cysticerci develop in muscles, heart, brain, skin, and other organs. The human being then becomes the intermediate host. Symptoms of the condition known as cysticercosis are mainly neurological.

Diphyllobothrium latum.   This is the largest of the tapeworms, measures up to 33 feet in length, and has over 3000 proglottides. The intermediate host is a fish, and the disease is most prevalent among the inhabitants of the fish-eating countries: Scandinavia, parts of Russia, and Asia.

Hydatid Disease.   *Echinococcus granulosus* is a small tapeworm found in the intestine of dogs, wolves, and other carnivorous animals. Ova are ingested by sheep, which constitute the usual intermediate host. The cysticercal forms, called *hydatid cysts,* develop in the liver, the lungs, and elsewhere (Fig. 14–4). Dogs become infected by eating infected sheep carcasses. Occasionally, humans ingest eggs and also develop hydatid cysts. These are commonest in the liver and lungs, but they may occur in any part of the body. The disease is particularly prevalent in the sheep-rearing areas of Australia.

The Nematodes or Roundworms

Ascaris lumbricoides.   The adult ascarides are 15 to 35 cm in length and live in the small intestine, where they usually cause no trouble except in those instances of a heavy infection, when their bulk causes obstruction (Fig. 14–5). Ova are passed in the stools and develop in soil into embryonated ova. When these are ingested, they hatch into larvae, which penetrate the gut wall and reach the lungs via the blood stream. They enter the alveoli, ascend the bronchi and trachea, and finally pass down the esophagus to reach the intestine. Why this parasite pursues this remarkable course is quite unknown. Perhaps its ancestors had a different life cycle (*i.e.,* like that of *Ancylostoma duodenale,* described below), and the migrating habit has been retained by the worm for no more useful purpose than as a reminder of its heritage. During the migratory phase, the patient may experience asthmatic attacks and develop patchy pneumonic consolidation. Blood eosinophilia is common, as it is in many helminthic infections, particularly when the parasites are migrating through the tissues.

Ancylostomiasis (Hookworm Disease).   This disease, which is of worldwide distribution, is caused by *Ancylostoma duodenale* in the Old World and *Necator americanus* in the New World. The worms attach themselves to the wall of the small intestine and cause bleeding. With a heavy infection, the blood loss may lead to a severe chronic iron deficiency anemia, which when combined with undernutrition is an important cause of chronic ill health in underdeveloped countries. Elsewhere, it is rare.

Eggs that are passed in the feces and hatch in the soil into larvae have the ability to penetrate the skin of a barefooted passerby. They migrate via the blood to the lungs, penetrate the alveoli, ascend the trachea, and finally reach the gut to develop into adult worms.

FIGURE 14–5. *Ascaris lumbricoides.*

This worm is the largest roundworm parasite of humans and superficially resembles an earthworm (from the Latin *lumbricus,* an "earthworm"). It ranges in length from 15 to 35 cm. The specimen above was approximately 20 cm (8 inches) in length. Other common roundworms are considerably smaller: *Trichuris trichiura,* 3 to 5 cm; *Enterobius vermicularis,* 8 to 13 mm; and *Ancylostoma duodenale,* up to 1.0 cm. (The scale above the roundworm shown is 1 cm.)

Enterobius vermicularis. The pinworm, or threadworm, is very common in all parts of the world and lives in the lower gut. The females deposit their fully infective eggs around the anus, particularly at night, when their host is asleep. In so doing they cause severe itching (*pruritus ani*); pinworm infection should always be suspected as a cause of this condition, particularly in children. Infection is acquired by swallowing the eggs, which develop into adult forms in the intestine. The worms have a short life span (one to two months), but continuous reinfection will maintain the infection unless strict personal hygiene is enforced. One cannot but admire the ingenuity of this worm: the severe anal itching demands scratching and results in deposition of eggs under the nails. How many small children can refrain from sucking their fingers at some stage during the day?

Trichuris trichiura (Whipworm). Infestation with the whipworm is extremely common, but it rarely causes any symptoms. Its life cycle is similar to that of the pinworm, except that the ova are passed in the feces, and infection is acquired by ingesting the ova in contaminated food or in water.

Trichinella spiralis. The ban on eating pork imposed by some religious groups and the tradition of eating only well-cooked meat by others probably originated with some understanding of the life cycle of this worm.

Trichinella spiralis is primarily a disease of rats. In the intestine the adult male worm dies after copulation — a fate that is not uncommon in the world of worms. The pregnant female burrows into the intestinal wall and discharges hundreds of larvae into the blood stream. When these reach skeletal muscle, they curl up and form small cysts. Those larvae that reach other tissues are less fortunate — they die. When rats eat infected rat muscle, the dormant, encysted parasites awaken and develop into adult worms. Pigs and bears become infected by eating the carcasses of diseased rats, and human beings acquire infection (trichinosis) by eating undercooked pork or bear.

The symptoms of trichinosis vary. Minor infection is common and there are no symptoms. With heavy infection the early symptoms are gastrointestinal; these are followed by systemic symptoms such as fever, generalized edema, and muscle pains. Involvement of the respiratory muscles or heart can, on occasion, cause death. In Canada this is an occasional sequel to an otherwise successful bear party.

FIGURE 14–6. *Filariasis.*

Section of a nodule from a patient with onchocerciasis. The lymphatic vessel contains adult worms shown in cross section. Numerous microfilariae (mf) are present in the body of the gravid female (× 250).

FILARIASIS

Filariasis is caused by a type of nematode that invades the subcutaneous tissues and lymphatics of man (Fig. 14–6). The female produces vast numbers of larvae or, *microfilariae,* which pass through the one intermediate host that transmits the infection to the human host.

Bancroft's Filariasis.   This disease, commonly referred to as "filariasis," is caused by *Wuchereria bancrofti,* which is a worm about 10 cm in length and residing in lymphatics. The females produce large numbers of microfilariae, which are liberated at night into the blood stream, where they can be sought for diagnosis. If an infected individual is bitten by a mosquito (also nocturnal), the mosquito becomes a carrier of the disease and infects persons it subsequently bites.

The adult forms of *Wuchereria bancrofti* produce little damage to lymphatics until they die. There then follows a severe chronic inflammatory reaction that results in lymphatic obstruction. The lymphatics most commonly affected are those of the groin; the leg consequently develops severe lymphatic edema. Marked overgrowth of the skin and subcutaneous tissues produces enormous swelling of the limb and sometimes the scrotum. The condition is called *elephantiasis* and occurs in many tropical and subtropical countries.

Three other filarial diseases are worthy of note:

Onchocerciasis. This is caused by *Onchocerca volvulus,* which in man usually resides in the skin and causes an inflammatory reaction that leads to subcutaneous nodule formation. The microfilariae produced by the females migrate into the adjacent tissues; the most serious complication of this migratory phase of the disease is produced when the eye is invaded. Involvement of the cornea, the vitreous humor, and the ciliary body can result in blindness. The disease is seen in Africa, Mexico, and Guatemala.

Loiasis. This is a form of filariasis restricted to tropical West Africa. The causative organism, *Loa loa,* is also known as the eyeworm. The adult worm occurs in the skin and at times invades the eye. In contrast to Bancroft's filariasis, the microfilariae of loiasis appear in the peripheral blood during the day. The disease is transmitted by a fly that bites during the daytime.

Dracunculiasis. This type of filariasis occurs in the Middle East, India, and parts of Africa. The parasite is known as *Dracunculus medinensis,* or the guinea worm. The adult male is small and dies after copulation. The female worm is about 1 meter in length and wanders about the subcutaneous tissues, particularly the legs. The worm burrows through the skin to produce a small papule, which finally develops into an ulcer through which its embryos are discharged. The embryos are taken up by a freshwater crustacean of the genus *Cyclops,* and after a period of maturation, the larvae are infective. Infection is acquired by swallowing the larvae.

The guinea worm is of interest, not because it is common, but because of its history. It is believed to be the oldest known parasite. The account of the fiery serpents sent by the Lord among the Israelites is believed to be an early description of dracunculiasis.*

The traditional treatment is to apply water to the area of ulceration of the leg so that the worm can be grasped and wound onto a stick. Steady pressure day by day results in extraction of the entire worm. Tradition has it that this is the origin of the serpent wound around the staff which is the emblem of the medical profession.

This account of human helminthic diseases has included only some examples of worms that affect persons in widespread areas of the world. Many other examples are known, some restricted to particular geographic areas. Thus, a localized outbreak of infection by *Capillaria philippinensis* has been described in the Philippine islands and is manifested as a type of enteritis with a high mortality. It is caused by a minute whipworm and is acquired by eating infected fish and crustaceans. The latter are often eaten alive in a form of "jumping salads"!

Review Questions

1. Describe two tapeworm infections in which man is the intermediate host.
2. Compare the life cycle of *Ancylostoma duodenale* with that of *Enterobius vermicularis.*

---

*Numbers, 21:6.

3. List the helminthic infections that can be acquired in the following ways:
   - (a) going barefooted
   - (b) eating undercooked or raw pork
   - (c) eating raw fish.
4. What helminthic infections would you suspect as a cause of the following conditions:
   - (a) pruritus ani
   - (b) muscle pains
   - (c) jaundice
   - (d) chronic lung damage with hemoptysis
   - (e) chronic iron-deficiency anemia
   - (f) elephantiasis
   - (g) hematuria.

Selected Readings

Jeffrey, H. C., and Leach, R. M.: Atlas of Medical Helminthology and Protozoology. 2nd ed. Edinburgh, Churchill Livingstone, 1975. An atlas giving the morphology, life cycle, and major effects of common parasites. Useful for parasite identification.

Robbins, S. L.: Pathologic Basis of Disease. Philadelphia, W. B. Saunders Company, 1974. See pp. 456–466 for a description of the pathological features of helminthic infections.

Wintrobe, M. M., et al. (Eds.): Harrison's Principles of Internal Medicine. 7th ed. New York, McGraw Hill Book Company, 1974. See Section 22, pp. 1035–1058, "Diseases Caused by Worms."

PROTOZOAL INFECTIONS

Chapter 15

After studying this chapter the student should be able to:

- Describe the clinical features of *amebiasis,* the nature of the causative organism, its mode of transmission, and the importance of carriers.
- Explain the worldwide importance of *malaria,* the life cycle of the organism, and the features of the disease in man.
- Discuss how *malaria* is diagnosed and the approaches available for its eradication.
- Discuss the mode of transmission of *trypanosomiasis* and the main features of the three forms of the disease in man.
- Compare and contrast the three types of *leishmaniasis* in man.
- Describe the importance of *trichomoniasis* as a vaginal pathogen.

    Protozoa are unicellular motile animals that have a well-defined nucleus. Some travel by ameboid movement, while others are ciliated or have a single flagellum. They are widely distributed in nature, but few species are pathogenic to man. Yet one of these causes malaria, which is currently the major infectious disease problem in the world.

AMEBIASIS

    The causative agent of amebiasis is *Entamoeba histolytica,* which exists in two forms: an active amebic trophozoite, which is present in active lesions of the disease, and a cyst, which develops when the organism is confronted by adverse conditions. It is by the swallowing of cysts that the disease is acquired. Cysts can withstand the acidity of the gastric juice and develop into active trophozoites, which by invading the mucosa of the large intestine cause ca-

240

PROTOZOAL INFECTIONS

tarrhal inflammation and ulceration. Following infection, symptoms are absent (in *asymptomatic carriers*), or they consist of intermittent diarrhea with the passage of blood and mucus *(chronic amebic dysentery)*, or sometimes the colitis is severe and has an abrupt onset. Fever, severe abdominal pain, and the passage of profuse blood-stained stools are the features of this *acute amebic dysentery*. Cases of the acute form occur sporadically, and almost always in the tropics. Why the ameba is so aggressive in some people but causes a symptomless state in the majority of patients is not known. The existence of virulent strains of *Entamoeba histolytica* has been postulated, but it seems more likely that a synergistic action exists between the ameba and the intestinal flora in certain individuals.

Entamoeba histolytica occasionally penetrates the portal venous circulation, and this leads to amebic hepatic abscess formation. A diagnosis of this condition is often difficult because the complication is seen more commonly in cases of asymptomatic infection of the colon than in patients with overt dysentery. The diagnosis of active amebic colitis depends on identification of the active trophozoites by microscopic examination of fresh warm stool.* In the absence of diarrhea, the trophozoites encyst before leaving the gut. The feces of asymptomatic carriers contain cysts only and are the chief source of infection. Outbreaks of amebic dysentery are generally water borne and are never as explosive as are those of bacillary dysentery (see Chapter 32).

MALARIA

Malaria is a protozoal disease caused by infection by a member of the genus *Plasmodium*. It is characterized by paroxysms of fever, each lasting 2 to 4 hours and initiated by a severe rigor. The paroxysm passes through the classic cold, hot, and sweating stages (Chapter 22). The infection is acquired from the bite of a female anopheline mosquito whose injected saliva contains sporozoites that travel via the blood stream to reach the liver cells, where they multiply (Fig. 15–1). This *exoerythrocytic stage* occurs during the incubation period of the disease. Finally, infective forms return to the blood stream, invade the red cells, and divide asexually to produce sporozoites, each of which breaks up into numerous merozoites. These are liberated as the red cell ruptures, and each merozoite invades another red cell. This asexual cycle (schizogony) takes 48 hours with *Plasmodium falciparum*. It is a remarkable fact

*Both trophozoites and cysts of *Entamoeba histolytica* must be distinguished from those of *Entamoeba coli*, which are part of the normal flora of the colon.

241

FIGURE 15–1. *Development of malaria parasites in humans.*

Infection begins with the bite of an infective mosquito. The injected sporozoites travel in the blood stream and enter the liver cells, where they develop. Infective forms are released into the blood, and the majority of these enter red cells, develop into ring forms, and mature to form trophozoites. The erythrocytic cycle is completed by the development of a schizont; with the subsequent destruction of the red cell, infective merozoites are released. Except in the case of *Plasmodium falciparum* some malaria parasites continue to multiply within liver cells and constitute the exoerythrocytic cycle that is responsible for the persistence of the malarial infection. The male and female gametocytes, which are formed by some parasites, do not develop further in the human host but must await the bite of another mosquito. The precise shape and form of the malarial parasites vary according to the species. In the diagram the forms approximate those of *Plasmodium vivax.* (After H. C. Jeffrey and R. M. Leach: Atlas of Medical Helminthology and Protozoology. 2nd ed. Edinburgh, Churchill Livingstone, Medical Division of Longman Group Ltd., 1975. Reproduced by permission. Drawing by Margot Mackay, Department of Art as Applied to Medicine, University of Toronto.)

that the maturation cycle of each parasite soon becomes synchronized. The release of merozoites is accompanied by the onset of a paroxysm—each third day with tertian malaria (due to *Plasmodium vivax* and *Plasmodium ovale*), and each fourth day with quartan malaria *(Plasmodium malariae)*. Paroxysms are more erratic with malignant malaria (due to *Plasmodium falciparum*). The last type of malaria is so named because it is the most severe and is accompanied by two serious complications.

CEREBRAL MALARIA.   A complication of malignant malaria, cerebral malaria is characterized by the rapid development of a high fever (hyperpyrexia), coma, and death. (See Fig. 22–2.)

BLACKWATER FEVER. In blackwater fever, a malarial paroxysm is followed by massive intravascular hemolysis, hemoglobinuria, cessation of urine formation (anuria), and frequently death. The pathogenesis is not understood, but this complication is usually seen in chronic falciparum malignant malaria treated episodically with quinine.

Course of Malaria. The first attacks of malaria are often severe, but as time goes by the episodes become more mild. Persistence of infection is due to the persistence of the exoerythrocytic forms in the liver. In endemic areas, reinfection constantly occurs, and a state of chronic infection ensues. This state is characterized by anemia, enlargement of the spleen (splenomegaly), debility, and cachexia, leaving the patient open to other infections. Tuberculosis, cholera, bacillary dysentery, and bronchopneumonia all take their toll in patients with chronic malaria.

Eradication of Malaria. The malarial parasites divide asexually in man, who is therefore the *intermediate host.* Gametocytes are formed in some infected red cells, but their maturation to form gametes and subsequent union to form zygotes only occurs in the female mosquito (Fig. 15–2). The anopheline mosquito is therefore the *definitive host.* The eradication of malaria involves mosquito control and the treatment of patients, who serve as the reservoir for the disease. Neither of these has proved to be easy. Mosquitoes have developed immunity to insecticides, and drug-resistant strains of plasmodia have emerged. Evolution, which designed the complex life cycle of the plasmodia, is not easily relinquishing such a prize.

Diagnosis of Malaria. The diagnosis of malaria rests on finding the parasite in a stained blood film. (See Figs. 15–2 and 22–2.)

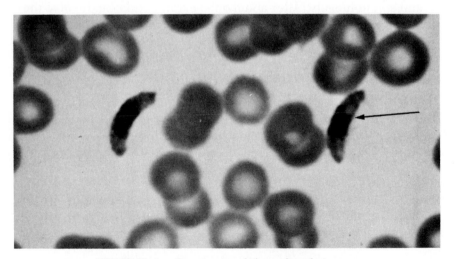

FIGURE 15–2. *Gametocytes of* Plasmodium faciparum.

The two gametocytes shown were found in a routine blood film of a Malayan soldier. He was asymptomatic at the time. The crescentic shape of the organism is characteristic of this species of malaria parasite. One gametocyte (arrow), which has a more pointed end, is male; the other is female. The patient had a history of previous attacks of malaria, but he evidently had developed sufficient immunity to remain as an asymptomatic carrier. After a host has been bitten by a mosquito, gametocytes develop into gametes, which fuse to form a zygote. This zygote develops further and ultimately produces vast numbers of sporozoites that are ready to be injected when the mosquito bites her next victim.

Table 15-1   TYPES OF TRYPANOSOMIASIS

TYPE	ORGANISM	VECTOR	LESIONS
African	*T. gambiense* *T. rhodesiense*	Tsetse fly Tsetse fly	Localized skin ulcer Generalized infection Brain
South American	*T. cruzi*	Kissing bug	Skin nodule Generalized infection Encephalitis Myocarditis

TRYPANOSOMIASIS

The trypanosomes are protozoa with a terminal flagellum and an undulating membrane. They cause infections of many animal species and pose a great economic problem in many parts of the world. Millions of acres in Africa are sparsely populated because of the impossibility of keeping domestic animals free of trypanosomiasis.

Three types of infection occur in man (Table 15-1).

AFRICAN TRYPANOSOMIASIS

Trypanosoma gambiense and *Trypanosoma rhodesiense* are transmitted by a bite of the tsetse fly, which injects infective forms with its saliva. A generalized infection occurs that is characterized by fever, skin rashes, lymphadenopathy, and splenomegaly. After about one year infection can involve the central nervous system, and the patient becomes lethargic and lapses into a coma. It is this latter feature that has given the disease its other name—*sleeping sickness.*

CHAGAS' DISEASE, OR SOUTH AMERICAN TRYPANOSOMIASIS

Trypanosoma cruzi is transmitted by the kissing bug, which tends to bite the face of the victim around the mouth, a habit that has earned it its name. A local nodule is followed by evidence of generalized parasitemia, with fever and involvement of many organs—skin, mucous membrane, lymph nodes, and the central nervous system.

Chronic Chagas' disease is characterized by parasitization of the heart muscle. This accounts for many cases of heart failure in some parts of South America. There is no treatment for it.

LEISHMANIASIS

The leishmania are protozoa that are transmitted by species of sandflies (genus, *Phlebotomus*). In the fly the organism has a flagellum, but in the lesions of man and other animal hosts, the organism is non motile (forming Leishman-Donovan bodies) and parasitizes macrophages (Fig. 15-3). Three main types of leishmaniasis are known (Table 15-2).

FIGURE 15–3. *Photomicrograph of stained bone marrow of patient with leishmaniasis.*

The specimen illustrated here was taken from a sternal puncture. In the center is a large macrophage stuffed with parasites. Each organism has one large nucleus and a smaller rod-shaped structure called a *kinetoplast.* The arrow points to a typical organism showing these two structures. The membrane surrounding each individual organism is not clearly seen in this photograph. For more information on the patient with leishmaniasis, see Case History I.

Table 15–2   TYPES OF LEISHMANIASIS

TYPE	ORGANISM	VECTOR	LESIONS
Kala-azar (Visceral leishmaniasis)	*L. donovani*	Sandfly (*Phlebotomus*)	Local skin ulcer in some types only
			Generalized infection of reticuloendothelial system
Cutaneous leishmaniasis (Oriental sore, Aleppo button, Baghdad boil, Delhi boil, and others)	*L. tropica*	Sandfly	Skin only
Mucocutaneous, or American, leishmaniasis	*L. braziliensis* and others	Sandfly	Skin and mucous membranes of mouth and nose

Case History I.   (See Figure 15–3.)   The patient was a 25-year-old Maltese male who was serving in the British Army in London. He had been complaining of general malaise for several weeks and was noted to be running a low-grade fever. His spleen was markedly enlarged and could be felt about four fingers' breadth below the left costal margin. There was also some enlargement of the liver. Lymph nodes in both axillae were enlarged. A blood count showed a mild anemia, reduction in platelet count, and a white count of 3500 cells per cu mm. The leukopenia was due to a reduction in the number of polymorphs (see Fig. 15–3 for a stained section of bone marrow).

The patient was treated with a pentavalent antimony compound and consequently made an uninterrupted recovery.

Visceral leishmaniasis, or kala-azar, in addition to being found in the Mediterranean, is found in China, Russia, India, Africa, and Central and South America.

KALA-AZAR, OR VISCERAL LEISHMANIASIS

Kala-azar is widely distributed, affecting the Far and Middle East, the area around the Mediterranean, particularly Malta and Greece, Africa, and to a lesser extent Central and South America.

Kala-azar is caused by *Leishmania donovani,* of which there are probably several species, since the disease shows considerable geographical variations. Generally there is no local lesion at the site of the sandfly bite, and the organism proliferates in the reticuloendothelial cells of the spleen, lymph nodes, liver, and bone marrow. Compensatory reticuloendothelial hyperplasia leads to enormous splenomegaly and hepatomegaly. Involvement of the marrow leads to anemia and low granulocyte count.

The mortality rate in untreated kala-azar is about 90 per cent, but the disease responds to treatment with antimony compounds.

CUTANEOUS LEISHMANIASIS, OR ORIENTAL SORE

Oriental sore, which is the least serious form of leishmaniasis, occurs in countries bordering the Eastern Mediterranean, in Asia Minor, and in India. The causative organism, *Leishmania tropica,* produces a local infection of the skin at the site of the sandfly bite. A chronic ulcer is formed, and this heals spontaneously after a protracted course.

MUCOCUTANEOUS, OR AMERICAN, LEISHMANIASIS

The best-known variant of this type of leishmaniasis is espundia due to *Leishmania braziliensis.* One or more cutaneous lesions first appear and resemble oriental sore. However, the organisms spread to involve the mucosa of the mouth and nose. Here, even after the skin lesions have been treated, the disease progresses and leads to great tissue destruction, secondary bacterial infection, and death.

TRICHOMONIASIS

Trichomonas vaginalis is the cause of a common vaginal infection that produces itching and a profuse, watery, yellow, frothy, vaginal discharge. The diagnosis is made by examining a fresh specimen of the discharge under the microscope and identifying the motile trichomonads. On the fixed smear stained by the Papanicolaou method the organisms can be seen, but often with difficulty.

In the male, a mild urethritis is the only evidence of infection. Usually the male carrier is symptomless. Transmission is by sexual contact, and both patient and sexual partners should be treated simultaneously.

Review Questions

1. A patient with kala-azar develops an acute gingivitis and an ulcerative pharyngitis. Can you suggest why?
2. Why is a polyclonal hypergammaglobulinemia, together with enlargement of the lymph nodes, liver, and especially spleen, so common in kala-azar?
3. Describe the possible after effects of eating a salad that has been washed in water contaminated by fecal material containing *Entamoeba histolytica*.
4. Outline the steps that can be taken in an attempt to eradicate malaria from a community.
5. Enumerate the organisms that might be responsible for a vaginal discharge. How could the diagnoses be confirmed?

Selected Readings

Baker, J. R.: Parasitic Protozoa. London, Hutchinson University Library, 1970.

Belding, D. L.: Textbook of Parasitology. 3rd ed. New York, Appleton-Century-Crofts, 1965.

Bruce-Chwatt, L. J.: Malaria eradication at the crossroads. Bulletin of the New York Academy of Medicine, 45:999–1012, 1969.

Faust, E. C., Russell, P. F., and Jung, R. C.: Clinical Parasitology. Philadelphia, Lea & Febiger, 1970.

Garnham, P. C. C.: Malaria Parasites and Other Haemosporidia. Oxford, Blackwell Scientific Publications, 1966.

Köberle, F.: Chagas' disease and Chagas' syndromes: The pathology of American trypanosomiasis. Advances in Parasitology, 6:63–116, 1968.

World Health Organization: Amoebiasis. World Health Organization Technical Report Series, 421, 1969.

World Health Organization: Parasitology of malaria. World Health Organization Technical Report Series, 433, 1969.

Elsden, R.: Amebiasis as a world problem. Bulletin of the New York Academy of Medicine, 47:438, 1971.

Juniper, K.: Amebiasis in the United States. Bulletin of the New York Academy of Medicine, 47:448, 1971.

Chapter 16

After studying this chapter the student should be able to:

- Describe the causes of developmental anomalies.
- List 10 types of malformation and give an example of each.
- Describe the lessons learned from the thalidomide tragedy.
- Compare and contrast hypertrophy with hyperplasia.
- Define the following terms: atrophy, hypoplasia, aplasia, metaplasia, dyscrasia, and dysplasia.
- Classify the causes of atrophy and give examples of each.
- Discuss the use of the term *dysplasia* as applied to diseases of the skin, cervix uteri, and breast.

INTRODUCTION

Disorders of growth and differentiation most commonly occur during the period of embryonic development. This is hardly surprising, since a single fertilized ovum can transform itself into an entire animal in a short space of time—21 days in the case of the mouse and 9 months in the case of human beings. Errors that occur during this period of marked change can result in gross defects. Postnatal development, on the other hand, is a relatively sedate affair, and the likelihood of an error occurring is correspondingly less.

Minor variations in development are so common that the resulting changes are regarded as normal. More serious errors in development result in the production of malformations that are usually present at birth but may not become evident until during the growing periods of childhood and adoles-

DISORDERS OF GROWTH

cence. Gross abnormalities are often incompatible with life and result in abortion, stillbirth, or neonatal death.

The changes that are described in this chapter concern the abnormalities of cell growth: too much, too little, or the wrong sort. Such changes form a heterogeneous group; they often appear to bear little relationship to each other. Nevertheless, the changes are worthy of study, for they form cellular or functional entities that are commonly encountered in many diseases processes.

It is convenient to divide the abnormalities of cell growth into two groups:

DEVELOPMENTAL ANOMALIES. These arise before the affected part has reached its mature, adult form.

ACQUIRED ANOMALIES. These arise in an organ or tissue after the mature configuration has been attained.

Inevitably, there is some overlap between these two groups, because it is sometimes difficult to decide at what point in time a particular organ does attain maturity. Nevertheless, the classification has some merit. A "developmental anomaly" is found in an organ that has never been normal. In contrast, an "acquired anomaly" occurs in an organ that has previously attained normal adult stature.

DEVELOPMENTAL ANOMALIES

CAUSES

Genetic Errors. Inherited conditions, such as achondroplasia, and gross chromosomal anomalies (see Chapter 3) are well-known causes of malformations. When one encounters a patient with a developmental anomaly, it is wise to carry out a chromosomal analysis and to investigate the family for a history of similar anomalies. Genetic counseling is a practical way of avoiding future mistakes.

Environmental Factors. It is becoming increasingly obvious that many external agents are capable of causing serious developmental anomalies if they act *in utero.* Infection transmitted from the mother to the fetus can cause serious damage, particularly if the transmission occurs during the first three months of pregnancy when the development of important organs, such as the heart, is proceeding rapidly. German measles has acquired a particularly evil reputation in this respect. Deformities occur in as many as 25 per cent of babies born to mothers who have had this infection during pregnancy. Congenital heart disease frequently occurs in children of women exposed to German measles. The first month of pregnancy is the most dangerous period to be exposed.

The tragedy that followed the administration of the sedative drug thalido-mide has highlighted the selective toxic effects that some drugs have on the de-veloping embryo. The most common anomalies found in the "thalidomide babies" were absence of limbs or parts of limbs, angiomatous malformations (see *hamartomas,* discussed later) of lips and nose, as well as other malforma-tions of the heart, alimentary tract, and genitourinary system. Since the dele-terious effects of a particular drug on the human fetus can be established only by testing the substance on pregnant women, it is current policy to avoid ad-ministration of any drug during pregnancy unless it is absolutely vital (see the following section).

Thalidomide: A Teratogenic Drug.   Thalidomide was first introduced in 1956 as a pleasant and safe hypnotic. During 1960 and 1961 an outbreak of *phocomelia,* or "seal extremity," occurred in West Germany. With this type of deformity the long bones of the limbs are defective, and rudimentary hands and feet arise from the trunk like the flippers of a seal. Viruses, radioactive fallout, food preservatives, and contraceptives were among the agents considered as possible causes, but thalidomide was finally in-criminated. Similar outbreaks were reported from other parts of the world; by the end of 1961 the drug had been withdrawn from the market. By that time, tragically, many thousands of babies had been affected. Approval for the drug was delayed by the Food and Drug Administration of the U. S. because of other side effects (*e.g.,* peripheral neu-ritis). Fortunately, its effects on the fetus became known and general distribution in the U.S.A. was avoided. Nevertheless, some thalidomide babies were born as a result of premarketing clinical trials. The tragedy has taught us some lessons:
1. New drugs must be tested on pregnant laboratory animals.
2. Pregnant women should avoid all unnecessary drugs, particularly during early pregnancy. The use of thalidomide is dangerous during the crucial period of from 37 to 54 days after the first day of the last menstrual period.
3. All adverse drug reactions should be reported to a central bureau for evaluation. It took five years to associate the striking birth deformities with thalidomide. Minor or subtle defects may never be recognized unless information is gathered and expertly analyzed.
4. New drugs are not necessarily the best drugs.

TYPES OF MALFORMATIONS

Malformations can affect any part of the body, and a large number have been described. It is convenient to group them under the following ten head-ings:

1. FAILURE OF DEVELOPMENT.   There may be a complete failure of a part to develop (*agenesis*), or the part may remain rudimentary and never attain a full mature size (*hypoplasia*). An example of this lack of or incomplete develop-ment has already been mentioned in the case of the thalidomide babies' limbs. Likewise, one or both kidneys can show either agenesis or hypoplasia. The possibility of this anomaly is important to the surgeon who is considering the removal of one kidney. It is essential to check that the other kidney is present and normal.

2. FAILURE OF FUSION.   During development many structures normally fuse together, and a failure to do so can result in abnormality. A harelip or cleft palate is a common example of this failure to fuse.

3. FAILURE OF SEPARATION. A good example of this malformation is the webbing that may persist between the fingers or toes (Fig. 16–1).

4. FAILURE OF CANALIZATION. Many channels in the body originate as solid cords and subsequently canalize. A failure in this process leads to a congenital obstruction, which is frequently termed *atresia*. Examples of this are esophageal atresia and imperforate anus (anal atresia).

5. ECTOPIA. Sometimes organs and tissues are found at abnormal sites. This is termed *ectopia, heterotopia,* or *aberrance.* An interesting example of this is the ectopic thyroid that develops at the base of the tongue. In such a case, no thyroid tissue is found in the normal location, *i.e.,* in the neck. Aberrant blood vessels are quite common. They may even be noticed by a patient and cause anxiety, such as when the radial artery runs a superficial course at the wrist and its pulsation can be seen. Aberrant renal arteries can be damaged by a careless surgeon who relies on the normality of the patient's anatomy.

6. HETEROPLASIA. Sometimes there is an anomalous differentiation of a particular tissue in an organ. For instance, tissue identical to gastric mucosa may be found in the esophagus. Sebaceous-gland formation may occur in the oral mucosa; the small white dots that this produces can be seen in the buccal mucosa of many otherwise normal individuals.

7. LOCAL GIGANTISM. Occasionally, there is a simple overgrowth of an organ or tissue. Thus there may be an enlarged limb in neurofibromatosis. Likewise, there may be enormous overdevelopment of the female breast or breasts at puberty.

8. SUPERNUMERARY ORGANS. Additional or supernumerary organs are not uncommon. A good example is hands or feet that exhibit six digits (polydactyly). Supernumerary nipples are not uncommon, and infrequently these are associated with breast tissue.

9. HAMARTOMAS. *A hamartoma is a tumorlike malformation in which*

FIGURE 16–1. *Syndactyly.*

The third and fourth fingers of the hand are joined together. This abnormality can easily pass unnoticed in a young baby. (Photograph courtesy of V. S. Brookes.)

FIGURE 16–2. *Hamartoma of the lung.*

In the center of the upper lobe there is a circumscribed, pearly-white, hard, round mass. It consists predominantly of mature cartilage, and there is no obvious capsule around it. (Specimen ER 22.1. Reproduced by permission of the President and Council of the R.C.S. Eng.)

the tissues of the particular part of the body are arranged haphazardly, usually with an excess of one or more components. The term was coined by Albrecht and is derived from the Greek word *hamartanein,* meaning "to err." The concept of the hamartoma is of great importance, because a large number of common lesions fall into this general category.

The best-known example of a hamartoma is a simple mole or melanotic nevus of the skin. The lesion is composed of an excess of melanocytes that subsequently change into nevus cells. This lesion is described in detail in Chapter 41.

Many hamartomas (both of the skin and elsewhere) are composed of vascular spaces. Like many other hamartomas, these vascular lesions are given a name resembling that given to a tumor (hemangioma), even though, strictly speaking, this is incorrect, since they are not tumors.

An uncommon but important hamartoma is found in the lung. This consists of a nodule of cartilage and a few spaces lined by a respiratory type of epithelium (Fig. 16–2). The lesion appears on a radiograph as a circumscribed opacity, commonly called a "coin lesion"; its discovery can lead to the mistaken diagnosis of cancer. Radical surgery for such a lesion is a medical catastrophe.

Some hamartomas tend to be multiple: Hemangiomas of the face can be associated with similar hemangiomas of the retina or brain. The skin lesions are thus pointers to the more serious underlying condition. Another well-known but distinctly uncommon example is neurofibromatosis (von Recklinghausen's disease, Fig. 3–2). This inherited autosomal dominant trait results in widespread hamartomatous overgrowths of nerve-sheath tissue. These lesions closely resemble tumors and are generally loosely described as "neurofibromas." There is sometimes localized regional overgrowth, and gross deformity can result.

10. PERSISTENCE OF NORMALLY VESTIGIAL STRUCTURES. During the course of development, many structures are formed that are of immediate importance to the developing embryo but that ultimately disappear and become obliterated by the time of birth or shortly thereafter. Occasionally, such structures persist and lead to trouble. The two most important complications are neoplasia and cyst formation. These tumors are considered in the next chapter. Persistent ductus arteriosus is described in Chapter 28.

A good example of a *developmental cyst* is the dermoid cyst. This is due to the sequestration and growth of a piece of skin beneath the surface and occurs when folds of skin fuse together during development. During the complex development of the face, various folds are formed and fuse. Dermoid cysts tend to occur along the lines of these fusions, such as at the angles of the eye or mouth. Another example is persistence of a segment of the thyroglossal duct, which results in a midline cystic swelling in the neck, known as a *thyroglossal cyst.*

ACQUIRED DISORDERS OF GROWTH

In the mature individual, all organs and tissues (with the notable exceptions of muscle fibers and neurons) show a steady turnover, with mitosis compensating for cell death. In some organs, such as the liver, the turnover is slow; in others, such as the lymphoid tissue, it is fast. The mechanism controlling this turnover is not understood, but the end-result is that most organs remain at a constant normal size. Furthermore, there is a considerable reserve of tissue that can be drawn upon whenever additional work is demanded of it. Therefore, under normal conditions, no structural adjustment is necessary other than that of regulating the blood flow through the organ. Thus, tissues at rest are maintained by an intermittent blood flow through their supplying capillaries. This mechanism results in an economical use of the circulation, and it explains why noxious substances spread by the blood stream may nevertheless produce spotty effects. When more work has to be performed, the shut-down vessels dilate, and the organ shows active hyperemia. This is well illustrated by the tremendous increase in blood flow that occurs in skeletal muscle during periods of activity and in the salivary glands during eating.

Under abnormal circumstances, organs and tissues may show a change in size that is due either to an increase or a decrease in the bulk of parenchymal cells. Abnormalities of cellular growth are found in virtually all tissues, and only a few examples will be given here.

Quantitative Abnormalities of Cellular Growth: Hyperplasia

An increase in the number of cells of a tissue or organ that results in enlargement is called *hyperplasia*. The cause is generally related to the overaction of a tangible stimulus, which is often a basically physiological one acting to excess. Hyperplasia is therefore often the result of an increased demand for function. Following blood loss, there is consequently an increased demand for red-cell production, and hyperplasia of the bone marrow ensues. Likewise, in chronic infection the draining lymph nodes are stimulated so that there is hyperplasia of their component reticuloendothelial and lymphoid cells. In bacteremia there is also reticuloendothelial hyperplasia of the spleen, causing this organ to become enlarged.

In passing, it should be noted that enlargement of an organ is commonly denoted by the use of the suffix -*megaly*. Thus, enlargement of the spleen is described as "splenomegaly." The term gives no indication of the cause of the enlargement; for example, it might be due to hyperplasia of the spleen's constituent cells, or it could equally well be caused by an abscess or a tumor. As always, since there are exceptions to any rule, enlargement of the lymph nodes is spoken of as "lymphadenopathy."

Hyperplasia is generally regarded as an adaptive mechanism by which an increased number of cells is produced as a useful response to a stimulus. Thus chronic physical irritation of the skin results in thickening of the epidermis; calloused hands are well suited to manual work. When the physical irritation is removed, the epidermis returns to normal. This response is different from that seen in neoplasia, in which withdrawal of the stimulus does not lead to a return to normal (see Chapter 17 for further discussion). Nevertheless, there are examples of cellular overgrowth in human disease that, although classified as hyperplasias, are neither produced by any known stimulus nor are necessarily self-limiting or useful. An example of this is the hyperplasia of the thyroid gland in Graves' disease (see Fig. 39–5). The precise stimulus for this hyperplasia is not known, but the gland shows enlargement with massive production of new cells and considerable overactivity, so that there is excessive production of thyroid hormones and the patient suffers from hyperthyroidism. Other examples of hyperplasias in which the cause is not known are the epithelial and connective tissue hyperplasias seen in mammary dysplasia in women (see Chapter 38) and in the extremely common condition of prostatic enlargement encountered in elderly men (see Chapter 36).

Hypertrophy

Hypertrophy is defined as the increase in size of an organ or tissue due solely to an increase in the size of its constituent specialized cells. In practice, this phenomenon applies only to muscle, and the stimulus for this enlargement is almost always a mechanical one.

Any muscle that is continually stimulated by overwork tends to show enlargement. This is commonly seen in skeletal muscle, in which the bulging muscles of the athlete contrast with the slender ones of the sedentary worker. Cardiac muscle, likewise, shows enlargement if the heart is constantly forced to overwork. This is seen when the heart has to force blood through a stenosed orifice (*e.g.*, when there is left ventricular hypertrophy in aortic stenosis; Fig. 16–3) or when it has to contract against a high blood pressure (*e.g.*, in patients with left ventricular hypertrophy in systemic hypertension).

It is noteworthy that the human heart at birth weighs approximately 30 gm,

FIGURE 16–3. *Hypertrophy of the left ventricle.*

This patient had aortic stenosis with enlargement of the heart (*cardiomegaly*) due to hypertrophy of the muscle of the left ventricle. It is convenient to assess the size of the heart by comparing the maximum width of the heart shadow (C) with the width of the chest cavity at the level of the highest point of the right side of the diaphragm (T). The cardiothoracic ratio, C/T, is normally less than 0.5. Here, of course, the ratio is greater than 0.5. (Photograph courtesy of Dr. D. E. Sanders.)

and thereafter no new cells are formed. The heart muscle cells steadily increase in size; by maturity, therefore, there has been a tenfold increase in weight and a tenfold increase in size of muscle fibers. Any further enlargement is due to additional increase in muscle size. Although these large fibers are initially capable of vigorous contraction, it is unfortunate that they ultimately fail. This appears to be due to an inadequate blood supply, since enlargement of muscle-fiber size is not accompanied by an increase in number of blood vessels. It follows that an enlarged heart (cardiomegaly) due to hypertrophy is a diseased heart, and one that will ultimately fail to function efficiently.

Hypertrophy of smooth muscle cells is seen in the muscular coats of hollow organs, which are forced to expel their contents against resistance. The muscular urinary bladder wall hypertrophies when the prostate gland enlarges and causes urethral obstruction (Fig. 36–1). The intestinal muscular wall undergoes hypertrophy proximal to any stenosis (*e.g.*, the stomach wall thickens in pyloric stenosis).

Atrophy

NOMENCLATURE. A small organ or tissue is often spoken of as *atrophic* when its diminution in size is due to a decrease in either the size or number of its constituent specialized cells. Only in muscle is the decrease in size of cells a major factor. In all other instances the number of cells is also reduced. Atrophy of the bone marrow is commonly called *hypoplasia,* whereas extreme atrophy is known as *aplasia.* This is unfortunate, because hypoplasia is also used by some pathologists in a different connotation indicating an imperfect development of an organ or tissue.

Physiological Atrophy. There are many examples of structures that are well developed at a certain time of life but subsequently undergo atrophy. Many fetal structures, such as the thyroglossal duct and the hyaloid artery, which supplies the developing lens, completely disappear before birth. Other structures, such as the ductus arteriosus, atrophy early in postuterine life. From adolescence the lymphoid tissues of the body undergo steady atrophy; after parturition the uterus undergoes atrophy (commonly called *involution*); in old age most tissues (particularly the sexual organs) sustain a generalized process of atrophy.

Pathological Atrophy. Generalized atrophy occurs in starvation and is

FIGURE 16–4. *Atrophy of the pancreas.*

This patient had chronic pancreatitis, which caused the formation of a hard mass in the head of the organ. The mass had obstructed the main pancreatic duct. The section illustrated was taken from the body of the organ and shows atrophy of the exocrine component of the gland. Many acini have disappeared; those that remain are small. The shrinkage of the exocrine portion of the gland has resulted in condensation of the islets of Langerhans, which are themselves unaffected. At least six are present in the field illustrated. Compare this with Figure 2–3. There is some increase in the amount of fibrous tissue and a sparse infiltration by small round cells, indicating a mild degree of chronic inflammation. This case illustrates the principle that if the duct of a secreting gland is obstructed, its parenchyma undergoes atrophy. It is of historical interest to note that Banting and Best ligated the pancreatic duct to remove the exocrine portion of the pancreas so that insulin could be extracted from the endocrine component without the complicating action of trypsin on their tissue extracts.

also a feature of the cachexia of malignant disease. Hypopituitarism, for example, results in atrophy of most of the endocrine glands. The widespread atrophy of bone, termed *osteoporosis*, is described in Chapter 40.

Local Atrophy. Local atrophy is usually the result of impaired blood supply (ischemia). As the blood vessels supplying the brain steadily become obstructed in many persons past middle age, the brain undergoes atrophy. This results in the rigidity of mind and loss of intellect that all too frequently accompany old age.

A particular variant of ischemic atrophy is that which is produced by local pressure. A steadily enlarging cyst or an expanding tumor produces pressure on adjacent tissues and leads to atrophy of the parenchyma. The fibrous tissue stroma tends to be more resistant; it persists and forms a capsule round the lesion.

DISUSE ATROPHY. It has been tritely stated that what a patient does not use, he loses. A striking example of this is the effects of immobilization of a limb. There is marked atrophy of bone, ligaments, and muscle following joint immobilization; it is the task of the physical therapist to prevent this. Similar atrophy occurs when a joint is fused *(ankylosed)* or when movement is prevented by pain. Thus, atrophy of muscles and ligaments is common around rheumatoid and tuberculous arthritic joints. Disuse atrophy of a gland following obstruction of its duct is illustrated in Figure 16–4.

There are a number of conditions in which tissues undergo atrophy for no obvious reason. Sometimes there appears to be a genetic defect; sometimes there appears to be an autoimmune mechanism; in most instances, however, there is no apparent cause. A distressing example of this is the atrophy of the brain that occurs prematurely in some people and leads to severe mental deterioration (dementia). Various types of this presenile dementia are known and are categorized under different names, *e.g.*, Alzheimer's disease. Idiopathic endocrine atrophy is seen in some cases of Addison's disease (see Chapter 39) and in hypothyroidism and cretinism.

Abnormalities of Cellular Differentiation

METAPLASIA

Metaplasia is a condition in which there is a change in one type of differentiated tissue such that it takes on the characteristics of another differentiated tissue. Two forms of this condition are described below.

Epithelial Metaplasia. It is quite common for the pseudostratified columnar ciliated epithelium of the trachea and bronchi to be replaced by a stratified squamous type of epithelium that may even undergo keratinization and resemble epidermis. This *squamous metaplasia* generally seems to be the result of chronic irritation. This condition is also found in the urinary tract, particularly in association with urinary stones and infection. Sometimes metaplasia can be more subtle. The bronchial lining can be replaced by a columnar epithelium in which simple mucus-secreting goblet cells predominate. This is extremely common in chronic bronchitis and is one of the factors that results in the excessive production of mucus that is continually coughed up (expectorated). The concept of metaplasia is important, because it helps to explain why tumors of the lung can resemble those normally arising in the skin (squamous-cell carcinoma) or in a mucus-secreting gland (adenocarcinoma).

Connective Tissue Metaplasia. The fibroblasts of connective tissue and scar tissue can sometimes take on the characteristics of osteoblasts and lead to the laying down of bone. Spicules of bone are often found in chronically inflamed tonsils, in old scars, and in the fibrous elements of goiters. Since these areas of bone formation are visible in radiographs, they are of importance in diagnostic radiography.

OTHER CELLULAR ABNORMALITIES

The term *dystrophy* is commonly used, but it is difficult to define. It is generally applied to any condition in which there is an alteration in the structure or function of an organ or tissue that does not readily fit into the other categories (*i.e.*, agenesis, atrophy, hypertrophy, or metaplasia). For example, in *corneal dystrophy* the cornea becomes opaque at about the time of puberty and ultimately results in blindness. Some varieties are inherited, and these appear to be degenerative. Dystrophy is also used to describe the crumbly, deformed nails affected by fungal infection or psoriasis. It is evident that the term dystrophy has no precise definition and is used in many specialties to describe diseases of widely differing nature.

The term *dyscrasia* is now used only by hematologists to describe some blood disorders of unknown cause and undetermined pathogenesis. The term serves no useful function and should be abandoned.

Dysplasia has been used to describe an abnormal development of tissue; like dystrophy, however, the term is also used by specialists in many fields to describe conditions of widely divergent nature. Thus, when applied to the breast (mammary dysplasia), dysplasia denotes a complex condition of unknown origin in which there is irregular hyperplasia and metaplasia of breast substance. In the cervix uteri, dysplasia has acquired a completely separate meaning. It is used to describe a type of epithelial overgrowth that is thought to progress steadily to *carcinoma-in-situ,* and ultimately to invasive cancer. In the skin, dysplasia is used in a similar context to describe the atypicality and irregular maturation seen in the epidermis in actinic keratoses and in Bowen's disease (see Figs. 17–17, 17–18, and 17–19). In these organs, therefore, the term "dysplasia" denotes a change that is thought to precede the onset of cancer.

From this short account, it is evident that the terms *dystrophy, dysplasia,* and *dyscrasia* are used quite arbitrarily to denote various types of condition, the nature of which is poorly understood.

In this chapter many different perversions of cell growth have been described. The one factor they all have in common is that they are self-limiting and reversible if the stimulus is removed. In the following chapter, *neoplasia* is discussed. With this condition the perversion of cell growth persists even when the stimulus that produced it is eliminated.

Review Questions

1. At what stage of gestation is a drug most likely to produce severe fetal abnormalities? Describe the steps that can be taken to protect the fetus against potentially harmful drug action.
2. Define *hamartoma* and give three examples of those affecting the skin.
3. Describe how metaplasia differs from heteroplasia and dysplasia.
4. Differentiate between regeneration and hyperplasia.
5. Describe the changes that might occur when a leg is encased in a plaster cast for three months.

Selected Readings

Gillis, L.: Thalidomide babies: management of limb defects. British Medical Journal, 2:647–651, 1962. See this article for pictures of thalidomide deformities.

Lawrence, D. R.: Clinical Pharmacology. 4th ed. Edinburgh, Churchill Livingstone, 1973, pp. 667–670. Provides a fascinating account of the thalidomide disaster.

Marymont, J. H., and Herrmann, K. L.: Rubella in pregnancy: review of current problems. Postgraduate Medicine, 56(4):167–172, 1974.

Speirs, A. L.: Thalidomide and congenital abnormalities. Lancet, 1:303–305, 1962. Also see the leading article in the same issue, pp. 307–308.

Taussig, H. B.: A study of the German outbreak of phocomelia. Journal of the American Medical Association, 180:1106–1114, 1962. See this article for pictures of the thalidomide deformities.

Ward, S. P.: Thalidomide and congenital abnormalities. British Medical Journal, 2:646–647, 1962.

Willis, R. A.: Some unusual developmental heterotopias. British Medical Journal, 3:267–272, 1968.

Chapter 17

TUMORS

After studying this chapter the student should be able to:

- Define a tumor.
- Give a classification of tumors in tabular form.
- Define the following terms: adenoma, papilloma, cystadenoma, fibroma, and leiomyoma.
- Define carcinoma, sarcoma, adenocarcinoma, squamous-cell carcinoma, anaplasia, teratoma, dormant cancer, carcinoma-in-situ, and metastasis.
- Describe the microscopic features of malignant tumors and compare them with those of a benign tumor.
- Discuss the effects of a malignant tumor and contrast them with those of a benign tumor.
- List the malignant tumors that commonly metastasize to bone.
- Describe what is meant by the staging of a tumor and indicate the value of the procedure.
- Give an account of the important features of
    - (a) squamous-cell carcinoma
    - (b) carcinoma arising from a glandular epithelium
    - (c) fibrosarcoma.
- Subdivide the lymphomas into three groups and describe their salient features.
- Illustrate the structure and behavior of an intermediate tumor, using basal-cell carcinoma as an example.
- Discuss the difficulties in classifying tumors in relation to tumors of melanocytes, placenta, and embryonic rests.
- Give examples of carcinogenic chemicals that cause tumors in human beings.
- Give examples of physical carcinogenic agents that affect humans.
- List the human tumors in which there is a hereditary predisposition.
- Discuss the relationship between hormones and cancer.
- Give examples of viruses that have been incriminated as a cause of cancer in animals. Indicate the relevance to human disease.
- Describe the development of cancer through the stages of dysplasia and carcinoma-in-situ.
- Discuss the evidence indicating that cancer starts in one cell rather than in many cells simultaneously.

INTRODUCTION

The presence of a lump or mass is a common clinical finding, and the term "tumor" was applied at one time to such a lesion; the suffix -*oma* was used to denote it. The practice of classifying all swellings as tumors became established long before the nature of the lesions was understood, and even today this relic of medical history persists in the use of names like "hematoma," "hamartoma," "tuberculoma," and "granuloma." In due course, the swellings of known origin, especially the infective ones, were excluded from the category of tumors, and a group of swellings of unknown cause, which apparently had arisen as a result of the unrestrained growth of the individual's own cells, was left. In all other pathological processes the growth of cells appears to be coordinated and under strict control. A tumor is regarded as resulting from a breakdown in this mechanism and has been defined by Willis as *an abnormal mass of tissue, the growth of which exceeds and is uncoordinated with that of the normal tissues and persists in the same excessive manner after cessation of the stimulus which evoked the change.* This definition is unsatisfactory in several respects. First, it implies that the stimulus producing a tumor need act only for a short time. Second, it implies that the regulating mechanism governing cell growth is abolished. Unfortunately, we do not know the nature of this regulating mechanism, and we are consequently not able to prove or disprove that it is nonfunctional.

Although the excessive growth of cells is often manifested by the production of a tumor mass, this does not always occur. Sometimes the migration of newly formed cells from the site of formation outweighs the bulk of abnormal proliferation and no swelling as such exists. One excellent example of this is the diffuse infiltrating carcinoma of the stomach; another is leukemia. *Neoplasia,* which literally means "new formation or new growth," is a more suitable term. It implies that there is an abnormal type of growth that may be evident not only in the intact animal but also in cells grown in culture.

Classification of Tumors

A tumor is regarded as resulting from an unrestrained growth of cells, and it follows that one possible classification can be based on the cell of origin. Since the tissues of the body have been divided into either epithelium or connective tissue, tumors can likewise be placed into one of two groups. Furthermore, each group can be subdivided. Thus, epithelial tumors can be grouped into those arising from stratified squamous epithelium, those from columnar epithelium, etc. This delineation, based on the cell type of origin, is an important component of our present-day classification. In itself, it is quite inadequate, since the effects of a tumor are determined not only by the tissue of origin but also by its biological behavior. In some tumors the dividing cells adhere to each other, and the neoplastic mass remains as a circumscribed lesion. Such a lesion is termed a *benign tumor,* and its behavior can be contrasted with that of tumors in which the cells do not adhere to one another and are thereby enabled to invade the surrounding tissues. These are the *malignant tumors,* or *cancers.* Tumor cells often enter natural channels such as lymphatics or blood vessels, and groups of tumor cells are carried as emboli to other parts of the body, where they grow and set up *secondary growths,* or *metastases.* Local invasion and embolic spread are the two characteristics of malignant tumors. The term "malignant" is particularly suitable for this type of tumor, since death is inevitable in untreated cases. Nevertheless, the rate of progression varies markedly from one tumor to another, as will be seen from some examples studied later.

In addition to the typical benign and malignant tumors, there are other types that show patterns of behavior not fitting into either group. Most important are the *intermediate tumors,* in which tumor cells invade locally but do not metastasize. These are best called "locally malignant" tumors. *Carcinoma-in-situ* and the phenomena of *spontaneous regression* and *dormant cancer* are considered later.

When the patient is first seen clinically, the organ of origin is the most striking feature of many tumors. If the cell type of origin and biological behavior of the tumor can be determined, a satisfactory diagnosis may be obtained. In practice, however, it is not possible to assess behavior by leaving the tumor alone and awaiting development. It has been found that behavior can frequently be related to the microscopic appearance of the tumor. The ultimate classification of a particular tumor is therefore attained by establishing its site of origin, its tissue of origin, its behavior, and its microscopic appearances. An outline of the classification in current use is shown in Table 17–1.

Cancer is often regarded as a unitary disease, and one frequently hears references to its cause and treatment. It should be evident from this short discussion on classification, however, that "cancer" does not constitute a single entity but rather encompasses a large number of separate diseases. At the present time, it would seem to be as futile to search for the cause or cure of cancer as it would be to look for the cause and cure of "infection."

BENIGN TUMORS

BENIGN EPITHELIAL TUMORS

These are of two main types. Benign neoplasia of the surface or lining epithelium produces a warty tumor called a *papilloma* (Fig. 17–1). In a compact gland, such as the breast or the thyroid, the tumor is embedded in the tissue and is called an *adenoma.*

Papillomas. Papillomas may occur on any epithelial surface. Some have a broad base and are described as *sessile,* whereas others become pedunculated and are called *polyps,* a morphological term applied to any pedunculated mass attached to a surface and not necessarily neoplastic. Papillomas are supplied by a core of connective tissue stroma containing blood vessels, lymphatics, and nerves. This is covered by a folded neoplastic epithelium composed of stratified squamous, transitional, or columnar cells, according to the type from which it has arisen. The cells show an orderly arrangement, and the basement membrane is intact unless there is distortion due to inflammation. The epithelial cells are entirely restricted to the surface and do not show invasion.

Table 17–1   CLASSIFICATION OF TUMORS

TISSUE OF ORIGIN	BEHAVIOR		
	Benign	*Intermediate*	*Malignant*°
EPITHELIUM			
Types			
1. Covering and protective			
(a) Squamous	Squamous-cell papilloma		Squamous-cell carcinoma
(b) Transitional	Transitional-cell papilloma		Transitional-cell carcinoma
(c) Columnar	Columnar-cell papilloma		Adenocarcinoma
2. Compact and secreting	Adenoma; if cystic, cystadenoma or papillary cystadenoma		Adenocarcinoma; if cystic, cystadeno-carcinoma
3. Others	Adenoma	Basal-cell carcinoma Pleomorphic salivary gland tumors Carcinoid tumor (argentaffinoma)	Carcinoma
CONNECTIVE TISSUE			
Fibrous	Fibroma		Fibrosarcoma
Nerve sheath	Neurofibroma		Neurofibrosarcoma
Adipose	Lipoma		Liposarcoma
Smooth muscle	Leiomyoma		Leiomyosarcoma
Striated muscle	Rhabdomyoma		Rhabdomyosarcoma
Synovial	Synovioma		Malignant synovioma
Cartilaginous	Chondroma		Chondrosarcoma
Bone osteoblast	Osteoma	Giant-cell tumor	Osteosarcoma
Blood vessels and lymphatics	Benign hemangioma and lymphangioma		Angiosarcoma
Neuroglia		Astrocytoma, Oligodendroglioma, and Ependymoma†	
FETAL TROPHOBLAST	Hydatidiform mole		Choriocarcinoma
EMBRYONIC TISSUE			
Totipotential cell	Benign teratoma		Malignant teratoma
Pluripotential cell Kidney			Nephroblastoma
Unipotential cell			
Retina			Retinoblastoma
Hindbrain			Medulloblastoma
Sympathetic ganglia and adrenal medulla	Ganglioneuroma		Neuroblastoma
HAMARTOMA			
Melanotic nevus			Malignant melanoma
Neurofibromatosis	Neurofibroma		Neurofibrosarcoma

°Any malignant tumor may be so undifferentiated that it must be classified on a histological basis, *e.g.,* carcinoma simplex, spindle-cell sarcoma. The lymphomas and many rare tumors are not included in this table.

†These tumors are difficult to classify. The common types are locally malignant, but some also metastasize within the central nervous system. Rarely, they appear to be benign in children.

FIGURE 17–1. *Tumors of the epidermis.*

Three types of neoplasia of a keratinizing strati-fied squamous epithelium (e.g., epidermis) are shown. A, Benign neoplasia results in an excessive production of regular epithelium, which is thrown into a com-plicated folded structure in order to be accom-modated. This formation is called a *papilloma.* The epidermal cells mature in an orderly way from the basal cells to the superficial squames. B, In *carcinoma-in-situ* there is excessive growth of epidermis, which thereby becomes thickened (acanthosis). Maturation of the cells is disorderly; foci of keratinization are found within the epidermis instead of being present only on the surface (dyskeratosis). C, In carcinoma the atypical epidermal cells break through the base-ment membrane and invade the underlying tissues. (Drawings by Margot Mackay, Department of Art as Applied to Medicine, University of Toronto.)

Stratified squamous-cell papillomas are common on the skin and are seen as warts (Fig. 17–2) and seborrheic keratoses (see Chapter 41).

Adenomas. An adenoma is composed of a mass of glandular tissue that closely resembles the structure of the parent tissue. Adenomas are quite com-mon in the colon, where they arise from the glands in the mucosa. As with papillomas, they frequently become polypoid (Fig. 32–10).

In some adenomas the glandular spaces enlarge to form cysts (causing a *cystadenoma)* and papillomas can grow into these cysts (causing a *papillary cystadenoma).* Such a tumor is common in the ovary.

BENIGN CONNECTIVE TISSUE TUMORS

A benign tumor, which can arise from any connective tissue, is composed of a mass of cells whose structure closely resembles that of the parent tissue. Common tumors in this group are lipomas derived from fat, leiomyomas derived from the smooth muscle (Fig. 17–3), neurofibromas (Schwannomas) derived from the Schwann cells of the nerve sheaths, and fibromas derived from fibroblasts. These tumors are generally well circumscribed.

GENERAL CONSIDERATIONS OF THE EFFECTS OF BENIGN TUMORS

The cells of a benign tumor show no tendency to invade the surrounding tissues but do produce an expanding mass that has two local effects:

FIGURE 17–2. *Verruca vulgaris.*

This patient has a common wart overlying the proximal interphalangeal joint of the left index finger. The lesion is a squamous-cell papilloma, which is caused by a papovavirus.

FIGURE 17–3. *Leiomyoma of the uterus.*

The tumor consists of spindle-shaped smooth muscle cells arranged in sheaves, some of which are cut longitudinally, while others are seen in transverse section. No mitoses can be seen in this benign tumor (× 250).

PRESSURE ATROPHY. The adjacent specialized parenchymatous tissue undergoes atrophy, while the more resistant connective tissue survives to form a capsule. *Benign tumors are therefore usually well encapsulated* and are not intimately connected with the surrounding tissues except at points of entry of the supplying blood vessels (see Fig. 37–2). Benign tumors can therefore be excised with relative ease; if local removal is complete, they do not recur. Nevertheless, a benign tumor cannot be dismissed as inconsequential. One within the skull or vertebral column can produce serious pressure effects and even death. The shape of a benign tumor is generally spherical, but it may be modified by firm local structures.

OBSTRUCTION. A benign tumor may obstruct a natural passage, causing extensive damage. Thus, blockage of a bronchus can lead to bronchiectasis and bronchopneumonia (Fig. 30–13). A tumor of the intestine can produce obstruction. Benign tumors generally grow slowly and rarely ulcerate on the surface. Hence, bleeding is uncommon as a symptom, except for certain vascular surface papillomatous growths such as those of the colon or bladder. Benign tumors of endocrine tissue occasionally produce an excess quantity of the associated hormone; this oversecretion of hormone can lead to serious and sometimes fatal effects. A good example of this is the adenoma of the islets of Langerhans, which can lead to fatal hypoglycemia as a result of the overproduction of insulin. It is therefore not true that benign tumors cannot cause death.

Microscopically, the cells of a benign tumor closely resemble those of the parent tissue. They are therefore described as being "well differentiated." The cells tend to be regular in size and uniform in staining and shape; mitoses are scanty and when present are of normal type. The tumor cells are supported and nourished by a network of host connective tissue that consists predominantly of blood vessels, fibroblasts, and a varying amount of collagen. This network is called the *stroma* and although an intimate part of the tumor, it is not considered to be involved in the neoplastic change.

MALIGNANT TUMORS

GENERAL CONSIDERATIONS

The cells of a malignant tumor infiltrate surrounding tissues, normal cells are enveloped and destroyed, and the edge of the tumor is poorly defined. Microscopic spread occurs beyond the naked-eye edge of the tumor, and complete excision by surgery is therefore difficult. Even if much surrounding, apparently normal, tissue is included in the excision, malignant cells can often remain behind; their continued growth results in a *local recurrence*. The invading malignant cells spread in the planes of least resistance: fingerlike processes extend outward from the main tumor mass, and the growth has a fanciful resemblance to the silhouette of a crab. It is from this mode of spread that the term "cancer," from the Latin word meaning *crab*, is derived. In lay language it is generally applied to all malignant tumors. In medical terminology it is often used as being synonymous with *carcinoma, which is defined as a malignant tumor of epithelial cells. A sarcoma is a malignant tumor derived from connective tissue cells.*

Embolic spread of tumor cells is responsible for the production of distant metastases. Local invasion and embolic spread are the two characteristics of malignant tumors. Both are related to the reduced cell adhesiveness that appears to be a fundamental characteristic of malignant cells, for this property is evident not only *in vivo* but also in tissue culture. The cells do not resist mechanical separation as well as do those of normal tissue (see cell transformation, later in this chapter). The power to invade and spread, combined with the capacity for progressive growth, makes the term "malignant" particularly suitable for this type of tumor. Death is inevitable in untreated cases, except for those very rare — though well-documented — cases of *spontaneous regression,* in which proven cancers have disappeared either with no treatment or with very limited palliative treatment.

GROSS CHARACTERISTICS

Malignant tumors do not possess a limiting capsule, although with some very rapidly proliferating growths, such as secondary tumors in the liver, they may appear circumscribed. Microscopy, however, shows tumor extension beyond the apparent edge of the growth. Malignant tumors tend to be irregular in shape and are usually larger than their benign counterparts. As would be expected from their destructive properties, they tend to ulcerate along a free surface. Hence, any area of ulceration that fails to heal within a reasonable time should be regarded as malignant until proved otherwise. Since tumors invade and destroy blood vessels, bleeding is a frequent symptom. Bleeding and ulceration are thus features of malignant tumors.

MICROSCOPIC FEATURES

Several important microscopic features should be noted. Tumor tissue may resemble the parent tissue to a considerable extent, but the similarity is not as great as with benign tumors. Differentiation is not so well developed, and recognition of the tissue of origin is often difficult or even impossible. Tumors showing little or no differentiation are called *undifferentiated.*

Malignant tumors usually show much mitotic activity. The synthesis of DNA prior to division results in nuclear enlargement and hyperchromatism. This synthesis, together with the formation of polypoid cells, accounts for the irregularity in size and shape *(pleomorphism)* and the mode of staining that is so characteristic of malignant tumors. Mitoses are not only numerous but they are also abnormal (Fig. 17–4). A number of cells may deviate from the normal complement of 46 chromosomes, and occasionally cells are seen to divide into three instead of two *(triradiate mitosis).*

Anaplasia is a term that at first was introduced to describe new cells deviating from normal and resembling those of embryonic origin. It was at one time thought that tumors were derived from rests of embryonic cells. This concept has been abandoned, but the term anaplasia is still used to describe those cellular changes that are found in malignant tumors. Therefore, a tumor said to

FIGURE 17–4. *Anaplastic carcinoma of lung.*

The tumor shows no evidence of differentiation, and its cells exhibit marked pleomorphism. One cell possesses two nuclei, each with a prominent nucleolus (Cell 1), whereas another has many hyperchromatic nuclei (Cell 2). In an atypical mitosis scattered chromosomes can be identified (mit) (× 550).

show a high degree of anaplasia has cells that are pleomorphic, poorly differentiated, scarcely reproducing the parent tissue, and exhibiting frequent and bizarre mitoses.

EFFECTS

Malignant tumors produce their ill-effects in a number of ways, which are described below:

MECHANICAL PRESSURE AND OBSTRUCTION. Like benign tumors, malignant tumors cause obstruction to natural passages and lead to serious consequences. Thus a tumor of the colon produces intestinal obstruction; a tumor of the bronchus leads to collapse and bronchopneumonia in the lung beyond it (see Fig. 30–14).

DESTRUCTION OF TISSUE. Both primary and secondary tumors infiltrate and destroy tissue. This is well illustrated in bone, in which destruction may be so marked that minimal trauma produces a fracture. This is known as a *pathological fracture* and may sometimes be the first symptom of a previously missed tumor.

HEMORRHAGE. Malignant tumors that involve any surface usually ulcerate and bleed. Repeated bleeding can cause anemia; occasionally, a fatal sudden hemorrhage can occur where a large vessel is eroded. Clinically unexplained bleeding from any site should be treated seriously, since it is a common symptom of cancer.

INFECTION.   All ulcerating cancers are bound to become secondarily infected with bacteria. Infection often follows in the wake of obstruction, such as bronchopneumonia with cancer of the lung and urinary infection with cancer of the bladder. Repeated bouts of infection in an organ should always lead to a suspicion of an underlying malignant tumor.

STARVATION.   Cancer of the mouth, pharynx, esophagus, and stomach can so obstruct the passage of food that direct starvation occurs.

ANEMIA.   Anemia is common and is due to a variety of causes. There may be direct blood loss from an ulcerating tumor, malabsorption of essential dietary components, or bone-marrow replacement if there are multiple bony metastases.

CACHEXIA.   The emaciated appearance of patients with advanced cancer is characteristic, but it is nevertheless not uncommon for some patients to remain obese. The cause of the weight loss and the generalized body atrophy in many patients with cancer has given rise to much speculation. At one time, a toxic product from the tumor was postulated, but this has never been substantiated. The present tendency is to attribute cachexia to secondary factors such as starvation, hemorrhage, infection, and liver damage.

In advanced malignancy there is usually fever, a raised erythrocyte sedimentation rate (E.S.R.), and a neutrophil leukocytosis. In part, these are effects of infection and in part they are due to the presence of necrotic tissue both in the tumor and in the surrounding tissues.

HORMONAL EFFECTS.   Malignant tumors of the endocrine glands can sometimes produce effects by over-production of the relevant hormone. This is less common than with benign tumors, as would be expected, since malignant tumors are less differentiated both in structure and in function.

CARCINOMATOUS SYNDROMES.   A variety of syndromes have been reported in association with tumors that are not explicable in terms of infiltration by either a primary tumor or its metastases. Muscle weakness, skin eruptions, signs of an intracranial tumor, and venous thrombosis are some examples of this. At necropsy no local tumor is found to explain these features. A possible explanation is the deposition of immune complexes containing tumor antigen. For the most part, however, these strange manifestations of cancer have not been explained.

Another curious phenomenon is the hormonal effect produced by tumors of nonendocrine origin, which are particularly common in cancer of the lung. The tumor appears to be able to secrete hormonelike substances, symptoms of hypercorticalism (Cushing's syndrome), hyperinsulinism, and hyperparathyroidism may occur. It is apparent that the atypical cells of malignant tumors can produce and secrete hormones or hormonelike substances into the circulation. This is an instance of abnormal differentiation of a malignant tumor.

SPREAD OF MALIGNANT TUMORS

Direct Spread.   Tumor cells spread into the surrounding tissues, particularly along tissue planes and natural spaces. This is a feature that is used by the pathologist as an aid to the microscopic diagnosis of malignancy. Clinically, local invasion is often evident by the way in which the tumor becomes attached to adjacent structures. Thus a carcinoma of the breast eventually becomes attached to the skin and the underlying pectoral muscles.

INVASION OF LYMPHATICS. Carcinoma, but not sarcoma, shows a particular tendency to invade lymphatic vessels at an early stage, and the cells may grow as a long, ever-extending cord. The process is called *lymphatic permeation*, and the lymphatic obstruction it produces can cause lymphatic edema (Fig. 17–5).

INVASION OF THE ARTERIES AND VEINS. This is a common event and may lead to thrombosis and obstruction.

FIGURE 17–5. *Spread of carcinoma by lymphatic permeation.*

Section of skin showing dilated lymphatic vessels filled with carcinoma. The specimen was taken from the skin of a woman with advanced carcinoma of the breast. Although the tumor is derived from a glandular structure, it shows no evidence of differentiation. The tumor may therefore be labeled an undifferentiated carcinoma, a polygonal-cell carcinoma, a spheroidal-cell carcinoma, or a carcinoma simplex (× 250).

FIGURE 17–6. *Lymph node metastases.*

The specimen shows a group of peripancreatic lymph nodes that are greatly enlarged by metastatic carcinoma. Several nodules of tumor are also present in the spleen (S). The primary growth was a small-cell (oat-cell) carcinoma of the lung. This tumor is highly malignant and metastasizes early and widely. Secondary deposits are infrequent in the spleen, but they are often found in patients with widespread metastases from oat-cell carcinoma of the lung or malignant melanoma.

The growths seen in these enlarged lymph nodes are not diagnostic of secondary carcinoma. An identical picture, including the splenic involvement, could be seen in a lymphoma such as Hodgkin's disease. (P, pancreas; S, spleen.)

Spread by Metastasis. Groups of malignant cells may become detached, travel in some natural passage to a distant site, become implanted, and finally grow to produce secondary deposits, or metastases. Spread via the lymphatics, blood vessels, and serous cavities are the most important examples.

LYMPHATIC SPREAD. Detached groups of tumor cells that have invaded lymphatic channels travel to the regional draining lymph nodes (Fig. 17–6). If the cells survive and grow, they replace the lymph node by tumor; the cells then move on to the next group of nodes. This is a common event with carcinoma and melanoma, but it is rare with sarcoma.

BLOOD SPREAD. The occurrence of blood-borne metastases is the feature of malignant disease that is responsible for death in most cases. It is the factor that limits the surgical and radiotherapeutic treatment of cancer. At first sight, the mode of production of secondary tumors is easy to understand. Malignant cells invade small venules, become detached, and are then carried in the blood stream until they become impacted in the next capillary network that they encounter. There the emboli take root, and the cells proliferate and develop into secondary tumors. A second route of blood-borne metastases is via the lymphatics, for all the lymph eventually drains into the venous circulation.

As would be expected, the lung is one of the commonest sites of metastasis for all tumors. Primary tumors arising in an area drained by the portal vein regularly metastasize to the liver. Purely mechanical factors seem to account for this distribution, but such an explanation seems untenable upon a closer examination of the facts.

Many tumors, *e.g.*, of the breast and the kidney, give rise not only to lung metastases but also to secondary growths in the liver, bones, and other organs; such systemic metastases sometimes occur without apparent deposits in the lung. It is possible that such deposits are, in fact, present but are missed at an inadequate necropsy examination. Alternatively, one can postulate that the cells pass through the lung capillaries and travel to the systemic circulation, where they lead to secondary deposit formation.

One might expect that the distribution of metastases would be related to the blood supply of each organ. Such is not the case. Cardiac and skeletal muscle have an abundant blood supply, and yet it is rare to find metastases in muscle. The spleen also has a very large blood supply, but splenic metastases are also quite uncommon.

There is considerable evidence that malignant cells often reach the blood stream where most of them die. Only a selected few are able to take root and grow into secondary deposits. The factors governing this response are not known. The "seed" may be widespread, but only in some organs is the "soil" suitable for growth to occur. *Selective metastasis* is the theory often used to account for this response; the following examples are worth noting.

Liver. The commonest organ in which blood-borne metastases are found is the liver, regardless of whether the primary tumor is in an area drained by the portal vein or not. Although massive enlargement of the liver is common, it is rare for liver failure to occur (Fig. 17–7).

Lung. This is the next most common site of metastases.

Bone. Carcinomas of the breast, lung, and prostate commonly metastasize to bone. Such spread is less frequently seen with other tumors (Fig. 17–8). *Pain* is a common presenting symptom, particularly when the spine is involved and nerves are compressed.

FIGURE 17–7. *Liver with metastatic carcinoma.*

The liver contains numerous white nodules of metastatic carcinoma from a primary tumor in the naso-pharynx. The nodules are of varying size; one of them is 13 cm in diameter.

FIGURE 17–8.   *Metastatic tumor in bone.*

The medullary cavity is packed with tumor. Some of the malignant cells contain clear spaces. A suitably stained frozen section of another specimen of tumor revealed that the clear spaces contain neutral fat. The primary tumor was a liposarcoma arising from the subcutaneous tissues of the back. Note how difficult it is to distinguish the tumor cells from those of the stroma. Compare this with a carcinoma, such as that in Figure 17–9. Sarcomas tend to have a poorly formed stroma, thereby accounting for their tendency to invade blood vessels and to metastasize early by this route. The section also shows a spicule of normal lamellar bone (× 250).

Brain.   Cancer of the lung is notorious for the frequency with which it metastasizes to brain. Indeed, secondary lung cancer is the commonest type of tumor to be found in the brain.

Adrenal Glands.   This is a frequent site for secondary lung and breast cancer, an infrequent site for other primary growths.

TRANSCELOMIC SPREAD.   When a malignant tumor invades the serosal layer of a viscus, it causes a local acute inflammatory response. This results in the formation of a serous inflammatory exudate in the cavity, and bleeding usually occurs. It follows that the presence of a blood-stained effusion into any serous cavity such as that of the pleura or peritoneum, should always arouse suspicion of malignancy. Withdrawal of some fluid and an examination for malignant cells will sometimes lead to a positive diagnosis. Cells that travel in the effusion can form the basis of numerous secondary seedling growths.

STAGING

Stages can be assigned to tumors, depending on the extent of their spread. The criteria used in this staging vary from one type of cancer to another, but a typical example is as follows:

STAGE 1. Tumor confined to the organ of origin.
STAGE 2. Growth extends to involve the regional lymph nodes.
STAGE 3. Tumor extends to the distant lymph nodes.
STAGE 4. Blood-borne metastases occur.

Staging of tumors is useful in that it describes how far a tumor has already spread at the time of diagnosis; it is therefore related to prognosis. A patient with a Stage 1 tumor, therefore, has a much better prognosis than one with a Stage 4 tumor.

DORMANCY

One difficulty with staging is the tendency for some metastases to appear many years after the primary tumor has apparently been treated successfully. Patients may remain well for 10, 20, or even 30 years after removal of a primary tumor and then suddenly develop multiple secondary deposits despite the absence of any local recurrence. It is assumed that tumor cells were present in the body during the entire period, but for reasons unknown they remained dormant. This is one of the most mystifying aspects of malignant disease, and were we to know the factors responsible for keeping cancer cells dormant, we might well have an adequate treatment for the disease. Carcinoma of the breast and kidney and melanoma of the eye are tumors that are notorious for this tendency toward metastases developing after a period of dormancy.

Malignant Epithelial Tumors

Malignant epithelial tumors are the *carcinomas*, the most common of all malignant tumors. Three types may be recognized:

(1) Squamous-cell carcinoma
(2) Glandular epithelial carcinoma
(3) Transitional-cell carcinoma

Squamous-Cell Carcinoma. This histological type of tumor arises at any site normally covered by stratified squamous epithelium — skin, mouth, esophagus, and other similar regions. Squamous-cell carcinoma arises via the invasion of the underlying connective tissues by the germinal cells situated in the basal layer of the epithelium. Malignant cells may infiltrate separately, but more usually they form clumps and columns as they proceed into the connective tissue. The cells tend to differentiate into prickle cells and form keratin, so that in a well-differentiated tumor, clumps of cells are seen with a central whorl of keratin (Fig. 17–9). This is called an *epithelial pearl* and is in effect an attempt by the malignant cells to reproduce the stratum corneum of the normal skin. Tumors that are less well differentiated form no keratin, but they do contain prickle cells. Poorly differentiated tumors show few recognizable structures and are difficult to distinguish from poorly differentiated tumors of other types. Purely descriptive terms are used to name such tumors: giant-cell carcinoma, oat-cell carcinoma, and large-cell carcinoma.

Squamous-cell carcinoma can also arise from columnar or transitional epithelium. This can occur in one of two ways. The normal epithelium can un-

FIGURE 17–9. *Squamous-cell carcinoma of skin.*

The dermis has been invaded by malignant cells which have grown to form clumps. In some areas the central tumor cells have differentiated into keratin and have formed cell nests or epithelial pearls. This is characteristic of a well-differentiated squamous-cell carcinoma. Note that the groups of tumor cells are sharply separated from the stroma (compare this with Figure 17–8).

dergo metaplasia to squamous epithelium, and tumor growth subsequently occurs in this. A second, and more likely, explanation is that the tumor arises in the epithelium first, and then the tumor cells show squamous differentiation. One of the most common tumors of lung, arising from the bronchial mucosa, is a squamous-cell carcinoma. Likewise, squamous-cell carcinoma is also found in the urinary bladders and less frequently in the gallbladder. It should be noted that the term "squamous-cell carcinoma" is used to describe a particular microscopic appearance of a tumor showing differentiation into a keratinizing squamous type of cell. It does not always mean a tumor arising from a squamous epithelium.

Glandular Epithelial Carcinoma. This type of carcinoma may arise from a surface secreting epithelium, such as that which lines the stomach, or from a solid gland, such as liver or breast. The pattern of invasion of neoplastic epithelial cells is similar to that already described with squamous cell carcinoma. In the case of the tumors arising from glandular epithelium, groups of cancer cells, instead of producing keratin, tend to arrange themselves into acinar structures containing a central lumen into which some secretion is poured (Figs. 17–10, 17–11, and 17–12). The well-differentiated cancers showing excellent acinus formation can closely mimic the original glandular structure. If differentiation is poor, the tumor is composed of masses of cells with only occasional tubule formation. A tumor derived from glandular epithelium and showing glandular differentiation is called an *adenocarcinoma.*

In poorly differentiated tumors there are merely clumps of cells surrounded by a stroma and no evidence of central cavitation to produce an acinus. The names *carcinoma simplex, spheroidal-cell carcinoma* or *polygonal-cell carcinoma* are applied to this type of cancer (Fig. 17–5). Such tumors are particularly common in the breast and stomach.

MUCOID CANCER.   Occasionally a carcinoma derived from glandular epithelium shows such excessive production of mucus, that to the naked eye the tumor appears as a gelatinous mass, and microscopically there are pools of mucus in which are floating malignant cells. Sometimes the cells contain one large droplet of mucus with the nucleus pushed to one side, giving the appearance of a signet ring. This type of tumor occurs in the stomach or large intestine.

Transitional-Cell Carcinoma.   This type of tumor occurs in the urinary tract and often shows areas of squamous differentiation.

STROMAL REACTION TO CARCINOMA.   The reaction to the invaded tissue to carcinoma cells varies; its growth may be so stimulated that a hard fibrotic or *scirrhous* type of tumor is produced. Most breast cancers are of this type. As

FIGURE 17–10. *Adenocarcinoma of the colon.*

At this magnification the mucosa appears normal. The section was taken from an area adjacent to a carcinoma; tumor has invaded the submucosa. Normally this layer consists of loose connective tissue similar to that seen in the small intestine (see Chapter 2) (× 60).

FIGURE 17–11.   *Adenocarcinoma of colon.*

Higher magnification of section shown in Figure 17–10. The clumps of tumor cells in the submucosa have differentiated to form glandular spaces, and the label adenocarcinoma is therefore warranted. One group of tumor cells (arrow) has invaded the mucosa and is separated from the main mass of growth by the muscularis mucosa (mm) (× 250).

with wounds, the dense fibrosis appears to be associated with a contracting tendency that is poorly understood. It is this effect that leads to obstruction with many carcinomas of the colon. The contraction causes a purse-string deformity.

When a tumor has little stroma in relation to the cell bulk, it is soft or brainlike and is described as *medullary,* or *encephaloid.*

Malignant Connective Tissue Tumors

These malignant tumors are called *sarcomas* and are much less common than carcinomas; like carcinomas, they occur at all ages. On the whole, sarcomas spread more rapidly than carcinomas, and the prognosis is correspondingly more grave. Early blood-borne metastases generally occur, and the lungs are often riddled with secondary deposits. Lymphatic involvement is very much less common than with carcinoma.

Fibrosarcoma.   Fibrosarcomas can arise in any fibrous connective tissue and can vary in their degree of differentiation. A well-differentiated tumor shows some cellular irregularity and good collagen formation; distinction from a fibroma can be extremely difficult. Poorly differentiated tumors show little or no collagen formation and are then termed *spindle-cell sarcomas.* A distinction from anaplastic carcinomas is sometimes difficult.

FIGURE 17–12.   *Adenocarcinoma of colon.*

This section is from a lymph node metastasis of the tumor shown in Figure 17–6. Although the growth is well differentiated, the pattern of glandular formation is quite different from the normal. Some malignant cells line large spaces, whereas others form solid clumps (× 250).

Osteosarcoma. This is one of the commonest forms of sarcoma and is further described in Chapter 40. Other types of sarcoma are known (Fig. 17–8). They arise from blood vessels *(angiosarcoma),* fat cells *(liposarcoma),* and smooth muscle cells *(leiomyosarcoma),* and are all uncommon.

TUMORS OF THE STEM CELL AND ITS DERIVATIVES

The neoplastic lesions of these cells are the *lymphomas* and tumors of the *hematopoietic tissues.*

Lymphoma. The lymphomas are all malignant tumors and arise from the cellular elements of the lymph nodes, bone marrow, and occasionally other organs having a reticuloendothelial content. They are the second most common malignant tumors; carcinomas occur most often. They generally start at one site — usually a lymph node — but spread to other lymph nodes and eventually become disseminated, with deposits being found in the spleen, liver, bone marrow, lungs, and elsewhere. Whether this represents metastasis or multicentric origin is debatable. Unlike other types of sarcoma, they are generally extremely radio-sensitive. Sometimes a local lesion can be cured by radiotherapy, but unfortunately recurrence and spread throughout the body are the rule. Three major types of lymphoma can be recognized; their subdivisions are the task of the expert.

RETICULUM-CELL LYMPHOMA OR RETICULUM-CELL SARCOMA. The cells of this tumor differentiate to form reticulum cells and to lay down reticulin fibers. The disease starts in a group of lymph nodes, and later spreads. It is usually a disease of later life.

LYMPHOCYTIC LYMPHOMA, OR LYMPHOSARCOMA. This is about twice as common as the reticulum cell sarcoma, and clinically the two are indistinguishable. The tumor is composed of lymphocytes that may either be small and appear mature or be large and resemble lymphoblasts. One particular variant of lymphocytic lymphoma is the *Burkitt tumor.* This is a lymphoma that occurs extensively and almost exclusively in the low-lying moist region of Central and West Africa. It is almost entirely confined to children between the ages of 2 and 14 years and affects the jaws, ovaries, lymph nodes, and kidneys. The usual mode of presentation is an enormous facial swelling with loosening of the affected teeth. The fascination of this tumor is that it is thought to be caused by the Epstein-Barr virus.

HODGKIN'S DISEASE. This is the commonest of the lymphomas and attacks young and middle-aged adults predominantly. Lymph nodes are first affected and are replaced by tumors that consist of reticulum cells together with lymphocytes, eosinophils, and plasma cells. There has been some argument as to whether the disease represents an infective granulomatous process; the consensus is that it is a type of lymphoma. If the disease is treated while it is still localized, the prognosis is quite good, but when the disease has become systemic, the outlook is poor. The prognosis also depends on the histological appearance of the tumor present. Various classifications are in vogue that relate histological appearance to prognosis.

Malignant Conditions of the Hematopoietic Tissue. The most important of these are the *leukemias*, in which the malignant cells are found circulating in the peripheral blood, and *multiple myeloma*, in which the bone marrow is replaced by plasma-cell tumors. Both conditions are considered in detail in later chapters.

INTERMEDIATE TUMORS

In their behavior, intermediate tumors are between the benign and the malignant groups. Since local invasion occurs, the tumors cannot be regarded as benign. Nevertheless, they do not show the steady, inexorable growth pattern of true malignant tumors. The victims do not inevitably die of the disease if left untreated. The most common tumor in this group is the *rodent ulcer*, or *basal-cell carcinoma*. This invades locally, but almost never metastasizes (Figs. 17–13 and 17–14).

Another tumor in this group is the pleomorphic salivary gland tumor. Histologically, this is an adenomatous growth and is unusual in that the stroma appears to consist of cartilage (see Fig. 31–7). The tumors often appear encapsulated, but the capsule is infiltrated by lateral extensions of growth. Simple enucleation is therefore followed by recurrence, and eventually blood-borne metastases may develop.

In this group of tumors with erratic behavior are the "adenoma of bronchus" (see Chapter 30), and the carcinoid tumors of the intestine (see Chapter 32).

FIGURE 17–13. *Basal-cell carcinoma.*

This badly neglected tumor involves a large area of the face and has invaded the orbit and nasal cavity. Tumor invasion has combined with infection to cause considerable tissue destruction. The basal-cell carcinoma almost never metastasizes. This particular tumor was cured by radiotherapy together with excision of the left eye. This picture should be remembered when one considers the effects of any invasive tumor that is not readily visible. From this picture one can appreciate how an ulcerated carcinoma of the stomach, colon, or bladder could be accompanied by tissue destruction, infection, and bleeding. (Photograph courtesy of Professor D. D. Smithers.)

FIGURE 17–14.   *Basal-cell carcinoma of the skin.*

Masses of tumor cells are seen to be arising from the basal layer of the epidermis. Some still maintain their attachment to the epidermis, while others have become detached and are spreading deep into the dermis. This is a typical basal-cell carcinoma and shows no tendency to form keratin (× 60).

Difficulties in Tumor Classification

Although it might seem that all malignant tumors could be classified as either carcinoma or sarcoma, there are certain instances in which this cannot be done.

TUMORS OF INDETERMINATE ORIGIN

The best example of such tumors is the melanoma of the skin (see Chapter 41). Some authorities have called the melanocyte an epithelial cell, and its tumors have been called *nevocarcinomas*. Others regard them as of connective-tissue origin and label the tumors *melanotic sarcomas*. In practice, the term *malignant melanoma* is used to avoid this problem.

PLACENTAL AND EMBRYONIC TUMORS

Tumors can arise from cells that are not normally present in the adult body. Two examples can be recognized:

(a) tumors of placental origin (*e.g., choriocarcinoma*); and (b) tumors of embryonic origin. These tumors arise from cells that, although present in the developing embryo, should normally have disappeared by the time of birth. Such tumors generally arise in children; the best-known examples are the following:

1. The *retinoblastoma*, which arises in the eye generally before the age of four.

2. The *neuroblastoma*, which is a malignant tumor derived from primitive neuroblasts. Note that nerve cells do not divide and therefore cannot give rise to tumors. Primitive neuroblasts, on the other hand, can divide and subsequently differentiate into nerve cells. Neoplastic neuroblasts may behave similarly, thereby explaining the occasional occurrence of a tumor that appears to be forming nerve cells. A well-differentiated tumor of this type is benign and is called a *ganglioneuroma*.

3. The *nephroblastoma*, which is one of the common malignant tumors of childhood, involves the kidney. The tumor, which is derived from a primitive kidney cell, shows differentiation not only into renal tubules but also into connective tissue elements such as fibroblasts and striated muscle cells.

TERATOMAS

The commonest tumor of the ovary in young women is a benign teratoma or "dermoid cyst." The lining consists of epidermis together with normal skin appendages, including hair. Thus, the cyst contains sebaceous material and matted hair. In its wall other structures can be found, including thyroid tissue, teeth, bone, brain, and spaces lined by a variety of different types of epithelia (Fig. 17–15). This tumor clearly contains derivatives of all three embryonic germinal layers and could have arisen only from a totipotent cell that was capable of differentiating into virtually any of the normal tissues of the body. Such a tumor is called a *teratoma*. A controversy exists as to whether the original totipotent cell is from one of the derivatives of the early divisions of the fertilized ovum of the individual or whether it represents a perverted division of an ovarian cell destined to become an ovum. The tumor is thus either an included twin or a deviant child of the patient. A similar type of tumor occurs in the testis, but here the various tissues are poorly formed, and the tumor is nearly always malignant (Fig. 17–16). The frequency of these tumors in the gonads suggests that both are derived from a type of parthenogenetic development of a primitive germ cell.

THE INCIDENCE AND CAUSE OF TUMORS

Observations on the incidence of tumors both in individuals and in ethnic and geographic groups have led to the unraveling of many factors that are involved in the production of tumors. These will be considered under the following headings:

1. External Carcinogenic Chemical Agents.
2. External Carcinogenic Physical Agents.
3. Hereditary Predisposition.
4. Hormonal Factors.
5. Viral Infections.
6. Following Chronic Disease.

FIGURE 17–15. *Teratoma of ovary.*

For five years, the patient had had occasional episodes of abdominal pain. At the age of 32 she experienced a particularly severe attack, which led to her being admitted to a hospital. A rounded swelling was palpated in the abdomen above the pubis. A cystic ovarian tumor was removed at laparotomy.

The specimen shows the opened cyst. It is lined by skin, and on one side a hard mass projects into the cavity. This is covered by spongy skin containing numerous sebaceous glands and from it is growing a tuft of hair. The mass contains bone in which a number of teeth are partially embedded. One of these is clearly shown in the photograph. The mass of tissue (Seb) contains hair but is otherwise lying free in the cyst cavity. It consists largely of sebaceous material and desquamated keratin. (Photograph of specimen courtesy of the Boyd Museum, University of Toronto.)

EXTERNAL CARCINOGENIC CHEMICAL AGENTS

The observation by Percivall Pott in 1775 that cancer of the scrotum was common in chimney sweeps led to the conclusion that soot and its derivatives cause cancer of the skin. It has been amply confirmed both in humans and in animals that certain chemicals, termed *carcinogens,* can lead to the formation of tumors. As would be expected, the first group of chemicals to be discovered were those derived from coal tar, and of these 1,2:5,6 dibenzanthracene and 3:4-benzpyrene are among the best known. When applied to the skin of animals, they cause squamous-cell carcinoma, and when injected into deeper tissues, they cause a variety of other tumors, including sarcomas. It has been found that when skin is painted with relatively small doses of carcinogen, no obvious change may be apparent. Nevertheless, if the skin is subsequently irritated by relatively nonspecific agents, such as croton oil, tumors can arise upon it. The supposition is that the carcinogen produced a change called *initiation,* such that relatively nonspecific stimuli can subsequently *promote* the formation of a malignant tumor. This two-stage mechanism in tumor production may well be of importance in human pathology. A carcinogen may not immediately cause a tumor to develop in patients subjected to its action, but many months

FIGURE 17–16. *Teratoma of the testis.*

This tumor has several components. *A,* Much of the growth is composed of oval connective tissue cells that resemble primitive mesenchyme. In one area there is differentiation into cartilage (Cart). *B,* The second area is from the same tumor and shows several spaces lined by columnar epithelium. The presence of neoplastic connective tissue and epithelial elements in the same tumor is characteristic of a teratoma. Both elements can metastasize (× 250).

or years later a relatively nonspecific irritant can precipitate the occurrence of malignancy.

The appreciation that chemicals can cause cancer has been of great importance in industry. Bladder tumors are known to be more frequent in workers who come into contact with betanaphthylamine. This agent is used in the rubber industry, and workers coming into contact with it have a particular propensity to develop cancer of the bladder. This has now been shown to be due to the local effect of one of the metabolic products, 2-amino-1-naphthol, which is a carcinogenic agent. This is a good example of remote carcinogenesis, in which an agent taken by mouth or absorbed from the skin produces an effect at some distant site — in this case, the bladder. Chemical agents that are thought to cause cancer in humans include asbestos (causing cancer of the lung and mesothelioma of the pleura) as well as agents in cigarette smoke that are responsible for much of the cancer of the lung that is so prevalent today. Vinyl chloride used in the manufacture of polyvinyl chloride plastic is one of the recently recognized carcinogens. It appears to cause angiosarcoma of the liver.

EXTERNAL CARCINOGENIC PHYSICAL AGENTS

The discovery of ionizing radiations was soon followed by an appreciation that these rays can cause cancer. Cancer of the skin occurred in the early radium workers and in those exposed to x-rays. The ingestion of radioactive compounds can lead to more widespread damage. The most famous example of this was recorded in female workers who painted luminous watch dials. They sucked their brushes to point them and thus ingested radioactive compounds used in the luminous paint; these compounds were deposited in the bones. The patients developed sarcoma of the bones as well as leukemia. The most recent demonstration of the carcinogenic activity of ionizing radiation has been the increased incidence of malignant disease in the survivors of the Hiroshima and Nagasaki bomb explosions. It is now appreciated that even diagnostic radiology carries a minor risk; consequently, all efforts are made to minimize the dosage received for essential radiographic procedures. Since it is believed that the embryo is particularly susceptible, the radiation of pregnant women is now carried out only for vital reasons.

Ultraviolet light is another carcinogenic agent; its effects are well seen on the exposed parts of the skin of fair complexioned people who work in tropical climates. The common lesions are solar keratoses and basal-cell carcinomas.

HEREDITARY PREDISPOSITION

It is possible to breed a strain of animals in which virtually all members of the strain will die of a particular cancer if they live long enough. It seems likely, therefore, that some hereditary predisposition is a factor in the development of tumors. Nevertheless, it is doubtful whether this is of any great importance in human pathology, since statistical surveys among relatives of cancer patients have not yielded convincing evidence of an increased incidence of tumors. Cancer of the breast is possibly more common in the relatives of affected women than in the population at large.

There are, however, a number of very uncommon neoplastic diseases that are inherited. The condition *polyposis coli* is transmitted as an autosomal dominant trait; sooner or later one of the lesions becomes malignant, and the patient dies of carcinoma of the colon, usually before the age of 40 years. The very uncommon tumor *retinoblastoma* (see Chapter 42) is also inherited as a Mendelian dominant trait. With these and a few other extremely rare exceptions, there is little evidence that the tendency to develop cancer is inherited.

HORMONAL FACTORS

The early observations that the administration of estrogens to mice led to an increased incidence of cancer of the breast was at first thought to indicate that hormonal imbalance could cause cancer in humans. However, it was soon appreciated that in mice cancer of the breast is due to a viral infection by the Bittner virus, and that the major effect of the estrogens was to allow the male mice to develop breasts in which cancer could develop. There have been similar instances in human pathology. Some men who have been deliberately castrated and undergone "sex change operations," and who have been administered estrogens for developing breasts, have subsequently developed cancer of the breast and have died of this disease. There is indeed little evidence that hormones play a major part in the cause of most human tumors. Nevertheless, hormones are related to tumors in various subtle ways. Some teenage girls whose mothers were given the synthetic estrogen *diethylstilbestrol* during pregnancy have subsequently developed *carcinoma of the vagina*. This disease is extremely rare under normal conditions. It seems that the effect of estrogens on the developing fetus is to allow certain vestigial structures to remain; these subsequently developed into tumors during the offspring's adolescence.

Hormone-Dependent Tumors. If hormones can seldom be directly incriminated in the cause of human cancer, they are undoubtedly of great importance in maintaining the growth of some tumors, which are called *hormone-dependent tumors*. The best example is carcinoma of the prostate.

Both the normal prostatic epithelium and the carcinoma derived from it are dependent for their integrity upon a supply of testosterone. If patients with cancer of the prostate are castrated, there is often a dramatic relief of symptoms and regression of both the primary tumor and its metastases. Both castration and the administration of estrogens are now used in the treatment of carcinoma of the prostate. Unfortunately, although there is some initial response, the patients ultimately die of the tumor since it seems to lose its hormonal dependency.

Carcinoma of the breast is another tumor that manifests hormone dependency in some patients. The picture is complicated, however, because the tumor seems to depend upon ovarian, adrenal, and pituitary hormones. The treatment is somewhat arbitrary; it is found that some patients are aided by the administration of estrogens, while others derive benefit from the removal of the ovaries, adrenal glands, or pituitary. In each instance the remission is unfortunately only temporary, for the treatment has an ameliorative effect but not a curative one.

VIRAL INFECTIONS

Fowl leukemia was shown to be transmissible by a virus in 1908 by Ellerman and Bang; a short time later fowl sarcoma was observed by Rous to be transmissible. Since then a number of animal tumors have been identified that can be transmitted by viruslike particles. One of the most interesting is the agent responsible for cancer of the breast in mice. This is known as the *Bittner factor* and is an agent that is secreted in the milk and infects the newborn suckling mice. The females that develop subsequently die of cancer of the breast. Infected males do not develop cancer unless given estrogens to encourage breast development.

The tumor-producing, or *oncogenic viruses*, which are now known fall into two groups:

DNA Oncogenic Viruses. The common wart in humans is caused by a papovavirus and may be regarded as a benign type of tumor. Rabbits suffer from a similar squamous-cell papilloma called the Shope papilloma; this ultimately becomes malignant and metastasizes as a squamous-cell carcinoma. This malignant propensity is not shown with human warts. The Epstein-Barr virus, which is associated with infectious mononucleosis, is thought to be a factor in the cause of the Burkitt lymphoma, but although the association is close, proof that it is the cause of the tumor is still lacking. Likewise, the herpes simplex virus appears to be more common in patients with cancer of the cervix; once again, the precise relationship is not clear.

Because viruses grow readily in cancer cells, it is difficult to be sure whether a virus found in association with a tumor is the cause of that tumor or merely a passenger that happened to be growing rather readily in the malignant cells. The *polyomavirus* is another oncogenic DNA virus that has been studied in great detail. It causes various types of tumors in many species of animals if injected into them. One of the curious features of this virus is that, having produced a tumor, it can no longer be found in the tumor cells. There is, however, evidence that parts of the viral genome are present. It seems that the DNA or part of the DNA of the virus becomes incorporated into the nuclear genetic material of the malignant or transformed cell (see below). The polyoma virus is closely related to a simian virus (SV-40), which is a common commensal found in monkey kidney cells. This emphasizes the danger of using animal tissue cultures when preparing vaccines for human use. Both the polyoma and the SV-40 viruses induce changes in cells growing in tissue culture. The cells show rapid, unruly, proliferation and when implanted into an animal behave like malignant cells. This change is called *cell transformation* and is the *in vitro* manifestation of the development of malignancy.

RNA Oncogenic Viruses. These viruses differ from the DNA tumor viruses in that they commonly appear to produce tumors in their natural host; furthermore, the transformed cells regularly produce large quantities of infectious virus. The Rous virus belongs to this group, as does the virus that causes fowl leukemia. The mode of action of the RNA viruses is fascinating. It seems that the viral RNA leads to the production of DNA by means of a process of reverse transcription (see Chapter 2). This DNA can then reproduce and finally become inserted into a host chromosome. The DNA, in fact, becomes part of the genetic make-up of the new cancer cell.

The Bittner virus is also an RNA virus, and contains an RNA-dependent DNA polymerase that catalyzes the synthesis of DNA. It has been found that the DNA synthesized by this virus is complementary to RNA extracted from human breast cancers. There is considerable evidence that human breast cancers contain an RNA oncogenic virus very similar to the Bittner factor. The precise relationship of the virus to the tumor is as yet undetermined.

CANCER FOLLOWING CHRONIC DISEASE

It has often been taught that cancer follows prolonged stimulation of a tissue through "chronic irritation." Now that carcinogenic chemicals and agents have been discovered, it seems unlikely that pure physical irritation, acting alone, can produce cancer. Nevertheless, there are a number of conditions which may be regarded as precancerous, since the development of tumors is more common in the lesions than it is in normal tissue. Chronic skin ulcers from whatever cause are sometimes complicated by the later development of squamous cell carcinoma. About 90 per cent of primary liver cell cancer in humans is superimposed on a previous cirrhosis (see Chapter 33). Other examples in other organs could be quoted, but they are all rare, and it must be accepted that the great majority of human tumors apparently arise in previously normal tissue.

Early Stages in the Development of Cancer

In some organs cancer does not develop suddenly. Cancer of the epithelia of the skin and uterine cervix illustrates this well (Fig. 17–17 to 17–19). The first stage results in irregular maturation of the epithelial cells, and this *dysplasia* steadily progresses until the whole epithelium is replaced by atypical, pleomorphic cells that have the cytological features of carcinoma. At this stage the basement membrane is still intact, and the condition is called *carcinoma-in-situ*. The final stage results in invasion of the underlying connective tissues and subsequent metastasis. The whole process probably takes several years.

The cells of the cervix uteri are shed into the vaginal secretions; a smear from these can be examined for the presence of atypical cells. This examination forms the basis of exfoliative cytology, which was pioneered by Papanicolaou. By regular examination of "Pap smears" of adult women the early stages in the development of carcinoma can be detected, and the occurrence of invasive cancer can be prevented.

Carcinoma in situ is now recognized in other organs and has been studied most extensively in the skin, which is so easily examined. Bowen's disease and actinic keratoses provide obvious examples (see Chapter 41).

The Nature of Cancer

Cancer is generally assumed to be due to a change in the character of the cells, which causes them to exhibit uncontrolled growth. The possibility that

FIGURE 17–17. *Epidermal dysplasia.*

The epidermis is seen to be markedly thickened; this acanthotic area ends abruptly where it becomes continuous with the normal epidermis. In addition to being abnormally thick the affected epidermis contains occasional atypical mitoses (mit). The cells are also somewhat larger than normal and show delay in maturation. This is an example of mild dysplasia. The tissue was from a person having Bowen's disease (intraepidermal squamous cell carcinoma) (× 250). Compare this photomicrograph with Figure 17–18.

FIGURE 17–18. *Epidermal dysplasia.*

The epidermis is acanthotic. Its cells are enlarged and show irregularity in size and shape. Mitoses can be identified (mit) and the keratin layer shows occasional remnants of nuclei, a condition termed parakeratosis (× 250). Compare the degree of dysplasia in this picture with that depicted in Figures 17–17 and 17–19.

FIGURE 17–19.   *Carcinoma-in-situ.*

The epidermis contains many large atypical cells and abnormal mitoses (arrows). Parakeratosis is marked, and the entire epidermis has been thrown into folds (papillomatosis). Although the epidermal cells resemble those of a squamous-cell carcinoma, there is no invasion of the dermis (× 250). Compare this figure with Figures 17–9 and 17–18.

the connective-tissue stroma plays some part cannot be entirely ignored, because there are many examples in the embryological development in which the epidermis relies on the connective tissue for its stimulation and maintenance, and vice versa. The possibility that the essential change in cancer lies in the connective tissue has not been completely excluded. Nevertheless, it is generally assumed that the essential changes are in the cancer cell itself. The results of years of research have given us a vast amount of knowledge concerning the properties of such cells. The pleomorphic and bizarre appearances of malignant cells have already been described, and it is known that their chemical activities differ considerably from the normal. The changes detected are quantitatively rather than qualitatively different from the normal. Sometimes cells produce substances normally found in embryonic cells, but this can be regarded as a reversion to an older mode of growth rather than an acquisition of a new property.

Whether a tumor commences in one cell or simultaneously begins in many cells has been argued for years. Recent studies of tumors in women have provided a partial answer. It has been found that, with most tumors, all the tumor cells contain either the paternal X chromosome or the maternal X (see Lyon's hypothesis, Chapter 2). If the malignant change spreads from cell to cell like an infection, one would expect both types of cell to be involved. Thus, a tumor appears to be a clone of cells derived either from one cell or from a limited number of cells in one area.

The immunological aspects of cancer have been extensively investigated. Some tumors appear to lose tissue-specific antigens because of their poor differentiation, and it has been proposed that they thereby escape the immunological surveillance activity of lymphocytes. There is indeed some increase in the incidence of malignant tumors in patients who are immunologically deficient, but in general there is little evidence of immunological incompetence in cancer patients, except as a terminal event.

Some tumors develop new transplantation antigens. These may be individual for the particular tumor, or they may be related to viral infection in those animal tumors that have been investigated. An immunological reaction to these new antigens may be the means for holding some tumors in check—sometimes for many years. The heavy lymphocytic infiltrate around some tumors suggests that the cell-mediated immune response is involved in limiting the spread of these growths. Circulating immunoglobulins have been demonstrated against tumors, and it has been postulated that immune-complex formation can occur and can account for some of the curious manifestations of cancer, such as those not directly explicable by the presence of the tumor cells themselves.

The concept that the development of cancer can be held in check by an immunological response has led to attempts to cure cancer by stimulating the immune response. The current vogue for administering BCG ("BCG" stands for bacille Calmette-Guérin) to patients with terminal cancer is a reflection of this. Although some success has been attained with particular tumors, the results on the whole are disappointing. The evidence that cancer is due to a breakdown in immunological surveillance has yet to be proved.

The present treatment for cancer consists of the radical removal of the tumor by using either surgical resection or radiotherapy. These measures are effective only when the tumor is localized, but there is much evidence that cancer is not simply a local disease. Even if removal of the entire area were feasible, the presence of secondary deposits would present an unknown hazard. Since these may remain dormant for many years, it is evident that an assessment of the effects of local treatment is very difficult. When the disease is clinically generalized, the cytotoxic drugs may be used as a means of attack. Hormone therapy can produce some alleviation of symptoms in particular cases.

The most successful approach to the control of cancer at the present time lies in its prevention. The many known physical and chemical carcinogenic agents have already been described, and their avoidance can appreciably reduce the incidence of cancer. Each tumor must be considered separately; for instance, a reduction in the amount of cigarette smoking and atmospheric pollution would undoubtedly reduce the incidence of lung cancer, and the avoidance of undue exposure to radiation would reduce the incidence of leukemia.

A second method of cancer prophylaxis is the treatment of known precancerous lesions. A regular Pap smear can reduce the incidence of uterine cancer; once again, each individual type of tumor must be considered separately.

Review Questions

1. Compare the properties of a benign tumor with those of a malignant one.
2. Predict the microscopic appearance and the effects of a carcinoma of the rectum. How would these affect the patient? Where would you expect to find metastases?
3. Distinguish between the following:
    (a) a malignant tumor of ectoderm and a carcinoma
    (b) a malignant tumor of mesoderm and a sarcoma.
4. Give three examples of a benign tumor that can cause death.
5. A patient who had had a mastectomy (removal of the breast) for carcinoma of the breast, develops metastatic carcinoma in the liver. Biopsy shows an adenocarcinoma. Postulate how this might have occurred.
6. Compare carcinoma with sarcoma.
7. Distinguish between a basal-cell carcinoma and
    (a) a squamous-cell carcinoma of the skin
    (b) a squamous-cell papilloma of the skin.
8. Discuss the structure of the following tumors and indicate their probable cell of origin:
    (a) ovarian teratoma
    (b) neuroblastoma
    (c) squamous-cell carcinoma of the bronchus.
9. How has the Lyon hypothesis been utilized in the investigation of the pathogenesis of tumors?
10. Compare the oncogenic DNA viruses with the oncogenic RNA viruses.

Selected Readings

Ackerman, L. V., and Rosai, J.: Surgical Pathology. 5th ed. St. Louis, The C. V. Mosby Company, 1974.
    A standard textbook covering the morphology of tumors and other aspects of surgical pathology.
Allen, D. W., and Cole, P.: Viruses and human cancer. New England Journal of Medicine, 286:70–82, 1972.
Editorial: Risk of cancer in ulcerative colitis. New England Journal of Medicine, 278:907, 1968.
Epstein, M. A.: The possible role of viruses in human cancer. Lancet, 1:1344–1347, 1971.
Fialkow, P. J.: The origin and development of human tumors studied with cell markers. New England Journal of Medicine, 291:26–35, 1974.
Gerald, P. S.: Origin of teratomas. New England Journal of Medicine, 292:103–104, 1975.
Herbst, A. L., Kusman, R. J., Scully, R. E., and Poskanzec, D. C.: Clear-cell adenocarcinoma of the genital tract in young females. New England Journal of Medicine, 287:1259–1264, 1972.
Leading Article: Circulating cancer cells. Lancet, 2:84–85, 1967.
Leading Article: Geography of primary liver cancer. British Medical Journal, 1:381–382, 1970.
Leading Article: E.B. virus, Burkitt lymphoma, and nasopharyngeal carcinoma. Lancet, 1:218–219, 1971.
Leading Article: Viruses and human breast cancer. Lancet, 1:359–360, 1972.
Leading Article: Herpesvirus and cancer of the uterine cervix. British Medical Journal, 1:671–672, 1976.
Ryser, H. J.-P.: Chemical carcinogenesis. New England Journal of Medicine, 285:721–734, 1971.
U.S. Armed Forces Institute of Pathology: Atlas of Tumor Pathology. Many fascicles have been published and each covers the tumors of a particular organ or system. Series 1–2, Washington, D.C., 1949–1976.

Chapter 18

After studying this chapter the student should be able to:

- Define the terms atomic number, mass number, and isotope.
- Describe in simple terms the atomic structure of hydrogen and its two isotopes.
- Describe alpha particles, beta particles, gamma rays, and x-rays with respect to their
    - (a) physical nature
    - (b) powers of penetration
    - (c) ability to produce ionization and tissue damage.
- Distinguish between the direct and indirect action of ionizing radiations.
- Describe the effects of irradiation on a cell and relate them to the stages of the mitotic cycle.
- Describe the relative sensitivities of cells when they are irradiated in the intact animal.
- Describe the effects of ionizing radiation on skin, gonads, lung, and bone.

294

IONIZING RADIATIONS AND THEIR EFFECTS

- Describe the immediate effects of total body irradiation with
    (a) 500 rads
    (b) 800 to 5000 rads
    (c) more than 5000 rads.
- Describe two important late effects of total body irradiation.
- List the factors that enable one to predict the radiosensitivity of a tumor.

INTRODUCTION

Although the damaging effects of ionizing radiation have been known since the discovery of x-rays and radium, it took the dramatic events of the atomic explosions at Hiroshima and Nagasaki to bring these to the fore. The effects of radiation vary from local tissue damage leading to ulceration that can terminate in cancer, to such disorders as leukemia and genetic damage. Since the physical properties of ionizing radiation have been well studied, it might be expected that the damage that the radiation produces and the mechanisms involved would be easy to explain. Such has not been the case, because the fundamental processes that occur in cells are poorly understood. Cancer produced by ionizing radiation is no easier to explain than that which evolves spontaneously or is produced by a chemical carcinogen.

Atoms are pictured as consisting of a nucleus containing closely packed protons and neutrons, around which are a number of orbiting electrons. Neutrons and protons are of equal mass, a proton having a unit positive charge, a neutron having no charge. An electron has a unit negative charge, and a mass of only 1/2000 of a proton. The *atomic number*, Z, of an element is defined as the number of protons in the nucleus; when the atom is in an electrically neutral state, the number of orbiting electrons is equal to the number of protons in the nucleus. The *mass number* of an element is the total number of protons and neutrons present in the nucleus (Fig. 18–1).

An element always has a particular atomic number, but various forms, or *isotopes*, can exist; these have differing mass numbers. Thus, the common form of hydrogen (mass number 1) has one proton in its nucleus and one orbiting electron. The isotope *deuterium* (mass number 2) has one proton and one neutron in its nucleus, whereas *tritium* (mass number 3) has one proton and two neutrons in its nucleus. Each has an atomic number of 1. Many other elements have isotopic forms, and exist in nature as mixtures of these isotopes.

The various isotopes of a particular element behave similarly in chemical reactions but differ in certain physical properties that are related to mass. Some

FIGURE 18–1. *Hydrogen and its isotopes.*

isotopes lose energy and mass spontaneously and emit radiations. Such *radio-active isotopes* are of great value in medicine. Some, such as radium, occur naturally, whereas others are man-made. Most of these radioactive isotopes give off three types of radiation:

1. *Alpha "rays."* These are particulate and consist of helium nuclei with two positive charges and a mass of 4.

2. *Beta "rays."* These are electrons of negligible mass but each having one negative charge.

3. *Gamma "rays."* These are electromagnetic waves of short wavelength. They are of a nature similar to x-rays.

X-rays are generated by allowing high-speed electrons to hit a target. Their energy is then changed into heat and electromagnetic waves of varying wavelengths, depending upon the voltage that is used to accelerate the electrons. When a low voltage, *e.g.,* 70 kilovolts (kV), is used, the x-rays have a long wavelength and a relatively poor penetrating power (they are said to be "soft"). X-rays of this nature are readily stopped by soft tissues and are used in diagnostic radiography. For cancer treatment, x-rays are generated at much higher voltage, are therefore of shorter wavelength, and penetrate the tissues of the body more readily.

CHANGES INDUCED IN MATTER BY PASSAGE OF IONIZING RADIATION

When ionizing radiation passes through matter, energy is absorbed. This leads to a variety of physicochemical events. Some molecules are excited, and ions and free radicals are formed. The changes vary with each particular variety of radiation.

Particulate Radiation. The density of ionization for charged particles is *directly proportional to the square of their charge and inversely proportional to their velocity.* Thus, electrons and protons of equal velocity produce the same ion density; as they slow down, however, the density increases. Alpha particles (with their double charge and slow velocity) produce very dense ionization—hence, more damage.

BETA PARTICLES.   Because of their charge and negligible mass, beta particles are rapidly slowed down and give up energy to atoms through which they pass. They therefore have little power of penetration and can be used in the treatment of superficial tumors. Beta particles or artificially produced beams of electrons are used therapeutically in certain forms of skin tumors. Electrons generated at 2 MeV (million electron volts) have a maximum range of about 1 cm in soft tissues.

ALPHA PARTICLES.   These have a double positive charge and a mass of 4. Their high charge and slow velocity means that they have little penetrating power. Alpha particles are readily stopped by the superficial layers of the epidermis; therefore, there is little danger of damage from an external radiating source. If taken internally, however, radioactive elements that emit alpha particles can cause serious damage.

Electromagnetic Radiation.   Gamma rays and x-rays have much greater penetrating power than the particulate radiations. The shorter the wavelengths, the greater their penetration. It should be noted that the particulate radiations have a definite range of penetration, whereas the electromagnetic radiations are merely reduced in quantity. Thus, a particular thickness of a sheet of material (the half-value thickness) will reduce the intensity by half, a further thickness will reduce it by another half, and so forth. When gamma and x-rays traverse matter, they give up a quantity of energy and cause atoms to emit high-velocity electrons, which then behave like beta particles. Gamma and x-rays of high energy (short wavelength) produce fewer ionizations than do low-energy x-rays. They are therefore less destructive, since damage is caused by energy that is absorbed.

Biological Effects of Ionizing Radiation

The net effects of these various changes is that molecules become more reactive, causing chemical changes to occur. Large molecules such as DNA and proteins can be affected by two separate processes:

DIRECT ACTION.   Chemical change may be caused by energy absorbed in the molecule itself.

INDIRECT ACTION.   Alternatively, chemical change may be induced in a large molecule from the action of an adjacent ion or radical that had been produced by the effect of ionizing radiation on a nearby water molecule. Many of the biological effects of ionizing radiation are due primarily to the effects on water. Highly reactive ions are formed, particularly in the presence of free oxygen.

It is generally supposed that ionizing radiations initially produce an intracellular chemical change and that this leads to a *biochemical lesion,* which in turn produces morphological and functional changes in the affected cells. The nature of this biochemical lesion is poorly understood.

EFFECTS ON THE CELL

Although it would be desirable to explain cellular damage in terms of known physicochemical changes, this is not yet possible. With very high dosages, *e.g.*, in the order of 10,000 rads* or more, cells die regardless of their stage in the mitotic cycle. With a lower dosage of radiation, DNA synthesis is inhibited and mitosis is delayed. When DNA synthesis is resumed, it may not be followed by mitosis, resulting in the formation of giant nuclei. When mitosis does occur, various chromosomal abnormalities become apparent. Breaks in chromosomes are characteristic, and the fragments may reunite in an abnormal way or join other chromosomes. Sometimes these abnormalities are incompatible with life, and the cell dies.

Fractionated doses of radiation do not produce a strictly cumulative effect, and an intracellular mechanism seems to exist to correct radiation damage.

The sensitivity of cells to damage varies according to the stage in the mitotic cycle at which the radiation is given. Maximum sensitivity occurs in most cell types during mitosis itself. It follows that normal tissues with a high mitotic rate, *e.g.*, lymphoid and hematopoietic, are more sensitive than are those in which mitosis rarely or never occurs, *e.g.*, skeletal and cardiac muscle. Likewise, as a general principle malignant tumors are more sensitive than either benign tumors or the parent tissue of origin.

Two main theories have been proposed to explain the mechanism of cellular damage:

THE TARGET THEORY. This supposes that damage to cells is related to injury of a specific sensitive spot in the cell. Attractive as it may be to visualize a chromosome or a particular organelle as a target, there is little evidence to support this theory.

THE POISON THEORY. This supposes that ionization leads to the production of poisonous substances — usually powerful oxidizing agents — that then cause the cellular damage. There is considerable evidence that oxidizing substances are indeed formed in irradiated tissues. Thus, chemicals with a reducing action, *e.g.*, cysteine, give some degree of protection against ionizing radiation if they are present at the time of the initial irradiation. Furthermore, if tissues are irradiated in the absence of oxygen, they show considerably more resistance. This is probably because free oxygen is necessary for the production of oxidizing substances by ionizing radiation. This observation is of some importance in clinical radiotherapy, because many areas of a tumor are relatively hypoxic and conceivably could be protected during radiation therapy. Attempts have been made to overcome this by allowing patients to breathe pure oxygen under pressure during the actual administration of radiotherapy.

EFFECTS ON THE INTACT ANIMAL

This important aspect of radiobiology is also the most difficult and least well understood. A remarkable feature is the delay in the appearance of radia-

---

*The original unit of measurement of radiation was the *Roentgen* (*r*), which was named after the discoverer of x-rays and was related to the number of ions produced in 1 ml of air. A more logical unit of measurement is the *rad*, which is related to the amount of energy absorbed per gram of substance radiated. "Rad" is an acronym for *r*adiation *a*bsorbed *d*ose.

tion lesions. The actual damage caused by radiation must be almost instantaneous, and yet the effects may not be apparent for days, months, or even years. An experiment with amphibians has helped to explain this phenomenon. Frogs can be given a dose of radiation that will kill them within six weeks. If irradiated animals are kept at 5° C, they remain alive for several months, but on being warmed up, they die within six weeks. The experiments indicate that radiation damage manifests itself only when cells are active. This lends strong support to the concept that a biochemical lesion is produced. Such a lesion is not in itself harmful, but it produces effects when cellular activity commences. This goes some way toward explaining two of the phenomena of radiation damage:

1. *Relative Sensitivity of Cells.* In the human, the germinal cells of the ovary are the most sensitive. Then, in order from most to least sensitive, are the seminiferous epithelium of the testis, the lymphocytes, the erythropoietic and myeloid marrow cells, the intestinal epithelium, the muscle cells, and the nerve cells. This order of sensitivity to some extent parallels the rate of mitoses seen in the various tissues. Thus, the highly active intestinal epithelium is sensitive, whereas neurons, which never divide, are relatively resistant.

2. *The Chronic Nature of Radiation Lesions.* When tissue is irradiated, several phases of damage occur. This is probably because different tissues have different rates of division and metabolic activity and therefore exhibit damage at different times. Hence, an irradiated area shows changes that persist for many weeks or months and have the characteristics of chronic inflammation. This inflammation can follow a single exposure of ionizing radiation.

When studying the action of radiation on any tissue, one must consider two main effects: (1) *the primary effect* of radiation on the tissue concerned; and (2) *the secondary effect,* which is due to damage to adjacent tissues. The most important example of this is damage to blood vessels, which generally results in thrombosis or gradual obliteration due to endarteritis obliterans. The ischemia that follows either event leads to necrosis. Some authorities attribute much of the beneficial effects of radiotherapy in cancer to this mechanism.

EFFECTS OF IRRADIATION ON INDIVIDUAL TISSUES

SKIN. Following a single ionizing radiation to the skin there is a phase of erythema beginning at about 10 days and showing all the features of acute inflammation. This phase is followed by pigmentation, due to melanin formation, causing the skin to acquire a dusky hue. With a heavy dosage, necrosis follows and an ulcer is produced. This heals slowly, and even when healed, the scar may subsequently break down, after only trivial injury. With a lower dose of irradiation of skin a smoldering chronic inflammation ensues. This is made evident by fibrosis and endarteritis obliterans. Giant fibroblasts are often seen in the dermis. The hair follicles and sebaceous glands are more sensitive than the epidermis, and these structures tend to disappear. After several years, the area of irradiation appears atrophic. There is disturbance of pigmentation, and the area—although ischemic—shows the presence of dilated blood vessels (telangiectasia). The disturbed pigmentation (areas of hyperpigmentation and hypopigmentation) combined with atrophy and telangiectasia is called

FIGURE 18–2. *Radiodermatitis and its complications.*

This patient has severe dermatitis as a result of repeated radiation treatments for atopic dermatitis. A new basal-cell carcinoma (BCC) is present just above the right upper lip. A chronic indolent ulcer (Ulc) is present on the left cheek. The black tissue in the base of the ulcer is necrotic facial bone. Several attempts to close this defect by skin grafting have failed. Note that part of the nose has been lost. For further information, see Case History I.

poikiloderma (Fig. 18–2). This is an unfortunate end-result, which is sometimes seen when a tumor such as a basal-cell carcinoma is treated by radiotherapy.

Case History I. (See Figure 18–2.) As a teenager and young woman, the patient had atopic dermatitis that was treated by local radiation and by many doctors. From repeated exposure to radiation, the patient developed severe radiodermatitis. During the previous 10 years several basal-cell carcinomas had appeared and had been treated by curettage or excision. The figure shows that a new tumor has developed and that necrotic facial bone is visible.

This patient's history illustrates many points:
1. It is dangerous to treat benign conditions with radiation, particularly in young people.
2. A patient can go from one physician to another, each being unaware of the treatment administered by the other. It was estimated that parts of this patient's face had received a total dose of over 11,000 rads. This is two to three times the dose commonly given to treat a malignant tumor.
3. Chronic ulceration is a feature of radiodermatitis.
4. Healing of radiation ulcers is slow, and skin grafting is often unsatisfactory because of the local ischemia.
5. Multiple tumors can develop in radiation-damaged tissues.

GONADS.   The ovaries and testes are particularly susceptible to irradiation damage, and with a dose of over 500 rads, the germinal cells are destroyed and permanent sterility results.

LUNGS.   Irradiation of lungs produces inflammatory changes that culminate in fibrosis. This is a complication of radiotherapy applied in the treatment of cancer of the lung or cancer of the breast (Fig. 18–3).

BONE.   Irradiation of bone produces inflammatory changes that can persist for years and be punctuated by episodes of painful radionecrosis. Doses of over

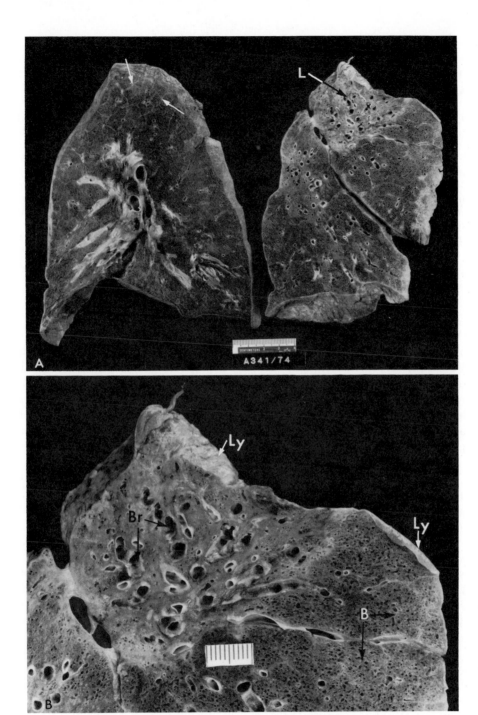

FIGURE 18–3. *Radiation fibrosis of lung.*

Specimens of lung taken at necropsy from a patient who had died of respiratory failure. *A,* The cut surface of both lungs. The right lung exhibits prominent septa (arrows) that outline the lung lobules. Microscopically, these septa are shown to contain tumor. The apex of the left lung (L) is shrunken. *B,* The lung parenchyma is seen to have been destroyed and replaced by fibrous tissue. The bronchi (Br) are dilated, a condition called *bronchiectasis.* Below this, the lung is consolidated, but some dilated bronchioles (B) can be seen. Lymphatic vessels (Ly) on the pleural surface contain tumor. (For a more complete description, see Case History II.)

301

1000 rads inhibit the growth of bone at the epiphyses, leading to stunted growth of the part affected.

Case History II. (See Figure 18–3.)   The patient was a 39-year-old woman whose left breast had been removed for carcinoma. Since several axillary lymph nodes had been found to contain metastatic tumor, postoperative radiotherapy was given. She remained well for two years but then began to experience fever, night sweats, and shortness of breath. A lung infection had been suspected, but in spite of extensive investigations, no definite diagnosis could be made. Thoracotomy and open-lung biopsy were performed in the hope that some treatable condition was present. The specimen (Fig. 18–3) showed extensive fibrosis consistent with radiation damage; in addition, however, carcinoma cells were present in lymphatic vessels. Death occurred three days later from respiratory failure. Necropsy revealed metastatic carcinoma in lungs, mediastinal lymph nodes, liver, and vertebrae. No tumor was present in the mastectomy scar or the right breast. Radiation damage was marked in the left upper lobe of the lung.

EFFECTS OF IRRADIATION ON THE WHOLE BODY

When the whole body is exposed to irradiation, the effect is the sum total of the damage to all tissues. This is called the *radiation syndrome.* It has been studied extensively in animals, but in humans experience is limited only to those occasional accidents that have occurred in atomic experiments and to those individuals involved in the Japanese atomic explosions. It is convenient to describe the effects of total body irradiation under two headings: (1) those occurring during the first two months (immediate effects) and, (2) those occurring later (late effects).

Immediate Effects of Total Body Irradiation

VERY HEAVY DOSAGE (over 5000 rads per single exposure).   Death usually occurs within a day or two, with the patient developing shock, convulsions, and coma. The effects are due to a direct action on the central nervous system, since a similar syndrome results when the head alone is irradiated.

MODERATE DOSAGE (800 to 5000 rads per single exposure).   An initial phase occurs shortly after irradiation and is manifested as loss of appetite, nausea, and vomiting. The explanation for this is not known. The symptoms usually abate, only to recur some two to three days later, with intractable severity. Vomiting and diarrhea dominate the picture, and death occurs from dehydration and shock. These serious effects are due to necrosis of the intestinal epithelium.

LOW DOSAGE (less than 800 rads per single exposure).   The initial phase of nausea and vomiting is less severe, and the subject may then appear to make a complete recovery. Two to three weeks later the results of bone-marrow aplasia become apparent. The serious effects of irradiation of this type are due to damage to the hematopoietic tissues. The granulocyte count falls after about one week and subsequently reaches very low levels. This predisposes the person to infection, particularly of the mouth and lungs. The lymphocytes show the earliest drop, and there is marked lymphopenia within a day or two. This is associated with an impaired immune response. The platelets also decrease in number, and there is marked thrombocytopenia within four weeks. This condition predisposes the victim to severe hemorrhage, often into the lungs. Although the red-cell precursors are highly radiosensitive, the mature red cells are resistant, and the effects of bone marrow aplasia on the peripheral count are delayed. Thus, the anemia is of gradual onset, and is maximal at six to eight weeks in those individuals who survive the effects of agranulocytosis and thrombocytopenia. If the patient survives, the blood counts return to normal over a period of many months. In humans, 450 rads is generally taken as the dose that will kill 50 per cent of those exposed.

Late Effects of Total Body Irradiation.   Those exposed to a sublethal dose may suffer from the following aftereffects:

THE CARCINOGENIC EFFECT.   Widespread irradiation of the bone marrow leads to an increased incidence of leukemia. This has been recorded in the survivors of the Nagasaki and Hiroshima atomic explosions, and in patients with ankylosing spondylitis treated with radiotherapy. Likewise, local irradiation is followed by an increased incidence of malignant tumors at that site. Thus, carcinoma of the skin was reported as early as 1902 in workers who handled radioactive material or who were exposed to x-rays. Other examples are carcinoma of the thyroid following accidental irradiation of the gland for treatment of mediastinal lesions and osteosarcoma following local irradiation of bone lesions. Tumors have also been reported after the ingestion of radioactive substances such as radium and mesothorium, which are stored in the bones.

GENETIC EFFECT.   The ability of ionizing radiation to increase the rate of mutation is well established in microorganisms, plants, and animals. Mutations in the germ cells are of potential significance, since the new factor is handed down to subsequent generations. In clinical practice it is usual to protect the genitalia as much as possible during routine radiography for this reason.

Radiotherapy

The destructive effects of ionizing radiation on living cells, particularly those in an active state, have led to their widespread use in the treatment of malignant disease. Radiotherapy plays an important part in the curative treatment of some primary cancers, as well as in the palliation of those that have metastasized and are beyond the scope of surgical removal.

FACTORS INFLUENCING RESPONSE

Tumors differ widely in their response to radiotherapy, and it is only after treatment has commenced that the effects can be assessed. Nevertheless, there are some guidelines that help one to predict the probable local results. The following factors are of importance.

Tissue of Origin.   The relative sensitivity of the normal tissue is often related to the radiosensitivities of the tumors derived from it. Thus the lymphomas, like the parent lymphoreticular system, tend to be highly radiosensitive. Fibrosarcomas, on the other hand, are relatively radioresistant, like the normal fibroblast.

Degree of Differentiation and Mitotic Activity.   It is generally taught that within any tumor group the most undifferentiated tumors are also the most radiosensitive. As a generalization this is true; nevertheless, the histological features of a tumor are no sure guide to its sensitivity in practice. Thus, a well-differentiated squamous-cell carcinoma of the tongue or skin is usually highly responsive to treatment.

The Tumor Bed.   The nature of the stroma supporting a tumor is also a factor of importance. If it is avascular as a result of previous radiation, the tumor tends to be more resistant. This has been attributed to the effects of hypoxia. It has been suggested that the stroma, particularly its lymphoid component, plays a part in restraining the growth of some tumors. Excessive irradiation, by destroying the stroma, might have a deleterious effect, since those tumor cells that survive are able to grow and subsequently metastasize.

Nature of the Individual Tumor.   In practice, it has been found that certain tumors respond well, while others are resistant. Thus, most basal-cell and squamous-cell carcinomas of the skin are sensitive to treatment, whereas squamous-cell carcinoma of the lung is less responsive.

THE CURE RATE

As with surgical treatment, the cure rate to be expected from radiotherapy must be considered in relation to the general properties of the tumor. Many malignant tumors (*e.g.,* the lymphomas) cannot be regarded as local diseases; although a tumor mass may respond remarkably well, the clinical course is characterized by the recurrence of the disease at other sites. Likewise, the oat-cell carcinoma of the lung is highly radiosensitive, and the local tumor masses in the chest melt with remarkable rapidity. Nevertheless, this tumor nearly always metastasizes widely, and death occurs from this generalized spread.

Radiotherapy is often effective as a palliative treatment, since it can reduce the size of a tumor mass and produce relief of symptoms. A mediastinal mass, such as that produced by oat-cell carcinoma or lymphoma, can obstruct the major blood vessels and trachea, producing grave respiratory difficulty: this condition can be alleviated by local irradiation. Bony metastases are often extremely painful, and the pain can be relieved by treatment. With relatively slow growing tumors (*e.g.,* cancer of the breast and Hodgkin's disease) radiotherapy can hold the disease in check for long periods and give the patient several years of useful life. It may well be that radiotherapy and surgery are both forms of palliation that allow the body to retard the growth of a tumor; depending upon whether the malignant cells stay dormant for a short or long period, one may speak of a "5-year cure," a "10-year cure," and so forth. It is doubtful, however, that any of our present modes of treatment of cancer can be regarded as curative, if by "cure" one means the complete eradication of all malignant cells.

Review Questions

1. A patient has a basal-cell carcinoma of the skin that forms a mass 1.0 cm in diameter and is about 0.25 cm thick. It is not attached to the underlying muscle. Would you expect this to be treated with
     (a) a beam of high-speed electrons
     (b) alpha particles

(c) x-rays generated at 60 to 140 kV

(d) x-rays generated at 2.0 MeV?

Give reasons for your choice.

2. Describe the changes that could be seen in the skin after the delivery of 1000 rads of x-rays (generated at 250 kV) to a rectangular area 4 × 5 cm after the following intervals of time:

(a) 1 hour

(b) 14 days

(c) 1 year

(d) many years.

3. List the following tissues in their order of sensitivity to radiation: germinal cells of the ovary, epidermis, muscle cells, intestinal epithelium, and lymphocytes.

4. A scientist is accidentally exposed to 250 rads of total body irradiation. What are the probable effects of this accident on the patient? Is he or she likely to survive? From what might the person die?

Selected Readings

Dalrymple, G. V., Gaulden, M. E., Kollmorgen, G. M., and Vogel, H. H., Jr.: Medical Radiation Biology. Philadelphia, W. B. Saunders Company, 1973. A reference book with an emphasis on the physico-chemical changes produced in biological systems.

Leading Article: Hyperbaric oxygen and radiotherapy. British Medical Journal, 2:368, 1972.

Pollard, E. C.: The biological action of ionizing radiation. American Scientist, 57:206–236, 1969.

Prasad, K. N.: Human Radiation Biology. New York, Harper & Row, Publishers, 1974. A comprehensive but readable account of the subject in 508 pages.

Tievsky, G.: Ionizing Radiation. Springfield, Ill., Charles C Thomas, Publisher, 1962. An elementary account in 154 pages.

Chapter 19

DISORDERS OF FLUID AND ELECTROLYTE BALANCE: EDEMA

After studying this chapter the student should be able to:

- Describe the three major fluid compartments of the body and indicate the volume of each in an average normal adult human being.
- List the important ions in each of the major compartments and describe the permeability of the membranes that separate the compartments.
- Discuss the value of expressing electrolyte concentrations in milliequivalents per liter.
- Give an account of the factors that maintain the body's content of water at a constant level.
- Describe the causes and effects of the following conditions:
    - (a) pure water deficiency
    - (b) pure water excess
    - (c) combined salt and water deficiency
    - (d) combined salt and water excess.
- Describe the causes and effects of potassium depletion and of potassium excess.
- Define "acid" and "base."
- Describe four important buffer systems in the blood.
- Contrast respiratory acidosis with metabolic acidosis in terms of these factors:
    - (a) causes
    - (b) plasma bicarbonate levels
    - (c) arterial PCO_2
    - (d) clinical effects.
- Contrast respiratory alkalosis with metabolic alkalosis in terms of these factors:
    - (a) causes
    - (b) plasma bicarbonate levels
    - (c) arterial PCO_2
    - (d) clinical effects.
- Define "ascites," "hydrothorax," and "anasarca."
- List the types and causes of localized edema.
- List the types and causes of generalized edema.

Water is the principal component of the body and forms about 70 per cent of the lean body weight. Since adipose tissue contains little water, it follows that the water content of the average person is about 60 per cent of the body weight. The body can be discussed in terms of three "compartments"(intracellular space, interstitial space, and plasma), that are illustrated in Figure 19–1. Water is freely diffusable across the barriers that separate these various compartments; the volume of each is preserved by the osmotic, electrochemical, and hydrostatic forces acting upon it. With regard to osmosis, potassium, phosphate, and protein are important in the intracellular compartment, whereas sodium, chloride, and bicarbonate are important in the interstitial and intravascular compartments.

Electrolytes

GENERAL CONSIDERATIONS

The biological effects of an electrolyte depend to a considerable extent on its equivalent concentration, *i.e.*, the number of particles present and the number of charges carried by each. It is therefore appropriate to describe the concentration of electrolytes in terms of milliequivalents per liter.*

Expressing Electrolyte Concentration *in Milliequivalents per Liter*
To convert concentration of ions from mg per 100 ml to mEq per liter, use this simple formula:

$$\left(\frac{\text{mg per 100 ml}}{\text{Equivalent Weight of Ion}}\right) \times 10 = \text{mEq per liter}$$

The equivalent weight is 23 for sodium, 39 for potassium, 22.4 for bicarbonate (as ml CO_2 per 100 ml), and 4.1 for protein. Expressing electrolyte concentrations in mEq per liter is more logical than expressing them in grams or milligrams per 100 ml. It allows the importance of each electrolyte to be readily appreciated. Furthermore, since any solution must contain the same concentration of cations as anions, a balance can be struck between the two. This is shown in Table 19–1, which gives the composition of normal plasma.

Table 19–1 COMPOSITION OF NORMAL PLASMA

CATIONS (in mEq per liter)		ANIONS (in mEq per liter)	
Na^+	142	Cl^-	104
K^+	5	HCO_3^-	27
Ca^{++}	5	Other anions	7
Mg^{++}	2	Protein	16
TOTAL	154	TOTAL	154

It is evident that sodium is the all-important cation in the extracellular fluids and is balanced mainly by the combined concentration of bicarbonate and chloride. The "other anions," which are not measured directly, include HPO_4^{--} and SO_4^{--} as well as keto acids. It should be noted that the combined chloride and bicarbonate (131) subtracted from the combined sodium and potassium (147) is 16. This "anion gap" is normal. It is a useful figure to calculate, because an increase indicates the presence of an abnormal acid, *e.g.*, keto acids in diabetic acidosis and lactic acid in shock.

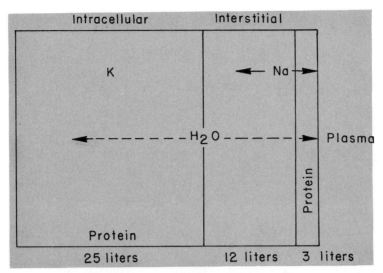

FIGURE 19–1. *The fluid compartments of the body.*

Diagrammatic representation of the three compartments in which the body's water is accommodated. An excess or deficiency of water, which is freely diffusible, produces the greatest effects in the largest compartment—the intracellular space. Changes in sodium affect mainly the interstitial compartment.

Fluid Balance

GENERAL CONSIDERATIONS

The total water content of the body is maintained at a constant level by balancing intake with output.

Water is derived mainly by drinking fluid; the amount of this varies according to individual custom and habit. Some water is contained in food, and about 300 ml is derived from the oxidative processes of metabolism. Fluid is lost in the urine (about 1500 ml per day); some is lost in the expired air (about 700 ml per day); some is lost in the feces (about 200 ml per day); and a moderate quantity is lost from the skin (300 to 500 ml per day). The mechanism by which fluid balance is attained can be considered under three headings.

1. Indirect Control. This includes the mechanisms that regulate sodium balance. Sodium cannot be retained without water (Fig. 19–2).

Aldosterone, a hormone secreted by the adrenal cortex, has the effect of increasing sodium reabsorption from the distal tubule of the kidney and thereby causes water retention as well. Sodium reabsorption from the proximal tubule is dependent to a large extent on the total glomerular filtrate. When the volume is reduced, as in shock and heart failure, sodium absorption is more complete, and water is also retained.

2. Renal Control. There are mechanisms that regulate the output of water by the kidney. The antidiuretic hormone (ADH) from the posterior lobe

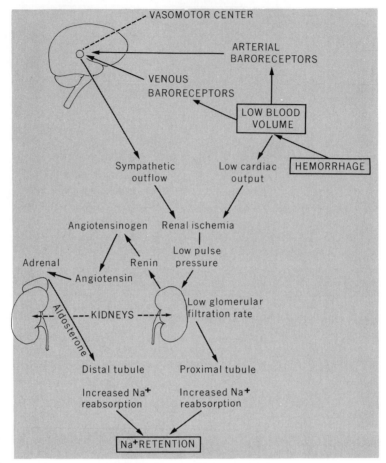

FIGURE 19–2. *Sodium retention.*

Diagrammatic representation of the means by which the body retains sodium after a sudden reduction in blood volume, *e.g.,* following a severe hemorrhage.

of the pituitary gland is important in this regulation. It acts by increasing water reabsorption from the collecting tubules of the kidney.

3. *Thirst.* Water intake is regulated by the sensation of thirst.

Water and sodium metabolism are so closely interrelated that it is convenient to consider them together.

DISTURBANCES IN WATER AND SODIUM BALANCE

Pure Water Deficiency. This condition follows deprivation of water. It is seen in enforced starvation and in patients who are unable to swallow because of dysphagia, esophageal obstruction, or coma. It may complicate diabetes insipidus, a disease due to lack of antidiuretic hormone (ADH). Patients with this disease pass enormous quantities of urine—often 20 liters a day—instead of the normal 1 to 1.5 liters.

EFFECTS. Since water can easily cross the membranes that separate the various fluid compartments, each is depleted in volume. The intracellular space, which is the largest compartment, is the most severely affected. Cellular dehydration causes intense thirst and eventually death.

Pure Water Excess. Excessive retention of water is called *water intoxication* and causes intracellular edema. It is encountered in patients who are given too much water too quickly. Rapid intravenous infusion of glucose solution is the common culprit, but even a large enema can lead to water intoxication in a susceptible patient, such as one in renal failure or in the immediate postoperative period, when water excretion is impaired. The effects of water excess are serious. Intracellular edema of brain and muscle causes vomiting, muscle cramps, headaches, convulsions, and—ultimately—death.

Combined Salt and Water Deficiency. Salt, or salt and water, deficiency is a common condition that is seen when there is a loss from any of the following:

(a) The gastrointestinal tract, such as following severe vomiting or diarrhea
(b) The skin, such as following prolonged excessive sweating (heat exhaustion)
(c) The kidney, such as following prolonged administration of diuretics for heart failure.

EFFECTS. The effect of salt—or salt and water—deficiency is a reduction in the volume of the extracellular fluids. The interstitial fluid volume is reduced in amount and the patient shows the clinical features of dehydration. The eyeballs are sunken, the skin is wrinkled, the tongue is dry, and the face is haggard. Surprisingly, thirst is often absent. The plasma volume is decreased, but vasoconstriction compensates for this. Since the veins are poorly filled, the blood pressure ultimately drops. Little urine is passed and renal failure may be superadded. The reduction in plasma volume is detectable by a rise in the hemoglobin concentration (hemoconcentration). Unless relieved, this condition rapidly terminates in circulatory failure.

Combined Salt and Water Excess. This is invariably an artificially induced condition that is seen in patients with defective renal function who are given excessive amounts of saline solution, such as during the early postoperative period or during the course of acute renal failure.

EFFECT. The excess fluid is distributed mainly in the extracellular compartments, which therefore expand. The manifestations of this are an increased venous pressure and edema, both systemic and pulmonary (see later).

DISTURBANCES OF POTASSIUM BALANCE

Potassium is an important intracellular ion; its level in the plasma is low (4.0 to 5.5 mEq per liter).

Potassium Depletion. Potassium can be lost from the body in the feces or in the urine. Chronic diarrhea, such as in ulcerative colitis, is a well-known cause of this depletion. Excess loss from the urine occurs in diabetes mellitus and following the use of certain diuretics (*e.g.*, chlorothiazide) in heart failure. Since cellular function is deranged, the effects of potassium deprivation are serious. In particular, the following structures are affected:

THE BRAIN.   Apathy, confusion, and coma can occur.

THE KIDNEY.   Degeneration of the tubules leads to polyuria and renal failure.

THE HEART.   Irregularity of the heart rate, hypotension, and heart failure can result.

MUSCLES.   Intense weakness of the muscles is characteristic. If death results from this ion depletion, it is generally due to respiratory failure caused by weakness of the muscles of respiration. Smooth muscle is also affected and paralytic ileus can follow.

Potassium Excess.   Retention of potassium is generally due to renal failure. Sometimes it is a complication of excessive potassium administration for potassium loss. The clinical manifestations of potassium retention are vague: mental confusion, apathy, and pains in the limbs. Although muscular weakness is also a feature, the most important complication is ventricular fibrillation; sudden death is not uncommon.

Acid-Base Balance

GENERAL CONSIDERATIONS

During metabolism, acidic substances are produced in large amounts. The most important of these is carbonic acid (H_2CO_3), which is the inevitable product of aerobic tissue activity. During anaerobic activity lactic acid is produced; phosphoric, sulfuric, and other acids are formed in smaller quantities. These acids are formed within cells and pass to the extracellular tissues where they tend to increase the acidity. Nevertheless, cellular activity can take place only within a narrow range of acidity. The regulatory mechanisms by which this range is maintained are an aspect of homeostasis, which is of vital importance. In order to understand this process, it is essential to have a working knowledge of acids, bases, and buffers.

An acid is a molecule or ion that is capable of giving up a hydrogen ion ($H+$, or proton). A base is a molecule or ion that is capable of receiving a hydrogen ion. Thus, in the equation

$$HB = H^+ + B^-$$

HB is an acid, whereas B^- is the base.

A strong acid is one that readily gives up its hydrogen ion. Thus, in the equation

$$HCl = H^+ + Cl^-$$

HCl is a strong acid and Cl^- is a weak base.

On the other hand, carbonic acid (H_2CO_3) is a weak acid:

$$H_2CO_3 = H^+ + HCO_3^-$$

The bicarbonate ion HCO_3^- is a strong base, because it accepts a hydrogen ion more readily than H_2CO_3 gives it up.

MAINTENANCE OF THE pH OF THE BLOOD*

The normal blood pH ranges from 7.36 to 7.44. Survival is not possible outside the range of 6.8 to 8.0. To prevent changes of pH as much as possible, the body is provided with a series of *buffer systems*. These are chemical systems that are capable of "mopping up" excess hydrogen ions if the pH falls and of contributing hydrogen ions if the pH rises.

A physiological buffer consists of a mixture of a strong base and a weak acid; thus, in the dissociation equation

$$HB = H^+ + B^-$$

If B^- is a strong base, an excess of H^+ combines with it to form more of the weak acid HB.

The most important buffer in the extracellular fluids is the bicarbonate–carbonic acid combination.

$$H^+ + HCO_3^- \rightleftharpoons H_2CO_3$$

If hydrogen ions are added to plasma, more H_2CO_3 is formed. This passes to the lungs, dissociates, and carbon dioxide (CO_2) diffuses into the alveolar gas and is eliminated. The great importance of the bicarbonate ion lies not only in its buffering capacity but also in the extreme volatility of carbonic acid and the ease with which CO_2 is eliminated by the lungs.

Two other buffer systems in the extracellular fluids should be noted: monohydrogen phosphate and the plasma proteins:

$$H^+ + HPO_4^- \rightleftharpoons H_2PO_4^-$$

$$H^+ + Protein^n \rightleftharpoons HProtein^{(n-1)-}$$

An important means of buffering carbonic acid within the blood is found within the red cells, which contain not only hemoglobin, which acts as a buffer, but also the enzyme carbonic anhydrase, which accelerates the following reversible reaction:

$$CO_2 + H_2O \rightleftharpoons H_2CO_3$$

The carbonic acid then dissociates into bicarbonate and hydrogen ions:

$$H_2CO_3 \rightarrow HCO_3^- + H^+$$

---

*The pH of a fluid is the negative logarithm of the hydrogen ion concentration of a solution. The form [H^+] is used to denote hydrogen ion concentration. In pure water at 25° C the following relationship exists:

$$[H^+] \times [OH^-] = 10^{-14}$$

$$\text{That is, } [H^+] = [OH^-] = 10^{-7}$$

Hence, pH $= 7.0$. At 37° C pH 6.8 corresponds to neutrality.

The hydrogen ions are largely buffered by the hemoglobin:

$$H^+ + Hb^- \rightleftharpoons HHb$$

The excess bicarbonate ions then diffuse into the plasma in exchange for chloride ions, which diffuse into the red cells. In this way the bicarbonate level in the plasma rises.

It is evident that the acids that are produced in the body or are ingested are eliminated by two routes: *the lungs,* as described above; and *the kidneys* (the cells of the distal tubules secrete H^+ ions).

ABNORMALITIES OF THE pH OF THE BLOOD

An increase in the hydrogen ion concentration of the blood (pH less than 7.36) is called *acidemia,* whereas a decrease (pH over 7.44) is called *alkalemia.* Although the terms *acidosis* and *alkalosis* are sometimes used synonymously with acidemia and alkalemia, it is preferable to restrict them to descriptions of conditions in which there would be an appropriate change in pH if there were no compensatory mechanisms.

Respiratory Acidosis and Alkalosis.   If there is hypoventilation of the lungs, CO_2 is retained and forms carbonic acid in the blood, which is a source of hydrogen ions. $[HCO_3^-]$ rises as well, but by a lesser amount. Hence, the pH of the blood decreases. This process is called *respiratory acidosis.* In like manner, if there is hyperventilation, excess CO_2 is eliminated, and both carbonic acid and bicarbonate are reduced in the blood causing an increase in the pH. This process is called *respiratory alkalosis.* It is evident that respiratory acidosis is directly related to hypoventilation of the lungs, with a resulting retention of CO_2 and a rise in the arterial P_{CO_2}. In respiratory alkalosis the reverse obtains and there is a drop in arterial P_{CO_2}. A measurement of the arterial P_{CO_2} is therefore an accurate and useful method of assessing the respiratory component of acid-base balance.

EFFECTS OF RESPIRATORY ACIDOSIS.   This condition results in vasodilatation, which is a direct effect of the raised P_{CO_2}. This vasodilatation may cause a rise in intracranial pressure. The level of plasma bicarbonate rises and the plasma chloride drops proportionally.

EFFECTS OF RESPIRATORY ALKALOSIS.   Respiratory alkalosis is seen during hysterical hyperventilation, during work at high temperatures or at a high altitude, or during anesthesia when muscle relaxants are used and excessively vigorous artificial ventilation is applied. Peripheral vasoconstriction causes pallor of the skin. The lack of stimulation of the respiratory center by CO_2 causes a tendency toward respiratory arrest. *Tetany* is characteristic. This physiological response is identical with that seen in hypocalcemia. The symptoms are those of increased neuromuscular excitability. The most characteristic is spontaneous spasms of the hand muscles so that the fingers are extended and the palm hollowed. Generalized convulsions can occur.

Metabolic Acidosis and Alkalosis.   If an excess of hydrogen ions is introduced into the blood, as a result of either ingestion or the production of acidic substances, the bicarbonate of the plasma is replaced by chloride and other anions. There is a secondary fall in the PCO_2 to match this low concentration of bicarbonate, an effect produced by the low pH stimulating the respiratory center and causing overventilation. This is *metabolic acidosis.* Excessive ingestion of sodium bicarbonate leads to a rise in both the $[HCO_3^-]$ and the pH of the plasma. This is *metabolic alkalosis.*

METABOLIC ACIDOSIS.   A fall in both pH and bicarbonate level of the plasma occurs under the following conditions:

(1) *in shock* and *following a cardiac arrest*, when underprofusion of tissue leads to anaerobic metabolism and production of lactic acid *(lactic acidosis)*; (2) *in severe diarrhea*, when there is a greater loss of hydroxyl (OH^-) ions than of hydrogen ions in the feces; (3) *in starvation* and *in uncontrolled diabetes mellitus*, when there is ketosis. The acetoacetic acids and β-hydroxybutyric acids provide the extra hydrogen ions, and (4) *in chronic renal disease*, and in conditions in which there is a failure of the distal tubules to excrete hydrogen ions (*e.g.*, renal tubular acidosis).

Clinical Effects.   The classic symptom of metabolic acidosis is "air hunger." Respirations are deep, rapid, and sighing. This is a compensatory mechanism, because it lowers the PCO_2 and thereby causes a respiratory alkalosis that tends to reverse the metabolic acidosis.

As the plasma bicarbonate falls, there is a corresponding rise in other plasma anions, particularly the chloride ions. In such cases there is a *hyperchloremic acidosis.*

Severe metabolic acidosis causes grave neurological symptoms that culminate in death. The heart's action is impaired, and a state of shock with low cardiac output and hypotension ensues. Metabolic acidosis is thought to potentiate traumatic and hemorrhagic shock, and it is one of the contributory factors in the development of irreversible shock (see Chapter 21).

METABOLIC ALKALOSIS.   Both blood pH and blood bicarbonate level rise in this condition. Metabolic alkalosis occurs when there is excessive ingestion of bicarbonate or when there is excessive loss of acid from the body. The most common cause of this is persistent vomiting, such as with pyloric stenosis, when the ensuing loss of acidic gastric juice causes the alkalosis.

Effects of Metabolic Alkalosis.   Tetany may occur. A fall in plasma chloride compensates for the rise in bicarbonate level.

CONCLUSION

It is evident from this brief account of electrolytes and acid-base balance that many abnormalities can occur in disease. With the aid of the modern clinical chemical laboratory the abnormalities can be measured and appropriate treatment can be instituted. In acute illness, serial estimations are often necessary to assess the effects of treatment. The "toxemias" that once afflicted patients having cholera, dysentery, and intestinal obstruction with vomiting are no longer mysterious, untreatable agents of death. Instead, these conditions are now known to be diagnosable, treatable upsets of the internal environment of the body.

Edema

As usually used, the term "edema" can be defined as an excessive accumulation of fluid in the interstitial tissues. It is particularly liable to occur in the various serous sacs, giving rise to *ascites, hydrothorax,* and *hydropericardium* (terms applied to effusions into the peritoneal, pleural, and pericardial sacs, respectively). When edema is generalized, it is called *dropsy* or *anasarca.* Of course, it is possible to have intracellular edema, as in hydropic degeneration of cells and in pure water intoxication. The remainder of this section, however, will be devoted to types of interstitial edema.

It is necessary first to understand the normal mechanisms regulating the distribution of fluid in the body.

NORMAL MECHANISM OF CONTROL IN THE SYSTEMIC CIRCULATION

Starling postulated that the movement of fluid between vessels and the extravascular spaces was determined by the balance of the hydrostatic and osmotic forces acting upon it (see Fig. 5–1).

FORCES TENDING TO MOVE FLUID OUT OF THE BLOOD VESSELS ARE THE FOLLOWING:

(a) *The hydrostatic pressure within the vessels*

(b) *The colloid osmotic pressure of the interstitial fluid*

Since the vascular wall is completely permeable to water and crystalloids, the only effective osmotic forces acting across the vessel wall are due to colloids — mainly protein — to which the vessel wall is not permeable. The interstitial fluids normally have a low protein content, and this is therefore an unimportant factor.

FORCES TENDING TO MOVE THE FLUID INTO THE BLOOD VESSELS ARE THE FOLLOWING:

(a) *The tissue tension.*   This is normally low (3 to 4 mg Hg). Tissue tension is important in determining the distribution of edema. Thus, edema readily occurs in lax tissues such as the eyelids, over the sacrum, and in the genital area. Tense tissues like the palms and soles do not readily become edematous. A rise in tissue tension is an important factor in limiting interstitial tissue fluid formation in the legs under normal conditions as well as in acutely inflamed parts.

(b) *The osmotic pressure of the plasma proteins.*   This pressure is normally about 25 mm Hg and is due mainly to albumin. Since albumin does not normally pass through the vessel walls, the vascular permeability is important in regulating the distribution of fluids between the intravascular and extravascular compartments. In the event of an increase in the permeability, such as that occurring in acute inflammation, an exudate rich in protein is formed.

There are two types of edema:

An exudate.   This is an accumulation of fluid in acute inflammation and is due to an increased vascular permeability. The fluid contains a high percentage of protein and has virtually the same composition as plasma.

A transudate.   This is an accumulation of fluid due to hydrostatic imbalance between the intravascular and extravascular compartments. Since it occurs in the presence of a normal vascular permeability, the protein content of the fluid is low.

The importance of the lymphatic vessels should be remembered in any discussion of edema. They form an elaborate closed network in most tissues, and their function is to drain away fluid and protein.

Types of Edema

When considering the cause of any type of edema, one should realize that the process is usually due to a combination of factors. Starling, who appreciated this, stated that dropsy was probably never due to the derangement of a single mechanism acting alone.

Edema can be classified into local and generalized types. The localized varieties are the simplest to understand, because there are fewer factors involved in their pathogenesis.

LOCAL EDEMA

ACUTE INFLAMMATORY EDEMA.   This condition has been described in Chapter 5.

HYPERSENSITIVITY.   Edema is present in all lesions of immediate hypersensitivity and in severe delayed hypersensitivity reactions. It is due to an increase in vascular permeability.

VENOUS OBSTRUCTION.   The rise in venous pressure leads to an increase in capillary pressure, which in turn results in the formation of a transudate. Thus, in phlebothrombosis of the leg veins, edema occurs but is rarely severe. Edema of the gut occurs in a strangulated hernia and in mesenteric venous thrombosis. It is this edema that causes further vascular impairment later resulting in infarction.

LYMPHATIC EDEMA.   Extensive lymphatic obstruction can produce an edema of high protein content. Because chronic lymphatic edema of the limbs stimulates connective tissue overgrowth, in due course there is such enlargement of the skin and subcutaneous tissues that the part becomes grossly distorted. This resulting grotesque deformity is called *elephantiasis.* It occurs in the legs as a complication of the lymphangitis from any cause, but is particularly severe in the lymphangitis associated with filariasis (see Chapter 14). A similar condition can occur as a result of congenitally deformed lymphatics. Lymphedema of an arm is occasionally encountered as a complication of cancer of the breast when the lymphatic vessels are blocked either by tumor or by the fibrosis induced by radiotherapy.

GENERALIZED EDEMA

CARDIAC EDEMA.   In congestive heart failure there is retention of sodium and water that is first evident as an increase in body weight and later as a detectable edema. The distribution of this fluid is influenced by gravity. When the patient is ambulant, the legs are affected first, and swelling of the ankles is often the initial symptom. When the patient is in bed, the edema appears in the sacral and genital areas. Firm pressure by a finger in an edematous area results in the formation of a pit that remains when the finger is removed. This "pitting edema" is characteristic of most forms of edema. Lymphedema is the major exception.

EDEMA IN THE NEPHROTIC SYNDROME. This condition resembles cardiac edema and is described in Chapter 35.

FAMINE EDEMA (NUTRITIONAL EDEMA). The edema that is seen after prolonged starvation is usually confined to the legs. At first sight, it would seem explicable in terms of the marked hypoalbuminemia that is usually present; on closer examination, however, one finds that there is no close correlation between the level of plasma proteins and the presence of edema. The precise explanation of famine edema is not known. An important factor appears to be loss of compact tissue — mostly fat — and its replacement by a loose connective tissue in which fluid can accumulate readily without any undue rise in tissue tension.

Marked edema is a feature of kwashiorkor (see Chapter 23).

UNEXPLAINED EDEMA

Generalized edema sometimes occurs in the absence of any known cause. Although such cases are uncommon, they indicate that factors other than those already discussed may operate even in the common types of edema. A well-recognized condition, *cyclical periodic edema,* presents with recurrent attacks of edema involving skin, mucous membranes, and even internal organs. When the area involved is delimited to the subcutaneous tissues, it is called *angioedema.* The immediate cause of edema appears to be an increase in vascular permeability, but the precise cause is not known. In chronic urticaria there is edema of the dermis; again, the cause is rarely discovered.

PULMONARY EDEMA

This condition is considered in Chapter 30.

CONCLUSION

Although dropsy has been recognized as a symptom of disease since the beginning of medical history, it is evident that the mode of its formation is complex and often incompletely understood.

Review Questions

1. What is meant by the term "anion gap"? Describe how it is estimated as well as the significance of a raised value.
2. A woman sustains an abdominal injury in a car accident; one kidney is damaged and has to be removed. On the third postoperative day she is given a large water enema for constipation. Predict the possible consequences of this.

3. What type of acid-base imbalance would be expected in a patient who has just been resuscitated following a cardiac arrest?
4. Predict the effects of voluntary hyperventilation in a normal subject. (Warning! Do not attempt to hyperventilate anyone without supervision.)
5. A patient has nonpitting edema of one leg. Suggest some possible causes and discuss the pathogenesis.
6. How may fluid retention be detected in a patient with heart failure?

Selected Readings

Campbell, E. J. M., Dickinson, C. J., and Slater, J. D. H.: Clinical Physiology. 4th ed. Oxford, Blackwell Scientific Publications Ltd., 1974. See, in particular, Chapter 1, "Body Fluids"; and Chapter 5, "Hydrogen Ion (Acid:Base) Regulation."
Davenport, H. W.: A B C of Acid-Base Chemistry: The Elements of Physiological Blood-Gas Chemistry for Medical Students and Physicians. 5th ed. Chicago, University of Chicago Press, 1969.
Robinson, J. R.: Fundamentals of Acid-Base Regulation. 5th ed. Oxford, Blackwell Scientific Publications Ltd., 1975.
Siggaard-Anderson, O.: The Acid-Base Status of the Blood. 4th ed. Baltimore, The Williams & Wilkins Company, 1975.

Chapter 20

After studying this chapter the student should be able to:

- Distinguish between platelet aggregation and platelet adhesiveness.
- Define *thrombosis* and distinguish it from blood clotting.
- Describe Virchow's triad.
- Describe the common causes of thrombosis in an artery and list the possible effects on the tissue supplied.
- Compare phlebothrombosis with thrombophlebitis in terms of their causes and effects.
- List the circumstances under which thrombosis can occur in the heart.
- Describe the possible fate of a thrombus.
- Define *hypoxia* and list the four types.
- Define *ischemia* and classify its causes.

320

DISORDERS OF THE CIRCULATION

- Define *embolus* and classify emboli according to their composition.
- Describe the syndrome of massive pulmonary embolism.
- Describe the effects of a small pulmonary embolus.
- Define *pyemia* and describe its causes and effects.
- Outline the causes and effects of fat embolism.
- Define *infarction* and describe the process as it occurs in the following organs:
    - (a) heart
    - (b) spleen
    - (c) brain
    - (d) intestine.
- Give examples of complications caused by arterial spasm.
- Distinguish between primary and secondary systemic hypertension.
- List the complications of systemic hypertension.
- Describe the main pathological and clinical features of malignant hypertension.

The publication of *De Motu Cordis* is generally conceded to be one of the great landmarks of medical research. In it, William Harvey propounded the theory of the circulation of the blood from the heart, through arteries, and to the veins. The missing link in this theory was the absence of any known connection between arteries and veins. Malpighi, who was born in the year of Harvey's publication, applied the compound microscope to the study of biological material and proved the existence of capillaries, thereby confirming Harvey's hypothesis. Today, although over 300 years of study have laid bare a wealth of information about the circulation, its disorders are still responsible for a vast amount of illness and death. Heart attacks and strokes are mounting in frequency, and so far there is no end in sight to this trend.

NORMAL FUNCTION

The function of the circulatory system is the maintenance of an adequate perfusion of blood to all tissues of the body. Each ventricular contraction ejects a quantity of blood into the aorta and causes a rise in systemic blood pressure. The aorta and its major branches are composed largely of elastic tissue; their expansion prevents an undue rise in pressure with each ventricular contraction (systole). The branches of these elastic vessels are the muscular arteries. It is by variation in the tone of their smooth-muscle walls that the amount of blood supplied to the various organs and tissues can be altered. The muscular arteries subdivide repeatedly, with blood next reaching the arterioles. These small muscular vessels provide the final mechanism by which blood is distributed to the tissues in response to their individual needs. The distribution of blood is in part regulated by the autonomic nervous system that acts on the smooth muscle of the arteries and arterioles, and in part by local mechanisms by which chemical agents, such as bradykinin, are released and act locally.

The blood flow in the major arteries is pulsatile. The elasticity of these vessels and the high resistance provided by the arterioles reduce the pulsation, so that in the capillaries and veins the blood flow is constant. It follows that blood escaping from damaged capillaries oozes out constantly, whereas blood from a cut artery spurts out.

Two obvious prerequisites of any circulation are the presence of a fluid and a means by which this fluid can be retained in the vessels should they be damaged. In the blood vascular system, a clotting mechanism helps to guard against the dangers of hemorrhage, and vascular damage is remedied by the deposition of platelets and fibrin on the vessel wall. This effectively patches any minor defect, and even severed vessels are soon sealed off. The control of platelet deposition and fibrin formation is an excellent example of a homeostatic mechanism designed to prevent bleeding. Unfortunately, the intravascular deposition can sometimes become excessive, leading to the complete obstruction of the damaged vessel. This process is called *thrombosis,* a subject that must be studied in some detail.

Thrombosis

The clotting mechanism is described fully in Chapter 26 and consists of the conversion of the plasma *fibrinogen* into a solid mass of *fibrin* by the action of *thrombin*. The clotting can be initiated by thromboplastin derived either from the blood (intrinsic system) or from the tissues (extrinsic system).

Platelets. Since platelets play an important role in thrombosis, their properties have been extensively studied. They are small nonnucleated structures present in the blood and have the property of sticking to each other (displaying *aggregation*) and of adhering to abnormal surfaces (showing *adhesiveness*).

PLATELET AGGREGATION. Platelets aggregate immediately in the presence of adenosine diphosphate (ADP). This mechanism may be demonstrated *in vitro* by the addition of ADP to a platelet-rich preparation of plasma that is kept agitated. The aggregation can be detected by measuring the ensuing decrease in optical density of the plasma. An important property of thrombin is that it causes the release of ADP from platelets, and it therefore soon causes aggregation.

PLATELET ADHESIVENESS. Experimentally, platelets are found to adhere to a variety of foreign surfaces. Thus, if a platelet-rich fluid is passed through a column containing glass beads, the platelets are found to adhere to the beads, and few are contained in the fluid that issues from the column. Since platelets also adhere to the walls of damaged blood vessels, it is believed that exposure of collagen in the vessel wall is an important factor in the ready adhesion of

FIGURE 20–1. *Thrombosis in aortic aneurysm.*

The aortic aneurysm has been opened to show adherent thrombus. The thrombus has a characteristic ribbed, or corrugated, appearance; this is quite different from the smooth, shiny surface of a postmortem clot.

these structures; platelets readily adhere to collagen when tested *in vitro*. The platelets that stick to an abnormal surface release a number of important chemical substances: ADP, a phospholipid (platelet factor 3), and 5-hydroxytryptamine (5-HT). The ADP causes platelet aggregation, so that a mass of them builds up at the site of damage in a vessel. *A solid mass formed by deposition of elements from the circulating blood is called a thrombus* (Figs. 20–1 and 20–2). The small platelet thrombus that first forms is quite unstable, for the platelets may break off and return to the circulation. Nevertheless, platelet factor 3 that is released aids the clotting system so that *fibrin is added to the thrombus and causes it to become stable.* The thrombin formed during the clotting process leads to further accumulation of platelets.

The formation of thrombi in the vessels serves several useful purposes. Small areas of damage are patched so that bleeding is prevented. The release of 5-HT causes contraction of the smooth muscle of the vessel wall, and this vasospasm also impedes bleeding. Diseased vessels that are lined by an irregular surface or that present a disturbed architecture have the normal streamlining of the blood flow restored by suitable thrombus formation (Fig. 20–4). A covering of endothelial cells soon forms so that the smooth lining of the vessel is restored and further deposition ceases. *Endothelialization* is therefore one checking mechanism that prevents the formation of too large a thrombus. Another process that limits thrombosis is the *activation of plasmin*, a fibrinolysin that dissolves fibrin (Fig. 20–3). Finally, the presence of a flowing blood stream carries away clotting factors before there is time for them to produce further platelet aggregation or clotting.

Under some conditions, vascular damage leads to the formation of a large thrombus; this abnormal event will be described in the following sections.

FIGURE 20–2. *The structure of a thrombus.*

This is a photomicrograph of a thrombus and includes its free surface on the right. The thrombus consists of pale platelet laminae between which there is coagulated blood. Many white cells are adherent to the platelet laminae. Retraction of the clot leaves the laminae projecting from the free surface, and this is responsible for the ribbed appearance noted in Figure 20–1. The organized structure, with platelet laminae alternating with coagulated blood, distinguishes a thrombus from a blood clot, because it indicates that the structure has been formed from the elements of a flowing stream of blood. (From Hadfield, G.: Annals of the Royal College of Surgeons of England, 6:219, 1950.)

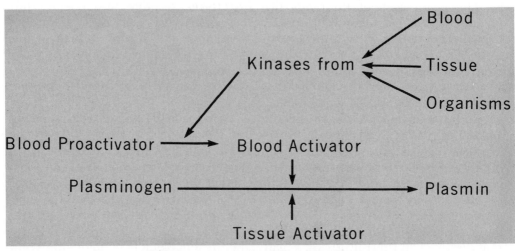

FIGURE 20–3. *The blood fibrinolytic system.*

Plasmin is a fibrinolytic enzyme that can be formed from plasminogen by the action of an activator. *Streptococcus pyogenes* is one organism that can produce a kinase (streptokinase). Other kinases are derived from tissue breakdown or from the blood itself. (Drawing by Frederick Lammerich, Department of Art as Applied to Science, University of Toronto.)

FIGURE 20–4. *Vascular abnormalities that lead to thrombosis.*

This diagram shows seven different causes of a disruption of the normal streamlining of the blood flow, and the manner by which platelets (shown in black) are laid down to restore the architecture. *A,* Bulging due to external pressure and spasm. *B,* Endothelial damage in inflammation, an area of intimal thickening (e.g., due to atheroma), and corrugation due to adjacent scarring. *C,* Aneurysm and a thickened, rigid valve. (From Hadfield, G.: Annals of the Royal College of Surgeons of England, 6:219, 1950.)

A   B   C

GENERAL CAUSES OF THROMBOSIS

Three factors *(Virchow's triad)* must be considered in regard to the mechanism of thrombosis:

(1) *The Vessel Wall.* The various types of anatomical changes in the vessel wall that may lead to thrombosis are depicted in Figure 20–4. In general, these abnormalities play an important part in thrombosis involving the heart valves and ventricles. In the arteries, atheroma is by far the most common cause of thrombosis. In the veins, changes in the vessel wall are usually of much less importance.

(2) *The Flow of Blood.* The formation of *eddy currents* is important, for whenever the stream of the blood is disturbed the flow becomes turbulent, and platelets are thrown against the vessel wall and are deposited as a thrombus. This mechanism is important in fast-moving streams, *e.g.,* over the heart valves and in arteries. Slowing of the blood, or *stasis,* is the most important cause of excessive thrombosis involving veins. It is also a factor in inducing thrombosis in the sac of an aneurysm as well as in the atria of the heart.

(3) *The Constituents of Blood.* An increase in the platelet count, an increase in platelet adhesiveness, and a decrease in the clotting time—events that occur after trauma and bleeding—are sometimes important in inducing thrombosis. Likewise, increased viscosity of the blood due to hemoconcentration or polycythemia also leads to thrombosis.

It should be noted that usually more than one factor is implicated in the cause of thrombosis. For instance, there is regional stasis and a high platelet count after a surgical operation. Atheroma acts both by causing a loss of the endothelium and by inducing eddy-current formation.

ARTERIAL THROMBOSIS

Thrombosis generally occurs in arteries as a complication of damage to the arterial wall; *atherosclerosis* is the most important cause, but *arteritis* also accounts for some cases. In an aneurysmal sac, thrombus deposition is a constant feature, and here stasis and eddy currents are important factors. These are considered in Chapter 29.

Effects of Arterial Thrombosis.   Except for the aorta and its very large branches, arterial thrombosis results in the complete blockage of the vessel. The effects of this depend upon the local architecture. The following are possibilities:

1. NO EFFECT.   When anastomoses are good, no ill-effect is noted. Thus, if the radial artery is blocked, the hand is supplied by the ulnar artery because branches of the two vessels are normally joined together by *anastomotic channels.* These channels enlarge so that a *collateral circulation* develops. Blockage of either artery alone, therefore, leads to no serious after-effects, provided the other vessel is not diseased.

2. FUNCTIONAL DISTURBANCES.   Blockage of a major vessel may render tissue ischemic only with exercise. In coronary occlusion, which is an example of this blockage, the effect is pain on exercise *(angina pectoris).* Likewise, occlusion of the mesenteric artery can lead to pain after meals when the intestine exhibits marked peristalsis. Occlusion of the femoral artery can lead to pain on walking. This is called *intermittent claudication.*

3. CELLULAR DEGENERATION.   Ischemia can induce enough hypoxia to cause the specialized cells of an organ to degenerate. This is a patchy affair and leads to atrophy. Often there is *replacement fibrosis (e.g.,* myocardial fibrosis); in the central nervous system there is *replacement gliosis.*

4. INFARCTION.   The ischemia may be so severe that the whole area undergoes necrosis. This effect is called *infarction* and is considered later in this chapter.

VENOUS THROMBOSIS

Although disease of the vessel walls is uncommon, stasis is particularly evident in the veins, especially those of the legs. Thrombosis with a large element of clotting is therefore common. Two distinct entities can be recognized: phlebothrombosis and thrombophlebitis.

Phlebothrombosis.   The commonest form of leg vein thrombosis is phlebothrombosis. This occurs in patients who are confined to bed, particularly if they have suffered heart failure or have been subjected to trauma, whether accidental or surgical. If the limb has been injured and immobilized *(e.g.,* a fractured femur), the stage is set for thrombosis, because the major cause is venous stasis (Fig. 20–5). A small thrombus forms at one site, perhaps where the vein has been injured by pressure such as that produced by a pillow behind the knee. The flow of blood stops in the vein proximal to the thrombus, and the entire column *clots* (Fig. 20–6). This process can extend, or propagate, up to the iliac vein; as the clot retracts, it has minimal attachment to the vessel wall. The great danger then is embolism, for should the clot become detached, it would travel in the circulation to the right side of the heart and subsequently be ejected into the pulmonary artery. Here it would block either the main pulmonary trunk or one of its major divisions, leading to sudden death or infarction of the lung (see a discussion of this later in the chapter).

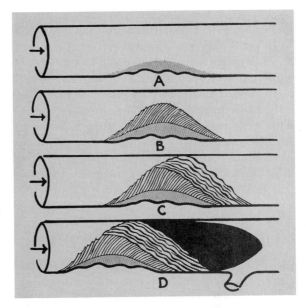

FIGURE 20–5. *The pathogenesis of phlebothrombosis.*

A, An area of intimal damage is covered by a pale platelet thrombus. In the presence of a sluggish stream, this initiates further thrombosis. *B,* Upstanding laminae of platelets with intervening clot constitute the main thrombus. *C,* The lumen is occluded by further thrombosis. *D,* Blood *clot* forms to the next tributary. (From Hadfield, G.): Annals of the Royal College of Surgeons of England, 6:219, 1950.)

Thrombophlebitis. Inflammation of a vein (phlebitis) can occur when there is an adjacent area of infection (*e.g.,* a boil). Thrombosis occurs *(thrombophlebitis)* and is confined to the inflamed area of vein. A propagated clot does not form, and the risk of embolism is slight unless the thrombus itself becomes infected (see "Pyemia," discussed later).

Thrombophlebitis affecting many veins at different times (called *migrating thrombophlebitis*) is an occasional manifestation of cancer, particularly cancer

FIGURE 20–6. *Propagation of clot in phlebothrombosis.*

A, Thrombus formation occurs at each entering tributary. This tends to anchor the clot. *B,* Clotting *en masse* in an extensive length of vein. This occurs when the circulation is very sluggish. The long propagated clot can easily become detached and lead to massive pulmonary embolism. (From Hadfield, G.: Annals of the Royal College of Surgeons of England, 6:219, 1950.)

of the pancreas. The pathogenesis is not understood. The first description of this condition is attributed to Trousseau, a French physician, who observed it in himself and subsequently died of pancreatic cancer.

Local Effects of Venous Thrombosis. In most tissues because the veins show extensive anastomoses, venous thrombosis produces few obstructive effects. There are some exceptions to this. Obstruction of the superior mesenteric vein leads to intense engorgement of the intestine and edema of the gut wall. This blockage can be so marked that further blood flow through the part becomes impossible, and the intestine undergoes infarction. In the leg, venous obstruction can lead to some elevation of the venous pressure of the limb, an effect particularly marked if the subject stands for long periods. The result of this is edema of the ankles.

CARDIAC THROMBOSIS

Thrombi may form in any of the chambers of the heart. The constant danger is their detachment and subsequent embolization. A common cause of atrial thrombosis is atrial dilatation secondary to mitral stenosis, atrial fibrillation, or heart failure. Ventricular thrombosis is most commonly encountered as a complication of myocardial infarction, either during the acute stage (see Fig. 28–6) or in an aneurysm that develops subsequently.

Thrombi on the heart valves (called *vegetations*) are a feature of acute rheumatic fever, infective endocarditis (see Fig. 28–3), and nonbacterial thrombotic endocarditis (see Chapter 28).

FATE OF THROMBI

Figure 20–7 summarizes the possible fate of a thrombus. These possibilities are further elaborated on below:

(a) Many thrombi undergo lysis and leave no trace of their previous existence. The fibrinolytic enzyme plasmin is probably important in removing thrombi (see Fig. 20–3).

(b) If an occluding thrombus in an artery or vein contains much clot, it retracts sufficiently for blood to pass by, in this way forming a new channel. It becomes endothelialized, and at that point *recanalization* is said to have occurred. In the pulmonary arteries a thin web of connective tissue may be all that remains of a previous life-threatening thromboembolism.

(c) A thrombus that is not removed may become organized into granulation tissue and subsequent scar tissue.

(d) Organized thrombi may become hyalinized and calcified. This response is common in the pelvic veins, and the *phleboliths* so produced may be seen on radiographic examination of the pelvis.

(e) Thrombi may be detached to form emboli – a process that is described later in this chapter.

Two important effects of thrombosis are occlusion of the lumen of the vessel involved and detachment from this to form an embolus. Vascular obstruction produces ischemia, which in turn leads to hypoxia.

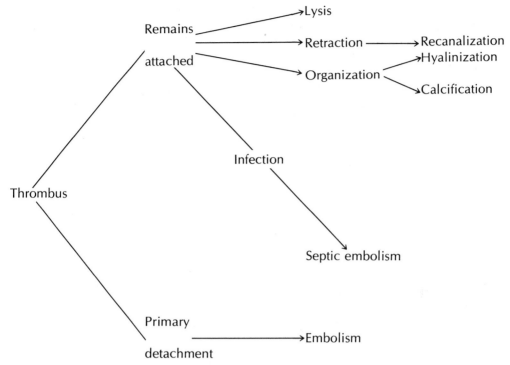

FIGURE 20–7. *Diagram illustrating the possible fate of a thrombus.*

Hypoxia

Hypoxia is a state of impaired oxygenation of the tissues.

Types. Four types are commonly described:

(1) *Hypoxic*, due to a low oxygen tension (PO_2) in the arterial blood. This form of hypoxia is a feature of some types of congenital heart disease and lung disease.

(2) *Anemic*, due to an inadequate level of hemoglobin, which carries the oxygen in the blood stream.

(3) *Stagnant*, or *ischemic*, due to an inadequate supply of blood to the tissues; this form of hypoxia may be due to a low cardiac output as in heart failure, or to some local vascular obstruction.

(4) *Histotoxic*, due to cellular poisoning, which prevents the uptake of oxygen (*e.g.*, cyanide poisoning).

Ischemia

Ischemia is a condition of inadequate blood supply to an area of tissue. It produces harmful effects in three ways:

HYPOXIA. A reduced oxygen supply is undoubtedly the most important factor in the production of damage in ischemic tissue. It is particularly important in active cells such as muscle and neurons. On the other hand, it plays no part in the lesions produced by pulmonary arterial obstruction because the alveolar walls derive their oxygen directly from the alveolar gas.

MALNUTRITION. This is probably a factor of little importance, because the blood contains more nutrients than could be metabolized with the amount of oxygen it contains.

FAILURE TO REMOVE WASTE PRODUCTS. The accumulation of metabolites is the most probable explanation of pain in ischemic muscles. The presence of waste products or the failure to maintain important electrolyte balances is probably a factor in the pathogenesis of pulmonary infarction.

CAUSES OF ISCHEMIA

General. Ischemia can be caused by an inadequate cardiac output. Not all tissues of the body are equally affected, because there is a redistribution of the available blood. The extremities — for instance, the fingertips and toes — tend to be most severely affected; in such cases the sluggish blood flow leads to peripheral cyanosis. (The term *cyanosis* refers to the blue color of tissues that is produced by the reduced hemoglobin in the vessels.)

Sudden cessation of the heart's action such as may occur during the induction of anesthesia, or as a result of coronary thrombosis, results in ischemia of all tissues in the body. The effects of this are confined to a single organ — the brain — which is particularly sensitive to hypoxia. If the arrest continues for 15 seconds, consciousness is lost; if the condition lasts for more than 3 minutes, irreparable damage is done. If the patient survives the neurons degenerate and are replaced by glial tissue. If cardiac arrest lasts for more than 8 minutes, death is inevitable. It follows that *all persons who deal with patients should be capable of diagnosing cardiac arrest (absent heart sounds) and of dealing with it by the maneuvers of external cardiac massage and assisted respiration.*

Local. By far, the most important cause of ischemia is obstruction to the arterial flow. Nevertheless, extensive venous and capillary obstruction can also produce ischemia.

ARTERIAL OBSTRUCTION. Most of the causes of obstruction have already been described. In review, they are:

THROMBOSIS.

EMBOLISM. The effects of an embolus are potentiated by the reflex spasm of the arterial wall and are completed by the rapid development of thrombus over the embolus.

SPASM. See later in this chapter.

ATHEROSCLEROSIS. See Chapter 29.

OCCLUSIVE PRESSURE FROM WITHOUT. Examples include tourniquets and ill-fitting casts.

VENOUS DISEASE. Extensive venous obstruction leads to engorgement of the area drained by the affected veins. This may reach such an intensity that blood flow is impeded and ischemia results.

CAPILLARY DAMAGE. See Chapter 29.

Embolism

An embolus is an abnormal mass of undissolved material that is transported from one part of the circulation to another. The most satisfactory classification is one based on the composition of the embolus.

TYPES OF EMBOLI

Four distinct types may be recognized: *thrombi* and *clot; gas; fat;* and *tumor;* a fifth category—*miscellaneous emboli*—is also discussed.

Thrombus or Clot Emboli

PULMONARY EMBOLISM.   The source of thromboemboli is generally one of the leg veins. If the embolus is large, it produces the syndrome of "massive pulmonary embolism." Either the main pulmonary trunk or many of its branches become plugged, so that the pulmonary circulation is greatly hindered (Fig. 20–8). The output of the right ventricle as well as that of the left ventricle drops precipitously. The effects of this drop are dramatic. The patient

FIGURE 20–8.   *Massive pulmonary embolism.*

The right ventricle and pulmonary trunk have been opened to reveal a large embolus. Part of the embolus is sitting astride the division of the pulmonary trunk and is blocking both pulmonary arteries. This condition is known as a *saddle embolus* and causes sudden death.

experiences sudden dyspnea and chest pain. Loss of consciousness and death may follow. The prevention of massive pulmonary embolism is the prevention of phlebothrombosis. A patient who is confined to bed must be given leg exercises to stimulate the venous circulation. Postoperative physical therapy and early ambulation have done much to reduce this complication of trauma and surgery. Anticoagulant drugs (*e.g.,* heparin) administered prior to surgery have been somewhat useful.

Small pulmonary emboli produce a different picture. If the subject is otherwise healthy, medium-sized pulmonary arteries can be obstructed without appreciable ill-effect. Since the lung derives much of its oxygen from the alveolar gas, the area beyond a blocked artery does not become hypoxic. Nevertheless, the altered gas tensions in the tissue can lead to bronchospasm, with the result that the area ceases to be ventilated and may collapse. This area can become reinflated within a few hours. The transient radiographic shadows that can be seen following pulmonary embolism may be explained on this basis. At other times, the area becomes edematous; hypoxia is added to ischemia, and necrosis ensues. The end-result is infarction of the lung.

The circumstances determining whether infarction will follow pulmonary embolism are not clearly understood, but patients who have experienced heart failure and are confined to bed seem to be most prone to this complication.

SYSTEMIC EMBOLISM. The embolus usually arises from the heart, either in one of its chambers or from a valve. Thrombi attached to atheromatous ulcers in the aorta sometimes embolize distally.

INFECTED EMBOLI. If a thrombus contains pyogenic organisms it tends to break up and produce multiple infected ("septic") emboli. Such a condition, which is called *pyemia,* is a complication of both acute endocarditis and thrombophlebitis in an area of suppurative inflammation (*e.g.,* acute appendicitis). If an infected embolus blocks a vessel supplying tissue that has a poor collateral circulation (*e.g.,* kidney), an infarct is produced, subsequently becomes infected, and a *septic infarct* results and soon suppurates. If the tissue has a good blood supply (*e.g.,* liver), no infarction occurs but a local infection leads to abscess formation—a *pyemic abscess.* Thus, a complication of acute appendicitis is portal pyemia and multiple pyemic abscesses in the liver.

Gas Emboli

AIR. Air may accidentally be introduced into a systemic vein during a surgical procedure. During operations on the head and neck, air may be sucked accidentally into the jugular vein and may then pass to the right side of the heart. Small quantities produce no adverse effect, but if a large quantity of air suddenly reaches the right ventricle, it becomes churned into a foamy mass that is compressed during systole but cannot be ejected. The cardiac output drops dramatically and sudden death ensues.

When a needle is introduced into the pleural cavity, as when fluid is aspirated, air may inadvertently be introduced into the pulmonary venous circulation and may reach the left side of the heart. From here it may travel to a coronary or cerebral vessel, occluding them. Even small quantities of air can produce serious, or even fatal, results in this manner.

Air embolism, either pulmonary or systemic, is a serious complication of open-heart surgery. All efforts must be made to exclude air from the circulation at the termination of the operation.

NITROGEN: THE DECOMPRESSION SYNDROME.   Bubbles of nitrogen appear in the circulation in those who, having been exposed to a high atmospheric pressure, are suddenly decompressed. This occurs in divers and tunnelers if they return to the surface too quickly. It is also seen in pilots if the cabin becomes decompressed at a high altitude. Nitrogen, being soluble in lipids, also appears as bubbles in the central nervous system. This particular effect may result in considerable damage to the spinal cord. The accompanying severe pain, which occurs most often in the joints, gives the condition its colloquial name "the bends." Permanent damage and death may ensue.

Fat Embolism.   Globules of fatty marrow may enter small veins in the area of a fracture of a long bone. With multiple injuries, this embolization can be quite extensive. Usually the emboli are trapped in the lungs, and because of the enormous capacity of the pulmonary vascular bed, can produce little harmful effect. Small areas of collapse can be detected radiographically. Occasionally fat emboli traverse the pulmonary capillaries and enter the systemic circulation where they produce the condition known as *systemic fat embolism.* Multiple emboli lodge in the kidneys, causing hematuria; in the brain, leading to severe neurological changes; and in the skin, causing petechial hemorrhages.

Tumor Emboli.   It is probable that all malignant tumors invade the local blood vessels at an early stage of the disease and that isolated malignant cells are a frequent occurrence in the circulation. The majority of these emboli become impacted and are destroyed. A small percentage develop into metastatic deposits. Occasionally, a large mass of tumor invades a major vessel and becomes detached. Thus, in lung cancer a tongue of tumor can invade a pulmonary vein, become detached, pass into the systemic circulation, and block a large artery such as the femoral artery. The event is uncommon.

Miscellaneous Emboli.   A variety of foreign bodies can act as emboli. For example, a portion of polyethylene tube may accidentally become detached and travel to the right side of the heart.

The condition described as *amniotic fluid embolism* is an occasional complication of pregnancy that follows escape of amniotic fluid into the veins of the uterus. It produces a syndrome characterized by shock and a generalized bleeding tendency. Although amniotic fluid does travel to the lungs, the syndrome is attributable not to embolism but rather to the initiation of intravascular clotting and fibrinolysis.

Infarction

Infarction is the circumscribed necrosis of tissue due to deprivation of its blood supply. The area of necrosis subsequently becomes organized into scar tissue. The process is as follows:

(a) Cells die in the area deprived of its blood supply. Blood, either from anastomotic vessels or from venous backflow, continues to seep into the devitalized area for a short time. Thus, most infarcts contain a greal deal of blood in the early stages and are swollen and red in color. The red cells entering the affected area escape from the damaged capillaries and lie free in the

FIGURE 20–9. *Pulmonary infarct.*

This vertical section through the lung shows an area of hemorrhagic infarction involving the apex of the lower lobe (arrow). Note how the surrounding uninvolved lung has collapsed postmortem; this has left the infarct standing out in relief. The specimen is from a patient who had carcinoma of the lung.

dead tissue. Infarcts of lax tissue such as the lung and intestine are much more engorged than those of compact organs such as the kidney and heart.

(b) The dead tissue undergoes necrosis. In solid organs, the associated swelling of the cells tends to squeeze blood out of the infarct, which then becomes pale. Infarcts of the spleen and kidneys characteristically show this color change and appear as pale, wedge-shaped areas of coagulative necrosis—the apex of such areas being a blocked supplying artery, the base being the capsule of the organ (Fig. 20–9). Infarcts of the heart are also pale, but their shape is more irregular owing to the arrangement of the vascular supply (see Fig. 28–4).

(c) Necrotic tissue undergoes progressive autolysis; red cells undergo hemolysis. Microscopically, the infarct shows a characteristic structured necrosis. The general outline of the cells is visible, but nuclei are either breaking up into fragments or have completely disappeared.

(d) At the same time the surrounding normal tissue shows an acute inflammatory reaction. Hyperemia gives the edge of the infarct a deep red color. Microscopic examination reveals an intense polymorph infiltration. Macrophages subsequently become the predominant cell and play an important part in removing the dead tissue.

(e) The infarct gradually shrinks and becomes replaced by granulation tissue that subsequently matures to scar tissue. The central portion of a large infarct may remain unorganized for many months and indeed may show dystrophic calcification and never become converted into scar tissue.

Infarcts in particular organs present certain characteristic features. For example, in the lung, the tissue is spongelike, and infarcts in it are always hemorrhagic. In the intestine, the necrotic bowel wall is soon invaded by putrefactive organisms and becomes gangrenous. In the limbs, sudden obstruction leads to infarction, which in turn is associated with infection and leads to *wet gangrene.*

In the central nervous system, on the other hand, the process of infarction is somewhat different, because the necrotic tissue immediately undergoes liquefactive necrosis. The affected area may collapse and eventually be replaced by a glial scar, but if the infarct is large, the end-result is the formation of a cyst lined by glial tissue.

Vascular Spasm

Although vascular occlusion is generally caused by an organic lesion, there are a number of conditions in which spasm of the vessel wall plays a most important part. Either veins or arteries can be affected by spasm, but it is debatable whether capillaries are capable of independent contraction.

FIGURE 20–10. *Splenic infarction.*

This section of spleen shows two pale areas of infarction. From a patient who died of bacterial endocarditis.

VENOUS SPASM

Trauma applied directly to the vessel wall can induce intense spasm. This may cause great difficulty during an inexpert venipuncture, *e.g.*, when a transfusion is set up or when blood is withdrawn from a vein. It is the reason why the novice has such difficulties in "taking blood."

Generalized venospasm occurs during hypovolemic shock, and it has also been postulated as occurring in heart failure.

ARTERIAL SPASM

Trauma to an artery produces localized spasm; at times, this may be lifesaving. There are many cases recorded in which whole limbs have been torn off (avulsed), and yet owing to the spasm of the main artery, the patient has not died of massive bleeding.

The ability of arteries and arterioles to contract can be used to advantage by a surgeon who is faced with severe bleeding during the course of an operation. It is a wise policy to pack the wound and await the onset of spasm rather than make heroic, though blind, efforts with a pair of hemostats. Indeed, *anyone faced with bleeding from a wound should apply local pressure and await vasospasm, rather than panic or apply a tourniquet.*

Although arterial spasm as a response to trauma may be beneficial, it may sometimes be detrimental. Trauma to an artery, *e.g.*, by the close proximity to a bullet path, or the jagged ends of a fractured bone, the pressure of a hematoma around a fracture, or the pressure of a plaster or tourniquet, may at times produce such persistent widespread spasm that the area involved becomes ischemic and infarcted. Because the process is often painless, the *pulse of a limb beyond an area of damage must always be carefully observed.* Absence of the pulse must be regarded seriously, and every effort should be made to relieve the spasm so that permanent damage will not occur.

Spasm of small arteries and arterioles is a feature of ergot poisoning and Raynaud's phenomenon (see Chapter 1). It may lead to gangrene of such extremities as the toes and fingertips. Widespread arteriolar spasm is a feature of shock (see Chapters 21 and 28). It has also been incriminated as a cause of primary hypertension, which is discussed below.

Systemic Hypertension

High blood pressure, or systemic hypertension, is a common condition that is often discovered accidentally during a routine medical examination. It is normal for the systemic blood pressure to rise as a response to emotion and physical exercise. If a raised pressure is discovered, it is wise to check the measurement after the patient has been at rest for some time and has grown accustomed to the surroundings. Another factor to consider is the age of the patient. As people get older, the aorta becomes less elastic, and with each ventricular contraction the systolic blood pressure rises rapidly. However, the blood drains away normally through the arterioles to the venous system, and the diastolic blood pressure remains normal. In systemic hypertension the diastolic blood pressure rises. A rough guideline is that the systolic blood pressure should be less than

100 mm Hg plus age in years, and the diastolic pressure should be under 100 mm Hg.

TYPES OF HYPERTENSION

For practical purposes two types of hypertension can be recognized: primary hypertension and secondary hypertension.

Primary, or Essential, Hypertension. This is the common form of high blood pressure, and its cause is unknown. It is a condition that is more common in women than men, and it is especially prevalent in North American Blacks. Primary renal or adrenal abnormalities have been postulated as causing this hypertension, but no conclusive evidence has been obtained.

Secondary Hypertension. Hypertension is a common complication of renal disease. It is a feature of pheochromocytoma, a rare tumor of the adrenal gland, and is due to the effects of epinephrine and norepinephrine, which are secreted by the tumor. The hypertension is characteristically episodic. Hypertension is also a feature of some adrenal cortical tumors (see Chapter 39).

PATHOGENESIS OF HYPERTENSION

It is generally assumed that the cause of the increased blood pressure is an increase in peripheral resistance to blood flow. Many experimental models have been investigated in attempts to elucidate the nature of this resistance to blood flow in essential hypertension.

The classic experiments of Goldblatt proved that in the dog an obstruction to the renal artery blood flow could produce hypertension. This response is due to the release from the ischemic kidney of a proteolytic enzyme (called *renin*), that acts on a plasma globulin, angiotensinogen, to convert it into angiotensin I. Another plasma enzyme converts angiotensin I into angiotensin II, a peptide that induces vascular spasm and produces hypertension.

In humans, hypertension sometimes, but not always, occurs in acute and chronic glomerulonephritis, pyelonephritis, and other renal diseases. The mechanism producing the hypertension may or may not be similar to that operating in the Goldblatt experiment; present evidence is against such a pathogenesis. Hypertension with unilateral renal lesions, such as obstruction to the renal artery, is sometimes relieved either by unilateral nephrectomy or by correction of the arterial stenosis. Unfortunately, this treatment is not always successful.

EFFECTS AND COMPLICATIONS OF HYPERTENSION

1. *Hemorrhage.* Weakened blood vessels tend to rupture more commonly in the hypertensive subject than in the normal; dissecting aneurysm of the aorta, ruptured berry aneurysm of the circle of Willis, and cerebral hemorrhage are all more common in the hypertensive subject.

2. *Arteriolosclerosis.* The small arteries of many organs show thickening of their walls, particularly the tunica intima, with hyaline material. This thickening is most marked in the arterioles of the renal glomeruli; gradually, as these vessels close down, the glomeruli and tubules that they supply become atrophic and are replaced by fibrous tissue. This scarring of the kidney is termed *nephrosclerosis.*

The arterioles of the retina share in this generalized process. The thickening of their walls together with ischemic changes in the retina constitutes the features of *hypertensive retinopathy* (see Chapter 42).

Arteriolosclerosis also affects the central nervous system. This sclerosis of the walls of the smaller arteries is presumed to be the cause of vague symptoms such as headache, lightheadedness, and giddiness. Personality changes and memory defects are also common. More severe lesions resulting from vascular occlusion or hemorrhage produce more definite effects, such as hemiplegia.

Heart Failure.   Systemic hypertension causes left ventricular hypertrophy and ultimately left ventricular failure (see Chapter 28).

MALIGNANT HYPERTENSION

Hypertension, whether primary or secondary, may occasionally evolve into a malignant phase. The blood pressure becomes very high, causing necrosis of the arteriolar walls. Two organs are especially affected: the kidney and the brain. In the *kidney* the vascular changes cause hematuria and culminate in uremia. In the *brain* the changes cause hemorrhage and edema. Swelling of the optic discs (papilledema) is a useful sign of raised intracranial pressure; symptoms include mental confusion and epileptiform fits. The syndrome of malignant hypertension usually progresses rapidly over a period of several weeks, and unless treated expeditiously, results in death either from uremia, from an intracranial vascular catastrophe, or from heart failure.

Review Questions

1. Describe the way in which a thrombus differs from a clot.
2. List the steps that can be taken to avoid death from massive pulmonary embolism.
3. Compare the process of infarction in the kidney with that which occurs in the intestine.
4. Describe the role of thrombin in the formation of a thrombus.
5. Discuss the possible effects of thrombosis of the femoral artery.
6. Describe the possible effects of pulmonary embolism.
7. A 50-year-old man is found to have a systolic blood pressure of 170 mm Hg. Discuss possible causes of this.
8. Discuss the relationship between systemic hypertension and the kidney.

Selected Readings

Fleischner, F. G.: Recurrent pulmonary embolism and cor pulmonale. New England Journal of Medicine, *276*:1213–1220, 1967.
Leading Article: Fat embolism. British Medical Journal, *3*:476–477, 1970.
Leading Article: Prevention of deep-vein thrombosis: the way ahead. Lancet, *2*:693–694, 1971.
Leading Article: Fat embolism. Lancet, *1*:672–673, 1972.
Leading Article: Ischaemia of the intestinal tract. British Medical Journal, *4*:566–567, 1972.
Salzman, E. W., Harris, W. H., and DeSanctis, R. W.: Reduction in venous thromboembolism by agents affecting platelet function. New England Journal of Medicine, *284*:1287–1292, 1971.
Sherry, S.: Thrombosis prevented. New England Journal of Medicine, *284*:1324–1326, 1971.
Walter, J. B., and Israel, M. S.: General Pathology. 4th ed. Edinburgh, Churchill Livingstone, 1974. See, in particular, Chapter 35, "General Features of Thrombosis and Its Occurrence in the Venous System"; Chapter 36, "Thrombosis in Arteries and in the Heart"; Chapter 37, "Embolism"; and Chapter 38, "Ischaemia and Infarction."

SHOCK AND HEMORRHAGE

Chapter 21

After studying this chapter the student should be able to:

- Describe the metabolic changes that follow injury.
- Describe the effects of an acute hemorrhage.
- Compare the clinical features of syncope with those of secondary shock.
- List seven important types of secondary shock and describe their pathogenesis.
- Discuss the concept of irreversible shock and describe its pathogenesis.
- List the organs that are frequently damaged in shock.
- Outline the treatment of shock.

METABOLIC CHANGES FOLLOWING INJURY

The body's response to injury is complex, for it involves a general reaction as well as the local phenomena of inflammation and repair.

Following any injury (except for the most trivial) there is a period of a day or two when energy requirements of the body are met by protein catabolism.

340

SHOCK AND HEMORRHAGE

The proteins of the muscles are broken down to amino acids, which are subsequently deaminated;* the nitrogen content is excreted, so that the body is temporarily in negative nitrogen balance. To some extent, this can be countered by the administration of glucose, and it is a common practice to give a sugar solution to injured patients. Administration of protein has no advantage, since in its turn it is deaminated and utilized for energy requirements. Following injury there is also a tendency for sodium and water to be retained, and the excessive administration of either of these substances can be dangerous. This initial catabolic phase is usually short-lived, but it is prolonged if complications such as infection supervene. Considerable loss of weight can then ensue.

The changes that occur following injury are not confined to protein metabolism. Potassium and nitrogen are lost, and there is retention of vitamin C in the body. The blood sugar tends to rise, and glycosuria is not uncommon. Likewise, a moderate rise in body temperature is frequent. The white cell count of the blood rises as a result of an increase in the number of neutrophil polymorphs, while at the same time the lymphocytes and eosinophils decrease in number. A thrombocytosis is characteristic, and together with a decreased clotting time is a factor that promotes thrombosis. An interesting feature of severe injury is the development of a progressive anemia. This is not due to iron deficiency or iron loss, but to the protein catabolism that is so characteristic of the reaction to injury.

The mechanism by which these metabolic changes take place is not clearly understood. There is over-action of the adrenal medulla and excess epinephrine secretion, which in part explain the hyperglycemia. The pituitary responds by an increased excretion of adrenocorticotropic hormone (ACTH), and the adrenal cortex produces more hydrocortisone, which plays an important part in the catabolic processes that follow injury. The sodium and water retention is related to an increased secretion of aldosterone and pituitary antidiuretic hormone (Fig. 21–1). These endocrine reactions to stress are responsible for some of the metabolic changes and are regarded as beneficial. Indeed, any patient who is receiving a maintenance dose of adrenal steroids, e.g., for pemphigus vulgaris or rheumatoid arthritis, must have the dose increased when he or she is subjected to injury, such as that of a surgical operation.

When protein catabolism and the other changes just described cease, convalescence is completed by an anabolic phase. There is reversal of the

---

*Amino acids are broken down in two ways: In deamination the amino group $(-NH_2)$ is removed as ammonia $(-NH_3)$, which is converted to urea in the liver. In transamination the $-NH_2$ group is transferred to a keto acid. This process can occur in most tissues and is catalyzed by transaminases.

341

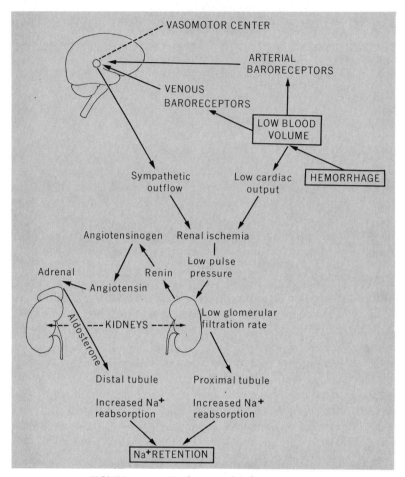

FIGURE 21–1. *Mechanism of sodium retention.*

Diagrammatic representation of the means by which the body retains sodium after a sudden reduction in blood volume, such as after severe hemorrhage.

changes, proteins are re-formed, and weight and health are restored. Severe injury is often followed by a state of *shock*, a name given to a clinical state in which the patient has tachycardia, and is pale, ashen, and sweating. The features are most easily understood by first considering the effects of acute hemorrhage.

Effects of Acute Hemorrhage

The vascular system contains about 5 liters of blood, which are kept in motion by the action of the heart so that all tissues are adequately perfused. The amount of blood reaching any area is determined by two factors: the diameter of the arterioles supplying it and the blood pressure.

The effects of blood loss depend on the quantity of blood lost and the speed at which the loss occurs. If a small quantity of blood is lost suddenly, there is scarcely any effect on the circulation because the large venous system acts as a reservoir for blood. Consequently, when a small amount is lost, an increase in venous tone reduces the capacity of the venous system, so that there is no reduction in the volume of blood reaching the heart (the venous return). Thus, there is no reduction in the cardiac output. When a larger volume of blood is suddenly withdrawn, this reserve mechanism of the venous reservoir is inadequate. The venous return is diminished, the cardiac output falls, and the blood pressure would also fall were there no other compensatory mechanisms available. The next response to hemorrhage is a series of actions designed to prevent any fall in blood pressure.

MECHANISMS FOR MAINTENANCE OF THE BLOOD PRESSURE

Following severe hemorrhage the fall in blood pressure is detected by the pressure-sensitive carotid sinus and other baroreceptors; these reflexly initiate a sympathetic outflow from the central nervous system (see Fig. 21–2). The

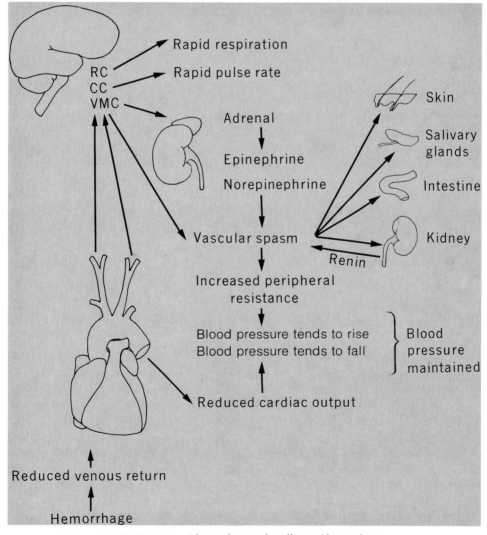

FIGURE 21–2. *The cardiovascular effects of hemorrhage.*

Abbreviations: RC, respiratory center; CC, cardiac center; VMC, vasomotor center.

result is an increase in heart rate and constriction of the arterioles of the *skin,* *kidneys,* and *splanchnic area* both by direct action and by the indirect action of the adrenal medulla, which is stimulated to secrete epinephrine and norepinephrine. In addition, the reduced blood pressure acts on the kidney directly and causes a release of renin (see Chapter 20). These mechanisms lead to an overall increase in the peripheral resistance, so that even with a reduced cardiac output, the systemic blood pressure is maintained at normal or near-normal levels. The maintenance of an adequate blood pressure allows the blood flow to the brain, the heart, and the respiratory muscles to remain virtually unaltered. However, the areas affected by arteriolar vasoconstriction tend to suffer; for example, the skin is cold and pale, the urine output falls, and salivary gland secretion decreases, resulting in dryness of the mouth. Thus, the vasomotor response to acute hemorrhage causes a redistribution of blood, a mechanism that may be regarded as an emergency measure designed to keep the essential organs supplied with blood.

RESTORATION OF BLOOD VOLUME

During the first few hours after bleeding the extravascular fluids pass into the blood stream, thereby restoring the blood volume. This can be demonstrated quite easily by checking the hemoglobin levels at intervals. Immediately after a sudden hemorrhage, the hemoglobin level is normal. During the next 8 hours it falls as dilution occurs. This process is largely complete by the end of 48 hours, by which time the hemoglobin level is a good guide to the extent of a previous blood loss. The transfer of extracellular fluid to the blood stream occurs as a result of the reduced capillary hydrostatic pressure, which is secondary to arteriolar vasoconstriction. Complete restoration of the plasma volume is dependent on replacement of the lost plasma proteins. These are manufactured for the most part in the liver and enter the circulation via the thoracic duct.

CHANGES IN THE BLOOD

Within a few minutes of bleeding, the clotting time is considerably decreased; during the next few hours, there is an increase in the level of platelets and neutrophils, which persists for several days. The restoration of the red cell count is a slow process, since the body has no reserve store of erythrocytes. New red cells have to be manufactured, and a normal count is not attained until four to six weeks later, regardless of the severity of the blood loss.

A normal adult can lose 500 ml of blood quite rapidly with little discomfort, a fact attested to by millions of blood donors. A sudden loss of 30 to 50 per cent of the blood volume (1.5 to 2.5 liters) can be fatal. However, such a loss spread over a day or so can be tolerated if the compensatory mechanism keeps pace with the blood loss. When the compensatory mechanisms are inadequate for this purpose, the patient sinks into a state described as shock, and this may be fatal.

Shock

Before the important subject of shock is discussed, the phenomenon of syncope will be described, since it has many features in common with shock and was at one time termed "primary shock."

SYNCOPE

Syncope, or a vasovagal attack, is better known as the common faint. The subject is invariably standing up; the initial symptoms are giddiness and light-headedness. Shortly after this, consciousness is lost and the subject falls to the ground. Pallor of the skin is a striking feature; the body is bathed in a cold sweat. The blood pressure is low, and the pulse is weak, with its rate either slowed or normal. Syncope can occur following blood loss, but it can also be caused by pain or psychological factors. The very thought of having an injection or having blood withdrawn is enough to send some people into a faint. It is believed that syncope is caused by sudden autonomic overactivity that leads to vasodilatation in the muscles and pooling of blood there. The venous return is suddenly reduced and with it the cardiac output, the blood pressure, and blood supply to the brain. The loss of consciousness in syncope is brief, and if the subject is laid horizontally, or attains that position spontaneously, he soon recovers. In rare cases death may occur—at least this is one suggestion for the rare cases of sudden death that occur unexpectedly, such as when a needle is introduced into the pleural cavity or during an attempted abortion. It has been reported that syncope occurring during induction of anesthesia may be fatal if the anesthetic is administered with the patient in the upright position, such as in a dental chair.

The remainder of this section deals with the much more serious condition of shock itself—or as it was once called, "secondary shock."

SHOCK

Shock is seen following many forms of injury; it may occur immediately, or it may happen after a period of comparative well-being. The patient lies still and listlessly; his temperature is subnormal, his skin cold and clammy, and his face ashen. Obvious cyanosis is often present, the blood pressure is low, and the pulse is rapid and thready. Little or no urine is passed.

In shock there is an inadequate blood supply to many tissues, leading to tissue hypoxia, metabolic acidosis, and defective function of the tissues concerned. Liver, lungs, heart, and kidneys are commonly affected, but under particular circumstances the effects of ischemia of other tissues (*e.g.,* retina, pituitary, and pancreas) may dominate the situation.

The clinical picture of shock may occur in a variety of conditions, and not surprisingly, these have all been assembled under the all-embracing title of "shock." Conditions that lead to a state of shock include:

Loss of blood
Following trauma
Loss of plasma (*e.g.,* following burns)

Loss of fluid and electrolytes
Overwhelming infection

Acute heart failure

Generalized anaphylaxis

The inclusion of so many diverse conditions under the one heading of shock has tended to obscure our understanding of the condition. They all produce a similar clinical picture, but it is hardly to be expected that the mechanisms involved would be the same in each case. Furthermore, a state of shock can occur as a terminal event under many other circumstances, *e.g.*, after electrocution, overdose of drugs, drowning, or massive total body irradiation. To attempt to understand shock one must consider each condition separately.

Hemorrhagic Shock.   If the compensatory mechanisms following bleeding are inadequate to maintain an effective perfusion of the tissues of the body, a state of shock ensues (Fig. 21–3). Recovery may occur spontaneously or as a result of efficient treatment, such as transfusion; such shock is therefore said to be *reversible*. Occasionally, in spite of efficient, vigorous treatment, the blood pressure continues to fall, the patient's clinical condition deteriorates, and death ensues. This response, termed *irreversible shock*, is considered later.

Traumatic Shock.   The circulatory changes following trauma are very similar to those seen following hemorrhage. The possible mechanisms are:

HEMORRHAGE.   It is often not appreciated that there is considerable bleeding into the tissues following any injury, even closed injuries such as a fractured femur. Much of the swelling that is seen around the fracture is due to blood that has poured into the adjacent tissues; some is due to inflammatory exudate.

INFECTION.   There is little doubt that the powerful exotoxins of the pathogenic clostridia exert a profound shocking effect. Gas gangrene, even in the absence of substantial tissue damage, causes shock and death.

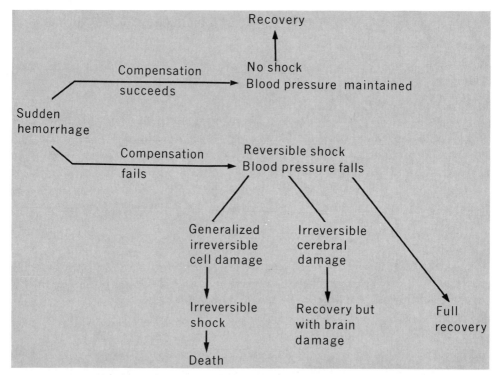

FIGURE 21–3.   *The possible end-results of a sudden hemorrhage.*

ENDOTOXIC FACTOR. The intravenous injection of endotoxins of the gram-negative bacilli leads to a shocklike state in animals. This is particularly marked following a second injection 24 hours after a previous one. The mechanism is not well understood, and the phenomenon is known as the Shwartzman phenomenon. Patients whose wounds are infected with gram-negative coliforms can suddenly develop shock as a result of endotoxemia or septicemia.

INFLAMMATORY EXUDATE FORMATION. The outpouring of fluid into inflamed tissues is responsible for some of the swelling around injured parts and adds its quota to that of bleeding as a cause of reduction in blood volume.

In summary, *blood loss is the single most important factor in causing traumatic shock.*

Shock Following Thermal Burns. The severe shock that follows burns is largely related to the tremendous loss of plasma in the inflammatory exudate. At a later stage, bacterial infection, such as that with *Pseudomonas pyocyanea* and other coliforms, may play a part. An important point of difference from hemorrhagic shock is that there is concentration, rather than dilution, of blood. The hemoglobin level therefore rises.

Shock Due to Loss of Fluid and Electrolytes. Loss of fluid or sodium can lead to such depletion of the extracellular tissue fluids that unless replacement therapy is instituted shock can develop as a result of an inadequate volume of circulating plasma. This condition is seen following persistent vomiting due to pyloric stenosis or intestinal obstruction, in cholera, in any severe diarrhea (particularly in children), and in dysentery.

Shock in Infection. Shock is seen in a variety of infections. It is prominent in infections with the toxic organisms of diphtheria and gas gangrene, and it is also a feature of many other severe infections: pneumonia, peritonitis, typhoid fever, typhus, and others of a similar nature. In recent years, a new syndrome — endotoxic shock — has been recognized; it is caused by the sudden entry of gram-negative coliform organisms or their endotoxins into the circulation. It is a complication of any coliform infection and is usually a sequel to urinary tract infection. There is a sudden onset of profound shock; unless treated expeditiously, it causes high mortality.

The shock of infection has a complex pathogenesis: at least three factors must be considered:

(1) *Pooling of blood.* Blood is sequestered in the splanchnic area because of vasodilatation. The effective blood volume is thereby reduced.

(2) *Loss of fluid in inflammatory exudate.* In gas gangrene the profuse loss of protein-rich exudate is in part responsible for the hemoconcentration and the reduction of blood volume.

(3) *Heart failure.* Some bacterial toxins (*e.g.*, diphtheria toxin) damage the myocardium, and an element of heart failure may further embarrass an already failing circulation.

Cardiogenic Shock. Extensive myocardial infection, sudden severe cardiac dysrhythmias, rupture of a valve cusp, and the sudden accumulation of fluid or blood in the pericardium can sometimes lead to a state of shock that resembles shock following trauma. This condition results from a low cardiac output, for it leads to underperfusion of tissues as an initial effect, and the resulting metabolic acidosis (see below) causes peripheral vasodilatation and pooling of blood. The shock that occurs following massive pulmonary embolism has a similar pathogenesis.

Anaphylactic Shock. Generalized anaphylaxis occurs when an individual, already sensitized by IgE, encounters the specific sensitizing antigen. See Chapter 9 for a more complete discussion.

THE METABOLIC UPSET DURING SHOCK

A patient in shock shows a profound reduction in metabolic rate (the nature of which is not well understood), but this reduction appears to be related to a block in carbohydrate utilization. In spite of cutaneous vasoconstriction — and therefore a reduction in heat loss — the patient's temperature tends to fall. An important effect of shock is that the underperfusion of tissues results in anaerobic glycolysis with the release of pyruvic and lactic acids into the circulation. A metabolic acidosis is characteristic of shock.

SUMMARY OF THE PATHOGENESIS OF SHOCK

It is evident that shock is essentially a state in which there is underperfusion of tissues. Shock may be caused by the following:

1. HYPOVOLEMIA. A low blood volume can occur after (a) hemorrhage (external or internal), (b) external loss of water and electrolytes (resulting from vomiting, diarrhea, diabetes insipidus, or the excess use of diuretics), (c) rapid accumulation of inflammatory exudate (from burns and infection), and (d) dehydration (heat exhaustion and inadequate fluid intake).

2. REDUCTION OF EFFECTIVE BLOOD VOLUME DUE TO INTERNAL SEQUESTRATION. Peripheral vasodilation can result in pooling of blood so that the effective volume of circulating blood is decreased. The splanchnic area and skeletal muscle are the sites where vasodilation commonly occurs. This state has been called *peripheral circulatory failure* and is encountered particularly in endotoxic shock and metabolic acidosis.

3. CARDIAC FACTORS. A state of low output can result from acute heart failure or from mechanical problems such as cardiac tamponade.

4. SLUDGING. If the flowing blood of a patient in shock is observed with a microscope, it will be seen that the red cells tend to flow in clumps rather than as individual cells. When this phenomenon was first described, the blood was said to be converted into a "mucklike sludge," from which comes the name *sludging*. The process differs from true agglutination in that the masses of red cells can be broken up mechanically *in vitro*. The cause of sludging appears to be an increase in the high-molecular-weight substance of the blood, and its effect is to impede the blood flow through tissues. Sludging therefore contributes to the poor perfusion of tissues in shock.

IRREVERSIBLE SHOCK

Some patients with shock recover either spontaneously or as a result of treatment. Others steadily deteriorate in spite of all efforts to save them. It is commonly believed that there is a stage from which recovery becomes impossible. This is called *irreversible shock*. The phenomenon can be demonstrated experimentally. If an animal is bled, it passes into a state of shock. It can be allowed to stay in a state of hypotensive hypovolemic shock for a few minutes and then be resuscitated by returning its own lost blood through a catheter. If the animal is allowed to stay in a state of shock for too long, the transfusion fails to reverse the shock, and its condition steadily deteriorates until death ensues.

The present concept of shock is that the major abnormality is the underperfusion of certain vital organs. If the state of shock is allowed to persist too long, there is permanent damage to tissues and recovery is therefore impossible. Organs that show damage are the following:

LIVER. It is common to find centrilobular necrosis in patients dying of shock.

HEART. Patchy myocardial infarction is common, and acute heart failure can be added to a state of shock produced by other mechanisms.

LUNG. Progressive pulmonary congestion, edema, and hemorrhages are common complications of shock. The precise pathogenesis of the "shock lung" is not known. It is probable that many factors are involved and the following have been suggested:

   (a) overtransfusion and fluid overload (see Chapter 26)
   (b) graft-versus-host reaction from transfused lymphocytes (see Chapter 9).
   (c) fat embolism (see Chapter 20).
   (d) oxygen toxicity (see Chapter 30).
   (e) bronchopneumonia.

The initial symptom is overventilation, which results in a low arterial P_{CO_2}. As respiratory function deteriorates, there is cyanosis and metabolic acidosis due to tissue hypoxia.

KIDNEY. Oliguria and anuria are characteristic of shock. Acute tubular necrosis, which can become extensive, may lead to irreversible renal damage (Fig. 21–4).

FIGURE 21–4. *Cortical necrosis of the kidney.*

Specimen from a 40-year-old woman who died in renal failure. The specimen shows necrosis of the outer two thirds to three fourths of the cortex. The inner layer of the cortex and the medulla are congested. This is the most severe type of ischemic renal damage encountered in shock. The condition affects both kidneys equally and is similar to the changes seen in the rabbit in the generalized Shwartzman phenomenon. For a more complete description, see Case History I.

Case History I. (See Figure 21–4.)   The patient was a 40-year-old woman who had had a normal pregnancy until the thirty-first week of gestation. She was then found to be hypertensive (blood pressure raised to 240/120); she also developed abdominal pain and began to bleed from the vagina. Her condition was diagnosed as abruptio placentae (premature detachment of the placenta). An emergency cesarean section was performed, but it failed to save the child; there was also considerable loss of blood during the operation. The patient went into shock, developed anuria, and in spite of peritoneal dialysis, experienced a rise in blood potassium to 7.0 mEq per liter (normal level is 3.5 to 5.5 mEq per liter). Her blood urea nitrogen also rose to 100 mg per 100 ml (normal level is 10 to 20 mg per 100 ml). She died in renal failure eight days after the onset of symptoms.

INTESTINE.   In the dog, shock leads to such ischemia of the gut that necrosis and gangrene occur. In the human, patchy mucosal necrosis can occur in both the large and the small intestine and can further complicate the situation clinically.

PITUITARY.   Infarction of the pituitary is best known as a complication of shock following labor.

EYE.   Retinal ischemia can result in blindness.

PANCREAS.   Patchy pancreatitis is not uncommon, but it is usually silent clinically.

It is evident that death from shock may occur for many reasons, either as a result of damage to some organ or from a metabolic upset secondary to this damage. From a practical point of view, the efficiency of treatment is of overriding importance because many of the potentially lethal causes and effects of shock can be counteracted. Irreversible shock must be regarded as being almost always due to inefficient treatment.

TREATMENT OF SHOCK

The treatment of shock is a complex affair but includes the following:

1. *Restoration of blood volume* by the administration of blood, water, or electrolytes, depending upon the circumstances. Fluid must be administered quickly, and the central venous pressure must be monitored with a catheter placed in one of the large systemic veins. A rise in venous pressure indicates overburdening of the heart and the necessity for reducing the speed of fluid input.

2. *Maintenance of renal function.*

3. *Correction of metabolic acidosis* by the intravenous administration of sodium bicarbonate solution.

4. *Maintenance of adequate pulmonary ventilation.* Avoidance of any obstruction of airways can be life-saving; the inhalation of 30 per cent oxygen is helpful.

5. *Administration of drugs.* It is worth remembering that in any form of shock a drug administered by the subcutaneous or intramuscular route is liable to be absorbed slowly owing to the poor state of the circulation. Failure to get a satisfactory clinical response can lead to the need to readminister the drug. This, in turn, could lead to the formation of a large depot of the drug which could subsequently be absorbed with fatal results.

Patients in shock are particularly sensitive to the effects of depressant drugs such as anesthetic agents. The place of morphine in shock should be limited to its use in alleviating severe pain and apprehension.

It was at one time recommended that norepinephrine and drugs with a similar action should be given with a view to causing vasoconstriction and a rise in blood pressure. Unfortunately this treatment further imperils the blood supply to various vital organs—particularly to the kidney and intestine—and the use of these drugs is not now recommended. Indeed, *vasodilator* drugs are sometimes given. There are some authorities who recommend their administration with massive doses of glucocorticoids, although the mode of action of the steroids is by no means clear. Perhaps they block the action of endogenous epinephrine, and thereby prevent vasospasm in vital organs.

6. *Treatment of Infection.* Although obvious enough in diseases like gas gangrene, infection following trauma may sometimes pass unnoticed and untreated.

7. *Treatment of Mechanical Complications.* The presence of shock may lead to a failure to appreciate the presence of remediable mechanical lesions such as a subdural hematoma, pneumothorax, and hemopericardium.

CONCLUSION

There are many features about shock that we do not understand. Nevertheless, vigorous, well-designed treatment can save many cases. "Shock" is not a diagnosis that should be accepted without qualification; it indicates that something is wrong—a low blood volume, metabolic acidosis, sludging, arterial desaturation, renal failure, pericardial hemorrhage, or some other drastic deviation from normal—all of which can be diagnosed and often treated. When a patient has very severe injuries, when shock has been present for some time, when patients are already ill with some other disease, and when a severe untreatable infection is present, death may be inevitable. The diagnosis of irreversible shock, however, should be made only after death has occurred.

Review Questions

1. A previously healthy 25-year-old man was involved in a brawl and was stabbed several times in the upper abdomen. He was admitted to the hospital and was given a laparotomy as part of his emergency treatment. The spleen was lacerated and had to be removed. Several puncture wounds of the intestine were located and were closed by sutures. The blood pressure, pulse rate, respiratory rate, and fluid balance were carefully monitored, and for 24 hours the patient did well. His condition then deteriorated, and he passed into a state of shock. Discuss the possible causes and indicate the investigations that might be helpful in managing this case.
2. Compare the general effects of a severe hemorrhage with those of a severe burn.
3. List the changes that occur in the constituents of the blood following the sudden loss of two pints of blood from a severed radial artery.

Selected Readings

Dowd, J., and Jenkins, L. C.: The lung in shock: a review. Canadian Anaesthetists' Society Journal, *19*:309–318, 1972.

Herman, C. M.: Advances and newer concepts in shock. *In* Copper, P., and Nyhus, L. M. (Eds.): Surgery Annual. Vol. 4. New York, Appleton-Century-Crofts, 1974, pp. 1–49.

Jacobson, E. D.: A physiologic approach to shock. New England Journal of Medicine, *278*:834–839, 1968.

Rutherford, R. B.: The pathophysiology of trauma and shock. *In* Ballinger, W. F., Rutherford, R. B., and Zuidema, G. D. (Eds.): The Management of Trauma. 2nd ed. Philadelphia, W. B. Saunders Company, 1973.

Sevitt, S., and Stoner, H. B. (Eds.): The pathology of trauma. Journal of Clinical Pathology (Suppl.), *23*: (Suppl. 4) 1–214, 1971. This publication contains articles covering many topics, including the metabolic changes caused by trauma, fat embolism, and changes in coagulation.

Various authors: Federation Proceedings, *29*:1832–1873, 1970. Report of a symposium entitled "Physiologic Basis of Circulatory Shock" in which various authors discuss different aspects of shock, including its treatment with glucocorticoids.

FEVER AND HYPOTHERMIA

Chapter 22

After studying this chapter the student should be able to:

- Describe the physiological mechanisms by which the body's temperature is maintained within narrow limits.
- Define fever and hyperpyrexia.
- List ten causes of fever.
- Describe the central heat-regulating center and outline its mode of action
   (a) under normal conditions
   (b) in a patient with pneumonia
   (c) in a patient with heat stroke.
- Compare bacterial pyrogens with endogenous pyrogens.

354

FEVER AND HYPOTHERMIA

- Describe the circumstances under which malignant hyperpyrexia is usually encountered.
- Define hypothermia and describe the common causes and effects in infants and in adults.
- Give two examples of the value of induced hypothermia in medicine.

A rise in the body's temperature is so commonly found in illness that this response has been recognized since ancient times. Indeed, the term "fever" is sometimes used as being synonymous with disease. "Hayfever" and "cat-scratch fever" bear witness to this association, because in neither disease is fever an important feature. To avoid this confusion, the term "pyrexia" is commonly used in clinical medicine.

Before considering fever itself, one must understand the normal body temperature and the mechanism of its control.

THE NORMAL BODY TEMPERATURE

The most reliable method of taking the body's temperature is by placing a thermometer under the tongue with the lips closed. The temperature taken in this way varies from 97° to 99° F (36.1° to 37.4° C). The maximum temperature is generally attained at about 6:00 P.M., whereas it is at its lowest at about 3:00 A.M. In women there is an elevation of the temperature during the middle of the menstrual cycle; its onset is thought to herald ovulation, and this rise in temperature has been utilized in the rhythm system of contraception. In unconscious patients it is convenient to take the temperature by placing a thermometer in the rectum; the readings obtained in this way are about 1°F higher than those taken by mouth. Measurement of temperature by placing the thermometer in the axilla or groin is quite unreliable, since the surface skin temperature fluctuates widely and may approximate that of the external environment.

The maintenance of a constant body temperature is one aspect of homeostasis, and in humans has obtained a high degree of efficiency. The importance of this is obvious when it is remembered that cellular activity involves many chemical reactions that are largely dependent upon enzymatic activity and therefore very susceptible to changes in temperature. The body's temperature is regulated by a central heat-regulating center that initiates the various mechanisms to increase or decrease heat loss.

Temperature Regulation

The constancy of the body's temperature is maintained by balancing the amount of heat produced in the body with that which is lost.

Sources of Heat.   The major source of heat is the body's metabolic activity. Heat production under fasting conditions with the individual at complete mental and physical rest is called the *basal metabolic rate* (BMR), which ranges from 1400 to 1800 calories per day. Under normal active conditions, additional heat is produced by exercise, which can be quite modest with sedentary workers (*e.g.*, 1000 calories) or rather high in those engaged in heavy manual labor (*e.g.*, 6000 calories). The heat produced by metabolism raises the temperature of the blood through the relevant organs. Thus, the blood leaving the brain and the liver is warmer than that entering it. Likewise, during manual work blood leaving the skeletal muscles is heated. The warm blood from these centers of heat production is distributed to the organs of heat loss. Of these the skin is the most important.

Areas of Heat Loss.   Heat is lost from the blood as it perfuses the skin. Convection, radiation, and evaporation of sweat all play a part in the loss of heat. The latter is particularly important when the ambient temperature exceeds that of the body. Since the blood supply to the skin is regulated by the sympathetic division of the autonomic nervous system, the latter plays a dominant role in the maintenance of a constant body temperature. Some heat is also lost from the respiratory tract and mouth. In humans, this is a relatively constant amount, but in animals it can be increased considerably by panting.

THE CENTRAL TEMPERATURE-SENSITIVE AREA

Situated in the anterior part of the hypothalamus, in the *preoptic area*, is a group of nerve cells that is sensitive to the temperature of the arterial blood reaching it. When the temperature of the blood changes, impulses pass from this area to other parts of the hypothalamus. There are two main areas: (1) an anterior *heat-losing center,* which when stimulated leads to changes in the rest of the body, causing increased heat loss, and (2) a posterior *heat-promoting center,* which when stimulated leads to increased heat production and conservation (Fig. 22–1).

Mechanism for Increasing Body Temperature.   The heat-promoting center acts mainly through the sympathetic division of the autonomic nervous system. Cutaneous vasoconstriction reduces the amount of heat lost from the skin, and blood diverted to the internal organs is insulated from the exterior by the subcutaneous fat. Furthermore, as the skin becomes cooler, the subject feels cold and may take appropriate voluntary action such as putting on extra clothing.

The increased sympathetic outflow causes an increased output of epinephrine and norepinephrine from the adrenal glands. These hormones increase the metabolic rate of all cells through a mechanism that is not well understood. Metabolism is further increased by a *generalized increase in muscle tone.* If these mechanisms are inadequate, muscle tone increases to the extent that stretch reflexes are elicited and *shivering* commences. As one group of muscles

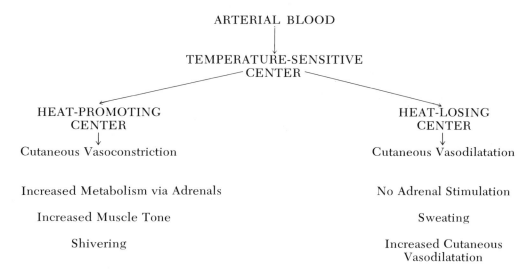

ARTERIAL BLOOD

TEMPERATURE-SENSITIVE
CENTER

HEAT-PROMOTING
CENTER

Cutaneous Vasoconstriction

Increased Metabolism via Adrenals

Increased Muscle Tone

Shivering

HEAT-LOSING
CENTER

Cutaneous Vasodilatation

No Adrenal Stimulation

Sweating

Increased Cutaneous
Vasodilatation

FIGURE 22–1.

Diagram to illustrate the principal heat-regulating mechanisms.

contracts, a stretch reflex of the antagonistic group is set in motion and initiates a fresh stretch reflex of the first group. This continuous shaking can increase the rate of heat production severalfold.

Mechanism of Decreasing Body Temperature. When the body's temperature tends to rise, there is a withdrawal of sympathetic vasoconstriction activity, the skin becomes warm and heat is lost. The subject feels hot and may remove clothing, retire to the shade, or take other appropriate action. If this regulating mechanism does not suffice, the heat-losing center initiates sweating from the eccrine glands. Evaporation of this fluid requires heat, but an additional effect of sweating is the local release of bradykinin from the glands. This induces further vasodilatation and heat loss.

PERIPHERAL TEMPERATURE RECEPTORS

The heat-regulating mechanism is also influenced by impulses received from the peripheral receptors in the skin. This influence can be demonstrated by an experiment in which the blood to one arm is occluded by a cuff and the arm is then immersed in cold water. Within seconds the skin of the opposite arm undergoes vasoconstriction, indicating that a nervous reflex is involved rather than a change in blood temperature. After a while, this vasoconstriction wanes, but on restoration of the circulation, a more prolonged period of vasoconstriction ensues as the cooled blood of the limb reaches the hypothalamus and activates the central mechanism directly.

Fever

Fever, or *pyrexia,* may be defined as an elevation of the body's temperature following a disturbance of the regulating mechanism. When the temperature reaches or exceeds 104°F (40.5°C), the condition is called "hyperpyrexia."

Heat Stroke.   Some rise in body temperature normally occurs during extreme exercise, because the heat-eliminating mechanisms cannot immediately keep pace with the excessive heat production in the muscles. When the environment is hot and humid, even mild exercise can cause a marked rise in body temperature. Sometimes the heat-regulating mechanism breaks down under these circumstances and the temperature rises. This is the condition of *heat stroke* or *sun stroke;* unless promptly treated, the temperature continues to rise, reaching 109°F (43°C) or even more. Patients become comatose, often have convulsions, and may have permanent brain damage if they survive. Heat stroke must therefore be treated most energetically with tepid sponging or immersion in cold water until the temperature approaches normal.

Infection.   Infection is the most common cause of fever; the pattern of the temperature chart is sometimes characteristic of a particular disease. The relapsing course of malaria and brucellosis are examples of this. So also are the two phases of fever that characterize dengue. With some acute infections, particularly if there is an initial septicemia as in urinary tract infections and lobar pneumonia, the onset of fever is sudden. The following stages are recognized:

THE COLD STAGE.   At the onset of the illness, the patient experiences an intense feeling of cold. There is peripheral constriction which is manifest by pallor, and the patient starts to shiver. The teeth chatter and the patient shakes all over with the familiar condition called a "rigor." The increased muscular activity combined with reduced heat loss causes the temperature to rise. The blood pressure and pulse rate also rise. In general, there is an increase in pulse rate of about 10 beats per minute for each 1° F rise in temperature (18 beats per minute per 1° C). In children, the rigor may be replaced by a convulsion.

THE HOT STAGE.   As the temperature approaches its peak, the peripheral vasoconstriction relaxes, and the patient feels dry and warm. The amount of heat lost now balances that formed and the temperature remains constant. It must be noticed that the thermostat of the heat-regulating mechanism is still under control but is geared to maintain the temperature at a higher level than normal. The normal daily variation in temperature is seen, so that the highest levels occur during the evening. This phase can last for several hours or days.

THE SWEATING PHASE.   The temperature begins to fall, and the patient soon experiences a sensation of intense heat. The patient feels the urge to throw off clothing, sweats profusely, and then the temperature returns to normal. When this phase occurs over a short period, the termination is described as "crisis." This is particularly characteristic of lobar pneumonia and attacks of malaria. In some illnesses, the pyrexia subsides slowly (such as in typhoid fever), and its termination is described as "lysis."

In old age and in debilitated subjects, no fever may occur even with severe infections. This absence of response is said to be of poor prognostic import. It is the opposite of childhood response to infection — with children, even a trivial infection can cause a high fever.

Chronic infections frequently cause fever, and the prolonged rise in metabolic rate combines with loss of appetite to produce wasting. Chronic pulmonary tuberculosis provides an example of this; the emaciated appearance of the patients earned the terms "consumption" and "phthisis" for the disease.

Infarction. A mild fever is commonly seen in patients with infarction, such as of the lung or the myocardium.

Tumors. Some tumors are particularly liable to produce pyrexia, even in the absence of a complicating infection. It is a well-known feature of Hodgkin's disease as well as of carcinoma of the kidney.

Hemorrhage. Fever may follow bleeding, particularly bleeding into the gastrointestinal tract or the peritoneal space. Sudden bleeding from a ruptured ectopic pregnancy, for example, can produce acute abdominal pain, distention, and fever, which might mimic an infection.

Brain Damage. Any cause of brain damage (*e.g.*, bleeding, infection, or infarction) can lead to an upset of the central heat-regulating mechanism, either by damaging the hypothalamus directly or by interfering with the outflow of autonomic nervous impulses.

Injury. Fever lasting for several days often follows mechanical trauma, such as a crushing injury.

Severe Anemia. During phases of acute hemolysis, fever is sometimes prominent.

Miscellaneous Conditions. Fever is a prominent feature of acute gout and some of the collagen diseases (*e.g.*, lupus erythematosus and rheumatic fever). An adverse reaction to a drug is an important cause. In most instances, the disease is accompanied by an inflammatory reaction, and the fever is probably related to this (see below).

DIAGNOSIS OF FEVER

Disease is so often accompanied by fever that the pyrexia itself is sometimes the presenting symptom.

Fever or pyrexia of unknown origin *(FUO or PUO)* is a common clinical problem, and accurate diagnosis demands considerable clinical skill combined with laboratory aids. A good history combined with a knowledge of epidemiology will sometimes suggest the correct diagnosis (see Case History 1 and Fig. 22–2).

Case History I. The patient was a 69-year-old man who had gone on an African safari for one month. While there, he had occasional attacks of diarrhea and had developed a chronic cough, which was productive of a large amount of sputum. He gave a history of having had such severe night sweats on several occasions that the whole bed had been soaked. Before leaving Africa, he developed a superficial skin infection between the fourth and fifth fingers of his right hand. Two days after arriving in Canada he was brought into the emergency ward, having collapsed at home while unpacking a suitcase. He had struck his head and had lost consciousness for about 20 minutes. He complained of a mild headache, had a temperature of 102° F, and had a laceration of the left frontal area of the scalp. Infection was noted on the hand, and the fever was attributed to this infection. He was given penicillin and sent home. The next day he felt quite well, but the following day he was found by a friend to be drowsy, although still responsive and able to watch a hockey game. The next morning he was found unconscious and was again admitted to a hospital—this time, in a coma. Blood and urine were obtained for culture, and numerous biochemical tests were ordered. In view of the history of cough and drenching night sweats, the possibility of pulmonary tuberculosis was considered; a radiograph of lung, however, revealed no evidence of disease. Cerebrospinal fluid was obtained by lumbar puncture and revealed an elevated protein content (56 mg per 100

FIGURE 22–2. *Blood film from patient with malignant tertian malaria.*

Numerous ring forms (small arrows) of *Plasmodium falciparum* are present in blood film. Particularly characteristic is the presence of two or more organisms in one red cell (large arrow). Blood film stained by Giemsa stain (× 1000).

ml). The patient was noted to be slightly jaundiced. Before the results of the various tests were obtainable, a blood film was examined and was found to contain a large number of malaria parasites (see Fig. 22–2). A diagnosis of malignant malaria with cerebral involvement was made, and emergency treatment with the antimalarial drug chloroquine was undertaken. Nevertheless, the patient rapidly deteriorated, developed hypotension, and died within four hours. This case illustrates how a good history and a knowledge of diseases endemic to particular geographic locations can help in arriving at a diagnosis. Attributing fever and loss of consciousness to a minor skin infection was a mistake that cost this patient his life.

A fever combined with a heart murmur suggests bacterial endocarditis; repeated blood cultures must be performed for an accurate diagnosis. Pulmonary tuberculosis can be remarkably silent but will be revealed by an x-ray. Fever in a patient past the age of 40 should lead to a search for occult cancer, fever in a child might suggest leukemia, and fever in a young adult might cause suspicion of infectious mononucleosis. In the diagnosis of PUO the physician's skills and knowledge can thus be taxed to the extreme (see Case History II).

Case History II. A 30-year-old male was admitted to the hospital for the investigation of fever. Five weeks before admission, he had developed severe pain in the back, which had been relieved by aspirin. Two weeks later, the pain recurred and radiated toward the sternum. Although a heart attack was suspected, an electrocardiogram showed no abnormality; his serum enzymes were also normal. He had several bouts of fever during the next three weeks. On examination in the hospital he was found to be a pale, sallow, somewhat overweight man, who was sweating profusely and in moderate distress. His temperature on admission was 105° F. and his pulse was 120 beats per minute; blood pressure was 115/65 mm Hg. A murmur was heard over the precordium, and bacterial endocarditis was considered a possible cause. Numerous blood cultures were performed, all of which were sterile. Analysis of the urine was normal; culture was sterile. No obvious site of infection could be found clinically. The fever dropped to 100°F with aspirin but recurred each evening while the patient was in the hospital. Numerous other investigations were performed, including radiographs of the chest and vertebrae and an intravenous pyelogram. Blood was taken for the Widal, Weil-Felix and brucella agglutination tests. Radiographs of the abdomen revealed no evidence of a sub-phrenic abscess such as might occur following a perforation of appendix, peptic ulcer, or diverticulum of the colon. All agglutination tests were negative as was the VDRL test. A blood count was, however, unusual. In spite of the patient's having a fever, he had a total white count of 4400 with 95 per cent neutrophils and 4 per cent band forms. The platelet count was 95,000. Systemic lupus erythematosus was first considered, but since no anti-DNA antibodies were present in the blood this condition was eliminated from consideration. In view of the unusual blood findings, a bone marrow puncture was performed, and the smear revealed almost complete replacement of normal marrow cells by primitive blast cells. There were a few normal erythroid precursors and virtually no megakaryocytes. In cases such as this, at times it is not possible to decide whether the cells are lymphoblasts or myeloblasts. The terms *stem cell leukemia* or *blast cell leukemia* are therefore convenient. About a week after admission, the patient still had a fever at night, and he developed ulceration of the mouth. He was treated with a variety of chemotherapeutic agents in courses over the next few months, but he died eight months after the first admission with bronchopneumonia. This case illustrates how malignant disease—in this case leukemia—can closely mimic infection by virtue of fever that is a presenting and constant feature.

PATHOGENESIS OF FEVER

The intravenous injection of gram-negative organisms produces a rigor and a sharp rise in temperature. This response appears to be due to lipopolysaccharide substances that are part of the bacterial body and are called *bacterial pyrogens*. They are thought to act indirectly by causing polymorphs to release an *endogenous pyrogen* that circulates in the blood and acts on the heat-regulating center. There is evidence that in humans, a similar pyrogen can be released from monocytes as well as from polymorphs. The actual mode of action of endogenous pyrogens is not known. It appears that the substance acts directly on the heat-regulating center and sets its thermostat to a higher level. It is clear that the common pathogenesis of fever is the release of endogenous pyrogens for inflammatory cells.

The bacterial pyrogens are heat stable and are of importance because they can produce febrile reactions if present in the fluids used in intravenous therapy, which though sterile, may still cause a sharp rigor (see Chapter 26). The fluids used for injection purposes must be carefully prepared by distillation to insure the exclusion of all bacterial products. Such pyrogen-free fluids must always be used.

The fact that fever often accompanies necrosis, such as in tumors, infarcts, and following hemolysis of red cells, suggests that dead tissue contains pyrogenic substances and that agents similar to those of bacteria have been isolated.

Certain steroid hormones can produce a rise in body temperature, and it is believed that the release of progesterone is responsible for the temperature rise that occurs during the menstrual cycle.

In the fully anesthetized patient, the heat-regulating mechanism is not functioning. The body therefore becomes poikilothermic (like the body of an amphibian) and takes up the temperature of the surrounding atmosphere. The patient must therefore be protected against hyperpyrexia as well as hypothermia.

Fulminating or *malignant hyperpyrexia* is a rare but important condition in which there is a rapid rise in temperature during the administration of general anesthesia. The progress of the pyrexia is extremely rapid and unless vigorous cooling is employed, the patient dies from hyperpyrexia and cardiac arrest. In most cases, the skeletal muscles show increased tension; it is believed that excess heat is produced in them. The precise cause of this condition is not known; in many instances, however, it is related to a type of muscle disease or myopathy that can be detected before surgery by finding an elevation of the serum levels of creatine phosphokinase, an enzyme that is released from damaged muscle. Sometimes there is a family history of myopathy.

Although recent work has shed some light on the mystery of fever, much has yet to be illuminated. It would be satisfying to believe that a rise in temperature in infection was a beneficial reaction designed to aid the body's defenses. There is, however, little evidence to support this. As yet, we must regard the maintenance of a normal temperature as an important homeostatic mechanism for the proper functioning of the body. Any marked departure from the normal appears to be, at best, of no value and, at worst, deleterious to well-being. There is some indication that fever is of benefit in virus infections. It seems that fever stimulates interferon production of infected cells and so may limit the course of the disease.

Hypothermia

Hypothermia may be defined as a body temperature below 95°F (35°C). It is an important cause of death in cold climates, especially of infants and the aged, and it has been utilized as an adjunct to anesthesia.

HYPOTHERMIA IN INFANTS

Newborn infants are particularly susceptible to cold, because of the relatively high ratio of surface area to body mass, the paucity of subcutaneous fat, and the low production of heat by physical means because of the inability to exercise or shiver. Furthermore, the thermoregulatory mechanism is relatively inefficient at birth and remains so for several hours.

During the first few weeks of life, infants need constant warmth, especially when ill. In cold countries open windows, lukewarm baths, and power cuts can cause inconvenience to adults but can be fatal to infants.

The early signs of cold injury are lethargy and difficulty in feeding. Indeed, the child has a still, serene appearance and the cheeks, nose, and extremities have a flush that deludes the onlooker into believing all is well. The cry is like a whimper, and the body feels cold. Later, bradycardia and edema of the eyelids and extremities occur. In the worst cases, the subcutaneous fat becomes hard.

HYPOTHERMIA IN ADULTS

Hypothermia can occur in adults in a number of circumstances. Immersion hypothermia is one of the lethal factors in shipwreck. Hypothermia is an important complication of myxedema and hypopituitarism, and it also occurs in patients with widespread eczema and generalized erythroderma. In widespread skin disease, the passive diffusion of water through the epidermis is greatly increased, and heat is lost both by evaporation and convection.

The most important example is the spontaneous hypothermia that occurs in old people — usually women — who live alone in poorly heated rooms and are poorly clothed. Undernutrition is often an additional factor; in persons who are in both calorie- and protein-deficient states, the basal metabolic rate is decreased. Hypothermia in the aged is sometimes a complication of senile dementia, or the effects of depressant drugs like alcohol and chlorpromazine that have dulled the mind. There is sometimes a severe precipitating infection such as pneumonia.

The patient with hypothermia looks ill. There is a corpselike chill of the body, and the rectal temperature can be as low as 70° F. The skin is pale, and the subcutaneous tissue is pliant and doughy. The patient remains still; muscles are rigid, and shivering is absent. The tendon reflexes are sluggish, and there is bradycardia, sometimes with atrial fibrillation. Since peripheral edema and puffiness of the eyelids are common, myxedema may be simulated. Oliguria (diminished urine output) is common, respiration is depressed, and death often occurs from cardiac arrest.

It is easy to overlook hypothermia, both in infancy and adults. Clinical thermometers that register as low as 75°F (24°C) should be available and used if the circumstances raise the possibility of hypothermia.

INDUCED HYPOTHERMIA

Some animals have acquired the ability to hibernate for long periods in a state of hypothermia as a useful adjunct to survival in winter. From experimental work carried out on small animals, it has been found that they can be cooled below 32°F (0°C) if they are made first to ingest propylene glycol. Mice can be kept in suspended animation for about one hour and then reanimated by artificial respiration and microwave diathermy. Larger animals do not tolerate this treatment so well and usually die within a few days. A lesser degree of hypothermia has been used as an adjunct to cardiac surgery. If the body's temperature is lowered, cardiac arrest can be tolerated for about one hour. The development of extracorporeal circulatory systems has allowed profound hypothermia to be used in open-heart surgery. In one method, the blood is cooled rapidly by passage through a heat exchanger and the circulation is maintained extracorporeally. At the temperature of 55 to 59° F (12.7 to 15° C), the circulation is stopped, and the heart is opened in a bloodless field. When the operation is finished, the blood is rewarmed, the heart is defibrillated and a normal circulation is restored. Extracorporeal circulations are now so efficient that hypothermia is less commonly used or is merely used as an adjunct to this procedure.

LOCAL HYPOTHERMIA

Extreme cold causes tissue damage; when the part is rewarmed, an acute inflammation follows and blisters occur. Direct damage to the capillaries is prominent, and vascular occlusion contributes to tissue necrosis. This type of cold injury is called "frost bite" and in cold climates is not uncommon following accidental exposure to cold. Usually, the toes, fingers, ears, and nose are affected. Deliberate application of extreme cold (cryosurgery) is used therapeutically in surgical practice. Solid carbon dioxide and liquid nitrogen are commonly applied to warts and other skin tumors. Various types of probes that are refrigerated by liquid nitrogen have been devised for applying cold to deeper tissues. They have been used to treat eye tumors as well as in intracranial surgery. At present, the use of cold is confined to special centers; the late effects are still being assessed.

Review Questions

1. Write an outline of the investigations that should be performed on a patient with pyrexia of unknown origin (PUO).
2. It is often assumed that fever indicates infection. Discuss this proposition, and give some examples of conditions in which fever is a manifestation of a noninfective process.
3. Compare the temperature-regulating mechanisms of an infant with those of an adult.
4. A patient develops a rigor following an intravenous injection of 500 ml of glucose solution. List the possible causes.

Selected Readings

Guyton, A. C.: Textbook of Medical Physiology. 5th ed. Philadelphia, W. B. Saunders Company, 1976. See in particular Chapter 72, "Body Temperature, Temperature Regulation, and Fever."
Petersdorf, R. B.: Alterations in body temperature. In Wintrobe, M. M., et al. (Eds.): Harrison's Principles of Internal Medicine. 7th ed. New York, McGraw-Hill Book Company, 1974, pp. 48–54.
Petersdorf, R. B.: Chills and fever. In Wintrobe, M. M., et al. (Eds.): Harrison's Principles of Internal Medicine. 7th ed. New York, McGraw-Hill Book Company, 1974, pp. 54–63.

DISORDERS OF NUTRITION

Chapter 23

After studying this chapter the student should be able to:

- Describe the metabolic effects of starvation.
- Distinguish between nutritional marasmus and kwashiorkor.
- Classify and list the vitamins that are required by humans.
- Describe the sources of vitamin A and discuss the effects of vitamin A deficiency and excess.
- Describe the sources of vitamin C and give an account of scurvy.
- Classify beriberi according to its several forms and describe the features of each type.
- Describe the effects of riboflavin deficiency.
- Outline the main features of pellagra.
- Describe the effects of pyridoxine deficiency.

STARVATION

With the world population expanding at an estimated rate of 70 million each year, it is likely that malnutrition will become increasingly common. The effects of total starvation will first be described.

METABOLIC CHANGES DURING STARVATION

The body's store of glucose and glycogen is sufficient for only one day's metabolic needs. The protein supply and the triacylglycerols of adipose tissue

366

provide enough energy for an additional three months in the average individual. For a fat person there are enough energy reserves for about one year's survival.

Immediate Changes in Starvation. The brain normally uses only glucose as fuel; after the first day of starvation the blood glucose level is maintained by new glucose formation in the liver, in which amino acids are used as fuel. The amino acids are provided by the breakdown of protein. Because the nitrogen component is excreted as urea, the body is therefore in negative nitrogen balance.

The triacylglycerols of adipose tissue are broken down to glycerol and fatty acids. Fatty acids are converted into ketone bodies in the liver, and these are used directly by most organs of the body instead of glucose.

Later Changes in Starvation. After the first week of starvation the breakdown of protein declines rapidly. A change occurs in the brain's metabolism such that it is able to utilize ketone bodies, particularly beta-hydroxybutyrate, instead of glucose. Starvation can now continue until all the stores of body fat are utilized. When the supply of fat has been exhausted, only protein remains. The muscle masses decline and death soon follows.

During starvation the body conserves energy by reducing energy output. The starved individual is apathetic and lacks interest in life. Hypothermia is a danger in cold climates. This picture of starvation differs from that of the patient with anorexia nervosa, who is usually restless (see Chapter 39).

Loss of water is a characteristic feature of early starvation. Its cause is unknown. For individuals who try weight reducing diets this loss provides false encouragement during the first few days of the regimen. In starvation the kidney is unable to concentrate urine and polyuria results.

The edema of starvation affects the dependent parts and appears to be due to the laxity of the subcutaneous tissues.

The wasted appearance of the starving person is all too familiar. The lax dry skin and wasted muscles are matched by wasting of the internal organs. In particular, with advanced starvation the intestine becomes increasingly thin; hence, when treating a starving patient one must give frequent small feedings if the person's life is to be saved.

Protein-Calorie Malnutrition in Childhood

Protein-calorie malnutrition is regarded as a spectrum of disease with marasmus at one end and kwashiorkor at the other end.

NUTRITIONAL MARASMUS

Marasmus is the name given to starvation in infants. It is due to deficiency of both protein and calories and is encountered in infants under one year of age. It is a common condition in the underdeveloped world and is usually due to cessation of breast feeding when the mother again becomes pregnant. The child exhibits the wasted appearance of starvation and in addition shows lack of growth. In those who survive, dwarfism is a frequent complication. As with starvation in adults, the marasmic child is more susceptible to infection; tuberculosis and dysentery often complete the lethal process initiated by starvation.

KWASHIORKOR

This is a syndrome observed in children between the ages of one and three years. Its name is derived from a local African word denoting illness in a child displaced from the breast by a subsequent pregnancy.

Kwashiorkor is due to a low protein intake and the presence of an adequate carbohydrate supply. It is characterized by a fatty liver and marked edema of the subcutaneous tissues. The inadequate protein supply leads to defective pigment formation; consequently, the hair becomes pale and even red in African children, and the skin is often depigmented and shows hyperkeratosis and flaking.

THE VITAMINS

Definition and Classification

Vitamins are organic substances that the body cannot manufacture and that are necessary for normal metabolism; only ten such substances are known. If these substances are present in insufficient quantity, disease results. The ten vitamins essential for good health are listed below in Table 23–1.

Causes and Effects of Individual Vitamin Deficiencies and Excesses

VITAMIN A (RETINOL)

Vitamin A is one of the fat-soluble vitamins. In herbivorous animals the colored pigments (carotenoids, such as carotene) of plants and vegetables are converted into vitamin A in the intestine, are absorbed, and subsequently are stored in the liver. Humans acquire their supply either directly from the carotenoids in vegetable matter (e.g., carrots, beet root, and green vegetables in

Table 23–1 THE ESSENTIAL VITAMINS

FAT-SOLUBLE	WATER-SOLUBLE
Vitamin A	Vitamin C
Vitamin D	Vitamin B Complex
Vitamin K	Thiamine
	Riboflavin
	Niacin
	Pyridoxine
	Cobalamin (B_{12})
	Folate

general) or indirectly from animal or dairy produce. The concurrent absorption of fat and the presence of bile salts in the intestine favor vitamin A absorption.

Causes of Vitamin A Deficiency. This is usually due to a deficient diet. This nutritional problem usually occurs in Indonesia, parts of Asia, India, the Middle East, and Latin America: it is almost unknown in North America and Europe. Vitamin A deficiency does, however, occur as a complication of the malabsorption syndrome; indeed, the blood level of carotene or vitamin A is used as a measure of the degree of malabsorption occurring.

Effects of Vitamin A Deficiency

THE EYE. Vitamin A forms an essential component of rhodopsin, a pigment in the rods of the retina. By absorbing light, rhodopsin initiates an electrical impulse that is transmitted to the brain and is interpreted as light. The first sign of vitamin A deficiency, therefore, is *night blindness.* Apart from this known biochemical action of vitamin A, its other functions remain a mystery in spite of much research. It is known that vitamin A regulates the structure of certain epithelial cells. In vitamin A deficiency, the epithelia of the genitourinary tract, the trachea, the nose, and the conjunctiva tend to undergo squamous metaplasia. The most important effect is in the eye. The conjunctival epithelium loses its mucus-secreting goblet cells and becomes keratinized, thereby taking on the characteristics of epidermis. The lacrimal ducts are affected in the same way, so that the eye becomes dry and subject to cracking and infection. The condition is called *xerophthalmia.* In due course the cornea becomes cloudy; with infection it can soften (*keratomalacia*), causing the globe to be perforated. The lens can be extruded and blindness results. Indeed, vitamin A deficiency is a leading cause of blindness in the world.*

OTHER EFFECTS. The replacement of respiratorylike epithelium (with its goblet cells and cilia) by keratinized squamous epithelium is a factor in the production of respiratory infections (see Fig. 30–8). Nevertheless, in the presence of a normal amount of vitamin A there is no evidence that an excessive intake can prevent respiratory infections. The time-honored tradition of administering children large quantities of vitamin A (in cod-liver oil) to prevent colds and respiratory infections appears to be quite ill-founded. Indeed, such a practice can cause toxic effects (see below).

In spite of the dramatic changes seen in epithelium in vitamin A deficiency, the biochemical nature of the defect is quite unknown. If a small piece of skin is grown in organ culture and is subjected to vitamin A deficiency, it soon shows hyperkeratosis. If an excess quantity of vitamin A is now added to the medium the epithelium changes to a goblet cell, mucus-secreting type. There is no evidence, however, that excess vitamin A in humans can convert normal keratinized epidermis into mucus-secreting epithelium.

Toxicity of Vitamin A. Very large doses of vitamin A are toxic and can cause an increase in intracranial pressure with headache, blurring of vision, and vomiting. This effect has been noticed by Arctic explorers when they ate polar-bear liver, which is a very rich source of vitamin A. Chronic poisoning can cause loss of hair, bone pains, and other symptoms.

---

*Other common causes are trachoma, diabetes mellitus, smallpox, onchocerciasis, gonococcal ophthalmia, injury through accidents, cataract, and glaucoma.

VITAMIN D

Vitamin D is present in all fat-containing animal products, but its richest source is cod-liver and halibut-liver oil. Vitamin D is also formed in the skin by the action of ultraviolet light on 7-dehydrocholesterol. Vitamin D exists in several forms. The most active compounds are formed by the liver and kidney.

The main action of vitamin D is to maintain calcium balance by aiding in the absorption of calcium from the intestine. The effects of hypovitaminosis D— that is, rickets and osteomalacia—are considered in Chapter 40.

Hypervitaminosis D. Toxic doses of vitamin D can cause hypercalcemia and metastatic calcification (see Chapter 40). Vomiting, diarrhea, drowsiness, and renal failure are the main clinical features.

VITAMIN K

Vitamin K is widely distributed in vegetable and animal foods. It is also synthesized by bacteria in the gut. Vitamin K deficiency is considered in Chapter 26.

VITAMIN E

Vitamin E includes a group of fat-soluble substances (tocopherols) that act as antioxidants. Various vitamin E deficiency states are recognized in animals. In humans, vitamin E deficiency has been described in premature infants and in patients having cystic fibrosis with severe steatorrhea (see Chapter 33). There is unfortunately no good evidence that excess vitamin E can ward off old age, coronary disease, or the other ills that are associated with the aging process.

VITAMIN C (ASCORBIC ACID)

Humans share with other primates and the guinea pig the feature of being one of the few mammals that cannot synthesize vitamin C. The main dietary sources are citrus fruits, currants, berries, green vegetables, and potatoes.

Vitamin C is needed for the synthesis of collagen; a deficiency of this vitamin causes *scurvy*. The effects in adults are different from those encountered in children.

Adult Scurvy. The outstanding feature is swelling and bleeding of the gums. This is seen only in those who have teeth, and it is associated with infection. Wound healing is impaired (see Chapter 7). Bleeding into the skin is characteristic and is first detected around the hair follicles. Bleeding may also occur into the joints, the gastrointestinal tract, and elsewhere.

In the past, scurvy has plagued sailors on long sea voyages. For example, Vasco da Gama is reported to have lost 100 men of his 160-man crew on his trip around the Cape of Good Hope (1497). Lind, a British naval surgeon, introduced oranges, limes, and lemons into his sailors' diet in 1747 and he thereby earned the nickname of "limey" for his countrymen.

Infantile Scurvy. Milk and milk products are often a poor source of vitamin C; consequently, scurvy can develop in infants at about the age of 8 months. There is impaired osteoid formation, and the epiphyses can become dislocated. An outstanding feature is subperiosteal hemorrhages, which are extremely painful. Bleeding can occur elsewhere, but gum lesions are not seen unless the teeth have erupted.

VITAMIN B COMPLEX

Thiamine. Thiamine is a coenzyme necessary for several steps in carbohydrate metabolism. In the absence of this vitamin, lactic and pyruvic acids accumulate rather than enter the Krebs cycle. The vitamin is widely distributed in foodstuffs. Thiamine deficiency was once prevalent in the Orient, where polished (highly milled) rice formed the staple diet (the process of milling removes most of the thiamine from the rice). Thiamine deficiency is now much less common in the world, but it is still encountered in the Orient, particularly in persons of all ages living in isolated communities, in infants, and in pregnant women. In North America it is sometimes encountered in chronic alcoholics.

EFFECTS OF THIAMINE DEFICIENCY. The early symptoms of thiamine deficiency (called beriberi) are vague: weakness, swelling of the ankles, "pins and needles" (paresthesia), and numbness of the legs. At any time, one of the two major severe forms may develop:

Wet Beriberi. In this form it is theorized that the accumulation of lactic acid and other vasodilator chemicals causes so much vasodilatation that a form of high-output heart failure develops. The outstanding feature is extensive edema and accumulation of fluid in the serous sacs. Sudden death from heart failure is not uncommon.

Dry Beriberi. The outstanding feature of this form is degeneration of nerve fibers, particularly of the peripheral nerves (polyneuropathy). Numbness and anesthesia are the result of sensory nerve damage, whereas weakness and muscle wasting are the effects of motor nerve involvement. The patient eventually becomes bedridden.

Two other effects of thiamine deficiency are noteworthy:

Infantile Beriberi. Infants with a low thiamine intake can develop acute beriberi between the ages of two and six months. The sudden development of heart failure, which is often fatal, is characteristic.

Wernicke's Encephalopathy and Korsakoff's Psychosis. These conditions, described in Chapter 44, may occur with other forms of beriberi, but in Europe and North America they are invariably encountered in alcoholics.

TREATMENT OF BERIBERI. Beriberi responds promptly to thiamine administration; with the wet form, early treatment is essential, since sudden death is common. Likewise, in Wernicke's encephalopathy, delay may lead to irreparable brain damage.

Riboflavin. Riboflavin is a constituent of many foods and is a component of several enzymes that play a vital role in metabolism. Yet the lesions associated with its deficiency are ill-defined. Inflammation of the angles of the mouth (*angular stomatitis*), of the lips (*cheilosis*), and *seborrheic dermatitis* are the best documented.

Niacin.   As with thiamine and riboflavin, niacin (nicotinic acid) is widely distributed in plant and animal food and is also a component of important enzymes. Deficiency of niacin causes *pellagra,* a disease so named because of the rough skin (from the Italian *pelle agra,* or "rough skin") that is present. Pellagra is a disease of poor peasants who subsist chiefly on maize (American corn). Although this cereal contains niacin, the vitamin is in a bound form. Furthermore, maize is deficient in tryptophan, an amino acid from which the body can manufacture niacin.

Pellagra was once common in Spain and Italy. It became widespread in the United States in the early 1900s but it has been largely swept away by improved economic circumstances. Nevertheless, it is still sometimes encountered in chronic alcoholics.

SYMPTOMS.   The symptoms of pellagra are most easily remembered as the *four D's:*

Dermatitis.   Erythema, superficially resembling a sunburn, is present on the sun-exposed areas. This may progress to blistering and a chronic type of dermatitis.

Diarrhea.   Diarrhea is common, as is a smooth, sore tongue of "raw beef" appearance.

Dementia.   Mental symptoms are common; they may be in the form of acute delirium or a chronic depression or dementia.

Death.   Death was a common end-result of pellagra before the advent of vitamin therapy.

Pyridoxine (Vitamin B₆).   Pyridoxine is also a component of important coenzymes. Dietary deficiencies are unusual, but pyridoxine deficiency has been reported as a complication of drug therapy — particularly with the administration of isoniazid, which is used in the treatment of tuberculosis. It has also been reported as a complication of taking the birth control pill.

It is evident from this short account that thiamine, riboflavin, niacin, and pyridoxine are widely distributed in food and that deficiencies are due to an unbalanced or inadequate diet. Such dietary deficiencies are generally the effect of poverty, ignorance, or alcoholism. It follows that multiple deficiencies are often present in the same patient. Hence, it is common and acceptable practice to treat a patient with a prescription containing a mixture of all members of the vitamin B complex.

Cobalamin (Vitamin B₁₂) and Folate.   These vitamins are necessary for red-cell maturation. The absence of these substances leads to a megaloblastic anemia (see Chapter 26).

Review Questions

1. Describe the changes that occur in the metabolism of the brain during starvation.
2. Describe the effects of vitamin deficiency on the skin and the mucous membranes.
3. Describe the effects of thiamine deficiency and indicate the circumstances under which it might be encountered in North America.

Selected Readings

Leading Article: Laboratory tests in protein-calorie malnutrition. Lancet, *1*:1041–1042, 1973.

Lehninger, A. L.: Biochemistry. 2nd ed. New York, Worth Publishers, Inc. See Chapter 13, pp. 335–360, for a description of the vitamins and pp. 840–845 for a description of starvation.

Mason, J. B., Hay, R. W., Leresche, J., et al.: Treatment of severe malnutrition in relief. Lancet, *1*:332–335, 1974.

Truswell, A. S., and Wright, F. J.: Nutritional factors in disease. *In* Macleod, J. (Ed.): Davidson's Principles and Practice of Medicine. 11th ed. Edinburgh, Churchill Livingstone, 1974, pp. 111–172.

Chapter 24

After studying this chapter the student should be able to:

- Describe how the level of blood glucose is regulated.
- List the hormones and their actions that are involved in glucose homeostasis.
- Describe the metabolic changes that occur in diabetes mellitus.
- Outline the etiology of diabetes mellitus.
- Distinguish between growth-onset diabetes and maturity-onset diabetes.
- Outline the laboratory tests used in the diagnosis of diabetes mellitus.
- List the complications of diabetes mellitus.
- Describe the causes and effects of hypoglycemia.
- Describe the clinical and pathological features of gout.
- Distinguish between primary gout and secondary gout.

GLUCOSE METABOLISM

The most important upset of glucose metabolism is diabetes mellitus. The frequency of this disease, which affects about 3 per cent of the population, has stimulated a vast amount of research into glucose metabolism. Yet even today there are many aspects of the disease that are incompletely understood.

Glucose is used as a fuel by many cells of the body and is the only substance used by the brain under normal circumstances. Hence, the maintenance of a blood-glucose level between narrow limits (70 to 110 mg per 100 ml in the fasting person)* is an important homeostatic mechanism. The blood level is regu-

---

*Various methods of estimating glucose are available and give slightly different results, depending on whether the method used estimates true glucose only or other substances as well. The figures quoted in this chapter refer to the results obtained with the autoanalyzer, a device used in most clinical biochemistry laboratories.

374

lated by the balanced production of insulin, which lowers the blood glucose level, and by four other hormones whose action is to raise it.

Insulin. This hormone is the secretion of the beta cells of the islets of Langerhans in the pancreas. It binds to specific receptors on its target cells (mainly muscle and fat cells) and causes the formation of cyclic GMP (guanosine 3′,5′-cyclic phosphate), which acts as a second messenger within the cell and is analogous to cyclic AMP. The effects on the cell include:

(a) enhancement of the entry of glucose into the cell by aiding its transport across the cell membrane

(b) enhancement of glycogen formation

(c) inhibition of the formation of glucose from noncarbohydrate sources in liver (gluconeogenesis)

(d) inhibition of lipid breakdown in fat cells.

Insulin therefore lowers the blood-glucose level; the stimulus for its release from the pancreas is a raised blood-glucose level. Thus, following a carbohydrate meal the glucose is absorbed into the blood stream and the blood level rises. Insulin is secreted, and the level of glucose returns to normal. This forms the basis of the *glucose tolerance test.* With this test 100 grams of glucose are taken by mouth, and then blood and urine samples are collected at intervals for the next three hours. The peak blood glucose should not exceed 170 mg per 100 ml, and glycosuria should not occur at any time.

Glucagon. This hormone is the secretion of the alpha cells of the islets of Langerhans. It is released whenever the blood glucose level drops below 80 mg per 100 ml. The main action of glucagon is to cause the liver to break down glycogen into glucose, which is then released into the blood. Therefore, glucagon counterbalances the action of insulin.

Epinephrine. The action of epinephrine is to raise the blood glucose level by causing the breakdown of glycogen in the liver and in the muscles.

Pituitary Growth Hormone. The action of this hormone is to oppose the actions of insulin and thereby raise the blood glucose level.

Adrenal Glucocorticoids. The glucocorticoids decrease glucose utilization in muscle and fat. Gluconeogenesis is stimulated in the liver and the blood glucose level rises.

Diabetes Mellitus

Diabetes mellitus may be defined as a disorder of carbohydrate and fat metabolism that is due to an absolute or relative lack of insulin.

METABOLIC CHANGES

The lack of insulin causes a rise in blood glucose level (*hyperglycemia*), and when this level exceeds 170 to 180 mg per 100 ml (the *threshold level*), glucose escapes into the urine (*glycosuria*). The presence of glucose leads to an increased secretion of urine in order to contain it, an effect called *osmotic diuresis*. This leads to a loss of water and electrolytes, and the patient becomes dehydrated and thirsty. Fluid intake is therefore increased (*polydipsia*).

Insulin deficiency prevents the entry of glucose into fat cells; synthesis of fatty acids ceases. Indeed, neutral fat is broken down to fatty acids, which are released into the blood stream and form a major source of energy in all tissues except for the brain. Most of the fatty acids are oxidized to carbon dioxide and water, but when there is a great excess, some of the fatty acids are converted by the liver into *ketone bodies,* e.g., acetone, acetoacetic acid, and beta-hydroxy-butyric acid. This condition of *diabetic ketosis* is extremely dangerous, because unless it is treated at once with insulin, the patient lapses into a state of severe metabolic acidosis and coma, which terminates rapidly in death.

In diabetes mellitus gluconeogenesis in the liver is accelerated. The major raw material for this process is amino acids that are derived from ingested protein or from the breakdown of tissue protein. It is evident that in diabetes mellitus the body's metabolism is geared to maintaining a high blood-glucose level even though this exceeds the renal threshold. The body literally starves in the midst of plenty, as fats and proteins are converted into glucose, only to be passed into the urine and lost from the body. Loss of weight and hunger are therefore characteristic symptoms of diabetes.

ETIOLOGY OF DIABETES MELLITUS

Three major forms of diabetes have been recognized:
1. *Hereditary diabetes,* by far the most common type
2. Diabetes associated with other endocrine disorders
3. Diabetes associated with destructive pancreatic disease.

Hereditary Diabetes. Although diabetes is a familial disease, the precise mode of inheritance is unknown. The disease does not fit into any simple pattern, because it is inherited neither as a simple dominant trait nor as a recessive trait. It is probable that the tendency to develop diabetes is inherited and that the onset of the disease is precipitated by other factors, *e.g.,* pregnancy, infection, or obesity.

Diabetes Associated with Other Endocrine Disorders. Diabetes is encountered in Cushing's syndrome, acromegaly, pheochromocytoma, and following glucocorticoid therapy. Under these circumstances the disease is due to the overabundance of the hormones that antagonize insulin.

Diabetes Associated with Pancreatic Disease. Diabetes is occasionally a complication of chronic pancreatitis and fibrocystic disease (see Chapter 34).

CLINICAL TYPES OF DIABETES MELLITUS

The disease occurs in two clinical forms:
Growth-Onset Diabetes. This form of the disease affects children and young adults and appears to be due to an absolute failure of the pancreas to secrete insulin. The disease is severe, wasting is marked, and without treatment the patients die in diabetic coma. Insulin is particularly valuable in saving the lives of these patients.

Maturity-Onset Diabetes.   This form occurs in the middle-aged and elderly and is usually associated with obesity. The amount of insulin in the blood is reduced, but it is not absent. Glucose utilization by adipose tissue is not abolished and fat tends to accumulate. These patients are usually obese, their diabetes is mild, and they can often be treated successfully by diet alone.

DIAGNOSIS OF DIABETES MELLITUS

Three stages of the disease are recognized:

Prediabetes.   The subject has the inherited tendency to develop the disease but has neither symptoms nor detectable biochemical abnormality. Diagnosis is impossible until after the subject has developed diabetes.

Chemical Diabetes.   Symptoms are absent, and the fasting blood-sugar level is normal. The glucose tolerance test is, however, abnormal. A random blood-glucose determination is of little value in diagnosis at this stage. To avoid the tedious three-hour glucose tolerance test, one may take a single blood sample two hours after a carbohydrate meal as a screening test.

Overt or Clinical Diabetes.   Symptoms are present, the fasting blood glucose is raised, and glycosuria is present.

COMPLICATIONS OF DIABETES MELLITUS

Diabetic Ketosis and Coma.   This is most common in the growth-onset type of the disease and may be precipitated by a diabetic patient's failure to administer his insulin. Vomiting and abdominal pain may be severe enough to mimic an abdominal emergency. *This mimicking of one condition by another underlines the need to perform a routine urine analysis in all ill patients.*

Hyperosmolar Coma.   Very high blood-glucose levels (*e.g.*, over 1000 mg per 100 ml) can produce such a diuresis and an elevation of blood osmolality that hypovolemic shock and cerebral dehydration lead to coma, even in the absence of ketosis. The condition is not common. It usually occurs in the maturity-onset type of diabetes.

Susceptibility to Infection.   Pyogenic, candidal, and tuberculous infections are common.

Vascular Disease.   Diabetics are liable to develop more severe atherosclerosis than are nondiabetic subjects of a like age. In addition, the small vessels show a characteristic thickening of the intima (*diabetic microangiopathy*). The combined effect is to produce ischemic changes in many tissues. This causes *myocardial infarction* and *peripheral vascular disease*, usually of the legs, which culminates in gangrene.

Renal Disease.   The glomerular lesions may be accompanied by the nephrotic syndrome, but ultimately chronic renal failure ensues. Indeed, renal failure is a common mode of death in diabetes mellitus. At present, there is little evidence that adequate control of the disease can prevent death from renal failure.

Retinal Disease.   Diabetic microangiopathy is a common cause of blindness. The development of cataracts is also a complication of diabetes.

Neuropathy.   Ischemic damage to peripheral nerves causes a variety of effects, *e.g.*, pain, loss of sensation, and paralysis.

SURGERY AND DIABETES MELLITUS

The balance between insulin and glucose requirements is easily upset by trauma and infection. Any diabetic patient who is subjected to surgery should therefore have skilled medical treatment.

Hypoglycemia

If the blood glucose is below 50 mg per 100 ml, particularly if its fall is rapid, symptoms of hypoglycemia develop. These consist of sweating, hunger, mental confusion, and—in severe cases—coma, convulsions, and death. Common causes of hypoglycemia include:

1. *Insulin Overdosage.*   All diabetic subjects on insulin therapy should be warned of the effects of hypoglycemia.

2. *Diabetes Mellitus.*   In the early stages in the development of diabetes mellitus, the hyperglycemia that follows a meal may lead to such a delayed and excessive secretion of insulin by the pancreas that hypoglycemia follows.

3. *Tumors of the Islets of Langerhans.*   An islet-cell tumor (adenoma or carcinoma) can cause periodic attacks of hypoglycemia.

PURINE METABOLISM

Gout

CLINICAL FEATURES

Gout is a disease of great antiquity and is characterized by hyperuricemia (high blood uric acid level) accompanied by recurrent attacks of acute arthritis. Deposits of urates are found in the joint cartilages, and these lead to chronic arthritis. Nodular deposits of urates are also found in connective tissues around the joints as well as in some nonarticular cartilages, particularly those of the external ear, where they are called *tophi*. The clinical features of gout were well recognized by Hippocrates; the classic features were described by Sydenham, who himself was a sufferer. The initial attack invariably affects the great toe and is characterized by the sudden onset of severe pain and inflammation. Rigors and fever accompany the attack, which usually subsides within a few days. It responds well to the administration of colchicine, a drug still used today and introduced into North America by Benjamin Franklin, who was yet another famous sufferer of gout. Repeated attacks of arthritis occur and affect other joints; ultimately, a chronic arthritis develops in all four limbs, particularly in the distal joints. Urates are also deposited in the kidney, leading to renal damage and ultimately to renal failure. About one third of the patients develop kidney stones composed of urates.

PATHOGENESIS

Uric acid is the end-product of the metabolism of the purines derived from nucleic acid. Most of this uric acid is of endogenous origin, but some is exogenous, being derived from the diet. Two types of gout are recognized:

Primary Gout.   This is a heterogeneous group of inborn errors of metabolism. In some types there is an overproduction of uric acid that is sometimes accompanied by a failure to recycle purines in the formation of new nucleic acid. In other types there is impaired renal excretion. Primary gout is familial and tends to affect males more often than females. The precise biochemical error causing most familial forms of gout is not generally understood. There are, however, some rare types of gout in which the enzyme defect is known.

Secondary Gout.   As in primary gout, the secondary variety can be due either to increased production of uric acid or to decreased excretion of uric acid. Widespread malignant disease, such as leukemia and polycythemia—particularly if treated with cytotoxic drugs—is a common cause of secondary gout; this is due to overproduction of uric acid. Chronic renal failure, particularly if it is due to hypertension, and chronic lead poisoning can lead to typical attacks of gout through retention of uric acid.

The precise reason for the deposition of urates in joints, tendons, and cartilages is not understood. The acute attacks are believed to be due to the deposition of urate crystals in the joint spaces. These crystals are phagocytosed by polymorphs. Lysosomal enzymes are then released and mediate the local inflammatory reaction as well as the rigors and fever.

Review Questions

1. Explain why thirst is a common symptom of diabetes mellitus.
2. A patient who is known to have diabetes mellitus is found unconscious. Discuss the possible causes and indicate the test that would help in the differential diagnosis.
3. A patient is suspected of having diabetes mellitus. After a long wait in the outpatient clinic, he is finally examined at 11:30 A.M., and blood and urine samples are taken. No glucose was found in the urine, and the blood-glucose level was subsequently reported as being 100 mg per 100 ml. Discuss the significance of these laboratory findings.
4. Describe the symptoms of gout and indicate why the disease sometimes occurs as a complication of leukemia.

Selected Readings

Baird, J. D., and Strong, J. A.: Diabetes mellitus. *In* Macleod, J. (Ed.): Davidson's Principles and Practice of Medicine. 11th ed. Edinburgh, Churchill Livingstone, 1975, pp. 675–712.

Cahill, G. F., and Soeldner, J. S.: Diabetes, glucagon, and growth hormone. New England Journal of Medicine, *291*:577–578, 1974.

Duthie, J. J. R., and McCormick, J. N.: Gout. *In* Macleod, J.: Davidson's Principles and Practice of Medicine. 11th ed. Edinburgh, Churchill Livingstone, 1975, pp. 783–786.

Leading Article: Pathogenesis of diabetes mellitus. British Medical Journal, *3*:594, 1971.

Lehninger, A. L.: Biochemistry. 2nd ed. New York, Worth Publishers, Inc., 1975, pp. 810–822, 845–849.

Steinke, J., and Thorn, G. W.: Diabetes mellitus. *In* Wintrobe, M. M., et al. (Eds.): Harrison's Principles of Internal Medicine. 7th ed. New York, McGraw-Hill Book Company, 1974, pp. 532–550.

Chapter 25

After studying this chapter the student should be able to:

- Describe five methods used to separate the plasma proteins.
- List the causes of hypoalbuminemia.
- Classify the types of hypergammaglobulinemia.
- Outline how the erythrocyte sedimentation rate (E.S.R.) is performed, give the normal values, and indicate the usefulness of the test.
- Classify amyloidosis and outline the main features of each group.
- Describe the effects of amyloid infiltration on the
  - (a) Heart
  - (b) Kidney
  - (c) Liver
- Outline what is known about the composition of amyloid.

380

THE PLASMA PROTEINS:
AMYLOIDOSIS

The Plasma Proteins

The blood stream forms the major route by which the secretions of one organ can travel to distant parts of the body and influence other organs and tissues. It is not surprising, therefore, that an analysis of the blood itself has proved to be a rewarding pursuit and has shed light on many bodily functions. The fluid and electrolyte components have already been discussed in Chapter 19; in this chapter, the plasma proteins will be described. One great advantage of investigating the plasma proteins rather than tissue proteins is that blood is readily available and can be obtained easily with little inconvenience to the patient.

METHODS OF SEPARATION

The plasma proteins have been classified in various ways; unfortunately, the terminology is quite complex. In order to understand the classification, it is essential to have an elementary knowledge of the physicochemical properties of the proteins, because the name attached to a particular member is often a reflection of the method used in its identification.

Knowledge of the evolution of the present rather complex system is instructive. *Fibrinogen* presents no great problem; it is a protein that forms an insoluble fibrin clot during coagulation. Until the middle of the last century the remaining serum was thought to contain a single protein called "albumin." It was then shown that by half-saturation of the serum with ammonium sulfate part of the protein could be precipitated (now called *globulin*) leaving the remainder in solution (the *albumin*). Estimation of these three fractions is a useful first step in clinical investigation. The normal levels are the following:

Albumin	4.0 to 5.7 grams/100 ml
Globulin	1.5 to 3.0 grams/100 ml
Fibrinogen	0.1 to 0.5 grams/100 ml
TOTAL	6.2 to 8.2 grams/100 ml

In aqueous solutions at a suitable pH, the proteins have a negative charge so that when they are placed in an electric field, they migrate toward the anode. Individual proteins move at a particular rate dependent, to a great extent, upon their size and electrical charge. The test, called *electrophoresis*, is conveniently performed on strips of filter paper, starch gel, or cellulose acetate;

FIGURE 25–1. *Cellulose acetate electrophoresis of serum.*

On the left electrophoretic strips from eight separate sera are shown. The anode is on the left and the dense band that has moved furthest to the left is due to albumen. No. 8 is normal serum, whereas Nos. 4 and 7 show a diffuse increase in the γ globulins. Each shows the picture of a polyclonal gammopathy. No. 1 shows a dense band in the γ-globulin area. The density of the bands of strip No. 1 is depicted in graphic form on the right. The various serum proteins are in the same relative positions on both the strip and the graph. The sharp spike in the γ region is characteristic of a monoclonal gammopathy. (From Hall, C. A.: Gammopathies. *In* Halsted, J. A. (Ed.): The Laboratory in Clinical Medicine. Philadelphia, W. B. Saunders Company, 1976, p. 493.)

an electric current is passed for a suitable time, the strip is dried and the separated proteins are stained (Fig. 25–1). When serum undergoes electrophoresis, the albumin travels fastest as one large band. The globulins on the other hand separate into three major groups which have been designated α globulin, β globulin, and γ globulin. In fact, each of these bands can be resolved into numerous smaller bands, each composed of a distinct protein. It is the separation and identification of the globulins that have presented the greatest challenge to the ingenuity of the biochemist. Immunoelectrophoresis, illustrated in Figure 25–2, is an invaluable technique. The protein fractions are separated by electrophoresis and then identified immunologically.

Another method of plasma protein separation uses a high-speed ultracentrifuge. Large molecules tend to settle quickly, whereas small ones can be spun down with greater difficulty. The various fractions that can be obtained are measured in *Svedberg units*. The large globulin molecules, termed *macroglobulins*, are spun down in the 19S fraction. This fraction contains an important group of antibodies, which are therefore designated IgM. The more abundant IgG forms the 7S fraction.

Some proteins precipitate out in the cold. These are called *cryoglobulins;* an abnormal increase in concentration *(cryoglobulinemia)* can cause trouble because of vascular obstruction when the hands are exposed in cold weather. Finally, some proteins contain either lipid or carbohydrate. The former are called *lipoproteins*, and the latter are termed *glycoproteins*.

It is evident that an individual chemical protein can be described in a number of ways. Thus, a single protein may be a macroglobulin in the 19S range, a γ globulin, and also a glycoprotein. This protein may also be an antibody and therefore an immunoglobulin. The function of a particular protein is yet another way in which it may be described.

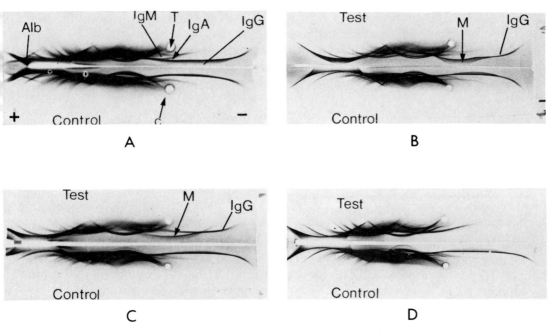

FIGURE 25–2. *Immunoelectrophoretic patterns in disease.*

The technique is illustrated in *A*. The test is performed in an agarose gel. Test serum is placed in well "T," and a control normal serum is placed in well "C." A current is passed for a suitable period, and then the proteins tend to migrate toward the anode (+). Albumen (Alb) migrates most quickly, whereas IgG moves most slowly; under the conditions of the test, some IgG actually moves towards the cathode. The separated plasma components are demonstrated by placing antiserum to whole plasma down the central strip. From there the antibodies diffuse to form precipitin lines with each separated protein. The sheet is stained and photographed. *A*, The IgG band is heavier than that of the control and is closer to the central strip. Serum tested here was from a patient who has systemic lupus erythematosus and a polyclonal hypergammaglobulinemia. The IgA and IgM bands are clearly shown. *B*, An M protein is present and distorts the normal IgG band. The serum is from a patient with multiple myelomatosis and an IgG M protein. *C*, An M protein is present and is in the position of the normal IgA band. Note how the normal IgG band crosses the M protein. The serum is from a patient with multiple myelomatosis producing an IgA M protein. *D*, Note the deficiency of the IgG band. From a patient with congenital hypogammaglobulinemia. (Courtesy of Dr. K. C. Carstairs.)

ALBUMIN

Albumin, like most of the plasma proteins (with the notable exception of the immunoglobulins), is produced in the liver.

Hypoalbuminemia. Chronic liver disease, especially in the terminal phases, is often accompanied by hypoalbuminemia resulting from underproduction of this protein. Similarly, during starvation the plasma albumin level tends to fall rather more quickly than the other plasma proteins. For reasons that are not well understood, the albumin level also falls during acute infections and following trauma or surgery. This appears to be due to increased catabolism and is accompanied by a rise in the α_2-globulins and fibrinogen. This has been termed the *acute reaction to stress*. Although the response is quite nonspecific—being mediated by the release of adrenal hormones—it forms the basis for a common pathological test—the erythrocytic sedimentation rate (ESR), which is discussed later in this chapter.

Hypoalbuminemia also occurs whenever there is excessive loss of albumin from the body. This is seen under several circumstances:

1. With the *nephrotic syndrome,* when large quantities are lost in the urine.

2. With *chronic loss of inflammatory exudate* from the body. Common examples are draining abscesses, extensive burns, and severe infected wounds.

3. With *protein-loss enteropathy,* which is an uncommon cause of hypoalbuminemia and is due to loss of protein into the intestine. This syndrome is associated with a variety of gastrointestinal lesions, including gastric cancer, Crohn's disease, and ulcerative colitis.

EFFECTS OF HYPOALBUMINEMIA.   Albumin is a small molecule (molecular weight: 70,000) and is in high concentration in the plasma. It therefore constitutes the major noncrystalloid component of plasma. As would be expected, hypoalbuminemia leads to edema (see Chapter 19).

Hyperalbuminemia.   This occurs whenever there is hemoconcentration, due either to lack of water intake or to excessive water loss. Fluid can be lost rapidly as a result of several mechanisms:

1. The rapid formation of inflammatory exudate (*e.g.,* in burns and gas gangrene).

2. The passage of a large volume of urine in a short time (polyuria), as in the recovery phase of acute renal damage or in chronic renal disease.

3. Acute addisonian crisis (see Chapter 39).

4. Severe vomiting or diarrhea.

THE GLOBULINS

The globulins include a wide array of plasma proteins. The immunoglobulins form a major component: mostly they are present in the gamma fraction, but they are also found to a lesser extent in the beta fraction. The normal level appears to be maintained by the body's contact with microorganisms, particularly those in the intestine. Thus in germ-free animals, the γ globulin level is maintained at about one fifth of normal. When the intestinal flora of such animals is restored, the plasma proteins return to normal.

Hypergammaglobulinemia.   Hypergammaglobulinemia is invariably due to an increase in the level of immunoglobulins. Two major patterns are described below:

POLYCLONAL GAMMOPATHY.   An increase in the gammaglobulins is seen in many chronic infections. Chronic tuberculosis and kala-azar can be singled out as typical examples. It is also characteristic of those diseases in which the production of autoantibodies is a major component. Systemic lupus erythematosus is the prototype of this type of disease. Hypergammaglobulinemia is also characteristic of sarcoidosis; the pathogenesis, however, is obscure. The electrophoretic pattern in these conditions is that of a broad-based elevation of the γ globulins. There is an elevation in the levels of all classes of immunoglobulins, and it is assumed that many clones of antibody-forming cells are stimulated. Hence, the term *polyclonal gammopathy.*

MONOCLONAL GAMMOPATHY. In some cases of hypergammaglobuline-mia, it is found that the increase in gammaglobulin is due entirely to an increase in one particular protein belonging to *one* of the major classes—IgA, IgG, IgE, IgM, or IgD—and furthermore consists of either the lambda or the kappa variety. The supposition is that the globulin is produced by one particular clone of antibody-forming cells. Monoclonal gammopathy is usually associated with malignancy of the lymphoreticular system. The most common example is that of Multiple Myelomatosis, which is described elsewhere, but it is also seen in a variety of other Malignant lymphomas and occasionally other Malignant tumors. The term *M protein* (derived from Multiple Myelomatosis; Malignant lymphoma; Malignant tumor) is therefore sometimes applied to an abnormal homogeneous protein, which appears as a spike on electrophoresis, in contrast to the broad-based increase seen in the polyclonal gammopathies (Fig. 25–1). The finding of such a spike in a case of hypergammaglobulinemia leads the physician to search for malignancy—particularly malignant lymphoma—in the patient.

THE LIPOPROTEINS

The lipoproteins form a complex group of proteins and have now been divided into five major types. Elevated levels of some of these types are associated with the development of atherosclerosis, particularly coronary atherosclerosis, which causes heart attacks. Some cases of hyperlipoproteinemia are familial and are therefore genetically determined. Nevertheless, in most instances the hyperlipoproteinemia appears to be secondary to some other disease, particularly diabetes mellitus, alcoholism, and the nephrotic syndrome. In addition, the precise pattern of an individual's lipoproteins is influenced by his diet. This complex subject is of tremendous interest, since it is possible that by detecting a dangerous pattern of hyperlipoproteinemia at an early stage, treatment by diet or drugs can correct the abnormality and avert or delay subsequent heart attacks.

The Erythrocyte Sedimentation Rate (ESR)

When a column of blood rendered incoagulable with an anticoagulant such as citrate or oxalate is allowed to stand vertically, the red cells steadily gravitate downward, because their density is greater than that of the plasma. The speed at which this sedimentation occurs is dependent on several factors, the most important of which are the degree of rouleaux formation and the extent of sludging. In *rouleaux formation*, the red cells pile one on the other like an orderly pile of plates; in *sludging*, the massing of red cells with mutual adhesion is much more irregular and more closely resembles that of agglutination except that the clumps of cells can be readily separated. Any increase in the plasma content of high-molecular-weight substances (*e.g.*, the macroglobulins and fibrinogen) is found to increase the ESR. The small molecular weight albumin *delays* red cell sedimentation. For this reason, a raised ESR is particularly characteristic of macroglobulinemia and hypoalbuminemia.

The ESR is normally higher in women than men, and it shows a significant rise with age. The upper limits of normal based on the commonly performed Westergren method* may be taken as 15 mm for men and 20 mm for women under the age of 50 years, and 20 mm and 30 mm, respectively, for those over that age. It is usually raised during infection and after tissue necrosis, *e.g.,* myocardial or pulmonary infarction. Presumably, an alteration in the balance between the plasma components is responsible, but the precise alterations concerned are ill-defined and rarely investigated. The nonspecific nature of the ESR limits its value in diagnosis; nevertheless, it is a useful investigation. It is of interest to note that the erythrocyte sedimentation rate was once introduced as a test for pregnancy, since ESR is elevated in this condition.

The presence of a raised ESR must always be taken to indicate disease, provided anemia and pregnancy are first excluded. Also administration of birth-control pills is reported to raise it slightly. However, a normal ESR does not rule out organic lesions. A patient with a small carcinoma of the breast or lung often has a normal ESR. The ESR is of value in following the course of a known disease, such as tuberculosis and rheumatoid arthritis. Sequential measurements provide a useful indication as to the activity of the disease and its response to treatment. In the Wintrobe method of measuring ESR, the tube contains 1 ml of undiluted oxalated blood and is graduated from 1 to 100. The method has the advantage that after the ESR is read, the tube can be centrifuged and the hematocrit (the volume percentage of erythrocytes in whole blood) can be measured. Normally it is about 45 per cent.

It should be noted that the precise values of the ESR depend very much on the technique employed. The Westergren and Wintrobe methods give different figures. When using a laboratory, one must learn to appreciate the normal range of its findings.

Amyloidosis

Amyloid is an eosinophilic, hyaline material, which is deposited in the extracellular spaces. It reacts with iodine in acid solutions to give a blue color; this superficial resemblance to starch led Virchow to call it starchlike or "amyloid." At a neutral pH it stains a mahogany-brown color with iodine.

Amyloid is not normally present in the body in detectable amounts; its deposition in the tissues constitutes the condition of amyloidosis.

GENERALIZED AMYLOIDOSIS

Four types are recognized, although the distinction between them is not rigid. In all of them there are deposits of amyloid in many tissues.

---

*In the Westergren method the column of citrated blood is 200 mm in height. As the red cells sediment, a clear zone of plasma appears on top of the red-cell mass. The ESR is reported as the distance from the top of the plasma to the top of the red-cell mass at the end of one hour. The Wintrobe method uses a smaller tube (100 mm in height) and oxalated blood. It is less accurate but has the advantage of permitting the hematocrit to be measured by centrifuging the tube after a reading of the ESR at one hour. Partial clotting of a blood sample and other errors in technique can influence the ESR. An unexpected result should always be checked by repeating the test.

FIGURE 25-3. *The spleen in amyloidosis.*

The patient had suffered from rheumatoid arthritis; during the last few months of her life, she developed the nephrotic syndrome (albuminuria, hypoalbuminemia, and edema). At necropsy, heavy deposits of amyloid were found in the liver, spleen, and kidneys. Smaller amounts were present in the intestine, lung, thyroid, and adrenal glands. The specimen pictured here is a cut surface of the spleen and has been treated with an iodine solution. Many dark, firm, semitranslucent nodules of amyloid material can be seen. These deposits have been likened to grains of sago. This type of splenic involvement, therefore, is commonly referred to as a "sago spleen."

Primary Amyloidosis. Generalized amyloidosis may occur as an idiopathic condition. The distribution is usually different from that of secondary amyloidosis (described below). Deposits tend to occur in mesenchymal tissues such as the tongue, respiratory tract, and heart. Liver, spleen, and kidney may be involved, although less extensively than with secondary amyloidosis. Amyloid is a rigid material, and its presence interferes with the mechanical activity of muscle. Hence, amyloidosis of the tongue interferes with swallowing, whereas the condition with cardiac involvement leads to intractable heart failure.

Secondary Amyloidosis. Deposits of amyloid are found beneath the endothelium of blood vessels and sinuses of liver, spleen, kidney, intestine, and many other organs but in smaller quantities (Figs. 25-3 and 25-4). The liver and spleen become enlarged and hard as the parenchyma is replaced by amyloid; such is the reserve of these organs that there is little functional derangement. The same response does not occur with the kidneys: the affected glomeruli leak protein (Fig. 25-5). The nephrotic syndrome (see Chapter 35) and renal failure result and prove fatal.

CAUSES. Generalized amyloidosis used to be encountered most frequently in patients with chronic suppurative infections (*e.g.,* chronic osteo-

FIGURE 25–4. *The liver in amyloidosis.*

There is extensive deposition of amyloid (Amy) around the liver sinusoids. This deposition has compressed the liver cells, many of which are small; others have disappeared completely. The liver cells around the central vein (CV) and the portal tract (PT) present a more normal appearance. A liver with this degree of involvement is enlarged, hard, and easily palpable. Nevertheless, clinical evidence of liver failure is generally lacking because of the reserve capacity of this organ (× 250).

myelitis and thoracic empyema), chronic tuberculosis, and tertiary syphilis with gummas. Presumably, the long-continued antigenic stimulation leads to the formation of amyloid. The presence of a soluble precursor in the blood would explain why amyloid is deposited in organs with a high reticuloendothelial cell content and in the kidney. Today generalized amyloidosis is associated with one of the following conditions: rheumatoid arthritis, lepromatous leprosy, and malignant disease (particularly Hodgkin's disease). It is also found in patients with large chronic bed sores associated with paraplegia and urinary tract infection.

Amyloidosis Associated with Multiple Myeloma. Amyloidosis is much more common in patients with multiple myelomas than with other malignant disease. Its distribution is similar to that of primary amyloidosis.

Heredofamilial Amyloidosis. Several hereditary syndromes are known. Each has characteristic features and affects particular organs, such as the heart or peripheral nerves.

LOCALIZED AMYLOIDOSIS

Amyloid can be deposited diffusely in one particular organ (*e.g.,* the heart, where it can lead to heart failure), or it can form tumorlike masses at any site (*e.g.,* lung, larynx, tongue, or bladder). Indeed, amyloidosis can mimic many

FIGURE 25–5. *Amyloidosis of kidney.*

Two glomeruli are shown, both of which are extensively replaced by amyloid. The proximal convoluted tubules (PCT) show numerous cytoplasmic granules composed of protein. The abnormal glomeruli leak protein, some of which is reabsorbed by the tubular cells and is formed into hyaline droplets. This patient had the nephrotic syndrome (× 250).

diseases, thereby underlining the need for obtaining histological confirmation of the diagnosis of any mass. One cannot assume that all masses are neoplasms.

THE COMPOSITION OF AMYLOID

Amyloid is a protein. In the past there was much discussion and disagreement as to its nature. It is now known that there are at least two separate types which are described below:

Amyloid of Immunoglobulin Origin. This type of amyloid is composed of segments of Ig short chains. It is present in cases of primary amyloidosis and that associated with multiple myeloma.

Amyloid of Unknown Origin. The amyloid that is found in cases of secondary amyloidosis is not formed of components of immunoglobulin molecules. At present, its origin is unknown.

Under the electron microscope all types of amyloid are seen to be made up of fibrils that have a characteristic appearance. The same type of fibril can be formed *in vitro* by many different proteins. Hence, at the present time amyloid is regarded as a fibrillar form of protein that can be derived from various sources. One of these sources is an immunoglobulin molecule; other sources have yet to be identified. The pathogenesis of amyloidosis remains a mystery, and the starchlike deposits noted by Virchow in the last century still present

FIGURE 25–6. *Immunoelectrophoresis of serum.*

The serum labeled "test" is from the patient described in question 2. A normal control serum is included for comparison.

modern medicine with a fascinating but unsolved problem. Even when we know what amyloid is, we may not know why it is formed.

Review Questions

1. An antibody to the red-cell antigen A may be described as a macroglobulin, an IgM protein, a glycoprotein, and a component in the 19S fraction. Explain what is meant by each of these descriptive terms.
2. An apparently healthy 54-year-old man was found to have an ESR of 75 mm. The result of immunoelectrophoresis of his serum is shown in Figure 25–6 together with that of a normal serum. Comment on these laboratory results and speculate on the diagnosis.
3. A patient is found to have albuminuria and a plasma albumin level of 1.5 grams/100 ml. A renal biopsy was attempted, but no suitable tissue was obtained. A biopsy of the rectal mucosa revealed infiltration by amyloid. Electrophoresis showed a spike in the γ region, and immunoelectrophoresis confirmed that this was an IgG protein. Discuss the diagnosis.
4. A 22-year-old married woman is found to have an ESR of 27 mm via the Westergren method. What significance should be attached to the results of the test?

Selected Readings

Glenner, G. G., and Page, D. L.: Amyloid, amyloidosis, and amyloidogenesis. International Review of Experimental Pathology, 15:2–92, 1976.

Halsted, J. A.: The Laboratory in Clinical Medicine. Philadelphia, W. B. Saunders Company, 1976. See pp. 409–412 for a description of the hyperlipidemias and pp. 509–512 for a discussion of the erythrocyte sedimentation rate.

Stirling, G. A.: Amyloidosis. In Harrison, C. V., and Weinbren, K. (Eds.): Recent Advances in Pathology, No. 9. Edinburgh, Churchill Livingstone, 1975, pp. 249–272.

DISORDERS OF THE BLOOD

Chapter 26

DISORDERS OF THE BLOOD

After studying this chapter the student should be able to:

- Outline the stages in the formation of the red cells and the white cells and indicate the sites of hematopoiesis.
- Describe the mature red cell and the abnormal forms that are encountered in disease.
- List the normal values of the red cell count, the hemoglobin content of blood, the packed cell volume (PCV), the mean corpuscular hemoglobin concentration (MCHC), and the white cell count.
- List the requirements for red-cell formation and describe the fate of old, worn-out red cells.
- Indicate the clinical features of anemia and describe the five main types of this condition (as outlined in this chapter) in terms of the following factors:
  - (a) causes
  - (b) blood picture
  - (c) pathological findings in organs other than the blood.
- Define polycythemia and distinguish between the primary and secondary forms.
- Define the following terms and give at least one cause of each: leukocytosis, leukopenia, neutropenia, lymphocytosis, monocytosis, eosinophilia, and pancytopenia.
- Classify the leukemias and describe the salient features of each type.
- Describe the outstanding features and important causes of the following conditions:
  - (a) bone-marrow aplasia
  - (b) hypersplenism
  - (c) leukoerythroblastic anemia.
- Describe the clotting mechanism and differentiate between the intrinsic system and the extrinsic system.
- Classify the bleeding diseases and give examples of each type.
- Briefly describe the following tests and indicate the value of each in assessing the cause of a bleeding disease:
  - (a) platelet count
  - (b) clotting time
  - (c) bleeding time
  - (d) capillary fragility test
  - (e) partial thromboplastin time
  - (f) prothrombin time.
- Describe the ABO and Rhesus blood groups and outline the way in which a sample of blood is typed.
- List the hazards of blood transfusion and indicate how they may be avoided.

The formed elements of the blood consist of the red cells (*erythrocytes*), the white cells (*leukocytes*), and the *platelets*. In the fetus, blood formation (*hematopoiesis*) takes place in the bone marrow (in the medullary cavity of the bones), liver, spleen, and other organs. After birth, the extramedullary sites disappear, so that within a few weeks blood formation occurs only in the bone marrow. As the child develops, the blood-forming tissue in the long bones is replaced by fatty marrow so that by the time adulthood is reached the main source of blood cells is the red marrow of the ribs and the vertebral column. The marrow of the long bones is available for extension of hematopoietic tissues should a need arise for increased production.

THE RED CELLS

DEVELOPMENT

The earliest recognizable precursor of the blood cells is a large cell with abundant basophilic cytoplasm and a nucleus containing one or more nucleoli. This cell is termed a *hemocytoblast*. The first recognizable red-cell precursor is termed a *proerythroblast;* its cytoplasm contains many ribosomes but no hemoglobin. As hemoglobin is formed, the cytoplasm becomes more eosinophilic and the nucleus becomes condensed (a process called pyknosis). Such a cell is termed a *normoblast;* early, intermediate, and late stages are recognized. Ultimately, the nucleus is extruded, and the cell assumes the flattened shape of the mature erythrocyte.

The Mature Erythrocyte.   The red cell is a biconcave disc and is conveniently examined by making a smear of blood on a glass slide and staining with one of the Romanowsky stains* (Fig. 26–1). The average diameter of a red cell when examined in this manner is 6.7 to 7.7 μm. Young red cells have a faint basophilia in the cytoplasm that is due to remnants of rough endoplasmic reticulum. Such cells are termed *reticulocytes*. Normally less than 2 per cent of

---

*These stains, which include Leishman, Jenner, and Giemsa, consist of blended mixtures of methylene blue and eosin.

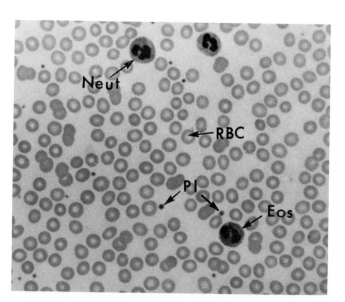

FIGURE 26–1. *Normal blood film.*

The red blood cells (RBC) are of uniform diameter and evenly stained. The central, pale-staining area is due to their biconcave shape. Also shown are two neutrophil polymorphs (Neut), one eosinophil (Eos), and several platelets (Pl) ($\times$ 600).

Table 26–1 CHARACTERISTICS OF THE NORMOCHROMIC RED BLOOD CELL

Diameter: 6.7 to 7.7 μm
Mean Corpuscular Hemoglobin Concentration: 32 to 36 per cent

the total red cells are reticulocytes, and an increase in their number generally indicates a more rapid production of cells such as occurs in hemolytic anemia or after a hemorrhage. Reticulocytosis is also seen whenever an anemia is treated successfully, such as when an iron-deficiency anemia is treated with iron. Under normal conditions the nucleated red cells are prevented from leaving the bone marrow; however, with extremely rapid erythropoiesis, particularly if it is occurring in abnormal sites such as the liver and spleen, nucleated red cells can appear in the circulation. A good example of this phenomenon is hemolytic disease of the newborn (see *erythroblastosis fetalis*).

EXAMINATION OF THE RED CELL. The normal red-cell count is 4.6 to 6.2 million per cu mm in males; the normal hemoglobin content is 14 to 18 grams per 100 ml. In women the red-cell count is half a million cells per cu mm less, and the hemoglobin level is 2 grams per 100 ml lower. A useful and accurate measurement is the *hematocrit reading,* or *packed cell volume* (PCV). In this test a thin, cylindrical, graduated Wintrobe tube is filled with blood and centrifuged for half an hour at 3000 revolutions per minute. In the adult male 40 to 54 per cent of the blood volume consists of red cells. The expression:

$$\frac{\text{Hemoglobin in grams per 100 ml}}{\text{Percentage packed cell volume}} \times 100$$

is known as the *mean corpuscular hemoglobin concentration (MCHC)* and is an index of the concentration of hemoglobin in the red cells. The normal range is 32 to 36 per cent. A value of less than 32 per cent indicates underhemoglobinization of the cells and suggests impaired hemoglobin synthesis, a condition often caused by iron deficiency.

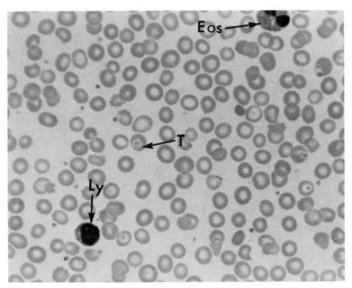

FIGURE 26–2. *Blood film from patient with iron-deficiency anemia.*

The red cells are hypochromic, and the central pale-staining area is more pronounced than normal. The cells that exhibit a central dot are called target cells (T). Also shown is an eosinophil (Eos) with a typical bilobed nucleus and a small lymphocyte (Ly) (×600).

With experience, it is possible to get a great deal of information merely by examining a well-stained blood film with a microscope. The normal red cell is described as *normocytic* and *normochromic*. If it is smaller than normal, it is called *microcytic;* if larger than normal, *macrocytic.* If the cell is poorly hemoglobinized, it looks pale and is termed *hypochromic.* The normal cell is fully saturated with hemoglobin and therefore hyperchromia cannot occur. If the cells vary greatly in size, the term *anisocytosis* is used. The presence of irregularly shaped cells is called *poikilocytosis. Burr cells* have projections or spikes arising from their surface; *sickle cells* have an elongated shape; *spherocytes* are spherical, rather than being flat discs. Spherocytes look abnormally small and stain darkly in a blood film. Another interesting pathological variant is the *target cell* in which a small central dot of hemoglobin is seen; this is separated from the outer rim by a wide clear area (Fig. 26–2).

REQUIREMENTS FOR RED-CELL FORMATION

Hemoglobin consists of protein (globin) combined with heme, an iron-containing porphyrin.

In starvation, inadequate globin production can result in anemia. Under most circumstances, however, it is the formation of heme and maturation of the cells that are most important for the formation of healthy red cells; for this the following components are required:

IRON.   Each heme molecule contains one atom of iron; without this, hemoglobin cannot be formed. Iron is absorbed from food in an ionic form by the mucosal cells of the duodenum and upper small bowel (see Fig. 2–7). It combines with an iron-free protein (termed *apoferritin*) to form ferritin, the storage form of iron in the body. Much of this is stored in the reticuloendothelial system, where it is available for hemoglobin and myoglobin synthesis.

VITAMINS.   The most important vitamins essential for blood formation belong to the B complex vitamins: *folic acid* and *vitamin B_{12}.* Both are necessary for the proper development of the normoblast. If either substance is deficient, the normoblast develops abnormally; that is, it remains large and the nucleus has an abnormal stippled appearance of its chromatin. Such a cell is termed a *megaloblast,* and the red cell which it produces is large (a *macrocyte*).

Table 26–2   REQUIREMENTS FOR RED-CELL FORMATION

| REQUIREMENT | RESULT OF DEFICIENCY | | |
	Marrow Changes	*Blood Changes*	*Other Changes*
Iron	Normoblastic hyperplasia	Hypochromic microcytic anemia	Oral mucosal atrophy
Folic acid	Megaloblastic hyperplasia	Normochromic macrocytic anemia	Oral mucosal atrophy
Vitamin B_{12}	Megaloblastic hyperplasia	Normochromic macrocytic anemia	Oral mucosal atrophy; subacute combined degeneration of cord

Both vitamins are present in the diet and are absorbed in the small bowel. The two vitamins differ in that folic acid is taken up directly, whereas vitamin B_{12} cannot be absorbed unless bound to a complex mucoprotein secreted by the gastric mucosa. This substance is called *intrinsic factor.* It follows that gastric secretion is essential for the absorption of vitamin B_{12}.

VITAMIN C.   Although this vitamin is also required for red-cell production, deficiency is rarely a factor in human disease.

OTHER SUBSTANCES.   These include copper, cobalt, and substances such as thyroxine, adrenocortical hormone, sex hormones, and erythropoietin. The latter is formed in the kidney as well as in other organs, and increased production leads to increased erythropoiesis. The stimulus for its formation is hypoxia.

DISPOSAL OF THE RED CELL

The normal life span of the red cell is about 120 days. As cells age, they become fragmented and are taken up by the reticuloendothelial cells (Fig. 26–3). Hemoglobin is split into globin and heme. The globin is degraded and returned to the body's pool of amino acids. The iron portion of the hemoglobin is split off and combined with apoferritin to form ferritin, which is stored for fur-

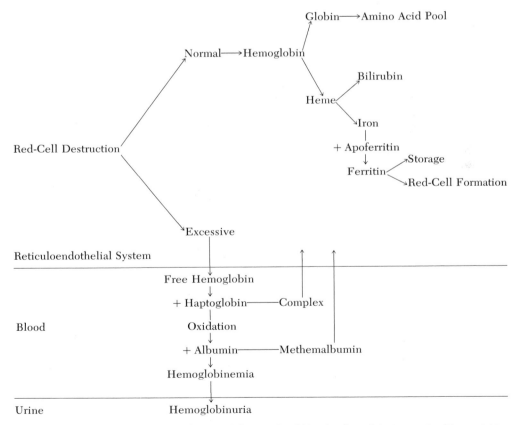

FIGURE 26–3. *Diagram showing the fate of destroyed red blood cells and their contained hemoglobin.*

ther use. The porphyrin nucleus is metabolized to bilirubin, which passes into the blood stream, becomes attached to albumin, and is excreted by the liver. Normally there is very little free hemoglobin in the plasma, and any that does appear is immediately removed by combination with a globulin component of the plasma called *haptoglobin.* Any large excess of hemoglobin in the circulation is oxidized and combined with albumin to form *methemalbumin.* Both the haptoglobin and the albumin complexes are removed by the reticuloendothelial cell so that none escapes into the urine. It is only when both these binding proteins are exhausted that free hemoglobin appears in the blood *(hemoglobinemia)* and in the urine *(hemoglobinuria).* Massive sudden destruction of red cells must occur before this is evident (see blackwater fever, Chapter 15).

The Anemias

Anemia is defined as a condition in which there is *a fall in the quantity of either red cells or hemoglobin in a unit volume of blood in the presence of a low or normal total blood volume.*

The main clinical features of anemia are the following:

1. *Pallor,* best detected in the conjunctiva, nail bed, or mucous membrane of the mouth. Pallor of the skin, particularly of the face, is a deceptive sign. It can be absent in some patients with anemia and yet present in many pale-skinned normal people.
2. *Tiredness, easy fatigability,* and *generalized muscular weakness* are common symptoms; the pathogenesis, however, is not clear. Such symptoms are also common in psychoneurotic patients who are not anemic.
3. *Shortness of breath* and *palpitations* are common. They are related to tissue hypoxia and an increased cardiac output. *Heart failure* can occur.
4. *Angina pectoris, intermittent claudication,* and *giddiness* are due to tissue hypoxia in organs in which the blood supply is already impaired by arterial disease.

The pathological effects of anemia are attributable to cellular hypoxia. At necropsy there is severe fatty change of the liver, heart, and kidneys, and death is usually attributed to heart failure.

The classification of the anemias is somewhat unsatisfactory, but for practical purposes the following groups can be recognized:

1. Acute posthemorrhagic anemia
2. Iron deficiency anemia
3. Megaloblastic anemia
4. Hemolytic anemia
5. Bone-marrow inadequacy anemia

Table 26–3   THE ANEMIAS

TYPE	BLOOD PICTURE	
Posthemorrhagic	Normochromic	Normocytic
Iron deficiency	Hypochromic	Microcytic
Megaloblastic	Normochromic	Macrocytic
Hemolytic	Normochromic	Normocytic
Bone-marrow deficiency	Normochromic	Normocytic

ACUTE POSTHEMORRHAGIC ANEMIA

The pathogenesis of the anemia that results from a sudden hemorrhage is described in Chapter 21. The anemia is normocytic and normochromic, provided the patient is not iron deficient as a result of previous blood loss or other disease. Within a few days a reticulocytosis occurs, and recovery proceeds to completion within six weeks.

IRON DEFICIENCY ANEMIA

Causes
CHRONIC BLOOD LOSS. This is the most important cause of iron deficiency anemia. Common examples are bleeding from a peptic ulcer, gastrointestinal cancer, or hemorrhoids. In women, menorrhagia is an important cause of blood loss, whereas in underdeveloped countries ankylostomiasis takes its toll.

DEFECTIVE IRON ABSORPTION. This may be secondary to dietary deficiency and is quite common in infants. It should be remembered that milk contains very little iron. Nutritional deficiency combined with the increased demand for iron by the growing fetus is a common cause of anemia in pregnancy. In the elderly an inadequate diet can also lead to iron deficiency anemia.

Defective iron absorption is a feature of the malabsorption syndrome (see Chapter 32). Thus, it accompanies many intestinal diseases and is also a common feature following gastrectomy because of the intestinal hurry that follows this operation.

Pathological Findings.
The bone marrow undergoes hyperplasia that is of the normal normoblastic type. Red marrow extends into the shafts of the long bones. In the peripheral blood there is a moderate anemia in which the red-cell count is relatively less reduced than the hemoglobin level. *The red cells are markedly microcytic and hypochromic*, and target cells may be present (see Fig. 26–2). The reticulocyte count is low, unless there has been a recent hemorrhage.

Two other features of iron deficiency sometimes accompany the anemia. The *nails* tend to become brittle and spoon-shaped; the most common *oral manifestation* is loss of the filiform papillae of the tongue, which consequently appears smooth and red. Mucosal atrophy can extend into the pharynx. Both in the mouth and pharynx this atrophy is sometimes complicated by the development of squamous-cell carcinoma.

MEGALOBLASTIC ANEMIA

Megaloblastic anemia is due to a deficiency of folic acid, vitamin B_{12}, or both. It is characterized by an abnormal type of erythropoiesis in the marrow.

Causes
DIETARY DEFICIENCY. This is quite common in underdeveloped countries, where the anemia is often due to an inadequate intake of folic acid.

PREGNANCY. Folic-acid deficiency resulting from poor diet is sometimes precipitated by the extra demands of the fetus in pregnant women.

GASTRIC DISEASE.   The intrinsic factor of the stomach is necessary for vitamin B_{12} absorption from the bowel. Therefore, total resection of the stomach must in time lead to vitamin-B_{12} deficiency. The most important gastric disease to produce megaloblastic anemia is *pernicious anemia,* an idiopathic condition in which there is progressive atrophy of the gastric mucosa. The stomach fails to secrete pepsin, hydrochloric acid and finally intrinsic factor itself. The disease is familial and appears to have an autoimmune component; autoantibodies against parietal cells of the gastric mucosa and against intrinsic factor itself are usually detectable in the patient's serum.

INTESTINAL MALABSORPTION.   Failure to absorb folic acid (occasionally vitamin B_{12}) is a feature of the malabsorption syndromes. The defect may be related either to the bowel disease itself or indirectly to an alteration in the intestinal flora (see Chapter 32).

Drugs.   Certain drugs, particularly anticonvulsants used in epilepsy treatment and the antimetabolites of the antifolic acid type used in cancer treatment (*e.g.,* methotrexate), can cause megaloblastic anemia if given over a prolonged period.

Pathological Changes.   The peripheral blood shows a severe anemia in which the *red-cell count is relatively more reduced than the hemoglobin level.* The red cells are conspicuously large (a condition called *macrocytosis*) and appear normally colored; they show marked *poikilocytosis* and *anisocytosis*. It is common to find both the white cells and platelets reduced in number. The bone marrow is markedly hyperplastic and contains many megaloblasts (Fig. 26–4).

The other effects depend on the cause of the anemia. Vitamin B_{12} is essential for the proper functioning of the central nervous system; without it, *subacute combined degeneration* of the spinal cord can occur. With this form of degeneration there is demyelination of the posterior and lateral columns of the cord. It does not occur in pure folic-acid deficiency.

There is sometimes a superficial stomatitis; the tongue is smooth and denuded of papillae, having a characteristic raw, beefy appearance.

HEMOLYTIC ANEMIA

The term *hemolytic anemia* is applied to those conditions in which there is an increased rate of red-cell destruction. This destruction is due either to an intrinsic defect in the red cells themselves or to some extracorpuscular factor acting on normal red cells. If the defect is primarily corpuscular, the red cells of a patient will not survive long when they are transfused into a healthy recipient; on the contrary, normal cells transfused into a patient's plasma will not be destroyed. If the cause of the hemolysis is extracorpuscular, normal red cells will be eliminated in the same way as those of the patient, whereas the patient's red cells will survive well in a normal recipient.

The increased red-cell destruction stimulates new red-cell formation, which is manifested by a reticulocytosis.

Causes

CORPUSCULAR DEFECTS.   In northern European races the most important cause is a spherical malformation of the red cells that causes the condition of

FIGURE 26–4. *Bone marrow smear from patient with megaloblastic anemia.*

The red cells show great variation in size. Some are large (Mac), whereas others are small and are irregularly shaped. The number of nucleated red-cell precursors is increased, and a group of megaloblasts is present (Meg). Also shown are a number of myelocytes (My) ($\times$ 600).

hereditary spherocytosis or *acholuric familial jaundice.* The abnormal cells are liable to become trapped and destroyed in the spleen so that splenectomy is usually effective in allaying the anemia while having no effect on the spherocytosis.

The Hemoglobinopathies. The hemoglobinopathies are a group of conditions in which the red cells contain an abnormal form of hemoglobin.

In *sickle cell anemia* the cells containing the abnormal hemoglobin HbS become sickle-shaped and are destroyed in the spleen when deprived of oxygen. This condition occurs almost exclusively in Blacks. Many other abnormal types of hemoglobin have been found—their presence sometimes leading to a hemolytic anemia. The best known is hemoglobin C, which leads to an anemia that is less severe than that of sickle cell disease.

In the *thalassemia syndromes* the red cells of a patient contain various types of hemoglobin that are normally present only in the fetus. The most common variant of the syndromes is *thalassemia major* in which the red cells contain much fetal hemoglobin (Hb-F). The disease is the common hemoglobinopathy of the Mediterranean races and causes severe anemia.

It should be noted that the hemoglobinopathies can occur in combination to produce complex syndromes. Thus, it is not uncommon to find sickle cell defect and hemoglobin C disease in the same person.

Enzyme Deficient Red Cells. It was the finding that some Black Americans were very liable to have a severe hemolytic anemia following the administration of certain drugs (*e.g.*, the antimalarial pamaquine) that led to the discovery that certain individuals have hereditary enzyme defects. The most important defect is a deficiency of glucose-6-phosphate dehydrogenase (G6PD) in their red cells. Many variants of G6PD deficiency have been described; these are inherited as dominant X-linked characteristics. Occasionally they lead to a chronic anemia, but more usually the defects become apparent as acute hemolytic anemia following ingestion of drugs or contact with a particular substance, such as the fava bean. The latter phenomenon is seen in some Mediterranean races; the anemia following contact with the bean is reputed to be the reason why Pythagoras counseled his followers never to walk in bean fields.

EXTRACORPUSCULAR DEFECTS

Autoantibodies. The most important antibodies that act on red cells are autoantibodies that usually occur idiopathically but may on occasion develop during the course of some other disease such as mycoplasmal pneumonia, lupus erythematosus, or a reticuloendothelial neoplasm. Two types of autoantibodies are described below:

Complete Autoantibodies. These antibodies agglutinate red cells directly in a saline suspension; they are termed *complete antibodies.* Most of these are not active at body temperature but become energized at room temperature. Such antibodies are therefore called *cold antibodies.* Although readily detectable in the laboratory, they have a feeble *in vivo* activity and consequently tend to cause comparatively mild hemolytic anemia.

Incomplete Autoantibodies. The most important autoantibodies do not agglutinate red cells in a saline suspension. They are, however, readily adsorbed onto the red cell surface, which thereby becomes coated with autoantibody. If an antihuman γ-globulin serum (obtained by immunizing a rabbit against human globulin) is added to a suspension of these coated cells, the cells undergo immediate agglutination. This antiglobulin technique is known as the *direct Coombs test.**

Most incomplete antibodies act maximally at 37° C, and are therefore also called *warm antibodies.* Although they do not hemolyze red cells *in vitro*, the coated red cells *in vivo* are damaged and are readily destroyed. Warm antibodies therefore lead to severe hemolytic anemia.

Alloantibodies.† The blood group antibodies can also cause a hemolytic anemia under special circumstances. For example, in Rh-hemolytic disease of the newborn, an Rh-negative woman married to an Rh-positive man produces an Rh-positive fetus. During the last part of pregnancy—and particularly during

---

*In the *direct Coombs test*, a sample of a *patient's red cells* that have been washed in saline is mixed with Coombs' reagent (antihuman γ-globulin). A positive test is indicated by agglutination due to the presence of a coating of antibody on the red cells. In the *indirect Coombs test*, a sample of a *patient's serum* is mixed with a suspension of suitable red cells. These are washed in saline and then mixed with Coombs' reagent. Agglutination indicates the patient's serum contains antibodies capable of adhering to the red cells. In Rh sensitization of pregnancy, the mother's serum is tested for antibodies (the indirect Coombs test), whereas the baby's cells are submitted to a direct Coombs test.

†An alloantibody is an antibody present in one member of the species, which is capable of reacting specifically with an antigen present in some other members of the same species. The term isoantibody was previously used in this connection, but it has been discarded so that the terms will parallel those used in transplantation immunology.

labor—a leak of fetal red cells into the maternal circulation is quite common. The mother is thereby stimulated to produce Rh antibodies. Although the first child escapes damage, future Rh-positive fetuses may be attacked by maternal Rh antibodies that cross the placenta. The fetus develops a severe hemolytic anemia, characterized by numerous nucleated red cells in its circulation (*erythroblastosis fetalis*). In severe cases the fetus is stillborn; generalized edema due to heart failure is a prominent feature. Less severely affected infants survive but are jaundiced and may suffer brain damage (see Kernicterus, Chapter 33).

Other important extracorpuscular factors that may lead to hemolytic anemia are the toxins of organisms such as *Clostridium welchii*, drugs such as sulfonamides, severe burns that damage the red cells locally, and finally the malarial parasite, which directly attacks the red cells.

Pathological Findings. *In hemolytic anemia the red cells are typically normochromic and normocytic. The outstanding feature of the disease is a high reticulocyte count,* which indicates active erythropoiesis. The reticulocyte count may even reach 30 per cent of the total cell count. The bone marrow shows marked normoblastic hyperplasia.

In hemolytic anemia there is overproduction of bilirubin; jaundice is present in most patients. When the hemolytic process is sudden and severe, hemoglobinemia may occur, leading to hemoglobinuria. This response is unusual, except in the most severe cases such as in patients having blackwater fever. The presence of much free hemoglobin in the blood, particularly when the hemolysis has been caused by an immunological reaction, may cause renal vasoconstriction, anuria, and renal failure.

BONE MARROW INADEQUACY ANEMIA

Anemia is frequent in many chronic diseases such as rheumatoid arthritis, leukemia, renal disease, and chronic suppurative infections. *The anemia* found with these diseases *is normocytic* and *normochromic* and is not attended by any significant reticulocytosis. Some deficiency or toxemia probably impairs red-cell production, but the mechanism is not known.

Two other types of anemia come into this category and are described later: bone marrow aplasia (aplastic anemia) and bone marrow replacement (leukoerythroblastic anemia).

Polycythemia

Polycythemia is a condition in which the red-cell count is raised in a unit volume of blood in the presence of an increased total blood volume. It must be distinguished from hemoconcentration, such as that occurring in burns, in which the red-cell count is increased because of a decrease in the plasma volume.

Polycythemia may be secondary to chronic hypoxia. It is therefore a feature of chronic lung disease and cyanotic congenital heart disease. Some degree of polycythemia is normal in those who live at a high altitude.

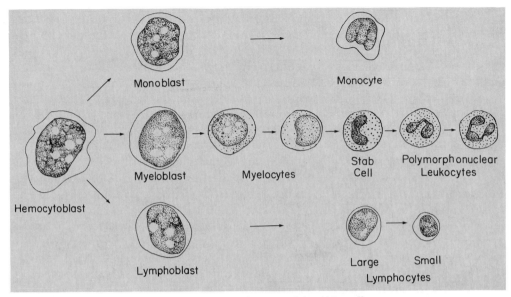

FIGURE 26–5. *Development of the white cells.*

The monoblast, myeloblast, and lymphoblast are depicted as being derived from a common pleuripotential cell called a *hemocytoblast*. The three blast cell types cannot be distinguished from each other on morphological grounds. The myelocyte matures to a stab- or band-form; the nucleus of the mature polymorph is formed by subsequent lobulation. (Drawn by Margot Mackay, Department of Art as Applied to Medicine, University of Toronto.)

As a primary condition *(polycythemia vera)*, the normoblastic proliferation of the erythropoietic element of the bone marrow appears to be of a neoplastic type. The red-cell count can reach 10 million cells per cubic millimeter, and there is often a considerable increase in both white cells and platelets, a change not encountered in secondary polycythemia. Indeed some cases terminate as myelocytic leukemia. Polycythemia vera is generally a disease of middle-aged or elderly people, and thrombotic complications are common because of the high viscosity of the blood. Mesenteric venous thrombosis, coronary artery thrombosis, and cerebral thrombosis are common terminal events.

THE WHITE CELLS

Important white cells are the granulocytes, the lymphocytes, and the monocytes (Figs. 26–5 and 26–6).

DEVELOPMENT

The precursor cell of the granulocyte is the *myeloblast*, a cell that closely resembles the hematocytoblast. As it matures, it loses its nucleoli and is then termed a *promyelocyte*. When specific cytoplasmic granules—neutrophils, eosinophils, or basophils—appear, the cell is called a *myelocyte*. The indented nucleus of the late or metamyelocyte is ultimately drawn out into two or more discrete lobes joined by fine chromatin threads. This is the mature *polymorphonuclear granulocyte* ("polymorph"), so called because of the shape

FIGURE 26–6. *Normal white cells in the peripheral blood.*

A, The neutrophil polymorph (Neut) has a typical lobed nucleus and fine cytoplasmic granules. The small lymphocyte (Ly) has a deeply staining nucleus and scanty cytoplasm. A number of platelets (Pl) are present. B, Typical small lymphocyte (see also Review Questions). C, Eosinophil with coarse granules (Eos). D, Monocyte (Mono). The cell is larger than a lymphocyte and has more abundant cytoplasm (× 960).

of its nucleus. Most granulocytes have fine lilac-colored granules and are called *neutrophils.* A few are *eosinophils,* which have large red granules, and the least common is the *basophil,* which has very large purple granules. The development of the granulocytes occurs in the bone marrow, and under normal conditions only mature cells appear in the peripheral blood.

The precursor cells of lymphocytes and monocytes are called *lymphoblasts* and *monoblasts.* As these cells mature, they lose their nucleoli; in the case of the lymphocyte, the cytoplasm becomes sparse as the nucleus condenses and becomes hyperchromatic.

NORMAL WHITE CELL COUNT AND ITS VARIATIONS

The total white cell count in the blood is 4 to 11 thousand per cubic millimeter. The range of the differential count is as follows:

Neutrophils—40 to 70 per cent (2500 to 7500 per cu mm)
Eosinophils—1 to 5 per cent (50 to 400 per cu mm)
Basophils—0 to 1 per cent (up to 100 per cu mm)
Lymphocytes—20 to 45 per cent (1500 to 3500 per cu mm)
Monocytes—3 to 7 per cent (200 to 600 per cu mm)

The suffix *-cytosis* implies an excess of cells, *e.g., leukocytosis* indicates an increased total white cell count, and *lymphocytosis* indicates an increase in the number of lymphocytes. The suffix *-penia* means a decrease in the relevant cells, *e.g., leukopenia* means a decrease in the number of white cells, and *lymphopenia* is a decrease in the number of lymphocytes. *Neutrophilia* is sometimes used as an alternative to neutrophil leukocytosis. Likewise, *neutropenia* denotes a reduction in the total number of neutrophil polymorphs, and the term *agranulocytosis* is commonly used as a synonym. The figures in parentheses in the range listed above indicate the absolute number of cells present. This is a more useful figure than the percentage. Thus, if there is a drop in the number of neutrophils the percentage of lymphocytes increases—a condition called a *relative lymphocytosis.* The term, however, is misleading, since the actual number of lymphocytes can remain unchanged. The main variations in the white-cell count are as follows:

NEUTROPHIL LEUKOCYTOSIS (NEUTROPHILIA). This common condition is usually due to infection. The highest counts are seen when the organism concerned is one of the pyogenic bacteria, *e.g.,* staphylococci, pneumonococci, and coliform.

Other important causes are massive tissue necrosis, such as after a myocardial infarct; uremia; acute gout; after severe hemorrhage and hemolysis; and rapidly growing malignant tumors and neoplastic disease of the marrow, such as chronic myelocytic leukemia and polycythemia vera.

NEUTROPENIA. A reduction in the number of neutrophils is seen in infections such as typhoid fever and malaria. It is also a common feature of the prodromal period of many viral diseases. Any overwhelming infection, whatever the cause, also reduces the neutrophil count.

Other causes of neutropenia are hypersplenism, bone marrow aplasia, and acute leukemia.

LYMPHOCYTOSIS.   An absolute lymphocytosis is not common. It is seen in *whooping cough* and in *infectious mononucleosis.* In the latter disease the lymphocytes are atypical and somewhat resemble monocytes. The disease, which is common in young adults, is thought to be caused by the Epstein-Barr virus. The illness usually commences with a sore throat, which is followed by enlargement of cervical lymph nodes, and later by the appearance of the characteristic cells in the blood. An interesting feature is the presence in the serum of antibodies that agglutinate sheep's red cells to high titer. The presence of these antibodies is confirmed by the Paul-Bunnell test. Another important cause of lymphocytosis is chronic lymphatic leukemia.

MONOCYTOSIS.   An increased number of monocytes are typically seen in some protozoal diseases, *e.g.,* malaria and leishmaniasis. It is a feature of monocytic leukemia and also of some chronic bacterial infections, *e.g.,* tuberculosis.

EOSINOPHILIA.   This condition, which is characterized by the formation and accumulation of a large number of eosinophils in the blood, is encountered in atopic conditions, particularly bronchial asthma, hay fever, and urticaria. It is also a feature of helminthic infections, particularly when the parasites are migrating through the blood stream and tissues.

The Leukemias

Leukemia is a condition in which there is a widespread proliferation of the white cells and their precursors throughout the tissues in the body. There is usually an increase in the number of circulating white cells also. The cause of leukemia is unknown, but it has been found that there is an increased incidence following exposure to ionizing radiation. In birds and mice the cause appears to be viral.

The leukemias are classified according to the rapidity of the disease and the type of cell involved:

Chronic Leukemia
(a) Chronic myelocytic leukemia (also called chronic myelogenous or myeloid leukemia)
(b) Chronic lymphocytic leukemia

Acute Leukemia
(a) Acute myeloblastic leukemia (also called acute myelogenous or myeloid leukemia)
(b) Acute lymphoblastic leukemia (also called acute lymphocytic leukemia)
(c) Acute monocytic leukemia

CHRONIC MYELOCYTIC LEUKEMIA

This is a disease of middle life and is characterized by an enormous leukocytosis, the white cell count reaching one million per cu mm on occasions. The predominant cell is the neutrophil polymorph, but metamyelocytes and myelocytes are also present. Coincidental with the leukocytosis is a progressive anemia and a gradual fall in the platelet count.

Clinically, the patient has immense enlargement of the spleen, and to a lesser extent, the liver. Death usually occurs within three to five years and may be heralded by an acute exacerbation in which the blood stream is flooded with myeloblasts.

CHRONIC LYMPHATIC LEUKEMIA

This is usually a disease of later life and there is a marked lymphocytosis with a total count ranging up to 250,000 per cu mm. Most of the cells in the blood stream are mature lymphocytes, but there are a varying number of lymphoblasts. There is a progressive anemia and thrombocytopenia.

Since the condition affects lymph nodes primarily, the patient usually presents with generalized lymphadenopathy. The spleen and liver are enlarged, but to a lesser extent than with myeloid leukemia. As with the latter disease, death usually occurs within five years and is due to anemia and secondary infection.

ACUTE LEUKEMIA

The three types of acute leukemia are best considered together because they resemble each other very closely. In the acute leukemias the white cell count may vary from less than 1000 per cu mm to over 100,000 per cu mm. When there is a raised count, the blood is invariably flooded with primitive blast cells; therefore, it is often difficult or even impossible to be sure whether these are myeloblasts, lymphoblasts, or monoblasts. In most cases there is also an increased number of more mature cells, thereby helping in the differential diagnosis.

In acute leukemia the primitive white cells replace the mature ones, and the polymorph count is invariably reduced (agranulocytosis). This leads to an impaired defense against infection, so that gingivitis and bronchopneumonia are common.

In acute leukemia there is rapidly progressive normocytic, normochromic anemia and severe thrombocytopenia.

Acute leukemia occurs at all ages. In childhood it is usually lymphoblastic, but in adult life the myeloblastic variety is more common. Monocytic leukemia is the least frequent, tending to occur in middle age. Clinically, it is not possible to distinguish between the three types. The onset is usually sudden, the main features being high fever, a generalized bleeding tendency, progressive anemia, and necrotic infective lesions of the mouth and throat.

Most patients with acute leukemia die within six months, usually as a result of infection or bleeding into vital areas such as the central nervous system. Treatment sometimes prolongs life to about one year; occasional cases go into remission, and some even appear to be cured.

Changes in the Organs in Leukemia.   The pathological course of leukemia is a monotonous infiltration of leukemic cells into numerous organs, which become enlarged, soft, and pale. Lymph nodes, spleen, and bone marrow are particularly involved and are crowded out by the responsible cells. No organ is exempt from this infiltration; massive local involvement is particularly characteristic of acute leukemia. Other changes found are those associated with infection and hemorrhage.

Bone Marrow Aplasia

When the bone marrow ceases to release mature elements into the circulation, there is a serious drop in the blood count, and the condition is described as *aplasia*. Sometimes the failure of division occurs at the "blast" stage; in such cases no mature elements are present either in the peripheral blood or in the bone marrow. At other times there is a failure in division at a later stage of hematopoiesis so that the marrow, although crowded with maturing cells, is unable to release them into the circulation. This is called *maturation arrest*.

Aplasia of the marrow may involve all three elements, thereby leading to a diminution of all cells of the blood *(pancytopenia)*, or it may affect only one of these elements. *Pure red-cell aplasia* is very uncommon, but aplasia of the granulocytes *(agranulocytosis)* is an important condition. *Platelet aplasia* is less common, but it does occur as an idiopathic condition in *primary thrombocytopenic purpura.*

PANCYTOPENIA

Aplasia affecting all the formed elements of the marrow can be due to ionizing radiations or drugs, of which the most important are chloramphenicol, the sulfonamides, and the cytotoxic drugs used in the treatment of cancer. It is also a rare complication of miliary tuberculosis. In some patients, no cause can be found, and the condition must be termed "idiopathic." Some instances of the last group eventually turn out to be leukemia. An occasional cause is hypersplenism, which is described later in this chapter.

Hematologically, there is an anemia with no reticulocytosis, a leukopenia, and a thrombocytopenia. If the bone marrow is found to be hypocellular, the prognosis is poor. On the other hand, cases of maturation arrest have a better prognosis.

AGRANULOCYTOSIS

Aplasia of the white-cell elements is a serious complication of therapy with certain drugs, particularly thiouracil (used in the treatment of thyrotoxicosis), phenylbutazone (used in treatment of arthritis), and chlorpromazine (used as a tranquilizer). Agranulocytosis also occurs as a result of the use of anticancer drugs. Some cases occur with hypersplenism, whereas others are idiopathic.

The chief effect of agranulocytosis is a tendency for infection to develop; consequently, ulcerating infective lesions occur in the mouth and throat, gastrointestinal tract, and vagina. Overwhelming infection with bronchopneumonia is the usual end-result.

HYPERSPLENISM

The function of the spleen in relation to blood formation is ill-understood. It is active in removing defective and aging red cells from the circulation, and it is possible that it exerts an inhibitory effect on the formation of white cells and platelets in the marrow.

Occasionally conditions leading to gross splenomegaly give rise either to marrow aplasia affecting any or all of the formed elements of the blood or to a hemolytic anemia. If the blood disorder abates after removal of the spleen, the condition is diagnosed as hypersplenism. The precise mechanism is not understood, and the condition is described in the splenomegaly of many conditions, *e.g.*, cirrhosis of the liver, schistosomiasis, and leishmaniasis.

BONE MARROW REPLACEMENT

The normal bone marrow is sometimes crowded out by foreign elements such as metastatic carcinoma or myeloma. This results in a typical blood picture of *leukoerythroblastic anemia*. In addition to the effects of anemia, nucleated red cells (normoblasts) are present in the blood, and there is a moderate polymorph leukocytosis with myelocytes present.

In a number of instances a leukoerythroblastic anemia is present in the face of fibrosis of the bone marrow. This condition has been grouped with polycythemia vera and leukemia under the all-embracing heading of *myeloproliferative disorder*.

THE PLATELETS AND CLOTTING FACTORS

Platelets are small discs devoid of a nucleus that are formed in the bone marrow by fragmentation of the cytoplasm of large multinucleate cells termed *megakaryocytes*. Platelet adhesion and aggregation have already been described in Chapter 20 in relation to thrombosis. In this section we shall consider the platelets and the clotting mechanism, particularly in relation to the defects that lead to a bleeding tendency.

The Clotting Mechanism

Blood clotting is a very complex mechanism and in essence consists of a conversion of fibrinogen (factor I) to fibrin by the action of thrombin (Fig. 26–7). This enzyme exists normally as an inert precursor, prothrombin (factor II), which is activated to thrombin by thromboplastin (factor III) in the presence of ionic calcium (factor IV). "Thromboplastin" is a vague, unsatisfactory term and refers to the total activity of the plasma in converting prothrombin to thrombin. No single substance can be identified as such.

Thromboplastic activity can be generated in two ways:

(1) In the *intrinsic system* contact with an abnormal surface leads to the sequential activation of factors XII, XI, IX, VIII, and X. Activated factor X, designated Xa, in conjunction with factor V and platelet factor 3 results in the formation of blood thromboplastin, also known as the intrinsic prothrombin activator. The early phases of the intrinsic system are slow to develop. Once thrombin has been formed, however, it potentiates the activation of factors V and VIII. Thrombin also causes platelets to aggregate, and thus it increases the amount of lipid factor 3. This mechanism is called the *autocatalytic action of thrombin*.

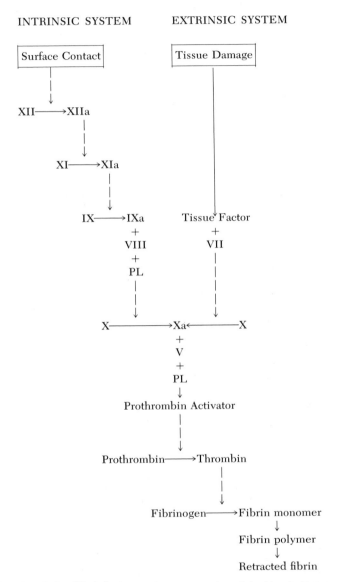

FIGURE 26–7. *A simplified diagrammatic representation of the blood-clotting mechanism.*

Solid lines indicate transformations; broken lines denote actions. *PL* denotes phospholipid, which in the formation of prothrombin activator via the intrinsic system is derived from platelets (factor 3). In the extrinsic system, phospholipid is derived from the tissues. Not shown in the diagram is the ionic calcium that is required for most of the steps shown. Factors are indicated by Roman numerals: XII, XIIa, VII, etc. (Modified from Marcus, A. J.: New England Journal of Medicine, *280:* 1213, 1969. Reprinted, by permission from the New England Journal of Medicine.)

(2) In the *extrinsic (tissue) system,* tissue damage results in release of tissue factor rich in phospholipid. In conjunction with factor VII, this activates factor X which (as in the intrinsic system) interacts with factors V and phospholipid to produce tissue thromboblastin, also known as extrinsic prothrombin activator. The first formed fibrin exists as a monomer. This subsequently polymerizes and retracts.

The Bleeding Diseases

When small blood vessels are damaged, platelets adhere to the damaged area and form an initial plug that stops bleeding. This plug is unstable, and it is only with the formation of fibrin that a stable hemostatic plug is formed. It is evident that diseases characterized by excessive bleeding fall into one of three groups:
1. *Deficiency of platelets*
2. *Deficiency of the coagulation system*
3. *Defects of the blood vessels*

BLEEDING DUE TO PLATELET DEFICIENCY

A low platelet count (thrombocytopenia) leads to spontaneous bleeding into the tissues with the production of small petechiae. In the skin the condition is called *purpura.* Spontaneous hemorrhage also occurs into the gastrointestinal and urinary tracts.

Thrombocytopenia may occur as an idiopathic condition *(primary thrombocytopenic purpura),* usually in young people. This appears to be a primary platelet aplasia, and the megakaryocytes in the marrow, although abundant, are abnormal and do not form platelets. Sometimes the condition remits spontaneously or following splenectomy, but relapses are common, and death not infrequent.

As a secondary condition, thrombocytopenia occurs in leukemia (especially the acute variety), marrow aplasia, hypersplenism, and following the administration of certain drugs.

BLEEDING DUE TO DEFECTS IN THE CLOTTING MECHANISM

Clotting mechanism defects are manifested by massive bleeding into the tissues and from the body orifices. Purpura is unusual, but intractable postoperative hemorrhage is characteristic and serious: fatal bleeding can occur even after a trivial operation such as dental extraction.

The following disorders are important:

HEMOPHILIA.   A hereditary disease characterized by spontaneous or traumatic hemorrhages, this is due to a deficiency of factor VIII. It affects only males, since it is inherited as an X-linked recessive trait (see Chapter 3). Bleeding is often severe; a special feature is bleeding into joints (hemarthrosis), which is usually recurrent and leads to extensive damage to the affected joints. The disease can now be treated by giving the patient preparations of plasma containing concentrated factor VIII.

CHRISTMAS DISEASE.　This condition is due to a deficiency of factor IX. Its mode of inheritance and clinical manifestations are indistinguishable from those of classical hemophilia.

DEFICIENCIES OF THE VITAMIN K–DEPENDENT COAGULATION FACTORS. The two common causes are liver failure and a deficiency of vitamin K. This vitamin is used by the liver for the synthesis of prothrombin as well as for the synthesis of other clotting factors. The vitamin is fat soluble, and its absorption is aided by the presence of bile salts. Consequently, it is poorly absorbed in obstructive jaundice, and this is one of the factors in the bleeding tendency that complicate obstructive jaundice and chronic liver disease.

Vitamin K deficiency also occurs in the newborn because of an inability of the infant to synthesize the vitamin in its bowel. If the mother's intake is also deficient, a serious bleeding state may occur—*hemorrhagic disease of the newborn*. Another cause of hypoprothrombinemia is the administration of dicumarol anticoagulants, which inhibit the synthesis of clotting factors in the liver. These drugs are used as a treatment of phlebothrombosis and myocardial infarction.

HYPOFIBRINOGINEMIA.　A deficiency of fibrinogen is usually acquired as a result of thromboplastic material entering the circulation. Such an event sets up intravascular clotting, causing the residual blood to become incoagulable. In addition, there is usually an activation of plasminogen so that fibrinolysis and fibrinogen destruction occur together with the clotting. The condition is called *disseminated intravascular coagulation,* or the *defibrination syndrome,* and is characterized by severe bleeding. It is encountered most commonly as a complication of pregnancy, when amniotic fluid enters the circulation and sets up both clotting and fibrinolysis. It also follows severe trauma, lung operations, and incompatible blood transfusions. The condition is a rather uncommon feature of widespread disseminated cancer.

BLEEDING DUE TO VASCULAR DISEASE

This type of bleeding usually takes the form of purpura, but more extensive bleeding can occur into the tissues as well as into organs to produce hematuria and hematemesis.

A common form of vascular damage is the vasculitis that is due to the deposition of immune complexes. This occurs in immune-complex disease and is also a feature of certain infections (*e.g.,* gonococcal) and other types of septicemia. Ingestion of drugs such as aspirin is another cause of vascular damage mediated by an immunological mechanism.

IMPORTANT TESTS IN BLEEDING DISEASES

1. PLATELET COUNT.　The normal platelet count is 150,000 to 400,000 cells per cu mm.

2. CLOTTING TIME.　This is the time taken for a specimen of whole blood to clot *in vitro* at 37° C. The normal time is 5 to 10 minutes. The clotting time is prolonged if there is a deficiency in any of the factors involved in the intrinsic clotting system or in the common pathway. It is therefore greatly prolonged in hemophilia and Christmas disease.

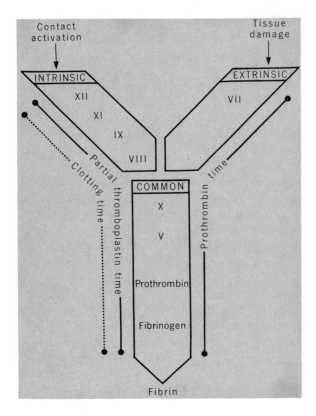

FIGURE 26–8. *The interpretation of screening tests of blood clotting.*

(Modified from Bithell, T. C., and Wintrobe, M. M. *In* Wintrobe, M. M., et al. (Eds.): Harrison's Principles of Internal Medicine, 7th ed. New York, McGraw-Hill Book Company, 1974. Copyright © 1974 by McGraw-Hill, Inc. Used by permission of McGraw-Hill Book Company.)

3. BLEEDING TIME. The time taken for a small skin puncture to stop bleeding is termed the *bleeding time.* It varies from 1 to 9 minutes and is prolonged when there is a lack of platelets. In hemophilia it is normal, but it is prolonged in thrombocytopenia.

4. CAPILLARY FRAGILITY TEST. A sphygmomanometer (blood pressure) cuff is placed around the arm and inflated to a pressure of 100 mm Hg for five minutes. If the test is positive, the skin of the arm below the cuff shows a petechial eruption. This test is positive when there is platelet deficiency as well as if the vessels themselves are abnormal, such as in scurvy.

5. PARTIAL THROMBOPLASTIN TIME (PTT). This is the time required for plasma to clot in a glass tube when an extract of brain, called *cephalin,* is added in the presence of calcium chloride. The cephalin provides excess phospholipid and makes the test independent of the platelet count. The PTT is a sensitive measure of the factors concerned in the intrinsic and common pathways.

6. PROTHROMBIN TIME (PT). In this test equal amounts of brain extract containing tissue factor, calcium chloride, and plasma are incubated, and the time required for clotting to occur is recorded. The test is measured against the time needed for a normal sample of plasma to clot. The prothrombin time is a measure of the factors concerned in the extrinsic system (factor VII) and in the common pathway (factors X, VII, and prothrombin). The intrinsic system is bypassed.

The PT and PTT together can give a fair indication of the nature of a clotting defect (Fig. 26–8 and Table 26–4). If both PTT and PT are normal, the defect

Table 26-4 THE BLEEDING DISEASES

DISEASE	PLATELET COUNT	CLOTTING TIME	BLEEDING TIME	CAPILLARY FRAGILITY TEST	PARTIAL THROMBO-PLASTIN TIME	PRO-THROMBIN TIME
Primary thrombocytopenic purpura	↓	N	↑	↑	N	N
Hemophilia	N	↑	N	N	↑	N
Christmas disease	N	↑	N	N	↑	N
Deficiency of the vitamin K-dependent coagulation factors	N	N	N	N	↑	↑
Disseminated intravascular coagulation	↓	↑	↑	↑	↑	↑

is probably in the vessels or in the platelets. If either PTT or PT is prolonged, there is probably a defect in the clotting system. If both PTT and PT are abnormal, the defect is most likely in the common pathway, whereas if the PTT is prolonged and the PT is normal, the defect is probably in the intrinsic system. The combination of a prolonged PT and a normal PTT is rare and indicates a deficiency of factor VII.

THE BLOOD GROUPS AND BLOOD TRANSFUSION

The red cells contain many antigens, but for practical purposes those concerned with the ABO and Rhesus blood groups are the most important.

THE ABO SYSTEM

Antigens of the ABO system are glycoproteins and are derived from a basic antigen called the H substance. Under the influence of the *A* or *B* gene, the H substance is converted into either A or B antigen. At birth there are no corresponding antibodies in the plasma, but within six months the antibodies corresponding to the antigens not present in the red cells make their appearance. These antibodies, called *alloantibodies,* are capable of agglutinating the red cells of normal people who are of a different blood group and of not agglutinating the red cells of persons having the same blood group as that of the individual tested. The following table describes the distribution of ABO antigens and antibodies:

BLOOD GROUP	ANTIBODIES NORMALLY PRESENT IN PLASMA
A	Anti-B
B	Anti-A
AB	None
O	Anti-A and Anti-B

These antibodies probably develop as a result of blood group–specific substances that are produced by bacteria in the intestine. The infant presumably forms antibodies against those antigens to which it is not immunologically tolerant.

To perform a blood grouping, one must treat a suspension of red cells with anti-A and anti-B sera, each derived from a donor with a high titer of these antibodies. If anti-A serum alone agglutinates the cells, the sample is of blood group A; if anti-B serum alone does it, the sample is of blood group B. If the cells are agglutinated by both anti-A and anti-B, the sample is of group AB, and if by neither anti-A nor anti-B, the sample is of group O. Similarly, with stock suspensions of cells of known blood group, it is possible to detect the appropriate antibodies in the patient's serum and to do the "reverse grouping."

THE RHESUS SYSTEM

About 85 per cent of the white population of the world has a red-cell antigen that was first noted in Rhesus monkey red cells. This is called the Rh antigen; cells containing it are called Rhesus positive (or Rh positive). Rh negative individuals do not normally have Rh antibodies in their plasma, but if they are immunized by Rh positive cells, they may form antibodies very easily. Such immunization can follow a mismatched blood transfusion or can occur after the pregnancy of an Rh negative woman bearing an Rh positive fetus. Many Rhesus antigens have been discovered: C, D, E, c, among others. The most important of these is D; cells containing it correspond to the original Rh positive cells.

OTHER BLOOD GROUPS

Human red cells contain many antigens other than those belonging to either the ABO or the Rh systems. At least 10 other blood group systems are known. Occasionally antibodies to these antigens are a cause of transfusion reaction.

Blood Transfusion

INDICATIONS

Blood transfusion is an essential and common procedure in clinical practice. Not only is it mandatory for restoring the blood volume after severe hemorrhage, but it is also used extensively in major operative procedures. In anemia packed cells should be given rather than whole blood, which contains unwanted plasma. Surplus plasma can always be used by blood banks for other purposes, such as the preparation of factor VIII concentrates. Whenever possible, it is desirable to treat anemia with the specific agent in short supply, *i.e.*, iron or vitamin B_{12}, unless the patient's life is in danger.

Various blood components are available from transfusion centers; these are useful in restoring deficient clotting factors, such as factor VIII in hemophilia.

CROSS MATCHING

The important elements to consider are the donor's red cells and the recipient's plasma. As a general rule, the donor's plasma is not important because, with rare exceptions, the antibodies it contains are so diluted by the recipient's plasma that they are not likely to react with the recipient's cells. It is always preferable to use the blood of exactly the same ABO and Rh groups as those of the recipient, but group O Rh-negative blood can be given in an emergency in which delay might lead to death from exsanguination (extensive blood loss). Under all other circumstances a cross matching is essential. To do this matching, cells of the donor are mixed with the serum of the recipient; no agglutination should occur.

HAZARDS OF BLOOD TRANSFUSION

Incompatible Reactions. These are usually due to the rapid destruction of the donor's red cells by the recipient's plasma such as when group A cells are transfused into a group O patient. The antigen-antibody reaction leads to agglu-tination of the red cells, causing blockage of capillaries and the release of vasoconstrictor substances and leading to widespread vascular phenomena. There is initial pain along the vein, followed by facial flushing, headache, a sense of constriction around the chest, and backache. In severe cases, renal vascular spasm combined with free hemoglobin in the blood lead to acute renal failure and death from uremia.

Bacterial Contamination of the Blood.   This is usually due to the acciden-tal introduction of coliform organisms in the transfusion fluid.

Diseases Introduced from the Donor.   The most important of these are viral hepatitis, syphilis, and malaria.

Febrile Reactions.   These are usually due to the presence in the recipient of anti–white cell antibodies that have been formed as a result of previous transfusions or pregnancy. This type of febrile reaction may be quite severe, but it generally responds to simple treatment such as the administration of aspirin. Although febrile reactions themselves are of little importance, each must be investigated; fever, although not dangerous in itself, may be a component of an incompatible transfusion. Future transfusions can be given with blood from which the white cells have been removed in order to avoid additional febrile reactions.

Febrile reactions may be also due to the presence of gram-negative endo-toxin present either in the transfusion fluid or in the apparatus. Modern disposable apparatus and properly prepared fluids have largely eliminated this complication.

Allergic Reactions.   These are usually urticarial and are due to some an-tigen present in the donor's plasma to which the recipient is hypersensitive.

Overloading the Circulation.   Transfusing an excess volume of blood can lead to heart failure and can be avoided by slow transfusion. Pulmonary edema is the usual manifestation of this complication.

Air Embolism.   With modern equipment this is a rare event.

Thrombophlebitis.   This response (inflammation of a vein with associated thrombus formation) follows the local irritation of the vein by the needle or cannula.

Transfusional Hemosiderosis.   Repeated transfusions are liable to lead to iron overload with hemosiderin deposited in many tissues, including the liver, where it may set up fibrosis.

Sensitization.   The transfusion of blood carrying antigens not present in the recipient may stimulate the production of alloantibodies against the foreign antigens. These alloantibodies to red cells, white cells, platelets, or plasma pro-tein antigens may complicate future transfusions or pregnancies (see also erythroblastosis fetalis, mentioned earlier).

In modern centers, blood transfusion is a life-saving procedure, but it must never be forgotten that the possible complications are numerous and occasion-ally fatal. Except under emergency conditions transfusion should never be at-tempted without expert supervision. Any patient receiving a blood transfusion must be carefully and repeatedly watched so that the early signs of any complication can be detected. The nursing attendants play a vital role in the teamwork that transfusion requires. A particular function which deserves special stress involves the correct identification of specimens. More serious complications of blood transfusion result from giving a unit of blood to the wrong patient than are due to errors of grouping or cross matching. The wrong Smith can soon become a dead Smith!

Review Questions

1. Distinguish between normoblastic and megaloblastic hyperplasia of the bone marrow.

2. A 45-year-old woman who had had indigestion for several months suddenly vomited about 250 ml of blood. This was repeated 12 hours later and she was admitted to a hospital shortly afterwards. Investigations revealed the following: hemoglobin, 8.5 grams per 100 ml; mean corpuscular hemoglobin concentration (MCHC) 25 per cent; and a reticulocyte count of 8 per cent. What conclusions can be drawn from these findings?

3. Describe the association of anemia with red cells containing:
     (a) An abnormal type of hemoglobin
     (b) An abnormal enzyme.

4. A woman gives birth to a child with generalized edema, severe anemia, and nucleated red cells in the peripheral blood. The direct Coombs test on the baby's blood is positive, and the mother's blood group is AB, Rh negative. Describe the pathogenesis of the baby's anemia assuming that:
     (a) It is the mother's second child
     (b) It is the mother's first child.

5. A 25-year-old man develops a sore throat, general malaise, and enlarged lymph nodes of the neck. Discuss the differential diagnosis if:
     (a) The total white-cell count is 2500 per cu mm and the neutrophil polymorphs constitute 25 per cent of the total.
     (b) The total white-cell count is 1000 per cu mm, and 20 per cent of the cells are large mononuclear forms with obvious nucleoli.
     (c) The total white-cell count is 15,000 per cu mm, and many of the cells are lymphocytes that are atypical but do not contain nucleoli.
     (d) The total white-cell count is 20,000 per cu mm and 90 per cent of the cells are polymorphs. No atypical cells are present.

6. Examine the red cells in Figure 26–6B. What type of anemia does the morphology of the cells suggest? What might be the cause of the anemia and how could the diagnosis be substantiated?

7. List the important steps that should be taken before a patient is given a blood transfusion.

Selected Readings

de Gruchy, G. C.: Clinical Haematology in Medical Practice. 3rd ed. Philadelphia, J. B. Lippincott Company, 1970, 800 pp.

Leeson, C. R., and Leeson, T. S.: Histology. 3rd ed. Philadelphia, W. B. Saunders Company, 1976. Note, in particular, Chapter 8, "Specialized Connective Tissue: Blood."

Silver, R. T.: Morphology of the Blood and Marrow. New York, Grune & Stratton, Inc., 1970, 125 pp. A well-illustrated, short account of common blood disorders.

Wintrobe, M. M., Lee, G. R., Boggs, D. R., Bithell, T. C., Athens, J. W., and Foerster, J.: Clinical Hematology. 7th ed. Philadelphia, Lea & Febiger, 1974. 1896 pp. Useful for reference.

THE COLLAGEN
VASCULAR DISEASES

Chapter 27

After studying this chapter the student should be able to:

- List the major collagen vascular diseases and discuss the validity of grouping them under one heading.
- Describe the main features of chronic discoid lupus erythematosus and systemic lupus erythematosus.
- List the autoantibodies that may be found in the various members of the collagen vascular diseases.
- Describe the lesions of dermatomyositis.
- Distinguish between morphea and progressive systemic sclerosis. Describe the main lesions of each disease.
- Describe the main features of
    - (a) The classical type of polyarteritis nodosa
    - (b) Three variants of polyarteritis.

    The term *collagen disease* was coined to describe a group of disorders in which the primary lesion appeared to be damage to collagen. *Lupus erythematosus, dermatomyositis, progressive systemic sclerosis,* and *polyarteritis* are now included in this group, and each will be described in this chapter. *Acute rheumatic fever* and *rheumatoid arthritis* can also be included, but they are described in Chapters 28 and 40.

    The evidence for these diseases being primary disorders of collagen is by no means convincing, but because they all possess certain features in common it is convenient to group them together. Since blood vessel involvement is as constant a feature as collagen damage the term *collagen vascular disease* is currently used.

422

THE COLLAGEN VASCULAR DISEASES

Lupus Erythematosus

CHRONIC DISCOID LUPUS ERYTHEMATOSUS (DLE)

This type of lupus erythematosus has been recognized for many years by clinical dermatologists as a skin condition that occurs particularly on the exposed areas of the body and is worsened by exposure to sunlight. The lesions consist of well-defined erythematous scaly papules and plaques. The epidermis shows atrophy, and as the lesions heal there is scarring. When the scalp is involved, there is loss of hair (alopecia). Indeed, lupus erythematosus is an important cause of alopecia with scarring; the lesions are very similar to those produced by scleroderma of the scalp. Chronic discoid lupus erythematosus may progress to the systemic disease, but this occurs only rarely.

SYSTEMIC LUPUS ERYTHEMATOSUS (SLE)

In systemic lupus erythematosus there are widespread lesions affecting many organs. The skin may show lesions identical to those of chronic discoid lupus erythematosus, or it may merely show erythema and edema of the sun-exposed areas. Typically, it affects the nose and both cheeks, thereby giving the classic "butterfly rash." Other important features of systemic lupus are arthritis, pericarditis (Fig. 5–6A), pleurisy, endocarditis, and glomerulonephritis. It is the kidney lesions which commonly cause the patient's death from renal failure (Fig. 35–3).

A prominent feature of SLE is the presence of many autoantibodies in the serum. Acute hemolytic anemia can occur, confirmed by a positive Coombs' test. The serological tests for syphilis are sometimes falsely positive. The rheumatoid factor is present in about 30 per cent of cases.

The important antibodies, from a diagnostic point of view, are those that react specifically with nuclear antigenic components. Antinuclear protein and anti-DNA antibodies can be demonstrated in most cases of the active disease. The antibodies may be detected by immunofluorescence: the patient's serum is applied to a section or smear of tissue, and the anti-DNA antibody that adheres to the nuclei is detected by subsequently applying fluorescein-labeled anti-IgG and examining the tissue by ultraviolet microscopy. A less sensitive method of detecting these antibodies is to search for the LE cell phenomenon. This was the first specific laboratory test described in the diagnosis of SLE. When normal human leukocytes are incubated for about two hours with the serum of a patient with SLE, some neutrophils are found to contain a homogenous

423

basophilic mass of nuclear material. Such neutrophils are called *LE cells*. The mass is derived from a necrotic leukocyte nucleus that has been acted upon by antinuclear antibody. Its subsequent phagocytosis by a polymorph produces the LE cell.

The cause and pathogenesis of SLE are not understood. A disease very similar to it, and encountered in Aleutian minks, is caused by a viral infection. Viruslike particles can be found in the lesions of human SLE, but they have not been cultured and their nature remains undetermined. There seems little doubt that SLE is a disease in which many autoantibodies are formed, particularly against nucleic acid, but whether the antigen is the patient's own nucleic acid or whether it is foreign—possibly viral—nucleic acid is not known. It is probable that the disease occurs in persons who are genetically susceptible, since there is an increased incidence of autoantibodies and autoimmune diseases in relatives of patients with SLE. It may well be that in these susceptible individuals various factors can trigger the formation of autoantibodies, and that the immune-complexes that are formed damage the blood vessels of the skin, kidney, and other organs to produce the syndrome of systemic lupus.

The precipitating factor may be a viral infection, administration of a drug (see Chapter 9), or exposure to sunlight.

The cutaneous lesions of chronic discoid lupus erythematosus cannot be distinguished from those found in some cases of SLE. Nevertheless, the two diseases appear to be distinct entities, but their inter-relationship remains to be clarified.

Dermatomyositis

The combination of muscle inflammation (myositis) causing progressive weakness of the proximal limb muscles and a variety of skin rashes constitutes this extraordinary disease. The occurrence of edema and erythema, particularly around the eyes, is characteristic. Skin and muscle biopsies help establish the diagnosis. The disease may run a fulminating, fatal course, or it may be chronic. In patients over the age of 40 years, dermatomyositis is often associated with a malignant tumor of some internal organ. Hence, a thorough search for carcinoma should be undertaken. Specific signs or symptoms may indicate where this might be; the common sites, however (*e.g.*, lung, gastrointestinal tract, and kidney), should always be investigated.

Scleroderma

Like lupus erythematosus, scleroderma can occur in two forms. The purely cutaneous disease is called *morphea*. The skin becomes thickened and ultimately densely fibrous. Small plaques may occur at any site, or the disease can be widespread and affect areas of skin. In the latter type, Raynaud's phenomenon is common (see Chapter 29).

In the systemic variety of scleroderma, called *progressive systemic sclerosis*, not only is the skin involved but so also are the internal organs. Particularly involved are the esophagus and other parts of the gastrointestinal tract, which show fibrosis and impaired peristalsis, thereby leading to obstruction. Fibrosis can occur in the lungs, and the condition is often associated with Raynaud's syndrome. Vascular involvement is usually not a feature except in the kidney, and in this organ progressive vascular obstruction leads to renal failure in a considerable number of patients.

Polyarteritis Nodosa

CLASSICAL POLYARTERITIS NODOSA

This type of polyarteritis, first described in the last century, usually affects middle-aged males and is characterized by an arteritis involving many organs. The inflamed arterial walls become necrotic and infiltrated with both inflammatory cells and fibrin, which gives the appearance of *fibrinoid necrosis*. The weakened vessel wall bulges and the aneurysms so formed are responsible for the designation "nodosa." The lumen of the affected vessels becomes obstructed by thrombus, and the disease is characterized by ischemia and infarction affecting many organs, particularly nerves, spleen, and kidney. Renal failure, often with hypertension, is a common end-result of this fatal disease.

VARIANTS OF POLYARTERITIS NODOSA

The classic polyarteritis nodosa described above is relatively uncommon, but many variants have been described recently. Often, when the vessels affected are small, the term *microscopic polyarteritis* has been applied to these lesions. In some of them, the precipitating cause appears to be an infection, whereas in others hypersensitivity to a drug has been implicated. In none of them is the pathogenesis at all clear; an immune complex type of vasculitis has been postulated, however. Some of the recognized syndromes are as follows:

Lethal Midline Granuloma. This disease usually affects young males. It commences with bleeding from the nose and is characterized by a vasculitis with much necrosis affecting the nose and nasopharynx. This terrible disease produces extensive necrosis and gangrene affecting the nose and nasopharynx. Death is invariable and results from local infection, massive bleeding, or bronchopneumonia.

Progressive Allergic Granulomatosis. This variant usually commences with asthmatic attacks and pneumonia. Infarcted areas, which are found in the lung, excite a granulomatous reaction that closely resembles tuberculosis histologically.

Wegener's Granulomatosis. This disease is defined as a microscopic polyarteritis affecting kidneys, lungs, and upper respiratory tract. In the last site, the lesions resemble those described in lethal midline granuloma. Death is usually due to renal failure.

It is not clear whether these variants of polyarteritis represent a single disease or are completely separate entities sharing one morphological component—namely, a necrotizing vasculitis. Certainly necrotizing vasculitis can occur in other conditions. Thus it is a prominent component of septicemia due to *Pseudomonas pyocyaneus* and gonococcal septicemia (Fig. 29–6). It is also a feature of the Arthus reaction, and it is encountered in rheumatoid arthritis, lupus erythematosus, and systemic sclerosis.

Summary

The validity of grouping these diseases under the heading of collagen vascular disease is dubious. Mixed cases occur and patients appear who exhibit features of several diseases. Thus some have lesions of scleroderma with vasculitis or lupus erythematosus with rheumatoid arthritis. The occurrence of these mixed connective tissue diseases suggests that there is a common mechanism, but it does not prove a common cause. The presence of autoantibodies is another feature that these diseases have in common, being the most striking in lupus erythematosus and the least evident in polyarteritis. Until the origin and pathogenesis of these diseases are discovered, it is convenient to refer to the group collectively as the "collagen vascular diseases" since they share many features. Thus, they all produce widespread lesions affecting many organs, and often they exhibit a marked constitutional effect such as fever, raised erythrocyte sedimentation rate (ESR), and hypergammaglobulinemia. This tendency is least marked in systemic sclerosis. All the diseases respond to glucocorticosteroid therapy as well as to other immunosuppressants such as azathioprine. Presumably, these act by suppressing autoantibody formation, thereby inhibiting the formation of new lesions. Once again progressive systemic sclerosis is the odd man out and is least responsive to therapy.

Review Questions

1. A young woman has developed an erythematous scaly rash on her face, the V of her neck, and forearms. She feels tired and generally unwell. What tests could usefully be carried out to substantiate a diagnosis of systemic lupus erythematosus (SLE)?
2. A 56-year-old man has developed marked weakness of his shoulder and back muscles. He cannot easily sit up in bed or stand without assistance. The illness began several weeks ago and has been accompanied by redness and swelling around the eyes and on the hands and forearms. What tests could be performed to help establish a diagnosis of dermatomyositis? What other examinations should be carried out?
3. What symptoms and pathological lesions can systemic lupus erythematosus and progressive systemic sclerosis have in common?

Selected Readings

Leading Article: Wegener's granulomatosis. Lancet, 2:519, 1972.
Peltier, A. P., and Estes, D.: Antinuclear antibodies. In Ioachim, H. L. (Ed.): Pathobiology Annual. Vol. 2. 1972, pp. 77–109.
Talbott, J. H.: Collagen-Vascular Diseases. New York, Grune & Stratton, 1974, 285 pp. All the topics mentioned in this chapter are described in detail in this book.

Part II

DISEASES OF
INDIVIDUAL ORGANS

Chapter 28

After studying this chapter the student should be able to:

- Relate the development of the heart to the common types of developmental heart disease.
- List the main features of Fallot's tetralogy and of coarctation of the aorta.
- Describe the main features of acute rheumatic fever and discuss the immediate and long-term effects of this disease on the heart.
- Indicate the importance of nonbacterial thrombotic endocarditis.
- Contrast acute infective endocarditis with subacute infective endocarditis.
- Describe calcareous aortic stenosis.
- Discuss the effects of myocardial ischemia and describe in detail the clinical and pathological features of myocardial infarction.
- List the causes and effects of stenosis and insufficiency of each of the four heart valves.

428

DISEASES OF THE HEART

- Describe the pathophysiology and effects of the major cardiac dysrhythmias. Draw a typical electrocardiogram of each type.
- List the cardiac reserves.
- Describe the causes and effects of left ventricular failure, right ventricular failure, and congestive heart failure.
- Describe what is meant by a "cardiomyopathy."

Diseases of the heart are a common cause of human ill-health and death. In the neonatal period, congenital disease accounts for many deaths, whereas a heart attack *(myocardial infarction)* is one of the chief causes of death in men between the ages of 30 and 50 years in the Western civilized world. The frequency of heart attacks has steadily increased—to the point that it has now attained almost epidemic proportions. The reason for this increase is not known, but one may anticipate that the trend will continue and, indeed, will spread to the underdeveloped countries as their inhabitants acquire Western habits.

Diseases of the heart may affect primarily the pericardium, the myocardium, or the endocardium—in particular, the endocardium that covers the valves. These structures may be attacked separately or in combination. The types and causes of heart disease are therefore many and varied; the effects, however, are few and stereotyped. Since the heart is a pump, it follows that the diseased and failing heart often pumps inefficiently. The consequences of this are circulatory disturbances that together constitute the syndrome of *heart failure*. This complex of disturbances will be described later, after individual diseases of the heart have been considered.

DEVELOPMENTAL ANOMALIES

The heart develops early in fetal life, and most of the developmental anomalies are therefore present at birth. This group of diseases is commonly called "congenital heart disease," and it is present in about 1 per cent of infants at birth. Without effective treatment at least 40 per cent of the infants so afflicted die during the first five years of life—most, in fact, during the first few months. Many developmental anomalies are known; until recently, however, their recognition was largely a matter of academic interest, particularly to the embryologist. Now, fortunately, since cardiac surgeons are able to offer a chance of cure, their interest is more than academic. Many techniques have been developed to assist in accurate diagnosis during life. Only a few of the common anomalies will be described.

SEPTAL DEFECTS

Since the heart develops from a single tube, a failure in the formation of the septa dividing the left and right chambers is not uncommon. In *atrial septal defects* some blood passes from the left atrium to the right atrium and from there into the right ventricle and the pulmonary circulation. The output of the right ventricle is several times greater than normal, but so long as it copes with this additional work, the patient is not seriously handicapped. This is indeed the most common congenital cardiac anomaly in adults and is not accompanied by cyanosis, as long as the shunt remains from left to right.

Ventricular septal defects are also common; if small, they cause little functional disturbance. With large defects the results are serious. There is a large left-to-right shunt that puts a strain on the left ventricle, because in addition to the shunted blood, it must eject an adequate amount of blood into the aorta if life is to be sustained. In time, the left ventricle fails. Furthermore, the right ventricle is subjected to the high pressure of blood coming from the left side so that the pulmonary circulation works at a high pressure. As long as the shunt is from left to right, the patient has no cyanosis. However, in response to the high pressure the pulmonary vessels become narrowed. The pulmonary resistance increases and the right ventricular pressure rises even higher. The shunt then changes from left-to-right to right-to-left, and cyanosis ensues. Ventricular septal defects illustrate one of the complexities of treatment in congenital heart disease. If the defect is closed when the patient is young, he may develop normally and live to old age. If treatment is delayed until the blood flow is from right-to-left because of increased pulmonary resistance, then closure of the defect causes rapid heart failure and death.

PULMONARY STENOSIS

An unequal division of the truncus arteriosus may result in the development of a large aorta and a correspondingly small pulmonary artery and valve (pulmonary stenosis).

TRANSPOSITION OF THE GREAT VESSELS

Owing to a failure of rotation, the aorta can arise from the right ventricle and the pulmonary artery can arise from the left ventricle. If this were the only anomaly, life would not be possible—a complementary defect must also be present. The patient's survival after birth depends upon there being some communication, *e.g.*, a septal defect, between the two sides of the heart. Transposition of the great vessels is one of the common fatal anomalies in children under one year of age.

DEXTROCARDIA

Occasionally the heart develops as a mirror-image of the normal. If this mirror-imaging involves all organs *(complete situs inversus),* the patient lives a normal life, since there are no other abnormalities. If only the heart is affected, the results are serious, because other defects are also present.

MULTIPLE DEFECTS

Developmental anomalies are often multiple. Malformations may be found not only in other organs but also in the heart itself. A common combination is the *tetralogy of Fallot,* which consists of the following:

(a) Pulmonary stenosis.

(b) Ventricular septal defect.

(c) Overriding of the interventricular septum by the aorta, so that blood from both the right and left ventricles enters the aorta.

(d) Hypertrophy of the right ventricle—this is compensatory.

The effects of Fallot's tetralogy illustrate many of the features of developmental heart disease and will be considered in some detail in the following paragraphs.

Murmurs. These are often loud and may be heard over the precordium with the aid of a stethoscope. They may even be felt as thrills.

Central Cyanosis. Since blood from the right ventricle enters the aorta directly, there is a considerable right-to-left shunt. The arterial blood is not fully oxygenated, and this causes central cyanosis. Patients with Fallot's tetralogy are born as "blue babies." Central cyanosis affects all tissues—skin, mucous membranes, tongue, and the others. Central cyanosis is also found in severe lung disease as well as in direct vascular shunts. It should be contrasted with peripheral cyanosis, which is due to stagnation of the blood in vessels of the skin. Peripheral cyanosis is never seen in the mucous membranes, which have an active blood supply, and this forms a useful clinical point of differentiation.

Polycythemia. This condition (an increase in the total red cell mass of the body) is due to hypoxia of the bone marrow.

Clubbing of the Fingers and Toes. This abnormality is generally seen when cyanosis is present and of long duration. The pathogenesis is obscure; it also occurs in other diseases, *e.g.,* chronic suppurative lung diseases, lung cancer, and bacterial endocarditis.

Underdevelopment. Unless the heart defects are corrected, the child shows poor physical development. Early death from infection or heart failure is usual.

Squatting. Patients tend to assume a squatting position after exertion, because this gives them relief from breathlessness.

Hypoxic Spells. A sudden increase in the amount of cyanosis can lead to cerebral hypoxia.

PATENT DUCTUS ARTERIOSUS

In the fetus, blood that reaches the right ventricle by-passes the unexpanded lungs because of the high resistance of the pulmonary circulation. The blood passes from the pulmonary artery into the aorta through the patent ductus arteriosus. After birth, as the pulmonary circulation opens up, the ductus normally becomes obliterated, but occasionally this fails to happen and it remains patent. This is an important site for infection in later life (see later in this chapter).

COARCTATION OF THE AORTA*

The process of obliteration that affects the ductus may involve the aorta and may then lead to the formation of a stricture. This generally occurs beyond the subclavian arteries, so that blood reaches the upper half of the body normally by the arch of the aorta and its major branches, but it arrives at the lower half of the body only via collateral vessels. This condition is important for two reasons: (1) the area of stenosis may become infected, and (2) systemic hypertension may occur in the upper part of the body, leading to left ventricular hypertrophy and failure. Unless it is treated, life is seldom prolonged over the age of 40 years.

The diagnosis of coarctation of the aorta should be suspected if systemic hypertension can be measured in the patient's arms, and yet no pulse can be felt in the femoral or other leg vessels.

ACQUIRED HEART DISEASE

RHEUMATIC HEART DISEASE

Acute rheumatic fever is a disease of childhood and generally affects those between 5 and 15 years of age. It typically occurs two to three weeks after a streptococcal sore throat and is currently believed to be due to an immune-complex reaction between large amounts of streptococcal antigen and antibody present in the patient's serum. The soluble antigen-antibody complexes appear to localize in the small blood vessels of the heart and joints and by activating complement lead to tissue damage. The reason for the localization of the lesions in rheumatic fever is not known.

The disease is characterized by *fever,* flitting *pains and swelling of the joints, subcutaneous nodules* (particularly over the bony prominences), and most important, *involvement of the heart.* Since *pericarditis* sometimes occurs, the two roughened surfaces of pericardium cause a characteristic rubbing noise that can be heard with a stethoscope. Some degree of heart failure is common and occasionally is fatal. At necropsy the heart is dilated, but the myocardium appears surprisingly normal. The characteristic lesion is a chronic inflammatory focus called an "Aschoff's nodule," which occurs between muscle bundles. Dilatation of the valve ring can lead to mitral regurgitation, which contributes to heart failure.

The most important lesions of acute rheumatic fever are those of the valves, which are swollen. Where the valve cusps meet there are depositions of thrombi on the endocardial surface—depositions called *vegetations,* which appear as small nodules along the line of valve closure. The mitral and aortic valves are most commonly affected by this *endocarditis.* Even though most other lesions of acute rheumatic fever undergo resolution, those of the valves do not. They tend to progress to a state of chronic inflammation, and the cusps become thickened, fibrosed, and contracted *(chronic rheumatic endocarditis).* Adjacent cusps adhere to each other, rendering the orifices stenotic, while the rigid leaflets and thickened chordae tendineae of the mitral valve lead to

---

*Although not strictly a disease of the heart, this topic is described here for convenience.

regurgitation (Figs. 28–1 and 28–2). If the aortic valve is affected, it is also rendered both stenotic and incompetent.

Not all patients who suffer from an attack of acute rheumatic fever have persistent heart valve damage. Nevertheless, the disease has a tendency to recur, and with each attack valvular damage increases. Since the disease is precipitated by streptococcal infection, long-term antibiotic therapy is often instituted as a prophylactic measure.

In those patients unfortunate enough to progress to chronic rheumatic heart disease, mitral stenosis is the commonest valvular lesion found. Blood is dammed back in the left atrium, which becomes dilated; its wall becomes hypertrophied. Stasis may lead to the formation of thrombus on the wall of the atrium, particularly if there is atrial fibrillation (see later in this chapter). Pul-

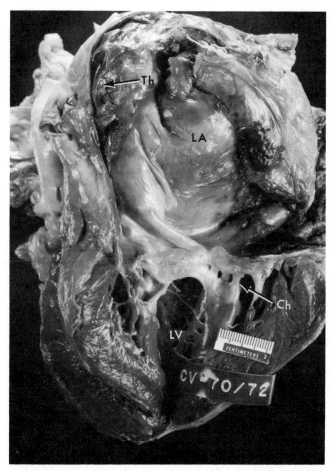

FIGURE 28–1. *Mitral stenosis due to chronic rheumatic disease.*

The heart has been opened by an incision passing from the left atrium (LA) to the apex of the left ventricle (LV). The left atrium is enormously dilated and thrombus (Th) is adherent to its walls. The mitral valve is markedly fibrosed, and its chordae (Ch) are greatly thickened and shortened. The left ventricle shows no abnormality, thereby indicating that the major function effect of the valvular lesion was that of stenosis. (Courtesy of Dr. M. D. Silver.)

FIGURE 28–2. *Mitral stenosis due to rheumatic heart disease.*

The mitral valve is viewed from the left atrium. Fusion of its cusps and fibrosis have combined to produce the characteristic rigid "fish mouth" or "buttonhole" stenotic deformity. (Courtesy of Dr. M. D. Silver.)

monary venous congestion follows. The effect of this is to make the lungs more rigid, so that breathing is more difficult and requires more effort. This alteration causes shortness of breath and distress *(dyspnea)*. Intra-alveolar bleeding leads to hemoptysis, and gradually to brown induration of the lungs (see later). In mitral stenosis the left ventricle is under no strain and is therefore small. However, should there be an additional factor of regurgitation or an aortic valvular lesion, the left ventricle would become enlarged and might subsequently fail. The back-pressure effect on the lungs eventually leads to pulmonary hypertension and right ventricular failure.

In chronic rheumatic heart disease the valves of the left side are much more frequently affected than are those of the right. Aortic lesions can occur alone or more commonly combined with mitral damage.

NONBACTERIAL THROMBOTIC ENDOCARDITIS

Small warty vegetations along the line of closure of the mitral or aortic valves are a fairly common finding at necropsy. These vegetations are sterile and are of importance in two respects. First, they occasionally become detached and embolize to the brain. About 10 per cent of cerebral embolism has been attributed to this mechanism. Second, the vegetations may form a focus (commonly called a *nidus*) for the development of infective endocarditis. Nonbacterial endocarditis has been called "terminal" or "cachectic" endocarditis, but of necessity, the lesions can be found only at necropsy. Probably they occur quite frequently.

INFECTIVE ENDOCARDITIS

In this condition the valve cusps are inflamed, covered by thrombus, and the whole area is invaded by organisms.

Acute Infective Endocarditis. During the course of septicemia, organisms may invade the heart valve and produce an endocarditis that is characterized by the deposition of large, friable thrombi on the valve surfaces (Fig. 28–3). The valves themselves may undergo destruction and then rupture. The clinical condition is generally overshadowed by a septicemia, but the presence of heart murmurs is characteristic: frequently, they change in character as vegetations form or the valves rupture. Pyemia occurs as fragments of infected thrombus become detached and enter the arterial circulation, usually the systemic. The infecting organism in acute infective endocarditis is generally *Staphylococcus aureus* or the pneumococcus. Unless vigorous and efficient antibiotic treatment is instituted early, acute bacterial endocarditis is invariably fatal.

Case History I. (See Figure 28–3.)   The patient was a 63-year-old man with a 15-year history of essential hypertension and a five-year history of intermittent claudication. Investigation revealed blockage of the bifurcation of the abdominal aorta. A by-pass operation was performed by insertion of an aortoiliac synthetic (Dacron) prosthesis. For the next four years the patient was able to walk without pain; then the claudication returned. Surgery was again performed, and the prosthesis was found to be obstructed by thrombus. The prosthesis was replaced. As a result of the previous surgery, many peritoneal adhesions were present. Unfortunately, the small bowel was accidentally opened during the operation. The tear was sutured, but the fecal contamination led to a postoperative wound infection. In spite of vigorous antibiotic therapy and surgical drainage of abscesses, the patient's condition steadily deteriorated and he died four months after the operation. On several occasions during the course of his illness *Escherichia coli* and *Candida* species had been isolated from the blood.

At necropsy septic infarcts and pyemic abscesses were found in the brain, myocardium, kidneys, and spleen. These were related to endocarditis involving the mitral valve (Fig. 28–3).

Subacute Infective Endocarditis.   The adjective "subacute," hallowed by tradition, is meaningless. The course of this disease is chronic.

The disease commonly affects a valve that has been previously abnormal

FIGURE 28–3. *Candida endocarditis.*

The heart has been opened to show the mitral valve, the left atrium (LA), and the left ventricle (LV). Friable vegetations (Veg) are present on the anterior cusp of the mitral valve; *Candida* was identified in the vegetations both by culture and in histological sections. The necropsy findings (see Case History I) indicate that this was an example of acute infective endocarditis. Nevertheless, the long clinical course was more suggestive of the subacute variety. Chemotherapy modifies the clinical and pathological findings; it is now more useful to describe endocarditis in terms of the infecting organism rather than as "acute" or "subacute." (Courtesy of Dr. M. D. Silver.)

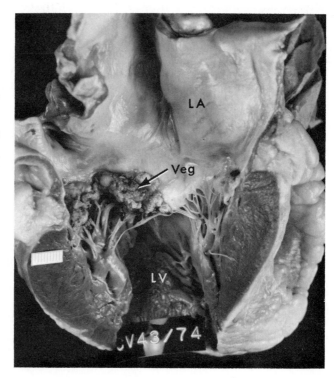

either as a result of rheumatic disease or congenital malformation. Any heart valve can be affected, but the mitral and aortic are most frequently involved. The valve is covered by large, red, friable vegetations that are liable to break off and embolize. Histologically, the thrombi contain numerous bacterial colonies that are well protected from the blood stream. Vegetations are attached to the valve by means of granulation tissue, which is neither profuse nor deeply penetrating into the vegetation. The organisms are once more beyond the reach of the blood. The poor vascularity of the valve cusp is probably the explanation for this inadequate organization. It is a good example of frustrated repair, and as such it is typical of chronic inflammation.

One of the curious features of this disease is that the organism is of relatively low virulence and is able to survive in the presence of a high degree of immunity. Its inaccessibility in the thrombus appears to be the explanation of this feature.

CLINICAL FEATURES.   The disease runs a chronic course; unless early, prolonged, and effective treatment is instituted, the patient dies within one year—usually of heart failure due to valvular destruction or cicatrization, or of a progressive glomerulonephritis, probably of an immune-complex type. Pyrexia of unknown origin is a common presentation of the disease; weight loss and anemia are constant features. The chronic bacteremia is responsible for reticuloendothelial hyperplasia, which accounts for the splenomegaly. Clubbing of the fingers is common, and multiple embolic phenomena are characteristic. Large emboli may cause infarction of the brain, intestine, kidney, or spleen, whereas smaller emboli produce kidney lesions that lead to hematuria. Petechial hemorrhages in the skin and under the nails are sometimes seen. Although the emboli contain bacteria, they behave as if they were sterile. When the infected thrombi leave the heart, the bactericidal action of the blood appears to be adequate to destroy the organisms.

A positive blood culture is necessary for a diagnosis of subacute bacterial endocarditis. *Streptococcus viridans* is the common causative organism. Nevertheless, because the disease is so serious, treatment should be commenced without waiting for bacteriological confirmation if the clinical picture suggests the condition.

Prior to the days of antibiotics, the disease was invariably fatal. With modern treatment, a cure is possible, but the healed valves are often grossly distorted, show calcification, and may require surgical excision to prevent the occurrence of heart failure.

ENDOCARDITIS FOLLOWING IMPLANTATION OF ARTIFICIAL VALVES.   The cardiovascular surgeon can now replace damaged valves by prosthetic valves of ball or flap design. The thrombus that forms around the rim of these devices, particularly where sutures are inserted, forms a nidus for infection. The endocarditis can cause local destruction, causing the artificial valve to become partially detached and to leak.

CALCAREOUS AORTIC STENOSIS

This condition usually affects elderly men and appears to be a degenerative condition arising in a congenitally abnormal valve. The aortic valve cusps become calcified and fused together, producing a tight stenosis. The left ventricle is hypertrophied, but in spite of the overaction of this chamber, an inadequate amount of blood is pumped into the aorta. In particular, the blood supply to the coronary vessels is impaired and these patients are in constant danger of sudden death. Surgical replacement of the diseased valve by a homograft or a plastic prosthesis is therefore indicated.

ARTERIOSCLEROTIC HEART DISEASE

Two coronary arteries supply the myocardium with blood. These vessels are particularly liable to be affected by atheroma, which causes narrowing of their lumina and subsequent myocardial ischemia.

Effects of Myocardial Ischemia

GRADUAL CORONARY OCCLUSION.   Slow occlusion of the coronary arteries leads to increasing ischemia; at first, this has no obvious effect on the heart. Some patients notice pain on exercise (called *angina pectoris*); characteristically, this is felt in the center of the chest and sometimes radiates into the neck and down the inner aspect of the left arm. The pain comes on with exercise, particularly in cold weather, and after a heavy meal. It can also be precipitated by emotional stress. The pain is thought to be due to accumulation of metabolic substances produced by muscle contracting under ischemic conditions. The type of pain experienced by a person suffering angina pectoris would be felt if the following occurred: If a blood pressure cuff is applied to the upper arm and the arterial supply to the limb is completely blocked, exercise of the forearm muscle would soon lead to such intolerable pain that the cuff must be released. What is not understood is why only some patients with coronary disease experience angina.

Invariably, the pain of angina pectoris is relieved by resting and by placing a tablet of nitroglycerin under the tongue. This drug is readily absorbed from the buccal mucosa and appears to act by causing peripheral vasodilatation, which lowers the systolic blood pressure and lessens the load on the left ventricle.

The morphological effects of myocardial ischemia are patchy necrosis of heart muscle and replacement fibrosis. At necropsy, the fibrosis is the most evident feature. Nevertheless, myocardial infarction can occur in the absence of complete coronary occlusion (see below).

SUDDEN CORONARY OCCLUSION.   *Myocardial infarction* or an acute fatal *dysrhythmia* is the common effect. These conditions are described below.

MYOCARDIAL INFARCTION

Extensive myocardial necrosis occurring suddenly is seen under the following circumstances:

1. *Following coronary artery thrombosis,* which is itself secondary to atherosclerosis. In the past it has often been assumed that nearly all myocardial infarcts were due to coronary thrombosis; the two terms (myocardial infarction and coronary thrombosis) are thus commonly used almost interchangeably. It is now realized that thrombosis is not always present, and it may even occur in the coronary artery after the infarction has already taken place.

2. *With coronary artery stenosis only.* When no thrombus can be found, it is assumed that some additional factor is concerned. Additional strain on the left ventricle may occur if blood pressure rises suddenly or if there is an increased heart rate (tachycardia). Sudden lowering of the blood pressure, as is seen in shock, is also a factor, since although it diminishes the load of the left ventricle, the blood flow through the coronary arteries is diminished even more so.

3. *With neither coronary artery stenosis nor coronary artery thrombosis.* Severe hypotension (as occurs in shock) and anemia may be present in some cases, but in others no explanation can be found. Multiple small platelet emboli or thrombi have been postulated, and their early dissipation can explain why they are not found at necropsy. It may come as a surprise to realize that in spite of the enormous amount of money and time spent in investigating myocardial infarction, the pathogenesis is still not understood. Perhaps this is why we have not yet found a means for decreasing its incidence.

Clinical Features of Myocardial Infarction. The sudden onset of severe pain in the center of the chest (retrosternal) is characteristic of myocardial infarction. The pain is not relieved by rest or nitroglycerin, and its severity may cause the patient to sweat. Although the typical heart attack is accompanied by severe pain, it is not uncommon for the pain to be relatively mild and atypical. Pain may be situated in the upper abdomen and therefore be mistaken for gastritis. It is not unknown for even well-trained physicians to complain of acute indigestion and subsequently to be found to have had a heart attack. Occasionally, the attack is not accompanied by any pain, and the presence of massive infarction comes as a surprise at necropsy of a patient who died of heart failure for unknown reasons.

Effects of Acute Myocardial Ischemia

ACUTE FUNCTIONAL DERANGEMENTS. Acute ischemia may cause sudden death. The left ventricle fibrillates in some cases, whereas in others ischemia of the conducting system causes heart block. Sudden death is most common during the first 24 hours after the onset of ischemia, and the value of acute coronary care units is that immediate external cardiac massage or defibrillation can save the life of a number of these patients.

HEART FAILURE. Acute heart failure, due directly to myocardial damage or to dysrhythmia, can produce a low cardiac output and a state of *shock* (see Chapter 21). Persistent low blood pressure *(hypotension)* is serious and may lead to renal ischemia, oliguria, renal failure, and fluid retention.

INFARCTION. If the patient survives, the ischemic muscle undergoes necrosis. The infarct appears as a firm, yellow area of coagulative necrosis with some surrounding hemorrhage and later inflammation (Figs. 28–4 and 28–5). Necrotic muscle releases its enzymes into the blood, and a rise of the level of certain enzymes (SGOT, LDH, CPK, and HBD; see Chapter 4) is a useful indication of myocardial infarction. Likewise, an increase in the white cell count and slight fever are manifestations of the inflammation.

Three early complications of myocardial infarction, described below, should be noted:

PERICARDITIS. This condition occurs if the infarct involves the pericardial surface.

FIGURE 28–4. *Recent myocardial infarction.*

The specimen shows part of the wall of the left ventricle. The recent infarct (Inf) is pale and has a hemorrhagic border. The lesion is about ten days old. Fibrosis in other areas (Fib) is the result of a previous heart heart attack.

FIGURE 28–5. *Myocardial infarction.*

The muscle fibers on the right-hand side are shrunken and show intense staining with eosin. Between the fibers there is an infiltration by polymorphonuclear leukocytes. A number of red cells are also seen extravasated in the interstitial tissue. Compare these fibers with the normal ones in the upper left part of the picture. This section was taken at autopsy from a man who eight days previously had sustained an intense crushing pain in the chest and shortly afterward had developed cardiac shock that was not alleviated by treatment (× 250).

FIGURE 28–6. *Myocardial infarction with extensive mural thrombosis.*

The dilated left ventricle has been opened, and part of its lateral wall has been swung over to the left. The anterior cusp of the mitral valve (Mit) is clearly shown. Part of the aorta is included in the specimen and the orifices of the two coronary arteries (Cor O) can be seen immediately above the three cusps of the aortic valve. There is extensive infarction (Inf) of the left ventricular wall immediately adjacent to the endocardium. Attached to the infarcted muscle there is dark mural thrombus. Both coronary arteries were markedly stenosed by atheroma, but no occluding thrombus was present. It is not uncommon to find this pattern of myocardial infarct in the absence of a thrombosed coronary artery.

MURAL THROMBOSIS.   This is seen if the infarct involves the endocardium (Fig. 28–6). Portions of this thrombus may break off and embolize to systemic organs (*e.g.*, the brain and the kidneys), thereby producing serious and sometimes fatal results.

RUPTURE.   Occasionally, the necrotic muscle ruptures, causing acute hemopericardium and sudden death. Both this complication and systemic embolism are likely to occur at the end of the first week. Rupture of an infarcted papillary muscle leads to sudden mitral insufficiency, heart failure, and death.

About 70 per cent of patients with coronary thrombosis survive their first attack. The infarct organizes to produce a fibrous scar (Fig. 28–7), which may later bulge and lead to an *aneurysm of the left ventricle.* The aneurysm itself may subsequently rupture, but this is an uncommon event. Usually the patient who has had a myocardial infarct is left with some heart damage, and further episodes of infarction are not uncommon.

In the past it has been customary to keep patients at rest for several weeks following myocardial infarction. At that time it was assumed that the heart needed rest for healing to occur. Medical personnel now realize that this rest is unnecessary. It is common practice to keep the patient in bed for two weeks only and then to allow increasing exercise. This program of moderate exercise has not increased the death rate and has diminished the incidence of complications of bed rest, *e.g.*, pulmonary embolism.

VALVULAR DISEASE OF THE HEART

It is convenient at this point to summarize the valvular defects. Details of these will be found in other parts of the book.

Mitral Valve Disease

MITRAL STENOSIS.   This defect is the most common valvular disease of the heart and is nearly always due to chronic rheumatic endocarditis (Figs. 28–1 and 28–2).

MITRAL INSUFFICIENCY.   Some degree of mitral insufficiency is common in chronic rheumatic mitral stenosis. It is also seen in heart failure when dilatation of the mitral ring leads to valve dysfunction. Occasionally, mitral insufficiency results from infarction of the papillary muscles holding the valve cusps. The insufficiency can be due to dysfunction or to actual rupture of the papillary muscles. Ulcerating endocarditis is a rare cause of mitral insufficiency.

Aortic Valve Disease.
Aortic stenosis is usually combined with aortic insufficiency in chronic rheumatic heart disease. Congenital stenosis can affect either the valve itself or, when the stenosis is produced by muscular hypertrophy (congenital subaortic muscular stenosis), the region below the valve. Calcified aortic stenosis is seen in old age, and most cases are probably the end-result of fibrosis in a congenitally bicuspid aortic valve. Some calcific aortic stenoses are probably examples of healed endocarditis.

AORTIC INSUFFICIENCY.   There are a number of conditions in which the

FIGURE 28–7.   *Myocardial fibrosis.*

The specimen is an oblique section through part of the wall of the left ventricle. White fibrous scar tissue has replaced much of the muscle in the lower part of the specimen. This was the end-result of an infarct several years prior to death.

elastic tissue of the aorta and the aortic ring are so weakened that the ring becomes dilated. The valve cusps fail to meet, causing severe insufficiency to result. Syphilitic aortitis and medionecrosis of the aorta fall into this group. Sufficient dilatation to cause regurgitation is also seen in hypertension.

Tricuspid Valve Disease. Tricuspid stenosis is generally of rheumatic origin, but it is rare. Tricuspid insufficiency, which is more common than stenosis, is generally due to dilatation of the valve ring in right-sided heart failure.

Pulmonary Valve Disease. Pulmonary stenosis is nearly always congenital in origin. Sufficient rheumatic endocarditis to cause deformity is rare.

CARDIAC DYSRHYTHMIAS

The term "dysrhythmia" is used to describe any condition in which the heart is beating either too quickly, too slowly, or irregularly. The impulse that initiates cardiac contraction commences in the sinoatrial (S-A) node in the right atrium, spreads throughout the atria to the atrioventricular (A-V) node, and then travels down the conducting bundle of His to reach the two ventricles via the two major branches of the bundle of His. This regular spread of electrical impulse can be interrupted in many ways by various pathological conditions. Only some of the most common disorders will be described here (Figs. 28–8 and 28–9).

Ectopic Beats. An ectopic beat arises prematurely from a site other than the S-A node. It may be in the atria, in the A-V node, or in the ventricle. Distinction between these types can be made only by study of the electrocardiogram. Following the ectopic beat there is a compensatory pause before the next normal heart beat. This sometimes produces the feeling of the heart "turn-

FIGURE 28–8. *The normal electrocardiogram (ECG).*

The electrocardiograph is a meter that amplifies and records the differences in electrical potential between two points (bipolar leads) on the surface of the body. Originally three standard leads were used (lead I, left arm – right arm, lead II, left leg – right arm, and lead III, left leg – left arm), but the "unipolar" or V leads are now commonly used. An exploratory electrode is placed on various parts of the chest wall; for example, VI lead is placed on the fourth right intercostal space near the sternum, and the second electrode is kept at zero potential.

The electrocardiogram is representative of the electrical activity in the heart, and this triggers muscular activity. P, the first wave, represents passage of activity through the atria (depolarization), and triggers atrial contraction. The QRS complex represents ventricular excitation corresponding to ventricular systole. The T waves represent ventricular recovery, or repolarization. The Q wave is a small negative deflection and is often absent. With the graph paper used for the standard electrocardiogram, each small square of the abscissa is 1 millimeter and represents 40 msec. The heart rate can be estimated by counting the number of millimeters between two consecutive R waves (or other portions of the complex) and dividing 1500 by this number. In the record shown above, the distance between each R wave is 29 or 30 millimeters, and this corresponds to a heart rate of just over 50 beats per minute. (Courtesy of Dr. R. S. Baigrie.)

FIGURE 28–9. *Abnormal electrocardiogram.*

A, Atrial flutter. Normal P waves are absent and are replaced by a flutter wave occurring at approximately 300 per minute. Some impulses reach the ventricles and lead to ventricular complexes. At point A, pressure was applied to the carotid sinus, and this produced reflex vagal activity. The effect of this was to produce a temporary heart block, and for a period there was ventricular standstill. *B, Atrial fibrillation.* In this electrocardiogram no P waves can be seen, and the irregular atrial fibrillation indicates chaotic atrial activity. The ventricles respond in an erratic manner, so that the heart rate in addition to being fast (95 beats per minute) is irregularly irregular. *C, Ectopic ventricular beats.* Two ectopic beats are shown in which the QRS complex is abnormal. This abnormality is a reflection of the beats arising within the ventricles themselves, and not being a response to normal stimulation from the atria. *D, Myocardial infarction.* The outstanding feature of this electrocardiograph is depression of the ST segment. This change was seen shortly after an acute myocardial infarction. In other leads there was ST segment elevation, and analysis of the changes in the standard leads can give a good indication of the site of the infarct. (Courtesy of Dr. R. S. Baigrie.)

ing over," but apart from this, ectopic beats produce no symptoms. They are common in normal people, but they can also be an indication of myocardial disease. This association with myocardial disease applies particularly to the ventricular ectopic beats, which are seen in patients with myocardial ischemia and in those who have taken too much digitalis.

Paroxysmal Tachycardia. In this condition there are attacks of rapid heart action resulting from a regular succession of ectopic beats that last for a few seconds or as long as several days. *Paroxysmal atrial tachycardia* is the most common type and is generally not associated with heart disease. The *ventricular type* is more usually seen in patients with ischemic disease; like ventricular ectopic beats, this condition may precede ventricular fibrillation in patients with myocardial infarction.

Atrial Fibrillation. This is a common and important disorder. It appears to be due to multiple ectopic foci discharging at variable rates in the atria. Rapid fibrillary waves take place rather than normal atrial contraction, and the multiple impulses that reach the A-V node (up to 600 per minute) cannot all be conducted to the ventricles. Approximately 100 to 160 reach the ventricles at a completely irregular rhythm. Because not all ventricular contractions are powerful enough to open the aortic and pulmonary valves, the pulse rate as felt at the wrist is less than that heard at the apex of the heart. Rheumatic heart disease, particularly mitral stenosis, is the most common cause of atrial fibrillation, but in older patients ischemic heart disease, systemic hypertension, and thyrotoxicosis are other important causes.

Atrial fibrillation is generally treated by the administration of digitalis, which acts by impairing conduction in the bundle of His. Fewer impulses reach the ventricles, causing them to be slowed, so that each contraction is more effective. The atrial fibrillation itself is not terminated. Indeed, to try to stop the fibrillation itself may precipitate detachment of a mural thrombus from the atrium.

ATRIAL FLUTTER. This form of dysrhythmia is less common than atrial fibrillation. The atria contract at a rate of about 300 beats per minute, being stimulated by a rapidly firing ectopic pacemaker. Atrioventricular block results in a slower ventricular rate (Fig. 28–9A).

VENTRICULAR FIBRILLATION. This is a most serious condition, and it is generally the immediate precursor of death in myocardial infarction. Immediate external electrical defibrillation is the most effective treatment if equipment is available.

HEART BLOCK. The term "heart block" is used to describe depression of conduction between the atria and the ventricles. In the early stages, the time required for the impulse to reach the ventricles is merely prolonged, but as the condition progresses, occasional impulses fail to reach the ventricles and a beat is dropped. When conduction is completely blocked, there is *complete heart block;* no impulses from the atria reach the ventricles, which then beat at their own intrinsic rate of about 40 beats per minute. The chief causes of heart block are ischemic heart disease and an overdose of digitalis. When complete heart block occurs suddenly, the ventricles may not start to beat for several minutes, and the patient rapidly loses consciousness and develops convulsions. These episodes are known as *Stokes-Adams attacks.*

Effects of Cardiac Dysrhythmias. Irregular or rapid cardiac contraction may lead to a sensation in the chest that is described as *palpitation.* If the heart rate is either very rapid (*e.g.,* over 160 beats per minute, as in paroxysmal tachycardia and atrial fibrillation) or very low (*e.g.,* below 40 beats per minute, as in complete heart block), the cardiac output is diminished, particularly on exercise. If the heart is otherwise normal, this change in rate may be of no immediate consequence, but if it is superadded to some other heart disease, the results can be serious. Tachycardia increases the heart's requirements for oxygen, and the energy expended is wastefully used by ineffective contractions. Furthermore, during tachycardia the coronary blood flow is decreased. Most of the coronary blood flow takes place during diastole, so that with tachycardia diastole is shortened and the blood flow is diminished. The heart muscle therefore has an increased need for oxygen at the same time that its supply is reduced. The ischemia that results further impairs myocardial activity and can lead to necrosis, either patchy or massive.

Heart Failure

The major contractile element of the heart is the muscular walls of the two ventricles. When the muscle is relaxed (*diastole*), blood flows into the ventricles; the flow is aided to some extent by atrial contraction. When the ventricular muscle contracts (*systole*), the atrioventricular valves close, and a volume of blood (the cardiac output) is forced past the pulmonary and aortic valves into the main arteries. At the end of systole some blood remains in the ventricles; this is called the *residual volume.* Under resting conditions the venous return to each ventricle is about 5 liters, but with exercise this increases to 25 liters or more. Cardiac output is correspondingly increased by utilizing the three *cardiac reserves* described below:

1. The increased filling of the ventricles stretches the heart muscle fibers, causing an increase in the force of the next contraction. This response is known as *Starling's law of the heart,* which states that *the energy of contraction is proportional to the initial length of the cardiac muscle fibers.* In spite of the increased venous return of exercise, the pressure of blood in the atria does not rise under normal circumstances.

2. Increased sympathetic tone causes an increase in the strength of cardiac contraction. This reduces the residual volume, and therefore increases the amount of blood ejected with each systole. A change in the force of contraction of the heart without a corresponding change in the initial length of the muscle is termed an *inotropic effect.* The alkaloids of digitalis are used in heart failure because they have an inotropic effect.

3. Increased sympathetic tone also causes an increase in heart rate, *e.g.,* from the normal 70 beats per minute to over double that figure.

The venous return to the right ventricle is the amount of blood draining from all the tissues of the body except the lungs, and this is directly related to the arterial supply to these tissues. The blood supply of a tissue is determined mainly by local self-regulatory mechanisms that are designed to ensure sufficient blood flow to satisfy the activity of the tissue at all times. The venous return, and hence the cardiac output, is governed mainly by extracardiac factors—namely, the metabolic requirements of the body as a whole. By using the reserves described above, the normal heart can cope with any normal load placed upon it. When it fails to do this, the result is heart failure, because in the presence of an adequate venous return it fails to supply the needs to the body. At first the effects of this are seen only during exercise, but as the failure increases, the effects are apparent even at rest. Either the left or the right ventricle may fail separately; more usually the heart fails as a whole. The condition is then called *congestive heart failure*.

EFFECTS OF RIGHT VENTRICULAR FAILURE

Rise in Central Venous Pressure.   A failure of the right ventricle to eject all the blood it receives leads to distension of the right atrium by a back-pressure effect. The pressure in the great veins rises, and the jugular veins are seen to be distended with blood when the patient sits up in bed. To some extent this aids heart function, because by stretching the heart muscle the raised pressure increases the force of contraction. Eventually, however, a point is reached beyond which increased stretching causes a *decrease* in cardiac contraction (Fig. 28–10). Exercise, by increasing the venous return, further reduces the cardiac output and forces the patient to be bedridden. Once past this critical point, therapeutic bleeding increases the cardiac output by reducing the venous pressure. (This is the basis of the time-honored practice of bleeding as a treatment of heart failure.) A similar effect can be obtained by applying tourniquets to the limbs to obstruct the venous return and to allow pooling of blood in the peripheral vessels. In right-sided heart failure all the organs of the body are congested because of the increased venous pressure. This effect is particularly evident in the liver, where the center of the lobules is congested and red. Congestion is also apparent in the skin, especially of the face.

Cyanosis.   The sluggish circulation allows the blood to become deoxygenated as it passes through the tissues; this response is apparent in the skin as a bluish discoloration known as cyanosis. Cyanosis is evident when the capillary blood contains more than 5 grams of reduced hemoglobin per 100 ml. Cyanosis due to stasis is known as *peripheral cyanosis*, and it should be contrasted with the type (central cyanosis) that occurs when venous blood is directly shunted into the systemic arterial system, as in some types of congenital heart disease. Peripheral cyanosis is not necessarily due to heart disease and occurs in other conditions when the circulation is sluggish. It is also seen in shock, whenever there is some local cause of venous obstruction, as well as when the blood becomes viscous. Stasis in the skin vessels sometimes occurs as a response to cold in people who are otherwise normal. Indeed, it is a common experience to see some degree of cyanosis of the ears, nose, and finger tips on a cold winter's morning.

Polycythemia.   An increased red cell count occurs as a result of bone marrow hypoxia.

Edema.   Edema of the dependent parts is a prominent sign of heart failure. If the patient is up and about, swelling of the ankles is first apparent, whereas if he is in bed, swelling of the tissues over the sacrum and external genitalia occurs most often. The pathogenesis of the edema is complex. In part

FIGURE 28–10. *Relationship of cardiac output to venous filling pressure (Starling's curve).*

(From Wood, P.: Diseases of the Heart and Circulation. 2nd ed. London, Eyre and Spottis Woode, 1956.)

it is due to the chronic passive venous congestion; this, in itself, is not the complete answer, however. It certainly helps to account for the *location* of the fluid accumulation—be it in the sacral region or legs—but it does not explain *why* the fluid accumulates. In right ventricular failure the output of the heart is inadequate for the needs of the body, and this results in peripheral vasocon-striction, which allows the blood to be most economically distributed. The mechanism is analogous to that which is seen in shock (see Chapter 21). The redistribution of blood appears particularly to affect the kidneys and results in a more complete reabsorption of sodium. This causes concurrent water retention and an increase in volume of the extracellular fluids. This increased volume ap-pears as edema. The importance of sodium retention in the pathogenesis of car-diac edema is reflected in treatment. Diuretics that cause excretion of sodium are of great use in treatment of cardiac edema. Likewise, a diet low in salt is frequently prescribed with advantage.

EFFECTS OF LEFT VENTRICULAR FAILURE

Rise in Pulmonary Venous Pressure. With the onset of left ventricular fail-ure the left atrial pressure increases, and the atrium together with the pulmo-nary vessels becomes distended with blood. As in mitral stenosis, dyspnea ensues. The rise in pulmonary venous pressure is extremely serious, because of the imminent danger of pulmonary edema. The edema of the lungs may ac-cumulate slowly, but sometimes acute attacks occur, particularly at night. This reaction, which is called *paroxysmal nocturnal dyspnea,* is a life-threatening event. The patient wakes up in the early hours of the morning with a sense of breathlessness and acute oppression of the chest. He becomes acutely distressed and coughs up the blood-stained watery sputum that is characteristic of severe acute pulmonary edema. Spasm of the bronchi is often a feature, and the condition resembles bronchial asthma to the extent that it sometimes is called *cardiac asthma.* The pathogenesis of acute paroxysmal dyspnea is only partially understood. It seems to be precipitated by a sudden sympathetic overactivity. Intense constriction of the peripheral systemic blood vessels drives the blood from the systemic circulation to the pulmonary circuit. The excess blood distends the pulmonary vessels, and there is a transudation of fluid into the alveoli to produce edema. Morphine quiets the patient and has a dramatic ameliorative effect, whereas epinephrine can be fatal. This effect is extremely important to remember, because in bronchial asthma epinephrine is helpful, whereas morphine is dangerous.

Chronic venous congestion of the lungs results in rupture of some capillaries, and blood-stained sputum (hemoptysis) is produced. Some of the extravasated blood is converted into hemosiderin, and the lungs become brown and slightly fibrotic (see Fig. 30–4). This is called "brown induration of the lungs," and it is characteristic of long-standing left ventricular failure (and mitral stenosis).

When considering the pathogenesis of heart failure (whether it is left or right), one must remember that the output of both ventricles is the same over any reasonable period of time. In left ventricular failure, the left ventricle is functioning with the aid of increased venous filling pressure, but the right ventricle, on the other hand, is working normally. This leads to a redistribution of blood, more being retained in the pulmonary circuit than is normal. As noted above, this produces congestion of the lungs, and ultimately there is a rise in pulmonary arterial pressure. Eventually this causes the right ventricle to fail as well, and congestive heart failure ensues.

CONGESTIVE HEART FAILURE

In congestive heart failure, both ventricles of the heart fail together, and the effects are a combination of those described under the separate headings of left and right ventricular failure. The inadequate output of the left ventricle leads to sympathetic overactivity with resultant peripheral vasoconstriction. In particular, the vessels of the skin tend to be constricted, causing stasis in the skin; this response leads to peripheral cyanosis. The lessened blood supply to the liver leads to atrophy and necrosis of the cells in the center of the classic liver lobules. This change contributes to the appearance of the characteristic "nutmeg" liver of heart failure (Figs. 28–11 and 28–12). The kidneys respond to the redistribution of blood by salt and water retention, but they show no morphological evidence of this malfunction. The brain receives an adequate supply of blood until the terminal stages of heart failure. Loss of consciousness tends to be a terminal event.

The Causes of Heart Failure.   Although the heart has adequate reserves that enable it to cope with any demand for additional work, it is not capable of maintaining a high output for any length of time. In the face of a continuous demand for additional work, it eventually fails. Thus, failure may be the result

FIGURE 28–11. *The liver in heart failure.*

This specimen shows the characteristic "nutmeg appearance" of chronic venous congestion in the liver. The insert shows how the pattern of the liver structure is situated. The dark areas consist of regions where liver cells have undergone necrosis and in which there is intense congestion. They are classically described as the center of the liver lobules, but in fact they correspond more accurately to the peripheral parts of the liver acinus (see Fig. 33–1).

of *overburdening due to a sustained increase in ventricular pressure.* This increase in pressure occurs in systemic and pulmonary hypertension and also in aortic and pulmonary stenosis.

Overburdening due to a sustained increase in cardiac output is another important cause of heart failure. In mitral regurgitation the left ventricle is forced to eject a large volume of blood, partly back into the left atrium and partly into the aorta. Aortic regurgitation also causes an increase in left ventricular output because during diastole blood from the aorta flows back into the left ventricle. With each ventricular systole a large volume of blood must be ejected so that the effective output remains normal. In time, both mitral and aortic regurgitation leads to left ventricular failure. Likewise, pulmonary and tricuspid valve regurgitation leads to right ventricular failure.

Another example of overburdening due to an increased cardiac output is seen in a group of diseases in which the resting cardiac output is above normal. This occurs under a variety of conditions. In *anemia,* for example, the tissues require an increased volume of blood to compensate for its low oxygen-carrying power. In *thyrotoxicosis* the metabolic needs of the tissues are increased. In cases in which a large *fistula* exists between an artery and a vein the shunt diverts so much blood that the cardiac output must be increased to meet the demands of the rest of the body. There are some common diseases (*e.g.,* *chronic lung disease* and *advanced liver disease*) in which the cardiac output even at rest is high for no very obvious reason. Whenever the resting cardiac

FIGURE 28–12. *The liver in congestive heart failure.*

Two portal triads are indicated by the arrows; radiating from them are columns of relatively normal liver cells. These are in Zone 1 of the Rappaport acinus. The liver cells in Zones 2 and 3 have undergone necrosis, and these zones are intensely congested. Correlate this appearance with Figure 28–11 (× 60).

output is increased, the heart copes with the load for a while, but it ultimately fails. Even in failure the output may be above that of the normal resting cardiac output, and for this type of condition the term *high-output failure* is used. Although the cardiac output is raised relative to the normal, it is still insufficient to meet the demands of the body. In the more common type of heart failure, termed *low-output failure,* the cardiac output is less than that of a normal person of similar stature.

MYOCARDIAL DISEASE

Myocardial ischemia is a common cause of heart failure. Acute infarction, described previously, may precipitate acute heart failure. Repeated infarcts, or gradual coronary occlusion causing fibrosis, may put such a strain on the remaining muscle fibers that failure ultimately occurs.

If one examines the heart muscle from a patient in failure due to hemodynamic conditions, it is disappointing to find that no abnormality can be detected. The muscle fibers may be hypertrophied, but this does not explain why they failed, nor does a biochemical examination elucidate the problem. We have to admit that the heart that fails in hypertension or valvular disease appears normal microscopically, but it does not behave normally. Obviously, our methods of examination are crude and not suited to detecting the lesion involved.

There are, however, many diseases in which the myocardium appears to be directly affected and which explain the cause of heart failure. The most important of these is when the muscle becomes hypoxic as a result of coronary artery disease; this has already been considered in detail. Some poisons seem to affect the heart directly: alcohol is one such poison. Likewise, various types of myocarditis and amyloid deposition disease are rare causes of heart failure. When all known causes have been eliminated from consideration, there remains a group of conditions in which the heart fails for no detectable reason. The heart is large, dilated, shows no valvular or coronary disease, and yet it fails. This is a fascinating residual group which, for want of a better name, is called *cardiomyopathy*. The diagnosis is one of exclusion. In some instances the disease seems to be the result of an inherited factor; for the most part, however, we must confess our complete ignorance as to its nature. When all the above morphological cardiac factors causing heart failure have been excluded, there remain four other very common contributory factors that do not themselves cause heart failure but rather enhance it when it is due to some other factor. These factors are *anxiety, pyrexia, pregnancy* and *dysrhythmias. Anxiety* raises the heart rate and blood pressure, thereby adding an additional burden to the left ventricle. By raising the metabolic rate *pyrexia* causes an increase in cardiac output. *Pregnancy* increases the strain as a result of an increased blood volume and the necessity for supplying blood to the fetus. The effects of *dysrhythmias* have been considered earlier in this chapter.

Review Questions

1. Describe the signs and symptoms leading you to suspect that a child might have a developmental heart lesion.
2. Compare *central cyanosis* with *peripheral cyanosis.*
3. Compare the effects of the emboli found in the following conditions:
    (a) nonbacterial thrombotic endocarditis
    (b) acute endocarditis
    (c) *Streptococcus viridans* endocarditis.
4. Where may thrombi be found in the heart? List the causes.
5. Describe the necropsy changes that would be expected in the heart of patients who had had the following:
    (a) angina pectoris
    (b) a myocardial infarct six months prior to examination
    (c) a myocardial infarct seven days prior to examination.
6. Describe the structural and functional effects of stenosis of the coronary arteries.
7. A patient who has had a recent myocardial infarct is being nursed in a coronary care unit. Pulse rate, blood pressure, ECG, respiration rate, and fluid balance are being carefully monitored. Discuss the signs or symptoms that would indicate that the patient's condition was deteriorating and that he might die.
8. Examine Figure 28–9A. What is the ventricular rate before carotid sinus pressure was applied? It is known that exercise has no influence on the rate of the fluttering

atria, but that it does decrease vagal activity. Predict the effect of exercise on the ventricular rate of contraction in this patient.

Selected Readings

Abelmann, W. H.: The cardiomyopathies. Hospital Practice, 6(3):101–112, 1971.

Braunwald, E.: Heart failure. *In* Wintrobe, M. M., et al. (Eds.): Harrison's Principles of Internal Medicine. 7th ed. New York, McGraw-Hill Book Company, 1974, Chapter 233.

Braunwald, E., and Sobel, B. E.: Cardiac dysrhythmias. *In* Wintrobe, M. M., et al. (Eds.): Harrison's Principles of Internal Medicine. 7th ed. New York, McGraw-Hill Book Company, 1974, Chapter 234.

Briller, S. A.: Electrocardiography. *In* Wintrobe, M. M., et al. (Eds.): Harrison's Principles of Internal Medicine. 7th ed. New York, McGraw-Hill Book Company, 1974, Chapter 229.

Brod, J.: Pathogenesis of cardiac oedema. British Medical Journal, 1:222–228, 1972.

Campbell, E. J. M., Dickinson, C. J., and Slater, J. D. H.: Clinical Physiology. 4th ed. Oxford, Blackwell Scientific Publications Ltd., 1974. See Chapter 2, "The Heart and Circulation."

Davis, J. O.: The mechanisms of salt and water retention in cardiac failure. Hospital Practice, 5(9):63–90 , 1970.

Perloff, J. K.: The clinical manifestations of cardiac failure in adults. Hospital Practice, 5(9):43–50, 1970.

Scully, R. E. (Ed.): Case records of the Massachusetts General Hospital. New England Journal of Medicine, 292:255–260, 1975. A case of staphylococcal endocarditis.

DISEASES OF
BLOOD VESSELS

Chapter 29

After studying this chapter the student should be able to:

- Describe the three layers of the arterial wall.
- Describe the changes that occur in Mönckeberg's sclerosis.
- List the causes of arteriolar sclerosis.
- Describe atherosclerosis with respect to the following factors:
    - (a) early lesions
    - (b) late and complicated lesions
    - (c) vessels affected
    - (d) etiology and pathogenesis
    - (e) complications.
- Classify the inflammatory diseases of arteries.
- List the causes of small-vessel obstruction.
- Describe the causes of acute vasculitis.

454

DISEASES OF BLOOD VESSELS

- Detail the pathological lesions that can cause peripheral vascular disease of a limb.
- Classify aneurysms according to their cause.
- List the ways in which aneurysms can produce damage.
- Describe the outstanding clinical and pathological effects of a dissecting aneurysm of the aorta.
- Give an account of the cause and effects of varicose veins of the leg.

DISEASES OF ARTERIES

Arterial disease and its complications are responsible for about 40 per cent of all deaths. Arteritis forms a distinct group, but the degenerative diseases (arteriosclerosis) are by far the most important. A knowledge of the structure of arteries is necessary in order to understand their diseases.

STRUCTURE OF ARTERIES

Arteries have three coats, which are described below:

THE INTIMA (TUNICA INTIMA). This layer consists of endothelium together with a small quantity of underlying connective tissue—collagen, occasional fibroblasts, and muscle cells.

THE MEDIA (TUNICA MEDIA). The media is the thickest layer and contains elastic fibers and smooth muscle cells, the proportion of each depending on the type of artery.

THE ADVENTITIA (TUNICA ADVENTITIA). This outer coat consists of loose connective tissue and small vessels (the *vasa vasorum*), which penetrate the media and supply it with blood.

ARTERIOSCLEROSIS

Arteriosclerosis, or *hardening of the arteries*, is a term applied to a group of disorders that appear to be degenerative in nature. Three conditions are included:

Mönckeberg's Medial Sclerosis. *This disease affects the muscular vessels, particularly those of the lower limbs.* The muscle coat becomes replaced by fibrous tissue, which subsequently calcifies and even ossifies. The thickened, pipe-stem arteries produce characteristic radiological findings; since the lumen of the affected vessels is not appreciably narrowed, however, the disease causes no ill-effects and is unimportant.

Arteriolar Sclerosis (Arteriolosclerosis). This condition involves *widespread thickening of the walls of small arteries and arterioles. It is an invariable accompaniment of systemic hypertension.* One effect is that the muscle coat shows hypertrophy, but the most striking change is fibrous thickening of the intima. The changes are most marked in the kidney, and the resultant ischemia leads to patchy degeneration followed by scarring. This is the pathogenesis of *nephrosclerosis* (Fig. 29–4).

Similar changes with intimal thickening of small vessels may occur as a localized event; such changes are not related to hypertension. It is found in the small vessels of the ovaries in postmenopausal women where it is a component of the aging process. It is common in mature scar tissue, is found in areas of chronic inflammation (*e.g.,* in the base of a chronic peptic ulcer), and is particularly marked in the fibrosis induced by ionizing radiation. Under these conditions the name *endarteritis obliterans* is applied.

Atherosclerosis. This is the most important component of arteriosclerosis and will be considered in detail in the following section.

Atherosclerosis

Atherosclerosis is the commonest killing disease of all highly advanced communities; its lesions are present to some extent in every adult of such societies. *The disease characteristically affects the large elastic arteries such as the aorta and its major branches. Of the medium-sized vessels, the coronary and cerebral arteries are the most commonly involved.* This is particularly unfortunate, since the tissues supplied by these vessels are vital to life. Indeed, it is the involvement of these arteries that accounts for the lethal effects of atherosclerosis. The disease may be considered as consisting of two types of lesion: type I and type II.

BASIC LESIONS OF ATHEROSCLEROSIS

Type I: Superficial Yellow Plaques in the Intima. Lipid-containing cells (probably muscle cells) accumulate in the subendothelial layer of the vessel and later break down to release their fatty content into the tunica intima. In this way are produced the yellow streaks that are a common necropsy finding in the aorta (Fig. 29–1). When the fatty deposits occur in small arteries, they do not produce appreciable narrowing of the lumen. These early yellow plaques are sometimes referred to as *atheroma.*

Type II: Accumulation of Fatty Material in the Intima with Additional Fibrosis. This is the common type of lesion seen in middle age and old age (Fig. 29–2). The lesions consist of intimal plaques and contain a central mass of fatty, yellow, porridgelike material (from the Greek *athere,* meaning "porridge") consisting predominantly of cholesterol and its esters. This material is covered by dense fibrous tissue, which gives the plaque a white, pearly appearance.

FIGURE 29–1. *Atheroma of the aorta.*

The abdominal aorta has been opened from behind to expose the intimal surface. The early lesions of atheroma are the bright, stippled areas and streaks that are seen in the lower part of the specimen. In the fresh state the lesions were bright yellow in color.

FIGURE 29–2. *Atherosclerosis of aorta.*

In addition to yellow streaks, the intimal surface shows raised plaques of fibrous tissue overlying the fatty atheromatous material.

FIGURE 29–3. *Atherosclerosis of the aorta.*

This aorta shows severe atherosclerosis. The arrow points to an area of ulceration that is covered by a thrombus.

ADVANCED AND COMPLICATED LESIONS OF ATHEROSCLEROSIS

Four further changes may be seen in the plaques as they progress:

(1) HEMORRHAGE. Proliferation of vessels from the vasa vasorum produces increased vascularity in the connective tissue surrounding the atheromatous plaque. Rupture of one of these vessels leads to bleeding into the plaque. In a small vessel such as the coronary artery, this bleeding produces acute obstruction.

(2) THROMBOSIS. Eddy currents around the plaque can lead to superadded thrombosis.

(3) ULCERATION. Sometimes the fibrous covering of the plaque becomes detached so that ulceration is combined with thrombosis (Fig. 29–3).

(4) CALCIFICATION. The fatty material in the atheromatous plaque undergoes dystrophic calcification.

ETIOLOGY AND PATHOGENESIS

The cause of atherosclerosis is not yet known, but genetic factors seem to play a part, since the disease sometimes appears in many members of a family. In some instances there are clues to the pathogenesis. Thus, atherosclerosis is more common in persons having diabetes, which is itself a familial disease. Likewise, there are some inherited conditions of abnormal lipid metabolism in which high blood lipid levels are associated with the early development of atheroma.

It is not known whether the lesions of type I atheroma progress to those of type II, or whether the two types are independent diseases. Experimentally, lesions resembling the human fatty streaks can be produced in animals by feeding them with an abnormal diet—usually one containing a high content of cholesterol. It is believed that certain types of diet predispose human beings to develop atheroma. Much of the cholesterol in the body is produced endogenously, but the level of plasma cholesterol is related to the types of lipid that are eaten. A diet high in saturated animal fats appears to predispose a person to atheroma.

Lesions resembling type II atherosclerosis can occur after the arterial wall has been injured. A thrombus forms and its subsequent degeneration and partial organization produce an atheromatous plaque. Either lipid deposition or thrombosis could be involved in the pathogenesis of human atheroma, and there is currently much controversy as to the relative importance of these two mechanisms. Furthermore, they are not mutually exclusive. Initial lipid lesions produced by dietary imbalance could progress by additional thrombosis. Injury and superadded thrombosis release chemicals (*e.g.*, histamine and 5-hydroxytryptamine) that could alter the endothelial permeability and allow plasma lipoproteins to enter the intima. Degradation of the lipoprotein together with failure to remove the lipid component is believed to be the mechanism of lipid accumulation in atheroma.

EFFECTS OF ATHEROSCLEROSIS

Gradual Obstruction. Atherosclerosis of small vessels such as the coronary or cerebral arteries produces intimal thickening and progressive occlusion of the lumen. This leads to ischemia of the area supplied (see Chapter 20).

Thrombosis. This leads to sudden complete obstruction and often to infarction (see Chapter 20).

Dilatation and Aneurysm Formation. The presence of an atherosclerotic plaque causes atrophy of the adjacent media. The wall consequently weakens, and the artery involved may show either a diffuse enlargement, termed *ectasia,* or a localized dilatation, termed an *aneurysm* (Fig. 29–4). These effects are seen most often in the aorta, in which the atherosclerosis is most severe. The lesions of atherosclerosis tend to be more advanced toward the more caudal regions of the aorta, and it is therefore in the abdominal portion that aneurysm formation is most common. The aneurysm is generally below the origin of the renal arteries, and rupture of such a lesion leads to exsanguination and death.

Case History I. (See Figure 29–4). The patient was a 71-year-old man who had had a 15-year history of hypertension. Five years prior to the examination he had been investigated for a possible aortic aneurysm. The findings were equivocal, however, and no treatment was advised. One year prior to his present admission he had noted the onset of angina pectoris and intermittent claudication. The angina was easily relieved by nitroglycerin tablets.

The patient's present complaint was that of pain in the abdomen. His blood pressure was 220/115 mm Hg and the blood urea nitrogen (BUN) was 50 mg per 100 ml (normal; 10 to 20 mg per 100 ml). A diagnosis of myocardial infarct was considered, but it was not confirmed by the electrocardiogram. The pain subsided for a few days but suddenly recurred with increased severity and was accompanied by signs of shock. The patient died before treatment for internal bleeding could be undertaken.

FIGURE 29–4. *Atheromatous aneurysm of the aorta.*

The aorta shows severe atheroma. An aneurysm, situated below the level of the renal arteries, is filled with thrombus, but has ruptured (arrow). The kidneys are reduced in size, and their surfaces are granular. This change is due to nephrosclerosis combined with many atheromatous emboli in the renal arterioles.

Necropsy revealed a ruptured aortic aneurysm, which is shown in Figure 29–4. There was extensive bleeding into the retroperitoneal tissues and into the peritoneum. The heart was enlarged (weight 850 grams, compared to 300 grams in a normal heart) due to marked left ventricular hypertrophy. The coronary vessels showed severe atherosclerosis with narrowing.

Embolism.   It is not uncommon for atheromatous material, or overlying thrombus, to become detached and embolize distally. Usually such emboli are small and are inapparent clinically. Nevertheless, the steady occlusion of many small vessels is probably a factor in peripheral ischemic disease of the lower leg as well as in the progressive ischemic renal disease that often accompanies atherosclerosis.

Inflammatory Diseases of Arteries

ACUTE INFECTIVE ARTERITIS

Arteritis may occur in pyogenic infections, and if the vessel wall undergoes necrosis, severe hemorrhage can result. A good example of this is the fatal hemorrhage from the lingual artery that sometimes ends the life of a patient with an ulcerating carcinoma of the tongue. Neoplastic invasion plays its part, but the major weakening effect is the result of infection. Similarly, destruction of an artery at the base of a gastric ulcer is a common cause of bleeding. Fortunately, in many chronic inflammatory lesions the artery responds by proliferation of its intimal lining so that the lumen becomes steadily occluded *(endarteritis obliterans)* and bleeding is restricted.

SYPHILITIC ARTERITIS

In tertiary syphilis an arteritis may occur, and it nearly always affects the aorta. A chronic inflammatory reaction is combined with destruction of the elastic coat and its replacement by fibrous tissue; the vessel becomes thickened, and at the same time is weakened. Either it dilates diffusely or an aneurysm (either fusiform or saccular) is formed. The thoracic part of the aorta is most severely affected; in the past, syphilis was the common cause of thoracic aortic aneurysms (Fig. 29–5). Today the disease is rare, and atheroma accounts for the majority of aortic aneurysms. Dilatation of the arch of the aorta and the aortic ring leads to separation of the aortic cusps so that in diastole they fail to meet and *aortic regurgitation* results.

FIGURE 29–5. *Syphilitic aneurysm of the aorta.*

The specimen shows part of the descending aorta from which a saccular aneurysm arises. Note the laminated thrombus in the aneurysmal sac and the wrinkled appearance of the aortic wall (arrow). This is characteristic of the syphilitic aortitis of tertiary syphilis. (Specimen from the Boyd Museum, University of Toronto.)

RHEUMATOID ARTERITIS

Rheumatoid aortitis, which is very similar to the aortitis of tertiary syphilis, is occasionally encountered in rheumatoid arthritis. It also leads to aortic insufficiency.

IDIOPATHIC INFLAMMATORY CONDITIONS

There are a number of diseases in which inflammation of the arterial wall leads to thrombosis.

Thromboangiitis Obliterans (Buerger's Disease). This disease occurs predominantly in young men and affects the arteries and veins of the legs. Thrombosis leads to ischemia and intermittent claudication; ultimately, gangrene of the toes sets in.

Giant-Cell Arteritis.   Giant-cell arteritis is a disease of elderly people. The affected artery shows thrombosis and a chronic inflammatory granulomatous reaction with many giant cells forming around disrupted elastic fibers. Since the disease commonly affects the temporal artery it is also called *temporal arteritis*. It is characterized by pain in the region of the artery and is important because it can affect the ophthalmic artery and lead to blindness.

Polyarteritis nodosa is described in Chapter 27.

DISEASES OF SMALL VESSELS

In consideration of vascular disease the capillaries and arterioles are usually forgotten. There are, nevertheless, many conditions in which so many vessels in an area are occluded that ischemia results. Because an additional effect is bleeding, petechial hemorrhages are a common feature of small vessel disease even though the extent of the occlusion is insufficient to lead to ischemia of the total area involved. Some causes of these diseases are briefly described below:

Frostbite.   The harmful effects of cold on exposed parts are due in large measure to small vessel damage. In mild cases there is an inflammatory reaction causing large blisters to form; if the damage is severe, the vessels become completely occluded by thrombus and gangrene occurs.

Occlusion of Capillaries by Red Cells.   This response occurs in severe sludging and is a component of shock.

Occlusion by Fibrin.   This occurs in disseminated intravascular coagulation (see Chapter 26). The kidney is the organ most affected.

Occlusion by Precipitated Cryoglobulins.   In cryoglobulinemia exposure of the extremities to cold leads to vascular occlusion and petechial hemorrhages.

Fat Embolism.   See Chapter 20.

Decompression Syndrome.   See Chapter 20.

External Pressure.   The best example of this is a bedsore. Continual pressure on one area produces such ischemia that necrosis of the skin and underlying tissues occurs. *It is a major duty of nurses to move nonambulatory patients often enough that no pressure sores develop.*

Occlusion by Antigen-Antibody Interaction.   This is a feature of such immune complex phenomena as the Arthus reaction (see Chapter 9).

Vasculitis.   The term vasculitis is used to describe an inflammatory reaction in the wall of small vessels. Typical lesions occur in the Arthus reaction; the immune complex deposition in the vessel wall causes damage associated with a marked polymorph infiltration and thrombosis (Fig. 29–6). This type of type III hypersensitivity is thought to occur in many drug reactions as well as in some infections. The petechial hemorrhages seen in the skin in septicemia (*e.g.*, gonococcal septicemia, see Fig. 10–2) and in infective endocarditis are explained on this basis. Internal organs are affected; the kidney appears to be the most vulnerable. In some examples of vasculitis no cause can be found. The disease then appears to be a component of polyarteritis nodosa (see Chapter 27).

PERIPHERAL VASCULAR DISEASE

"Peripheral vascular disease" is an inclusive term that is used to describe all those conditions in which the blood supply to the limbs is impaired. Usually it is the legs that suffer. The following diseases all play their part:

FIGURE 29–6.   *Acute gonococcal vasculitis.*

This section of dermis shows an arteriole that is obstructed by thrombus (Th). The vessel wall has undergone necrosis, and there is a heavy infiltration of polymorphs (Poly). The presence of many red cells (rbc) in the interstitial tissues indicates that the vessel has ruptured. This biopsy was taken from the patient shown in Figure 10–2.

FIGURE 29–7. *Types of aortic aneurysm.*

A, Shows two aneurysms. One is saccular and has arisen from the ascending aorta. It is filled with laminated thrombus. Fifty years ago this type of aneurysm invariably was due to tertiary syphilis, but today this form of the disease is so uncommon that atheroma is the usual cause. The abdominal aorta shows a fusiform aneurysm that is lined by thrombus. This type of aneurysm is usually due to atheroma and invariably affects the aorta below the origins of the renal arteries. B, Shows a dissecting aneurysm. It is thought to arise as a result of bleeding into the media of a weakened aortic wall. An intramural hematoma is formed, and this ruptures into the lumen of the aorta, usually in the ascending portion. Blood is then forced into the tear, and dissection occurs into the media. A false aneurysmal sac encases the aorta and can involve the entire length of the vessel as well as extending along some of its branches. Some branches are obstructed, and the effects of this account for the clinical signs and symptoms. Thus, in the aneurysm illustrated, the left femoral pulse would be weaker than the right and the ischemia of the right kidney has led to infarction. Dissecting aneurysm usually terminates by rupture of the external coat; bleeding into the pericardium, mediastinum, or retroperitoneal space causes death. Very occasionally the aneurysm ruptures internally into the aortic lumen, and the patient survives with no treatment. This accounts for the double-barreled aorta that is occasionally found as an unexpected necropsy finding. (Drawing by Margot Mackay, Department of Art as Applied to Medicine, University of Toronto.)

(1) ATHEROSCLEROSIS.   This tends to affect the large vessels such as the iliac and femoral arteries.

(2) THROMBOSIS.   This may be secondary to atherosclerosis.

(3) EMBOLISM.   Emboli may be large thromboemboli or small clumps of atheromatous material.

(4) SMALL VESSEL DISEASE.   Arteriolar sclerosis associated with hypertension and diabetic microangiopathy (see Chapter 24) are the most important.

Effects of Peripheral Diseases.   The effects are serious and disabling. The ischemia of the leg leads to atrophy of many structures, including the bones (osteoporosis) and the skin. Trivial injury can lead to chronic, persistent, and extremely painful ulceration. Ischemia of the muscle leads to pain on walking (intermittent claudication) and, ultimately, to pain at rest. Dry gangrene leading to loss of the limb is the all-too-frequent end-result.

Aneurysms

An *aneurysm* is a local dilatation of an artery or a chamber of the heart and is due to weakening of its walls. It may be saccular or fusiform (Fig. 29–7).

CAUSES OF ANEURYSMS

Weakening of the wall may be due to any of the following:

(1) CONGENITAL DEFICIENCY. A good example is a berry aneurysm of the circle of Willis (see Chapter 44).

(2) TRAUMA. Sometimes an injury can damage not only an artery but also an adjacent vein, thereby establishing a connection. This formation is termed an *arteriovenous aneurysm,* or fistula. It is important, because so much blood can be diverted from the peripheral tissues that heart failure ensues.

(3) INFLAMMATION. Syphilitic aortitis is a good example.

(4) DEGENERATION. Atheromatous degeneration is by far the most common cause of aortic aneurysm.

EFFECTS OF ANEURYSMS

An aneurysm can produce its effect in a number of ways:

(1) *Pressure.* An aneurysm of the thoracic aorta may press on the esophagus and cause difficulty in swallowing, or it may press on the recurrent laryngeal nerve and lead to changes of voice.

(2) *Thrombosis.* The sac and aneurysm soon become filled by laminated thrombus. This effect is due in part to damage of the endothelial lining, but it is mostly the result of local stasis and eddy-current formation.

(3) *Hemorrhage.* Rupture of an aneurysm leads to bleeding; for a while this can be quite trivial because of the plugging effect of the thrombus lining the sac. Nevertheless, when an aneurysm, such as one of the abdominal aorta, has begun to bleed, it is not long before massive hemorrhage follows and the patient dies of exsanguination.

(4) *Ischemia.* This is due to blockage of the branches of the artery at the site of the aneurysm, an effect produced either by local pressure or by thrombotic occlusion.

DISSECTING ANEURYSM OF THE AORTA

The basic defect in this condition is a degeneration of the media (medionecrosis), the cause of which is unknown. The pathogenesis is described in Figure 29–7. The condition is quite common and is usually heralded by the sudden onset of severe chest pain. As blood is forced into the wall of the aorta, there is blockage of the ostia of important branches. The consequences vary considerably from case to case. Thus, the coronary arteries may be occluded and myocardial infarction results. There is a varying degree of obstruction to the arteries supplying the upper limbs so that the pulses at the wrist are often either weak or unequal. Blockage of the renal arteries leads to infarction and anuria. The outer coat of the aneurysm usually ruptures, causing fatal hemorrhage into the pericardium, the mediastinum, the retroperitoneal space, or the peritoneal cavity.

DISEASES OF VEINS

Phlebothrombosis and its important complications of embolism and pulmonary infarction are described in Chapter 20. Inflammation of veins (phlebitis) is a common event in any inflammatory process. The overlying thrombosis that accompanies it is not important as a source of embolism, since the thrombus is firmly adherent to the wall of the damaged vessel. Only if the thrombus is invaded by pyogenic organisms is embolism a hazard. Under these circumstances emboli containing bacteria are thrown off and pyemia results (see Chapter 20).

VARICOSE VEINS

Elongation and irregular dilatation of veins is known as *varicosity*. It is generally assumed that persistent increase in pressure is a cause of this; esophageal varices can certainly be explained in this manner (see Chapter 33). Nevertheless, the common condition of varicose veins of the legs is not well understood. An inherited defect of the venous walls or valves has been postulated. There also seems to be a familial factor in the incidence of this common disease. Other suggested causes are standing for long periods over many years that is required in some occupations and the lack of support for the walls of the veins that is seen in fat people. Because pregnancy seems to initiate varicose vein formation, the disease is more common at an earlier age in women. Once varicose veins have formed, their valves become incompetent, so that on standing the full hydrostatic pressure of blood is applied to the vessel wall and further dilatation ensues. The extremely sluggish blood flow through the veins can predispose a person to thrombus formation, but embolism from this is extremely rare. The major effect of varicose veins is to produce venous stasis. The increased hydrostatic pressure leads to edema, and the skin exhibits *stasis dermatitis*. Trivial injuries lead to persistent ulcerations that characteristically overlie the medial malleoli. Even though these ulcers can enlarge, they are not painful. In this respect they contrast with the ulceration caused by arterial disease (ischemic ulcers).

Two particular circumstances under which venous thrombosis occurs are worthy of special note:

(1) *Thrombophlebitis Migrans.*   Migratory thrombophlebitis is described in Chapter 20.

(2) *Painful White Leg (Phlegmasia Alba Dolens).*   The painful white leg that is seen in pregnant women in the third trimester — or more often immediately following delivery — is due to ileofemoral venous thrombosis. It is thought that inflammation also involves lymphatics and that this contributes to the formation of such massive edema.

Review Questions

1. Describe the complications of atherosclerosis with particular reference to the changes encountered in the coronary arteries and in the aorta.
2. List the inflammatory lesions that may affect the following:
   (a) the aorta
   (b) medium-sized arteries
   (c) arterioles.
3. Describe briefly the diseases that may contribute to intermittent claudication.
4. Classify the causes of aneurysm formation.
5. Compare cutaneous stasis ulcers with ischemic ulcers with respect to these factors:
   (a) cause
   (b) site
   (c) symptoms.
6. Give examples of the relationship between lipid metabolism and the development of human atherosclerosis.

Selected Readings

Robbins, S. L.: Pathologic Basis of Disease. Philadelphia, W. B. Saunders Company, 1974. See Chapter 15, "Blood Vessels."

Ross, R., and Glomset, J. A.: The pathogenesis of atherosclerosis. New England Journal of Medicine, 295:369–377; 420–425, 1976.

Spaet, T. H.: Optimism in the control of atherosclerosis. New England Journal of Medicine, 291:576–577, 1974.

Chapter 30

After studying this chapter the student should be able to:

- Define respiratory failure.
- Compare the causes and effects of ventilatory failure with those of impaired alveolar–arterial gas exchange.
- Discuss the causes of dyspnea.
- Describe the causes and effects of bronchial obstruction.

DISEASES OF THE RESPIRATORY TRACT

- Give an account of the pathogenesis, clinical features, and the pathological findings of lobar pneumonia.
- Classify the causes of bronchopneumonia.
- Describe the causes of pulmonary edema.
- Define the term pneumoconiosis and give three examples of the condition.
- Give an account of chronic bronchitis.
- Define pulmonary emphysema as well as describe the lesions and effects of the destructive form of this disease.
- Compare bronchial asthma with cardiac asthma.
- Give an account of "adenoma" of the lung.
- Describe carcinoma of the lung with respect to the following factors:
    - (a) known causes
    - (b) gross appearances and types
    - (c) diagnosis
    - (d) histological types
    - (e) spread
- Distinguish between a transudate and an exudate with reference to hydrothorax.
- Describe the types and common causes of pleuritis.
- Define empyema and pneumothorax. Give at least one cause of each.

Normal Function

The function of the respiratory system is to enable gaseous exchange to occur between the blood and the atmosphere. The upper respiratory tract functions as an air conditioner for the lungs, the inspired air being filtered and humidified as it passes through the nose, nasopharynx, larynx, and trachea. Air eventually reaches the small air sacs, or alveoli, of the lung, where it comes into close contact with blood in the capillaries and where conditions for gaseous exchange are ideal (Fig. 30–1). Oxygen is added to the blood, and the carbon dioxide that is removed is exhaled. The gas in the alveoli is maintained at a fairly constant composition by the act of breathing, a process that has two components: *ventilation* and *distribution.*

VENTILATION.   This is the bellowslike action of the chest, by which fresh air is inspired and stale air is expired. The volume is approximately 7.5 liters per minute in the adult at rest.

DISTRIBUTION.   The inspired air is distributed in such a way in relation to

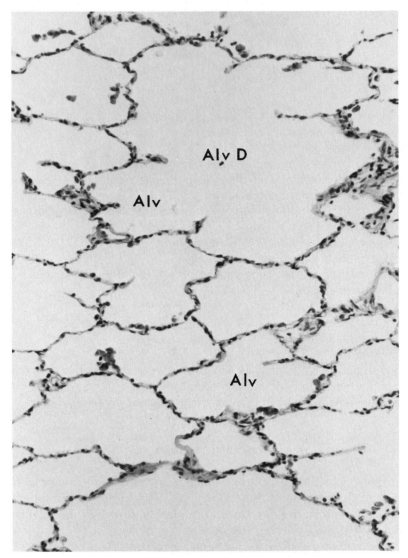

FIGURE 30–1. *Normal lung.*

This section shows a number of alveoli (Alv) and an alveolar duct (Alv D) from which some of them have arisen. Note how thin the alveolar walls are (× 60).

the volume of blood perfusing the lung that the composition of the alveolar gas is maintained at a constant level. Since the arterial blood, as it leaves the lung, is in equilibrium with the alveolar gas, it follows that the gaseous tensions of oxygen and carbon dioxide in the arterial blood are also maintained at this same constant level (Fig. 30–2).

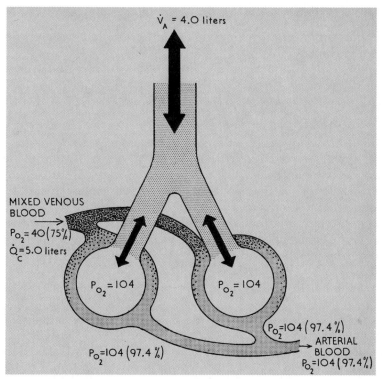

FIGURE 30–2. *Physiological relationships within lung.*

Diagrammatic representation of the lung, showing two alveoli with ideal $\dfrac{\text{Ventilation}}{\text{Blood Flow}}$ relationships. This relationship is generally written $\dfrac{\dot{V}_A}{\dot{Q}_C}$, the dot indicating that the volumes of alveolar ventilation (V_A) and capillary blood flow (Q_C) are in unit time. Thus, for the lung as a whole in a normal subject at rest:

$$\frac{\dot{V}_A}{\dot{Q}_C} = \frac{4 \text{ liters per minute}}{5 \text{ liters per minute}} = 0.8$$

In the diagram, the oxygen tensions are in mm Hg, and the figures in brackets are the percentage saturation of oxygen in the blood.

The partial pressure of a gas in a mixture is the contribution that the gas makes toward the total pressure. Thus, for moist air at sea level the total pressure is about 760 mm Hg. Water vapor contributes about 24 mm Hg, and the remaining 736 mm Hg is contributed by oxygen (20 per cent) and nitrogen (80 per cent) approximately. Hence, the partial pressure of oxygen (P_{O_2}) is 20 per cent of 736 mm Hg or about 147 mm Hg. As fresh air is drawn into the lungs, it mixes with expired gases. Under normal conditions the gas in the alveoli has an oxygen tension of about 100 mm Hg. (After Comroe, J. H., et al.: The Lung: Clinical Physiology and Pulmonary Function Tests. 2nd ed. Chicago, Year Book Medical Publishers, 1963.)

Respiratory Failure

If through dysfunction of the lungs there is oxygen lack or CO_2 retention, the condition is called *respiratory failure.* In the arterial blood under normal conditions, the partial pressure of oxygen, usually written PO_2, is about 100 mm Hg, and the partial pressure of carbon dioxide, written PCO_2, is about 40 mm Hg. In respiratory failure the PO_2 is under 60 mm Hg, and the PCO_2 is over 49 mm Hg.

Types of Respiratory Failure

Two main types can be recognized:

(1) *ventilatory failure,* which is due to an inadequate volume of inspired air available for exchange.

(2) *impaired alveolar-arterial gas exchange,* which is due to failure of distribution or diffusion.

VENTILATORY FAILURE (HYPOXIA WITH HYPERCAPNIA)

This condition is caused by the following factors:

(a) airway obstruction, which is usually due to chronic bronchitis, emphysema, or asthma—topics that are considered later in this chapter.

(b) restriction of thoracic movement such as that resulting from the presence of a pneumothorax or a large pleural effusion.

(c) neuromuscular impairment such as that found in infantile paralysis.

(d) disturbance of the brain, such as that due to injury or to overdose of a depressant drug (*e.g.,* a barbiturate).

Effects

Since

$$PCO_2 \text{ (arterial)} \propto \frac{CO_2 \text{ Production}}{\text{Alveolar Ventilation}}$$

and at rest the CO_2 production is constant, it follows that when alveolar ventilation is reduced, there is an increase in the arterial PCO_2 and an arithmetically equivalent decrease in PO_2. Thus, if the PCO_2 rises from 40 to 60 mm Hg, then the PO_2 falls from 100 to 80 mm Hg. A drop of this magnitude in the PO_2 does not greatly affect the amount of oxygen present in arterial blood, since hemoglobin has great affinity for oxygen. Desaturation of blood with subsequent cyanosis is a late event in ventilatory failure.

The main effect is a raised arterial PCO_2 *(hypercapnia),* and symptoms are related to this response. The pulse is rapid and the hands are moist and warm. The pupils are small and the blood pressure is raised. If there is severe CO_2 retention, then confusion, drowsiness, tremors, and coma may ensue. Carbon dioxide is a vasodilator, and severe CO_2 retention causes cerebral edema, which is the explanation of the nervous phenomena and can be detected clinically by the occurrence of papilledema. Finally, the plasma bicarbonate level is high and the patient has respiratory acidosis (see Chapter 19).

IMPAIRED ALVEOLAR-ARTERIAL GAS EXCHANGE (HYPOXIA WITHOUT HYPERCAPNIA)

In this type of failure there is a reduction of alveolar-capillary surface available for gas exchange. This reduction may occur as a result of lung destruction but more commonly it is due to an imbalance in the distribution of perfusion and ventilation. Frequently, these factors are combined; of the two, however, maldistribution is much more important, and it becomes prominent in all progressive lung disease.

Impaired alveolar-arterial gas exchange occurs in emphysema and severe chronic bronchitis, especially postoperatively, when there is mucous plugging of bronchi. It is a feature of pulmonary embolism.

Effects

Oxygen uptake is interfered with and the venous blood becomes more desaturated during exercise; increasing arterial desaturation also occurs. The patient develops central cyanosis.

Although impaired alveolar-arterial gas exchange leads to a severe interference with O_2 uptake, it interferes little with CO_2 elimination. In the distribution failure group some alveoli are underventilated relative to alveolar perfusion with blood. This situation is remedied by overventilation of the remaining lung. Overventilation serves to eliminate more CO_2 from the blood, but it cannot compensate for any unequal oxygen uptake, because it does not produce an appreciable increase above the normal level in the amount of oxygen taken up by the blood (Fig. 30–3).

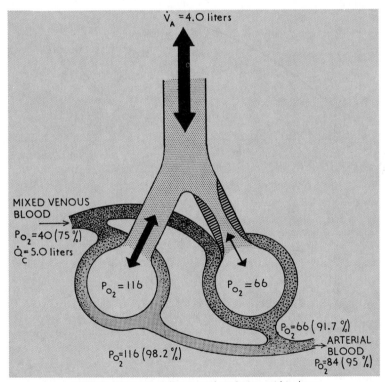

FIGURE 30–3. *Ventilation and perfusion within lung.*

Diagrammatic representation of the lung showing two alveoli that are unevenly ventilated but uniformly perfused. Note how the overventilation of one alveolus does not compensate for the underventilation of the other, with the result that some arterial desaturation occurs and the P_{O_2} is considerably reduced. (After Comroe, J. H., et al.: The Lung: Clinical Physiology and Pulmonary Function Tests. 2nd ed. Chicago, Year Book Medical Publishers, 1963.)

FIGURE 30–4. *Congestion of lung in heart failure.*

A small branch of the pulmonary artery (Art) is shown; the alveoli adjacent to it contain scattered red cells and many macrophages that are called "heart failure cells." Note that the alveolar walls are widened because of the presence of dilated capillaries. It is this congestion that makes the lung rigid and renders breathing more difficult. This rigidity accounts for the dyspnea of heart failure ($\times$ 250).

Dyspnea

In a healthy person, the rate and depth of respiration are so regulated that the individual is unaware of the movements involved in breathing. *Tachypnea* is an increased rate of respiration. Rapid, shallow breathing is seen when pain restricts respiratory movement, as in pleurisy or in increasing rigidity of the lungs, as in congestion (Fig. 30–4) or fibrosis. Tachypnea is sometimes accompanied by an increase in depth of breathing; the term *hyperpnea* includes both conditions. *Dyspnea* is a state in which the act of breathing causes distress. It occurs under two main circumstances:

(1) *when tachypnea or hyperpnea are excessive*

(2) *when the movement of the chest on inspiration is small in comparison with the muscular effort needed to produce it.* This occurs in any disease interfering with the respiratory excursions of the lung, such as fibrosis or congestion. Obstruction to the major air passages—whether due to pulmonary disease like chronic bronchitis or to strangulation—has a similar effect and produces intense dyspnea. Psychological factors also play a part. Thus, the sudden blockage of a tube through which a person is breathing can cause intense dyspnea. However, if the subject is asked to block the tube himself the maneuver causes no immediate discomfort.

Bronchial Obstruction

Causes. The common causes of bronchial obstruction are the following: (1) *tenacious mucus,* which is not expelled from the respiratory passages, as in asthma; (2) *chronic bronchitis;* (3) *inhaled foreign bodies,* such as roots of teeth, peas, and others; and (4) *tumors,* usually carcinoma.

Effects. The effects of obstruction depend on whether the obstruction is partial or complete.

PARTIAL OBSTRUCTION. The partial obstruction of a bronchus impedes the ventilation of the lung distal to the obstruction. It follows therefore that the blood perfusing that part of the lung is inadequately oxygenated, and that in effect a quantity of venous blood is shunted directly into the pulmonary veins and from there to the left side of the heart. Since the blood leaving the lungs is normally fully saturated with oxygen, it follows that no amount of overventilation of the unaffected lung can compensate for this shunt effect (Fig. 30–3). The arterial PO_2 is therefore lowered *(hypoxemia).* A very important example of partial obstruction of the bronchi occurs in chronic bronchitis, especially after a surgical operation requiring general anesthesia.

Widespread partial bronchial obstruction leads to overinflation of the lungs in asthma (see Fig. 30–12).

Infection commonly follows persistent bronchial obstruction. Organisms that are inhaled into the affected lung segment become trapped in the mucus, their expulsion is impaired, and bronchopneumonia follows. The infection also involves the bronchial walls; chronic infection will destroy the muscular and cartilaginous components of the walls, so that they are weakened and dilatation ensues *(bronchiectasis).* This effect is frequently seen distal to the obstruction caused by a carcinoma or a foreign body. Quite often, bronchiectasis occurs in several parts of the lung as an idiopathic condition; it might be the result of obstruction by mucus during some previous infection, such as measles or whooping cough. This type of bronchiectasis causes a chronic cough with expectoration of sputum. Recurrent attacks of pneumonia are common, and progressive lung destruction follows. Bronchiectasis is a common cause of hemoptysis, but if it is localized to one segment of the lung—particularly in an adult—the possibility of an underlying carcinoma must always be considered.

COMPLETE OBSTRUCTION. Where there is complete obstruction of a large bronchus, the lung distal to it shows a progressive absorption of its gas content

FIGURE 30–5. *Lobar pneumonia.*

The lower lobe is completely consolidated, whereas the upper lobe is unaffected. Note the sharp division between the two lobes. (R30.2, Reproduced by permission of the President and Council of the Royal College of Surgeons of England.)

until it becomes completely airless or collapses (*i.e.,* a *collapsed* lung). A plug of mucus sometimes causes this postoperative complication. Physical therapists can help to prevent this by encouraging the patient to breathe deeply and bring up sputum.

Pneumonia

Pneumonia is defined as "an inflammation in the alveolar parenchyma of the lung." Exudate usually fills the alveoli, which are thereby rendered airless and solid. This called *consolidation.* Sometimes, however, the inflammatory exudate is restricted to the alveolar wall. This is often called *interstitial pneumonia,* but *pneumonitis* is a term also used. Two main types of pneumonia (described below) are recognized; they are differentiated on the basis of the gross appearance of the lesions that result.

LOBAR PNEUMONIA

Healthy individuals are often affected by this disease, but an underlying debilitating disease, particularly chronic alcoholism, predisposes one to it. The infecting organism is invariably a highly virulent pneumococcus that is acquired by inhalation from another victim or a convalescent carrier. The disease has a sudden onset and is accompanied by rigors, fever, and pain in the chest. The organisms that reach the lung produce a rapidly spreading inflammatory edema that soon implicates a whole lobe or, at times, several lobes (Fig. 30–5).

Pathogenesis. The fact that infection spreads so rapidly in a gigantic wave of edematous exudate suggests that allergy is involved in the process. Perhaps the patient has already had a minor pneumococcal infection sufficient to produce an immune response. When now attacked a second time, the patient experiences a hypersensitivity reaction that accompanies the inflammatory response and renders it more intense. An alternative explanation is that lobar pneumonia is a primary infection. When the organisms reach the lungs, they pass on rapidly to the blood stream, proliferate in the reticuloendothelial system, and then escape into the blood to produce a septicemia. When they reach the lungs again, an allergic response occurs because of their interaction with recently formed local antibodies. This mechanism would be analogous to that described in typhoid fever and in syphilis.

Whatever the mechanism, there is no doubt that during the initial stage of the disease there is a septicemia. Sometimes the pneumococci may become localized not only in the lungs but also in the meninges, peritoneum, joints, and elsewhere. During the first few days of illness the patient is desperately ill and may die; the lobe of lung affected is *congested* and shows *inflammatory edema*. It is teeming with pneumococci.

In the next stage the lung shows complete consolidation and has a solid appearance that has been likened to a liver. Hence, it is sometimes called *hepatization*. The alveoli are filled with typical inflammatory exudate, with fibrin and polymorphs abounding.

The last stage of the disease is that of *resolution*. Macrophages replace the polymorphs, the inflammatory exudate is removed, and the lung returns to normal. This is an excellent example of complete resolution following acute inflammation.

During the acute stage of lobar pneumonia the overlying pleura shows acute inflammation *(pleurisy)* and is covered with a fibrinous exudate. This exudate is responsible for the creaking *pleural rub*, which may be heard with a stethoscope, and for the severe pain that occurs on inspiration.

Clinical Course. Following the acute onset, the patient remains seriously ill for 7 to 10 days with high fever. Death may occur during this stage. As suddenly as the disease started, it terminates. Sweating occurs, the temperature drops, and there is a sense of well-being. This is termed the *crisis*. In practice these stages are rarely seen today, since antibiotics rapidly terminate the course of the disease.

Complications. Lung abscess, pulmonary fibrosis, and empyema may occur but are uncommon, even in the untreated patient.

BRONCHOPNEUMONIA

In bronchopneumonia, unlike lobar pneumonia, there are discrete foci of inflammation around terminal bronchioles. Patches of consolidation are scattered throughout several lobes of the lung, and the condition is usually bilat-

FIGURE 30–6. *Staphylococcal bronchopneumonia.*

There are many discrete foci of consolidation scattered throughout the lung. Compare this with Figure 30–5, which shows lobar pneumonia. (R29.3, Reproduced by permission of the President and Council of the Royal College of Surgeons of England.)

eral (Fig. 30–6). The wildfire spread seen in lobar pneumonia is not present. There are many varieties of bronchopneumonia. They are best considered under two headings:

ENDOGENOUS BRONCHOPNEUMONIA.   The organisms are derived from the normal flora of the upper respiratory tract.

EXOGENOUS BRONCHOPNEUMONIA.   The organisms are derived from the exterior.

ENDOGENOUS BRONCHOPNEUMONIA

This type of bronchopneumonia is due to infection by commensal organisms normally resident in the upper respiratory passages. Of these organisms, the commensal pneumococci of low-grade virulence are by far the most important. *They cause infection whenever the defense mechanisms of the host are impaired.* The antagonists are therefore a weakly virulent endogenous organism and an enfeebled host. This situation contrasts sharply with lobar pneumonia, in which the contending parties are a highly virulent organism and a relatively healthy host.

Causes

The conditions leading to endogenous bronchopneumonia may be considered under two headings:

GENERAL FACTORS

Extremes of Age.   Bronchopneumonia is commonest in infancy and old age.

General Debilitating Illness. It is a common terminal event in cancer, cerebrovascular accidents, and uremia.

Impaired Immune Response. It may occur with agammaglobulinemia, agranulocytosis, and as a complication of glucocorticoid therapy.

LOCAL FACTORS. Any local condition interfering with ciliary action and the upward movement of mucus is liable to be followed by bronchopneumonia. Possible causes are listed below:

Pre-existing Acute Respiratory Disease. Bronchopneumonia often complicates influenza, measles, and whooping cough. In these infections the ciliated bronchial epithelium is shed, and organisms that gain access to the lung cannot be removed.

Local Obstruction. The trapped secretions form an admirable medium for bacterial growth, and bronchopneumonia is localized to the segment distal to the obstruction. Foreign bodies and tumors of the bronchi are well-known examples.

Chronic Bronchitis and Bronchiectasis. These are important predisposing causes of bronchopneumonia. Two factors are involved. First, the ciliated epithelium may be replaced by goblet cells or squamous cells, thereby impeding the upward flow of mucus. Second, the mucus itself is often of viscid consistency, and it cannot easily be removed. An excessive secretion of mucus accompanies the chronic venous congestion of heart failure because of the additional fluid contributed by transudation.

Pulmonary Edema. In edematous lung tissue the alveolar macrophages are unable to perform their normal protective function. Bronchopneumonia is a common terminal event in congestive heart failure and indeed is a common sequel to edema from whatever cause. The basal edema that occurs in debilitated, bedridden patients, in those who are unconscious, and in those who have just undergone surgery often progresses to pneumonia; this is called *hypostatic pneumonia.* Good nursing and physical therapy can do much to prevent this complication.

Bronchopneumonia is of much longer duration than lobar pneumonia. If the primary condition is incurable, the pneumonia is merely a welcome terminal event, and obviously little attempt is made at healing. Even in the childhood bronchopneumonias that follow measles and whooping cough, a prolonged course is the rule. The course of the disease is often punctuated by relapses and remissions, depending upon whether the organism or the host is gaining the upper hand. Both the onset and the termination of the disease are gradual.

Lesions of Bronchopneumonia

The disease is usually basal, posterior in distribution, and bilateral. If an area of bronchopneumonia is examined microscopically, it is found to consist of acutely inflamed bronchioles full of pus (Fig. 30–7). Some of the surrounding alveoli contain edema fluid in which there are macrophages and polymorphs, whereas others contain a dense, fibrinous exudate in which there are innumerable polymorphs. Some are collapsed as the result of the absorption of air distal to the blocked bronchioles, whereas neighboring alveoli are empty and distended because of compensatory dilatation. In contrast to lobar pneumonia, in which all alveoli in a lobe are at about the same stage of the inflammatory process, in bronchopneumonia there is a very varied picture.

FIGURE 30–7. *Bronchopneumonia.*

Part of a terminal bronchiole (Term Br) is shown with its lining of ciliated columnar epithelium. The bronchiole contains a mass of inflammatory cells, the majority of which are polymorphs. Alveoli (Alv) adjacent to the bronchiole also contain inflammatory exudate with polymorphs and fibrin. An alveolus further away from the bronchiole merely contains edema fluid.

Sequelae of Bronchopneumonia

RESOLUTION.   This is much less frequent than in lobar pneumonia.

PROGRESSIVE FIBROSIS OF THE LUNG.   This is correspondingly more frequent. The fibrosis is due to organization of the inflammatory exudate in the alveoli. In addition, there is often a continuance of the inflammatory process, so that more and more lung tissue is destroyed and converted into fibrous tissue. This is, of course, the condition of chronic inflammation, and bronchopneumonia often becomes chronic. In due course the infection spreads, and the muscle and elastic tissue of the adjacent bronchi are destroyed and replaced by granulation tissue. Consequently there is widening of the lumina, and eventually the dilatation becomes extensive. This is the pathogenesis of *bronchiectasis*, which is both a sequel of bronchopneumonia and a predisposing cause of further attacks (Fig. 30–8).

SUPPURATION.   Abscess formation is not uncommon, particularly when the host's resistance is exceptionally poor and the causal organism is *Staphylococcus aureus*.

EXOGENOUS BRONCHOPNEUMONIA

When inhaled a variety of virulent organisms may lead to severe bronchopneumonia. The host may be either healthy or enfeebled as a result of a previous disease. Examples of virulent organisms causing exogenous bronchopneumonia are listed below:

Staphylococcus aureus. The bronchopneumonia may come as a result of hospital cross-infection.

Streptococcus pyogenes. Bronchopneumonia from this source was particularly common in the 1918 influenza pandemic.

Mycobacterium tuberculosis and the deep-seated fungus diseases. This type of disease is quite distinct, since the lesions produced are characteristically chronic. They are described in Chapter 10.

Mycoplasma pneumoniae. See Chapter 11.

Viruses. Many types of viruses can cause pneumonia, *e.g.,* Coxsackie viruses, ECHO viruses, and myxoviruses (see Chapter 12). The histology of this group of pneumonias is poorly defined, since death from the uncomplicated disease is rare. There is usually a lymphocytic and macrophagic infiltrate in the alveolar walls so that the lesion may be described as an *interstitial pneumonia.* There is a variable amount of exudate in the alveoli themselves, and the fibrin component often becomes compressed against the alveolar walls as an eosinophilic lining, or *hyaline membrane.*

Pulmonary Edema

The systolic pressure in the pulmonary artery is 15 to 25 mm Hg; being much lower than that in the systemic vessels, it follows that there is less ten-

FIGURE 30–8. *Bronchiectasis with chronic lung infection.*

Since the age of 7 years, this patient had had repeated attacks of pneumonia. When he was 24 years of age, a diagnosis of cystic fibrosis of the pancreas was made. He was treated with vitamins and pancreatic enzymes by mouth but continued to be plagued by repeated lung infections. The terminal event was an overwhelming infection with *Pseudomonas pyocyanea.* The patient died at the age of 32 years. This specimen shows the effects of repeated bronchopneumonia. Toward the base of the lung there are several areas of bronchopneumonia (Bp), and the discrete areas of consolidation have fused together to become confluent. Nevertheless, the appearances are not those of lobar pneumonia. In another area the pneumonia has progressed to abscess formation (Ab). Toward the upper part of the lung there is tremendous dilatation of bronchi, and the upper lobe shows the typical appearances of advanced bronchiectasis (Bronch). Much of the intervening lung tissue has been destroyed.

dency to edema formation (see Fig. 5–1). The osmotic effect of the plasma proteins is relatively unopposed. Nevertheless, when edema does occur, two factors tend to ensure that it persists and even spreads:

(1) The loose nature of the lung prevents any immediate appreciable rise in tissue tension, a fact that in most tissues limits the extent of edema formation.

(2) When the lungs have become edematous, ventilation ceases, the vessel walls become hypoxic, and their permeability to protein increases. It follows that in all examples of pulmonary edema, the fluid has a high protein content. Therefore, it is not possible to distinguish between transudates and exudates, as in other tissues.

CAUSES OF PULMONARY EDEMA

ACUTE INFLAMMATION.   Edema occurs in the early stages of pneumonia; it is particularly marked in acute lobar pneumonia. It was a prominent feature in the bronchopneumonia that complicated the influenza of the 1918 pandemic. The lungs were described as showing acute hemorrhagic edema rather than bronchopneumonia of the classical type. Such a picture is also encountered in poisoning with certain gases, e.g., phosgene, chlorine, and nitrogen peroxide. Acute pulmonary edema also follows the inhalation of gastric juice such as may occur if a patient vomits during the inexpert administration of a general anesthetic.

HEART FAILURE.   Acute pulmonary edema is a frequent complication of left ventricular failure and mitral stenosis. Although increased pulmonary venous pressure is the usual explanation offered for this complication, it is unlikely that this is the major cause of pulmonary edema in heart failure. More important is the effect of a *redistribution of the blood volume;* attacks of acute pulmonary edema (*cardiac asthma*) occur quite suddenly (sometimes at night), and they are probably initiated by peripheral vasoconstriction. The amount of blood in the peripheral circulation is thus diminished, and the excess volume is displaced into the pulmonary circulation in which it appears as edema fluid. Support for this contention is the observation that acute pulmonary edema is a well-known hazard of epinephrine administration. This drug causes peripheral vasoconstriction. It must never be given to patients with acute pulmonary edema of cardiac origin. In bronchial asthma this drug is beneficial, but in cardiac asthma it can be lethal.

The terms *cardiac asthma* and *paroxysmal nocturnal dyspnea* are often applied to these attacks of acute pulmonary edema. The patient wakes up gasping for breath, with a sense of oppression in the chest. He sits up, but the dyspnea increases. Mounting restlessness drives him out of bed to seek the fresh air at the window. The sense of suffocation becomes intense, and with it there is profound distress. The skin has an ashen color because of the vasoconstriction combined with cyanosis, and there is also profuse sweating. The patient may cough up copious blood-stained sputum owing to a rapidly spreading pulmonary edema. In severe cases death ensues.

OVERLOADING THE CIRCULATION.   If an excessive volume of fluid is administered intravenously, some of the excess is accommodated in the great veins, but the remainder is diverted to the pulmonary circulation and leads to edema formation. It is obvious that patients already undergoing heart failure are particularly prone to this complication (see Chapter 26).

CEREBRAL DAMAGE. Acute pulmonary edema sometimes complicates damage to the brain, *e.g.*, trauma or cerebral hemorrhage. The most likely explanation is that increased sympathetic nervous impulses from the brain lead to peripheral vasoconstriction and cause diversion of the circulating fluid to the lungs as described above.

The Pneumoconioses

This group of diseases, produced by the *inhalation of dust*, is mostly occupational in origin. The most important condition is *silicosis*, which occurs in miners and in those whose work entails exposure to silica dust. Following the inhalation of this dust, a chronic inflammatory condition develops and eventually leads to marked fibrosis. Numerous *silicotic nodules* of dense fibrous tissue are formed that are readily demonstrable on a radiograph (Fig. 30–9). Silicosis predisposes one to pulmonary tuberculosis.

Asbestosis is another important pneumoconiosis. It affects workers who fabricate asbestos fibers; it does not affect the miners who quarry it. Asbestosis is important in predisposing the patient to cancer of the lung and to mesothelioma of the pleura.

FIGURE 30–9. *Silicosis.*

This radiograph shows numerous dense silicotic nodules scattered throughout the lung fields. Since there is a tendency to spare the bases of the lung, in this respect silicosis resembles the other pneumoconioses. Asbestosis is the only exception to this rule, because the large heavy asbestos fibers tend to gravitate to the bases of the lungs. (Courtesy of Dr. D. E. Sanders.)

Anthracosis, which is due to the inhalation of carbon, is the most common of the dust diseases, because to some extent it affects all city dwellers. The disease often severely affects coal miners, but since carbon induces little inflammatory reaction or fibrosis, the miners experience no ill-effects unless there is coexistent silicosis.

Chronic Bronchitis, Emphysema, and Bronchial Asthma

In the past, chronic bronchitis, pulmonary emphysema, and bronchial asthma have often been grouped together as *chronic nonspecific lung disease* or *chronic obstructive pulmonary disease*, since they are frequently diagnosed together and have many clinical and pathological features in common. Nevertheless, these conditions are often found separately. Since the origin of these diseases is poorly understood, it is advisable to consider each of them as a separate entity rather than to try to group them under one heading.

CHRONIC BRONCHITIS

Definition and Lesions.   Chronic bronchitis is best defined as a condition in which there is a chronic or recurrent increase in the volume of bronchial mucus—that is, enough to cause expectoration—and which is not due to localized bronchopulmonary disease. It is much commoner in tobacco smokers than in nonsmokers, and it is very prevalent in England, although less so in North America. The bronchial mucosa is thickened by hyperplasia of the mucous glands, and there is an increase in the number of goblet cells in the lining epithelium. True chronic inflammation is not a feature of this disease; consequently, Laennec's "bronchial catarrh" would be a more suitable name.

Recurrent inflammation is a common complication and may be due to infection or the effects of irritant chemicals—smog is particularly dangerous in this respect.

Effects.   Shortness of breath, dyspnea, and a chronic cough with expectoration are the outstanding clinical features. Symptoms tend to be worse during the winter, and severe attacks can be precipitated by a respiratory viral infection such as influenza or a common cold. The sputum is clear and mucoid in the early stages but becomes purulent during exacerbations.

The thickened mucosa leads to impaired ventilation of the lungs. CO_2 retention therefore occurs (see "Ventilatory Failure"). During attacks, bronchial spasm contributes to the bronchial narrowing, and combined with mucus, impedes uniform ventilation. Thus, arterial desaturation and cyanosis are added to the hypercapnia.

Polycythemia and *right heart failure* ensue. The patients, typically short and fat, are cyanosed and dyspneic. Since heart failure causes venous congestion and edema, they have aptly been described as "blue and bloated."

Patients with chronic bronchitis, having a raised arterial P_{CO_2} and lowered P_{O_2}, often tolerate these abnormal blood gas tensions remarkably well, and any sudden change can lead to serious consequences. Thus, if the hypoxemia (low P_{O_2}) is relieved by oxygen therapy, ventilation can become so depressed that CO_2 retention with coma ensues. Alternatively, vigorous artificial ventilation can relieve the hypercapnia to the extent that the low arterial P_{CO_2} causes vaso-constriction and cerebral ischemia.

The administration of general anesthetics to chronic bronchitics is particularly hazardous, since any further increase in mucus production or spasm of the bronchi is liable to precipitate respiratory failure.

Course.   The course of chronic bronchitis is a fluctuating one with recurrent acute episodes of infection, respiratory failure, and heart failure. Treatment can tide the patient over these exacerbations of the illness, but the single most important aspect of therapy is to *stop the patient from smoking tobacco.*

FIGURE 30–10. *Pulmonary emphysema.*

This thin section of a whole lung shows severe destructive emphysema. The lesions are so severe in the upper parts of the lung that light can be transmitted through the slice where there are bullae. (From Heard, B. E.: Pathology of Chronic Bronchitis and Emphysema. London, Churchill Livingstone, 1969. Reproduced by permission.)

FIGURE 30–11. *Pulmonary emphysema.*

Higher magnification of the center of the upper lobe of the specimen shown in Figure 30–10. Note the tremendous destruction of alveolar tissue. (From Heard, B. E.: Pathology of Chronic Bronchitis and Emphysema. London, Churchill Livingstone, 1969. Reproduced by permission.)

PULMONARY EMPHYSEMA

Definition. The word "emphysema," introduced by Laennec, is derived from the Greek, meaning an "inflation." It is defined as a condition in which there is an increase beyond the normal in the size of the terminal air passages. Two distinct types, which are described below, occur:

Dilatatory Emphysema. Emphysema due to dilatation of the air passages occurs as a compensatory phenomenon following the removal, collapse, or destruction of the adjacent lung. It is of no importance as a cause of respiratory failure.

Destructive Emphysema. This is of great clinical importance; the unqualified term "emphysema" is generally taken to mean this condition. There is destruction of the alveoli in the walls of the terminal air passages, which are therefore widened (Figs. 30–10 and 30–11). Sometimes large air-filled sacs, or *bullae*, are formed, and little lung parenchyma remains.

Effects. The effect of this lung destruction is to impair gaseous exchange. CO_2 can escape more easily than O_2 can be taken up. Nevertheless, hyperventilation (with dyspnea) is so marked that at rest the arterial P_{O_2} is maintained at a sufficiently high level to prevent cyanosis. The patients may be described as "pink and puffing." With exercise, the arterial P_{O_2} falls and cyanosis develops. CO_2 retention is not a feature.

Course.   The course of pulmonary emphysema is slow and unrelenting as more and more lung tissue is destroyed.

BRONCHIAL ASTHMA

Asthma may be defined as a condition of extensive narrowing of the bronchial airways; it *changes in severity over short periods of time* either spontaneously or under treatment and is not due to cardiovascular disease. It is characterized by *paroxysms of wheezing dyspnea.* The bronchial obstruction is caused partly by spasm of the bronchial muscle and partly by the presence of viscid mucus (Fig. 30–12). The disease often has a hereditary basis and is one of the manifestations of atopy. Its pathogenesis is complex: attacks may be the result of hypersensitivity to some inhaled antigen, but they may also be aggravated by psychological and other factors.

Pulmonary Tumors

The vast majority of lung tumors are epithelial in origin.

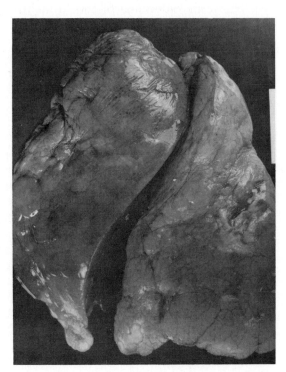

FIGURE 30–12.   *Bronchial asthma.*

This specimen is from a 28-year-old woman who had had a long history of bronchial asthma. She had an acute attack that became progressively more severe as dyspnea developed. She became cyanosed and finally unconscious. Despite vigorous resuscitation attempts she had a cardiac arrest and died 9 hours after the onset of the attack. The specimen shows the lung to be greatly overinflated. This is because bronchi are plugged with thick, tenacious mucus. In life this allows some air to enter the lung because on inspiration the bronchi dilate. However, the patient cannot expel air so easily, and the lungs become overinflated.

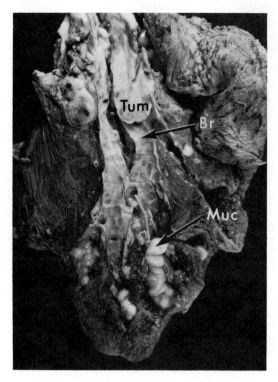

FIGURE 30–13.   *Carcinoid tumor of bronchus.*

This patient developed a patch of broncho-pneumonia that did not clear completely with chemotherapy. Bronchoscopy revealed a tumor obstructing a bronchus in the lower lobe. Biopsy showed that it was a carcinoid type of tumor. A lobectomy was performed, and the patient made a satisfactory recovery. The specimen shows the tumor (Tum), which is growing into and obstruct-ing a bronchus (Br). Distal to the tumor the bron-chus is widely dilated and contains thick muco-purulent material (Muc). Bronchiectasis distal to an obstructing tumor is characteristic.

ADENOMA

The term "adenoma of the bronchus" has been used to describe several distinct tumors. The commonest is the carcinoid tumor that arises in the wall of a large bronchus and causes partial – finally complete – obstruction. Distal *bronchopneumonia* and *bronchiectasis,* often with hemoptysis, are frequent (Fig. 30–13). The tumor is of the intermediate type; it invades locally but does not commonly metastasize. Hence, lobectomy or pneumonectomy is usually curative.

CARCINOMA

Cancer of the lung now ranks as the commonest lethal cancer in males, and it is also prevalent in females. Cigarette smoking is a major cause. Atmospheric pollution and asbestosis are other etiological factors.

Gross Appearance.   Two common types of tumor may be recognized:

Peripheral lung cancers.   These tumors presumably arise in one of the small bronchi or bronchioles and appear as fairly discrete tumor masses in the lung parenchyma. Symptoms are often absent until the pleura and chest wall are invaded, or until distant metastases appear.

Central lung cancers.   These tumors arise in one of the major bronchi and therefore cause early obstruction with resulting collapse, bronchopneu-monia, and bronchiectasis (Fig. 30–14). Frequently, the patient presents with fever and symptoms of pneumonia. Hemoptysis is common, the bleeding being either from the ulcerated tumor itself or – more often – from the inflamed dilated bronchi beyond.

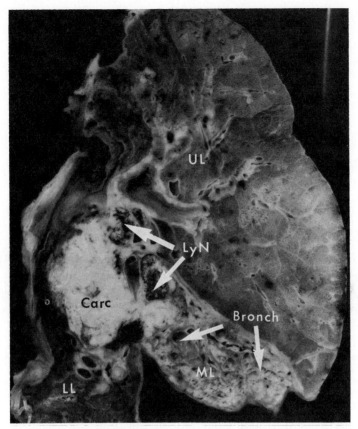

FIGURE 30–14. *Carcinoma of the lung.*

This section through lung shows a large carcinomatous mass (Carc) in which an obstructed bronchus is embedded. The main effect of this is seen in the middle lobe (ML) where much of the lung substance has been destroyed and replaced by fibrous tissue. Bronchiectasis (Bronch) is well developed. Tumor is seen to be extending into the lower lobe (LL), but the upper lobe (UL) is unaffected. Several hilar lymph nodes (Ly N) are invaded by growth and have fused with the tumor to form one large mass. The black material in the lymph nodes is carbon. This degree of anthracosis is common in city dwellers.

Diagnosis. *Hemoptysis, recurrent or "unresolved" pneumonia, or a persistent shadow on the radiograph should always lead to thorough investigation, particularly if the patient is a smoker* (Fig. 30–15). *Sputum examination* may reveal malignant cells. The tumor may be seen and biopsied at the time of *bronchoscopy.* Even if the tumor is beyond the range of the bronchoscope, mucus or pus may be aspirated from individual bronchi. The finding of malignant cells in a specimen will then localize the tumor. *Mediastinoscopy* is a useful procedure in which the mediastinum is examined with an instrument that is inserted through a small incision in the neck. Enlarged lymph nodes may be detected and biopsied. This investigation also gives the surgeon an indication of whether the tumor is operable. If these investigations are negative, thoracotomy and direct biopsy may be necessary, since a policy of "wait and see" is rarely justifiable.

Spread. Lung cancer spreads by all the classic routes:

LOCAL SPREAD. This can involve lung parenchyma, pleura, bronchi, arteries, and veins.

FIGURE 30–15. *Carcinoma of the lung.*

This radiograph shows a hilar mass (arrow) that is produced by the tumor. The linear shadow extending outward toward the chest wall is due to secondary changes — namely, collapse, infection, and bronchiectasis. This portion of the lung might well appear like the middle lobe in Figure 30–14. (Courtesy of Dr. D. E. Sanders.)

LYMPHATIC SPREAD.   The hilar and mediastinal nodes can be involved. This usually occurs early and is most marked with the oat-cell tumors. Supraclavicular and other lymph nodes are involved as the disease progresses.

BLOOD-BORNE METASTASES.   Secondary tumors are common in the *liver, bones, adrenals,* and *brain.* Even the spleen and bowel (organs not commonly the site of metastases from other tumors) may be involved. It is the frequency of distant spread that makes the prognosis so poor.

Histological Types.   Although arising from a mucus-secreting epithelium, cancers of the lung are remarkable for their histological variations.

SQUAMOUS-CELL CARCINOMA.   Microscopically this resembles squamous-cell carcinoma arising elsewhere, except that well-differentiated examples are not common. The tumors arise either in areas of squamous metaplasia or in an adenocarcinoma by tumor metaplasia; the latter explanation is the more likely. These tumors may be either central or peripheral, and they have the most favorable prognosis.

ADENOCARCINOMA.   These tumors are almost always peripheral and tend to be more frequent in females. Areas of squamous metaplasia are common.

ANAPLASTIC CARCINOMA.   These tumors show little or no differentiation; two variants are recognized.

Large-cell Tumors.   These are most probably tumors at the anaplastic end of the scale of squamous-cell carcinoma or adenocarcinoma.

Small-cell, or Oat-cell, Carcinoma.   Oat-cell carcinoma of the lung appears to be a distinct tumor, which is probably derived from neurosecretory cells of the bronchial mucosa that are akin to the argentaffin cells of the intestine. In this respect it shares a common origin with the carcinoid tumor. The tumor is composed of small, darkly staining cells, which may form small rosettes and may be round or oat-shaped (Fig. 30–16). Frequently the tumors are large, and their origin is difficult to determine. They metastasize early and widely. An enormous mediastinal mass may be produced that can impede the heart's action by directly invading the pericardium and myocardium and by compressing the great vessels. Although the tumors are very radiosensitive, the prognosis is extremely bad.

The Pleura

The pleural cavities are normally potential spaces situated between the visceral and parietal pleura, each lined by flattened mesothelial cells. An accumulation of fluid in the pleural space is termed a *hydrothorax,* or *pleural effusion.* There are two types, which are described as follows:

A TRANSUDATE.   The fluid has a low protein content and few cells. The most common causes are congestive heart failure and the nephrotic syndrome.

AN EXUDATE.   An exudate is formed as a result of inflammation or neoplasia involving the pleura. The protein content approximates that of plasma; inflammatory or neoplastic cells are present in the fluid.

PLEURISY

Inflammation of the pleura (pleurisy or pleuritis) is usually secondary to underlying inflammatory or neoplastic lung disease. This may be apparent as in

FIGURE   30–16.   *Oat-cell carcinoma of lung.*

The constituent cells are small, fusiform in shape, and have prominent darkly staining nuclei. Their shape has given rise to the descriptive term "oat cell" (× 500).

FIGURE 30–17. *Empyema and chronic lung abscess.*

This section of lung shows the meeting point between the upper lobe (UL), the middle lobe (ML), and the lower lobe (LL). The lower lobe shows a chronic lung abscess (Ab) and infection has evidently spread through the pleura to involve the pleural cavity. The space (Emp) was filled with pus, and this lesion is therefore a localized form of empyema.

acute lobar pneumonia or in a large area of infarction, or it may be inapparent, as in the pleurisy that accompanies a small tuberculous lesion. Occasionally, the cause of pleurisy is to be found below the diaphragm, *e.g.*, a subphrenic abscess.

 Fibrinous Pleurisy. "Dry pleurisy" is associated with an audible friction rub and can be extremely painful, particularly when the affected person takes a deep breath. Organization of the exudate leads to the formation of fibrous pleural adhesions.

 Serous or Serofibrinous Pleurisy. "Pleurisy with effusion" can lead to the accumulation of so much fluid that the affected lung is collapsed. Persistent pleural effusion should always be adequately investigated. Fluid can be withdrawn through a needle and sent for bacteriological and cytological examination. Tuberculosis and carcinoma (primary or metastatic) are two causes that must be considered.

EMPYEMA

 The presence of pus in the pleural cavity is termed an "empyema." It is generally formed as an extension of infection from a contiguous structure, *e.g.*, a lung abscess or subphrenic abscess (Fig. 30–17).

PNEUMOTHORAX

 The presence of air in the pleural cavity is termed a "pneumothorax." It may arise suddenly in an apparently healthy person (spontaneous pneumothorax), and it is usually due to rupture of a small subpleural emphysematous bulla. The onset is sudden, with severe pain in one side of the chest. Dyspnea and cyanosis follow, and their severity depends on the amount of air that escapes into the pleural cavity. The condition tends to recur.

PLEURAL TUMORS

The only common primary malignant tumor of the pleura is the mesothelioma. This tumor, which is related to asbestosis, forms an encasing mass around the lung.

Metastatic tumors, particularly from carcinoma of the breast and lung, are frequent in the pleural cavity.

Review Questions

1. Compare the pathogenesis and lesions of lobar pneumonia with those of a bronchopneumonia due to a pneumococcus of low virulence.
2. Give an account of the causes and pathogenesis of bronchiectasis.
3. Explain why patients with chronic bronchitis may develop respiratory failure after being administered a general anesthetic.
4. Describe the lung lesions in which the inhalation of asbestos fibers is believed to be an etiological factor.
5. Following a surgical operation performed under general anesthesia, a patient's radiograph shows areas of abnormal density that were not present before the procedure. Discuss the possible nature of these lesions.
6. A 56-year-old man states that he has coughed up blood-stained sputum on several occasions during the past four weeks. Indicate the investigations that are required to arrive at a diagnosis.
7. Describe the possible effects of a head injury on the lungs and on respiratory function.
8. Describe the signs and symptoms that would indicate a person might have cancer of the lung.
9. What lung lesions could cause an acute pain in the chest?

Selected Readings

Ashley, D. J., and Davies, H. D.: Cancer of the lung. Histology and biological behavior. Cancer, 20:165–174, 1967.

Comroe, J. H., Jr., et al.: The Lung: Clinical Physiology and Pulmonary Function Tests. 2nd ed. Chicago, Year Book Medical Publishers, Inc., 1962.

Fritts, H. W., and Thomas, H. M.: Dyspnea. In Wintrobe, M. M., et al. (Eds.): Harrison's Principles of Internal Medicine. 7th ed. New York, McGraw-Hill Book Company, 1974, Chapter 28.

Jones, N. L., and Campbell, E. J. M.: Chronic airway obstruction due to asthma, bronchitis, and emphysema. In Wintrobe, M. M., et al. (Eds.): Harrison's Principles of Internal Medicine. 7th ed. New York, McGraw-Hill Book Company, 1974, Chapter 252.

Kreyberg, L., Liebow, A. A., and Uehlinger, E. A.: Histological Typing of Lung Tumours. International Histological Classification of Tumours. No. 1. Geneva, World Health Organization, 1967.

Leading Article: Cancer and asbestos. British Medical Journal, 3: 448–449, 1968.

Leading Article: Enzymes and emphysema. British Medical Journal, 1:1–2, 1973.

Ochsner, A.: Bronchogenic carcinoma, a largely preventable lesion assuming epidemic proportions. Chest, 59:358–359, 1971.

Spencer, H.: The Lung. 2nd ed. New York, The Macmillan Company, 1968. A detailed reference book.

Staub, N. C.: The pathophysiology of pulmonary edema. Human Pathology, 1:419–432, 1970.

Wyatt, J. P.: Occupational lung diseases and inferential relationships to general population hazards. American Journal of Pathology, 64:197–216, 1971.

Chapter 31

After studying this chapter the student should be able to:

- Describe the mechanism of swallowing.
- Define dysphagia, classify its causes, and give a brief account of each.
- Distinguish between oropharyngeal dysphagia and esophageal dysphagia.
- List the causes of ulceration in the mouth and describe aphthous ulceration in detail.
- Describe the types of white lesions (leukoplakia) sometimes found in the mouth.

DISEASES OF THE UPPER ALIMENTARY TRACT

- State the clinical features, differential diagnosis, and complications of acute streptococcal sore throat.
- Compare and contrast carcinoma of the lips, carcinoma of the tongue, and carcinoma of the pharynx.
- Describe the pathogenesis and complications of dental caries.
- Describe the structures that constitute the periodontium.
- Give an account of the pathogenesis and complications of periodontitis.
- Describe the types and complications of hiatus hernia.
- Outline the main features of carcinoma of the esophagus with respect to the following:
  - (a) known predisposing causes
  - (b) site of occurrence
  - (c) symptoms
  - (d) prognosis.
- Give two examples of acute sialoadenitis.
- Describe pleomorphic salivary gland tumors with respect to these factors:
  - (a) common site of occurrence
  - (b) microscopic appearance
  - (c) invasive properties
  - (d) prognosis.

The alimentary tract is usually regarded as being within the body, but it is, in fact, a long tube exposed at each end to the exterior. Its contents, ranging from food in the mouth to feces in the rectum, are never within the body proper. This is an ideal arrangement, because within the lumen the chemical changes necessary for the digestion of food can occur under conditions that could not be tolerated inside the body itself. One effect of this arrangement is that many liters of digestive fluids are poured into the alimentary tract each day. Most of this is reabsorbed, but it can readily be appreciated that if much escapes to the exterior, the volume of fluid lost could reach alarming proportions. Diarrhea and vomiting (discussed in Chapter 21) are indeed potent causes of water and electrolyte loss.

The Mouth and Pharynx

In the mouth, food is masticated and mixed with saliva. By virtue of its mucus content, saliva performs a lubricating action in addition to initiating carbohydrate digestion by the enzyme ptyalin.

Swallowing (*deglutition*) is triggered by the voluntary contraction of the

495

pharyngeal and buccal muscles. By raising the larynx and tongue, the process of swallowing throws the bolus of food against the posterior pharyngeal wall. Thereafter, an involuntary wave of peristalsis sweeps the bolus down the muscular eosophagus, and as the cardiac sphincter relaxes, the bolus enters the stomach. Difficulty in swallowing *(dysphagia)* is described later in this chapter.

LESIONS OF THE ORAL MUCOSA

The oral mucosa shares many diseases with the skin. In *lichen planus** a white lacy appearance of the buccal mucosa is characteristic and may be the first—or, indeed, the only—manifestation of the disease. Likewise, *Pemphigus vulgaris* may first appear in the mouth. The severe ulcerations of the oral mucous membranes seen in the *Stevens-Johnson syndrome* are described in Chapter 41.

The rash of some acute systemic *viral infections* affects the mucosa, where it is called the *enanthem,* before becoming clinically apparent on the skin, where it is called the *exanthem.* Thus, the vesicles of chickenpox may first appear on the palate. The *Koplik's spots* of measles, which occur during the prodromal stage of the disease, are reliable forerunners of the skin rash that appears within a day or two. Koplik's spots are minute white ulcers with an erythematous base and can be described as resembling small grains of salt, each having a red halo.

The primary infection with herpes simplex virus can occur in the mouth, particularly in children. An acute gingivitis, which is the usual manifestation, appears as vesicles that soon ulcerate to produce multiple shallow ulcers.

The common *aphthous ulcers,* or canker sores, are not due to a viral infection. They have been estimated to affect between 20 and 50 per cent of the population and are invariably recurrent. Sometimes a single ulcer is present, but often several appear either at the same time or shortly after one another. They occur on the mucosal surface of the lips or buccal mucosa and appear as very painful, shallow ulcers covered by necrotic slough and surrounded by a bright erythematous zone. Healing generally occurs within a week or two, but in a few patients the lesions enlarge and persist. These may be accompanied by similar ulcerations of the genital mucosa and by recurrent uveitis *(Behcet's syndrome).* It is evident that an examination of the oral cavity can provide essential clues in the diagnosis of other diseases; such a procedure should never be neglected.

Leukoplakia. This term is applied by some authorities to any white patch of the oral mucosa. It includes the following entities:

Hyperkeratosis. This condition, which is hypertrophy of the corneous layer of the skin, can be due to smoking or to chronic trauma—such as that produced by persistent biting of the buccal mucosa or by the rubbing of an ill-fitting denture. A lesion of this type is not precancerous.

Lichen planus. The lesions of lichen planus show some tendency to become malignant, but this is not a serious threat.

---

*Lichen planus is a generalized papulosquamous skin disease of unknown cause. The characteristic lesions are flat-topped, violaceous papules, which are extremely itchy.

DYSPLASIA OF THE ORAL EPITHELIUM. Some authorities confine the term leukoplakia to the variety occurring in the mouth. The lesions appear as white patches that microscopically show dysplasia, either mild or sufficiently severe to warrant the term *carcinoma-in-situ*. It is this type of "leukoplakia" that is premalignant and must be regarded seriously. Obviously, any persistent white patch of the oral mucosa should be biopsied to determine its nature and malignant potentiality.

ACUTE STREPTOCOCCAL SORE THROAT

This is an acute infection of the tonsils and adjacent pharynx by *Streptococcus pyogenes*. The onset is sudden, and the sore throat is accompanied by fever, leukocytosis, and malaise. The tonsils and adjacent pharynx are swollen and red, and a white inflammatory exudate is seen on the surface. If the strain of streptococcus produces abundant erythrogenic exotoxin, and if the patient has no immunity to this toxin, the sore throat is shortly followed by an erythematous skin rash. At that stage the disease is called *scarlet fever*.

Streptococcal sore throat is an important disease, because in a number of patients it is followed by acute glomerulonephritis or acute rheumatic fever—conditions that are considered elsewhere in this book.

It should not be assumed that every sore throat, even if accompanied by tonsillar exudate, is due to the streptococcus. Viral infections, for instance those caused by adenovirus and the causative agent of infectious mononucleosis, can have a very similar clinical appearance, although the onset is generally more insidious. In the past it was essential to consider diphtheria in the differential diagnosis; now, however, the disease is extremely uncommon in the Western world. The diagnosis of diphtheria rests on obtaining a positive culture from a throat swab.

TUMORS OF THE ORAL CAVITY

Benign tumors (*e.g.*, papilloma and fibroma) of the oral cavity are not uncommon; since they are usually small and unimportant, however, they will not be considered further. The important tumor is carcinoma, which varies in character according to its site of origin.

Carcinoma of the Lips. Squamous cell carcinoma of the lips nearly always affects the lower lip and is more common in men than women. Predisposing causes are thought to be pipe and cigarette smoking often combined with exposure to sunlight. The tumor usually starts as a nonhealing crack in the lower lip to one side of the midline. Provided treatment is undertaken reasonably early the prognosis for this tumor is good, since the growth is well differentiated and lymph node metastases are late in appearing.

Carcinoma of the Tongue. This is the most frequent intraoral malignant tumor. Although it is more common in men, the tumor also affects women, particularly in association with the Plummer-Vinson syndrome, described later in this chapter. Cancer of the tongue appears as a nodule that soon ulcerates. Any nonhealing ulcer of the tongue, particularly if its edges are indurated, must be biopsied. Even with early treatment, cancer of the tongue has a less favorable prognosis than cancer of the lips. Approximately 60 per cent of patients live for five years following surgery or radiotherapy. If lymph node metastases are already present, the figure is reduced to about 30 per cent.

Squamous-cell carcinoma can occur in other parts of the mouth and oral pharynx. A tumor of the pharynx is often poorly differentiated and highly malignant. Even though the primary tumor is quite small, the lesion first manifests itself as enlargement of cervical lymph nodes due to metastasis. The prognosis is poor.

The Teeth

CARIES

Dental caries, commonly known as tooth decay or "cavities," is the most common affliction of mankind. Although it has been recognized since prehistoric times, the precise cause is not known. It is principally a disease of childhood, adolescence, and young adult life, affecting deciduous and permanent teeth alike. Tooth decay is particularly frequent in the Western world, where it is presumed to be due to dietary factors. Poor oral hygiene and a diet containing much refined carbohydrate appear to be the major factors.

Caries usually starts in pits, fissures, and other areas, such as the cervical parts of the tooth that are not self-cleansing. Bacterial colonies growing on the tooth surface (and forming *dental plaque*) combine with food debris to form a suitable focus for further bacterial growth. Organisms enter the small fissures in the enamel of the teeth, and ferment the carbohydrate, thus leading to the production of acid. This process steadily erodes the calcific material of the enamel and later of the dentine so that a deep cavity appears; this cavity is often much larger than would be suspected from an examination of the external appearance of the fissure. When a cavity has formed, infection can spread to involve the pulp *(pulpitis)*. Pulpitis can be acute and extremely painful; chronic pulpitis, on the other hand, can lead to the formation of a chronic apical abscess that is often remarkably silent clinically. It is believed that the abscess can act as a focus (or *nidus*) of infection and can lead to periodic episodes of bacteremia. This mechanism is an important factor in the pathogenesis of bacterial endocarditis.

Although dental caries appears to be related to infection, no one particular organism has been incriminated, since the bacteria that have been isolated from lesions are those constituting the normal flora of the mouth.

PERIODONTAL DISEASE

Inflammation of the periodontium *(periodontitis)* is a widespread disease affecting many children and almost the total adult world population. It causes halitosis and is second to caries as a cause of tooth loss. A knowledge of the normal anatomy of the periodontium is essential for a proper understanding of the disease (Figs. 31–1, 31–2, and 31–3).

Periodontitis. Unless meticulous dental hygiene is practiced, colonies of bacteria become attached to the surface of the teeth and form *dental plaque*. If

FIGURE 31–1. *Normal gingiva.*

   This photograph of the anterior part of the mouth shows a normal, healthy gingival condition. The free gingiva (FG) is not attached to the underlying enamel but is separated from it by the gingival crevice. The attached gingiva (AG) is firmly adherent to the underlying alveolar bone. (Courtesy of H. D. Glenwright, M.D.S., and the Department of Clinical Illustration, Birmingham Dental School, England.)

FIGURE 31–2. *Radiograph of a normal mouth.*

   Note how the teeth are deeply embedded in their bony sockets. (Courtesy of H. D. Glenwright, M.D.S., and the Department of Clinical Illustration, Birmingham Dental School, England.)

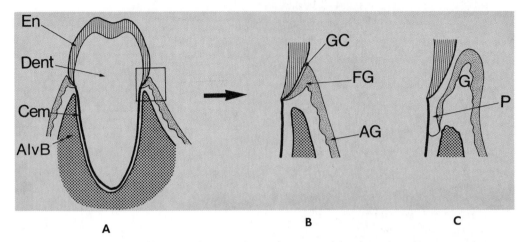

A   B   C

FIGURE 31–3. *Diagrams illustrating the normal periodontium and the changes in chronic periodontitis.*

A and *B* illustrate the normal periodontium, which consists of (1) alveolar bone (Alv B); (2) cementum (Cem); (3) the periodontal membrane, consisting of fibers running between bone and cementum; and (4) the gingiva, including the free gingiva (FG) and the attached gingiva (AG). Note how the gingival crevice (GC) is the space between the free gingiva and the enamel of the tooth (En). Note: Dent = dentine. *C,* The changes in chronic periodontitis. There is loss of alveolar bone and the associated periodontal membrane. Extension of the gingival crevice has resulted in the formation of a pocket (P), and this is partially lined by gingival epithelium which has grown in. The gingiva (G) is inflamed and swollen.

FIGURE 31–4. *Chronic periodontal disease.*

The gingiva is inflamed, swollen, and has lost its normal granular surface. The changes are most marked between the teeth. Deep pockets are present, because a probe can be passed between the gingivae and the roots of the teeth. One tooth is obviously carious. (Courtesy of H. G. Glenwright, M.D.S., and the Department of Clinical Illustration, Birmingham Dental School, England.)

FIGURE 31–5. *Chronic periodontal disease.*

This radiograph shows marked resorption of the alveolar bone. Some teeth have lost most of their bony support and are loose. They will be shed shortly. (Courtesy of H. G. Glenwright, M.D.S., and the Department of Clinical Illustration, Birmingham Dental School, England.)

this is allowed to remain, it calcifies to form *dental calculus* ("tartar"). Food debris, plaque, and calculus in the region of the gingival crevice predispose the gingiva to inflammation. This *gingivitis* is the first stage in the pathogenesis of periodontitis. With this condition the gingivae become red and swollen and tend to bleed, particularly after the teeth have been brushed. The inflammation leads to resorption of the alveolar bone (Figs. 31–3C, 31–4, and 31–5). The fibers of the periodontal membrane are also destroyed. Although the precise mechanism of this destruction is not understood, the process does lead to the formation of a pocket between the gingiva and the cementum of the tooth. Further accumulation of calculus and debris helps to perpetuate the inflammation; the pocket deepens. At the same time, gingival epithelium migrates into the pocket, and the process extends as more and more of the alveolar bone is destroyed. The teeth become loose and rock, even when they are subjected to normal forces during eating. The excessive movement further damages the attachments that remain, and loss of the teeth—one by one—is merely a matter of time.

The Esophagus

The esophagus or gullet is a muscular tube through which food is propelled to the stomach by peristalsis. Although there is some debate about the existence of an anatomical sphincter at its lower end (the cardiac sphincter), from a functional point of view there is little doubt that a working sphincter exists, because the contents of the stomach do not readily re-enter the esophagus. This phenomenon can be attested to by witnessing the gyrations of the acrobat and by noting that the bat (which has a structurally similar esophagus) can spend half its life upside down with no ill-effect.

ACHALASIA OF THE CARDIA

In this condition there is degeneration of the ganglion nerve cells of the lower esophagus, resulting in disturbed peristalsis and a failure of relaxation of the cardiac sphincter. The patients are generally middle-aged and complain of a sensation of food sticking beneath the lower end of the sternum. Often pain is a prominent symptom. The obstruction leads to great dilatation of the esophagus.

ESOPHAGEAL WEBS

Folds or webs of the esophageal mucosa are quite frequently demonstrated by radiologists, but their significance as a cause of dysphagia is debatable. Often the lesions cannot be detected at necropsy. Webs of the upper part of the esophagus are found in the *Plummer-Vinson syndrome* in which there is the triad of *iron deficiency anemia, dysphagia,* and atrophy of the mucosa covering the tongue *(atrophic glossitis).* The disease is virtually confined to women and is associated with an increased incidence of carcinoma of the oral cavity and upper esophagus.

HIATUS HERNIA

The two types of hiatus hernia are illustrated in Figure 31–6. Impaired function of the cardiac sphincter leads to regurgitation of gastric contents; in turn, this leads to an associated esophagitis and peptic ulceration of the lower esophagus. The fibrosis that is associated with the healing of these ulcers can culminate in the formation of a benign stricture.

ESOPHAGITIS

Inflammation of the lower esophagus can be due to regurgitation of gastric contents, which causes pain (heartburn). Esophagitis can result from the ingestion of irritating foods such as hot spicy meals and strong alcoholic beverages. The deliberate or accidental ingestion of corrosive acids and alkalies (*e.g.,* lye) can lead to severe esophagitis. If the patient survives, marked fibrosis with cicatrization results in an incapacitating stenosis.

Normal   "Sliding"   "Rolling"

FIGURE 31–6. *Hiatus hernia.*

ESOPHAGEAL VARICES

An important cause of hematemesis, esophageal varices are described in Chapter 33.

TUMORS OF THE ESOPHAGUS

The most important tumor of the esophagus is carcinoma. Squamous-cell carcinoma is most common in the lower– or middle–one third of the esophagus. It is more frequent in males and in those who smoke excessively or who ingest alcohol to excess. The tumor steadily obstructs the esophagus, causing the patient to experience increasing difficulty in swallowing—at first of solid foods and later of liquids. The onset is insidious, and although the tumor tends to invade locally and to metastasize late, by the time the diagnosis has been achieved, resection is often difficult or even impossible. The prognosis is therefore bad. The end-stages of this disease are particularly unpleasant, since the patient is unable to swallow anything, including saliva. Constant regurgitation from the mouth, inhalation of saliva and food, and starvation combine to terminate the illness. Bronchopneumonia generally relieves the patient of his misery.

DIFFICULTY IN SWALLOWING (DYSPHAGIA)

This condition is caused by a great variety of lesions, as follows:

1. PAINFUL CONDITIONS. These inhibit the voluntary initiation of swallowing. Aphthous ulceration and acute tonsillitis may be cited as examples.

2. MECHANICAL INTERFERENCE WITH SWALLOWING. Infiltration of the tongue or pharynx by scirrhous carcinoma is an example of this type of lesion.

3. MECHANICAL OBSTRUCTION. This usually occurs in the esophagus and is caused by a stricture that is either benign or carcinomatous. Dysphagia of the Plummer-Vinson syndrome, for example, is associated with obstruction of the upper end of the esophagus.

4. PARALYSIS OF THE MUSCLES OF DEGLUTITION. This occurs in poliomyelitis when it affects the brain stem, as well as in pseudobulbar palsy (see Chapter 44).

5. NEUROMUSCULAR INCOORDINATION. In elderly persons incoordination of peristalsis combined with muscular spasm may produce a sensation of obstruction and severe pain. Achalasia of the cardia has already been described.

6. PSYCHOSOMATIC RESPONSE. Difficulty in swallowing and a sensation of a foreign body in the throat are familiar accompaniments of fear and anxiety.

Clinical Classification of Dysphagia

For clinical purposes dysphagia may be divided into two groups:

OROPHARYNGEAL DYSPHAGIA. In this group attempted swallowing leads to the inhalation of food or its regurgitation through the nose.

ESOPHAGEAL DYSPHAGIA. The common symptom of this type is a sensation of obstruction in the chest during swallowing. Carcinoma of the esophagus is the lesion most to be feared, especially if the symptoms are progressive and difficulty in swallowing affects first solids and finally liquids.

The Salivary Glands

The three pairs of major salivary glands (parotid, submaxillary, and sublingual) can be afflicted by many diseases. With the exception of certain inflammations and one tumor, however, they are uncommon.

INFLAMMATION (SIALOADENITIS)

Mumps.   A painful swelling at the angle of the jaw is often the first indication of *mumps*, which is due to an acute nonsuppurative parotitis. The disease is caused by a myxovirus, has a long incubation period (18 to 21 days), and becomes bilateral in about two thirds of cases. Fever and mild malaise accompany the parotitis, and resolution occurs within one week. The most common complication of the disease in adult men is an acute orchitis (see Chapter 36). Acute pancreatitis, meningitis, and encephalitis are occasionally encountered.

Acute Suppurative Inflammation.   This condition is characterized by sudden swelling of the parotid gland, followed by abscess formation. Such an inflammation is encountered in patients who are either dehydrated or in shock and whose level of consciousness is decreased. Poor oral hygiene and a decreased flow of saliva combine to aid the migration of bacteria from the mouth, up the excretory duct, and finally to the parotid gland. It is to prevent this complication that careful cleansing of the mouth is an important component of the nursing care of severely ill patients.

Chronic Sialoadenitis.   Recurrent attacks of acute sialoadenitis and chronic inflammation are generally encountered in a submaxillary gland and are often related to obstruction of the duct by a stone (sialolithiasis).

TUMORS OF THE SALIVARY GLAND

The common tumor of the salivary gland is a pleomorphic tumor of the parotid. This tumor grows slowly to produce a painless mass in front of the external ear. Microscopically, it consists of epithelial elements forming tubules and stroma containing extravasated mucus and isolated cells (Fig. 31–7). The appearance of the stroma sometimes bears a remarkable resemblance to cartilage; indeed, by metaplasia cartilage itself can sometimes be formed. The presence of a connective, as well as an epithelial element, leads to the tumor being called a "mixed parotid tumor." Current belief is that the tumor is purely epithelial and the stromal change is secondary.

Although the tumor may appear to be encapsulated, small outgrowths are present. It is from these that growth recurs following a simple enucleation of the tumor. The current treatment is to excise not only the tumor but also the surrounding parotid gland. The recurrence rate is low and the prognosis is good. Unfortunately, the facial nerve travels through this gland and damage to the nerve sometimes follows. Some pleomorphic salivary gland tumors show local invasion, and in a few instances there is metastasis to lymph nodes or to the blood stream. The tumor is therefore best not classified as a simple adenoma but rather as one of the intermediate group.

Pleomorphic tumors occur in the other salivary glands but are much less common than those in the parotid gland.

FIGURE 31-7. *Pleomorphic salivary gland tumor.*

The tumor shows many clumps of obvious epithelial cells (Ep). In some areas mucin has accumulated in the stroma to produce a pseudocartilaginous appearance (PsC) ($\times$ 300).

Review Questions

1. A 22-year-old nurse complains of recurrent painful ulcers in the mouth. The ulcers developed over a five-day period and then healed within two weeks. Discuss the diagnosis.
2. Describe how an examination of the mouth can help in the diagnosis of systemic diseases. In particular, refer to those diseases that affect the skin or the blood.
3. List the causes of esophageal obstruction.
4. Give an account of the complications of poor oral hygiene.
5. Describe the causes of enlargement of a salivary gland and indicate the features by which each condition may be recognized.
6. Explain why the terms "mixed parotid tumor" and "adenoma of the salivary gland" have been abandoned in favor of "pleomorphic salivary gland tumor."

Selected Readings

Glickman, I., Glickman, V. A., and Less, W. C.: The oral cavity. *In* Robbins, S. L. (Ed.): Pathologic Basis of Disease. Philadelphia, W. B. Saunders Company, 1974. See Chapter 20, "The Oral Cavity" and Chapter 21, "The Gastrointestinal Tract."

Macphee, T., and Cowley, G.: Essentials of Periodontology and Periodontics. Oxford, Blackwell Scientific Publications Ltd., 1972. See, in particular, Chapters 1 to 4.

Morson, B. C., and Dawson, I. M. P.: Gastrointestinal Pathology. Oxford, Blackwell Scientific Publications Ltd., 1972. See section 1, "Oesophagus."

Chapter 32

After studying this chapter the student should be able to:

- Describe chronic peptic ulceration with respect to the following:
  (a) site of occurrence
  (b) pathogenesis
  (c) complications.
- Give an account of acute gastroduodenal ulcers and their complications.
- Describe carcinoma of the stomach and indicate its prognosis.
- Classify the causes of food poisoning.
- Describe the cause, course, and pathogenesis of cholera.
- Describe the lesions and complications of Crohn's disease.

506

DISEASES OF THE
GASTROINTESTINAL TRACT

- List the features of the carcinoid syndrome.
- Classify the causes and effects of the malabsorption syndrome.
- Describe the causes, pathological findings, and clinical features of bacillary dysentery.
- Describe the lesions, effects, and complications of
    - (a) idiopathic ulcerative colitis
    - (b) diverticular disease of the colon.
- Outline the incidence and pathological effects of carcinoma of the colon.
- Describe acute appendicitis with respect to the following factors:
    - (a) incidence
    - (b) pathological findings
    - (c) clinical features
    - (d) complications.
- Outline the causes of peritonitis.
- Distinguish a volvulus from an intussusception.
- List the common sites for a hernia and describe the complications.
- Distinguish between the mechanical and the nonmechanical types of intestinal obstruction. Describe the main causes and effects of each.
- Outline the common causes of an "acute abdomen."

The lower alimentary, or gastrointestinal, tract consists of the stomach, the small intestine, and the large intestine. Its functions are concerned mainly with digestion and absorption. Each region will be considered separately.

The Stomach

In the stomach the masticated food is softened, moistened, lubricated, and partially digested by the gastric juice. The food is kneaded by strong muscular contractions into a semiliquid mass called *chyme*, which passes steadily into the duodenum.

The gastric juice has four major active components:
1. *Mucus*, which has a lubricating action.
2. *Intrinsic factor*, which is necessary for the absorption of vitamin B_{12}.
3. *Pepsin*, which commences protein digestion.
4. *Hydrochloric acid*, which has an important bactericidal action and also provides the correct pH for the action of pepsin. Its presence is important in the pathogenesis of one of the common disabling human afflictions – peptic ulceration.

Whenever gastric juice comes into contact with non-acid-secreting mucosa, peptic ulceration is liable to occur. It is seen therefore at the pyloric end of the stomach, along the lesser curvature of the stomach, in the first part of the duodenum, at the lower end of the esophagus, and at the site of anastomosis between the·stomach and small intestine following the operation of gastroenterostomy.

CHRONIC PEPTIC ULCER

Chronic peptic ulcers are usually solitary and present a characteristic appearance (Fig. 32–1). Not only is the mucosa lost but also the underlying muscle layers are often destroyed, thereby producing a deep round or oval, punched-out ulcer with straight edges. For reasons that are not yet known, regeneration of the mucosal epithelium is inhibited, and chronic inflammation ensues. The floor of the ulcer consists of inflamed vascular granulation tissue covered by necrotic material that forms a slough. Bleeding is common, therefore. Deeper in the base of the ulcer the granulation tissue matures to form dense scar tissue that ultimately replaces the muscular walls.

Clinical Features.   Pain in the epigastrium is common and is related to the gastric acidity and muscle spasm. It is usually relieved by eating food or, in particular, by the administration of alkali.

Complications

HEMORRHAGE.   Repeated bleeding is a common cause of iron-deficiency anemia. Sometimes the ulcer penetrates adjacent structures, particularly the pancreas, and a large artery is eroded. When this occurs, there is massive

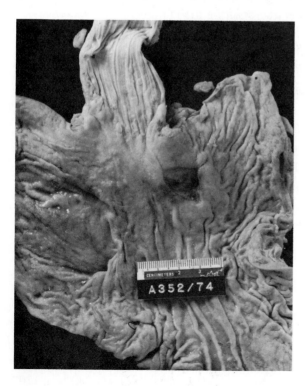

FIGURE 32–1.   *Chronic gastric ulcer.*

The stomach has been opened along its greater curvature to show the mucosal surface. There is a typical chronic peptic ulcer on the lesser curvature about 2 cm from the cardioesophageal junction.· Note the folds of mucosa (rugae) that are normal.

hematemesis and melena (altered blood in the feces, with the stools appearing black and tarry).

PERFORATION.   When the ulcer penetrates the peritoneal surface, it produces a localized fibrinous inflammation that may cause adjacent structures to adhere to it. If adhesions do not form, the ulcer may perforate, and the gastric or duodenal contents may then be poured into the peritoneal cavity. The patient immediately experiences severe pain, and generalized peritonitis soon develops.

CICATRIZATION.   As an ulcer heals, scar tissue tends to cicatrize and cause stenosis. Pyloric ulcers are particularly susceptible to develop this complication; the resulting *pyloric stenosis* causes persistent severe vomiting. This can lead to dehydration, starvation, and metabolic alkalosis resulting from loss of acid gastric juices.

Etiology.   Remarkably little is known about the cause of peptic ulceration. Without the acid content of the gastric juice, peptic ulceration cannot occur, but hypersecretion of acid *(hyperchlorhydria)* is not always related to ulcer formation. Hyperchlorhydria is usually associated with duodenal ulcers but not with gastric ulcers. Other factors that may play a part in the formation of ulcers are a demanding occupation, overwork, smoking, and emotional stress. Genetic factors have also been incriminated; thus, gastric ulceration is more common in patients who are of blood group O. All of these factors, however, appear to be secondary — the precise pathogenesis of the ulceration is not known.

ACUTE ULCERATION

Acute shallow ulcers, commonly called *erosions,* often occur in the stomach (Fig. 32–2). They are usually multiple and appear to be caused by dietary indiscretion, alcohol, and the action of irritant drugs, particularly aspirin. The ulcers are shallow and involve little more than the covering epithelium. Slight bleeding is common, but occasionally severe hematemesis may occur. Healing is generally rapid and complete.

Acute ulceration of the stomach or duodenum is also a complication of burns and any severe injury. The ulcers are usually multiple and generally heal rapidly with minimal scarring. Occasionally they erode a large vessel or perforate into the peritoneal cavity, giving rise to severe hemorrhage or peritonitis. Sometimes severe bleeding occurs from the stomach and no actual point of ulceration can be found. It appears that the entire stomach mucosa is congested and oozes blood. This condition is generally encountered as a complication of a severe injury or a major surgical operation.

CARCINOMA OF THE STOMACH

Gastric carcinoma is not uncommon in Northern European communities, but its incidence is now lower than that of colonic carcinoma. It is a common tumor in the Japanese, and in European communities it is more frequent in the lower social echelons than in the social elite. The tumor appears either as a fungating, cauliflower type of growth (Figs. 32–3 and 32–4), or as a typical malignant ulceration. In some instances the tumor cells invade the stomach wall so diffusely that no definite mass exists. Instead, the entire stomach wall is diffusely

FIGURE 32–2. *Acute erosions of the stomach.*

The mucosal surface of the stomach shows many shallow erosions up to 1 cm in diameter (arrows). The patient had cirrhosis of the liver and died of bleeding from esophageal varices. Multiple erosions are a common complication of any severe stress (e.g., major surgery) or in this case, severe bleeding.

FIGURE 32–3. *Carcinoma of the stomach.*

The stomach has been bisected, and both halves are shown. The wall is thickened, partly by tumor invasion, and partly by the muscular hypertrophy that the tumor has caused. The mucosa is obviously invaded (compare with previous two figures), and a polypoid mass of growth is present (arrow). This is shown more clearly in Figure 32–4.

510

FIGURE 32–4. *Carcinoma of the stomach.*
Note the cauliflowerlike mass of tumor. This is the same case as in Figure 32–3. Microscopically the tumor is a poorly differentiated adenocarcinoma.

thickened by tumor cells and by the dense fibrous stroma that develops in response to them. This formation is called a diffuse infiltrating carcinoma of the stomach, or *linitis plastica.*

The symptoms of carcinoma of the stomach are often vague: they include indigestion, pain not relieved by food or alkalis, and weight loss. Bleeding that causes an obscure anemia is common. Blood may be present in altered form in the vomitus ("coffee-ground vomit"), and melena may occur.

Histologically, cancer of the stomach is a poorly differentiated adenocarcinoma. The prognosis is extremely bad, and even with early excision few patients survive for more than five years. Metastasis is to the regional lymph nodes and by blood spread to the liver and elsewhere.

The Small Intestine

The small intestine consists of the duodenum, the jejunum, and the ileum and, in all, is about 20 feet long. The chyme that leaves the stomach is acted upon by bile, the pancreatic enzymes, and the intestinal secretion *(succus entericus).* The latter contains few enzymes; the most important of these is *enterokinase,* which converts trypsinogen to trypsin—a conversion that is an essential step in the activation of pancreatic enzymes. The function of the small intestine is therefore the final breakdown of fat, carbohydrate, and protein, as well as the absorption of the products formed. The complex structure of the mucosa with its numerous villi is well adapted to this function. Likewise, the microvilli of each luminal cell are designed for absorption of the products of digestion. The glycocalyx (Fig. 2–8) is thought to contain enzymes, including the important disaccharidases. These are responsible for splitting disaccharides (*e.g.*, sucrose and lactose) into monosaccharides (*e.g.*, fructose and glucose); in this form these sugars can be absorbed.

From this brief account of the functions of the small intestine it is evident that any derangement caused by disease can easily by accompanied either by malabsorption or by the loss of large quantities of fluid and electrolytes.

ACUTE INFLAMMATIONS OF THE SMALL INTESTINE

Food Poisoning.   *Acute enteritis* is often accompanied by inflammation of the stomach. Such an acute *gastroenteritis* produces vomiting, diarrhea, and abdominal pain; it may be severe, but it is rarely fatal. Many causes of gastroenteritis can be recognized:

(a) *Chemicals.*   Poisoning may be deliberate (*e.g.*, by ingestion of arsenic) or accidental (*e.g.*, by ingestion of poisonous mushrooms and spoiled potatoes).

(b) *Bacterial Toxins.*   If *Staphylococcus aureus* or *Clostridium welchii* are allowed to grow in food, such as in a meat pie, they produce toxin that causes acute gastroenteritis when ingested.

(c) *Bacterial Infection.*   Many strains of *Salmonella* are recognized that produce an acute, but fleeting, infection of the small intestine. Enteropathic strains of *Escherichia coli* cause some cases of infantile diarrhea as well as some examples of traveler's diarrhea (variously known as "Delhi belly," "gypsy tummy," "Montezuma's revenge," etc).

(d) *Viral Infection.*   Causative agents include enteroviruses, hepatitis viruses, and rotaviruses.

(e) *Idiopathic.*   No agent can be incriminated in many cases.

Typhoid Fever.   Typhoid fever is a specific type of enteritis and is described in Chapter 6.

Cholera.   Cholera has often been described as an acute enteritis, when in fact its pathogenesis is quite different from that of a simple inflammation. The disease, which is caused by a vibrio, has been responsible in the past for several pandemics that have originated in the Bengal basin. The disease is characterized by the sudden onset of intense vomiting and diarrhea, which rapidly leads to dehydration and hypovolemic shock, to be followed by death within two or three days in about one third of the cases. With efficient treatment by fluid and electrolyte administration, the mortality can be reduced to under 1 per cent. At a time when the disease appeared to be declining in the world, a new strain became prominent (the *El Tor* type); this appeared to have originated in Indonesia in 1961. It subsequently spread to involve large areas of the Far East, India, and Africa.

Cholera is acquired by ingesting the organism. The bacteria are not killed by the acid in the stomach and thus pass into the small intestine where they multiply and elaborate enterotoxin that acts on the plasma membrane of the intestinal epithelial cells. Cyclic AMP (adenosine 3':5'-cyclic phosphate) is formed and induces a tremendous outpouring of water and electrolytes into the intestinal lumen. A large quantity of fluid flows into the colon, which is unable to absorb the load. The result is a severe diarrhea with watery stools ("rice-water stools").

CROHN'S DISEASE (REGIONAL ENTERITIS)

Crohn's disease is a chronic inflammatory disease that can affect any part of the bowel but is usually most obvious in the lower small intestine (see Case History I). With this condition the bowel shows a chronic inflammatory response that involves its entire wall. The lumen becomes narrowed, causing the patient to develop intestinal obstruction (Fig. 32–5). Constipation alternates with diarrhea. An outstanding feature of the disease is that small abscesses form on the mucosal surface; since these penetrate the muscularis, the serosa is affected. The inflammatory reaction leads to local peritonitis and to adhesions between the abdominal organs (Fig. 32–6). Sinuses and fistulae develop so that communication is established between adjacent loops of intestine, the colon, the bladder, and the skin surface. The cause of this disease, which tends to affect young adults, is still unknown. Treatment by resection of the affected bowel is sometimes successful, but recurrence in other areas is quite common. The course is therefore protracted and presents great problems both to patient and attendants.

Case History I. (See Figure 32–6.)   The patient was a 30-year-old male who was admitted to a hospital with a complaint of abdominal pain and frequency of stool discharge for one year. The pain, which was colicky in nature, began between one and two hours after meals. It was relieved by having a bowel movement, which showed stools that were bulky, light brown, and foul-smelling. They floated in the toilet bowl because of their fat and gas content. Pathological examination of the feces showed the presence of pus cells, blood, and an increased amount of fat. A barium meal showed narrowing and

FIGURE 32–5. *Crohn's disease of the small intestine.*

The mucosa of the affected area is thickened and presents a hyperemic cobblestone appearance. Note the thickening of the intestinal wall (arrow); when marked, this can cause stenosis of the lumen. Note the sharp line of demarcation between the diseased bowel and the normal intestine. In this patient other areas of small intestine were affected; it is characteristic of the disease for there to be normal "skip areas" between them.

FIGURE 32–6. *Crohn's disease of the small intestine.*

This portion of small intestine shows hyperemia and thickening of the peritoneal surface. Focal white areas of inflammation are present, and this loop of intestine has become adherent to adjacent structures. The fat at the mesenteric border of the intestine (arrow) is prominent and is "creeping" over the gut wall. (See Case History I for additional clinical details.)

irregularity of the bowel wall involving two or three loops of ileum. Such findings were suggestive of Crohn's disease. Since the patient was thought to have signs of subacute intestinal obstruction, a laparotomy was performed. About 20 inches of small gut were resected. The disease started about eight inches from the ileocecal junction and extended upward. Two skip areas were noted between the lesions. The sigmoid colon also showed thickening, which was interpreted as Crohn's disease. Since there was no sign of obstruction, the colon was not resected. The postoperative course was uneventful. Part of the resected specimen is shown in Figure 32–6. Postoperatively, the patient continued to have three or four bowel movements daily, but he felt reasonably well. He noticed the occasional passage of blood. It was felt that his Crohn's disease was still present but stable.

Tuberculosis of the Intestine.   This disease is now extremely uncommon.

TUMORS OF THE SMALL INTESTINE

Small leiomyomas are not uncommon but rarely produce symptoms; carcinomas are rare. The most frequently encountered malignant tumor is the *carcinoid*. This tumor is characterized by the development of a considerable stromal reaction that causes a stricture to develop. The tumor grows slowly, but it ultimately metastasizes to lymph nodes and liver. These metastases sometimes lead to the *carcinoid syndrome*—diarrhea, valvular lesions of the right side of the heart, asthmatic attacks, and periodic flushing of the face. The pathogenesis of this syndrome is not clear, but the release of 5-hydroxytryptamine by the tumor, the activation of plasma kinin, and the deposition of platelets on the heart valves are all involved. Carcinoid tumors also occur in other parts of the intestine—the appendix, in particular. In the latter situation the tumor is usually small and does not spread.

THE MALABSORPTION SYNDROME

If the functions of the small intestine are impaired, a state of severe undernutrition results; this condition is called the *malabsorption syndrome.*

Causes

Common causes appear below:

LACK OF BILE SALTS OR DIGESTIVE ENZYMES. Obstructive jaundice and pancreatic disease, such as chronic pancreatitis, are examples of diseases having these deficiencies.

LACK OF ABSORPTIVE AREA. This problem usually follows extensive intestinal resections such as those performed following gunshot wounds to the abdomen or performed for Crohn's disease.

THE BLIND LOOP SYNDROME. Multiple diverticulae of the small intestine (which is a very uncommon condition), fistulae between adjacent loops, and blind loops caused by surgical procedures sometimes lead to the malabsorption syndrome. The precise mechanism of this syndrome is not clearly understood, but it is believed to be related to an upset in the intestinal flora.

INTRINSIC DISEASE OF THE INTESTINE ITSELF. A good example of an intestinal disease that leads to severe malabsorption is *sprue.* The intestinal villi show atrophy, but the cause is not known (Fig. 32–7). Two types of sprue, listed below, can be recognized:

(1) *Tropical sprue*

(2) *Gluten-induced enteropathy*

In children, gluten-induced enteropathy is called *celiac disease;* in adults it is known as *nontropical sprue.* The intestinal lesions and the symptoms can be relieved by a diet that is low in gluten. The way in which gluten (a protein contained in flour) produces the disease is not understood. Since there is a marked familial incidence, the disease is probably inherited as an autosomal dominant trait with incomplete penetrance.

Effects of Malabsorption. The lack of absorption produces some effects that are similar to those of starvation, *e.g.,* the effects following the dysphagia of esophageal cancer. Thus, there is loss of weight and generalized body atrophy.

Fat absorption is usually severely affected; therefore much fat—some of it undigested—is passed in the feces, which are pale and bulky. Excess fat in the stools is termed *steatorrhea.* There is often poor carbohydrate absorption, and the excess carbohydrate is fermented by bacteria in the bowel. The resulting gas causes the stools to be frothy and offensive.

In addition to the generalized wasting, there are the effects of specific dietary deficiencies (*e.g.,* deficiencies of the vitamin B complex, the fat-soluble vitamins A and D, and calcium). Calcium is poorly absorbed because it is bound by the fatty acids in the bowel. This results in a negative calcium balance with mild hypocalcemia and a tendency to develop tetany. A deficiency of vitamin D aggravates matters, causing osteomalacia to develop (Chapter 40). A deficiency of vitamin K leads to a low plasma prothrombin and a bleeding ten-

FIGURE 32–7.   *Gluten-induced enteropathy.*

This section is from a jejunal biopsy. Note the flat surface and absence of villi (compare this with normal intestine illustrated in Chapter 2). The lamina propria is heavily infiltrated with lymphocytes and plasma cells (× 250).

dency (Chapter 26). Dermatitis, peripheral neuropathy, and inflammation of the tongue (glossitis) may all be found and may be attributable to vitamin deficiencies. A failure to absorb iron, vitamin B$_{12}$, and folic acid leads to severe anemia. The effects of malabsorption from the small intestine are both widespread and serious, and their occurrence is a reflection of the importance of this part of the digestive tract.

The Colon

The colon has two main functions: (1) absorbing water and electrolytes, and (2) providing a convenient receptacle for feces, so that they may be discharged at the individual's convenience. Acute inflammation of the colon results in a derangement of its functions, and the diarrhea that results causes great inconvenience as well as a considerable loss of water and electrolytes. Two severe infections, described below, are recognized:

Bacillary Dysentery.   This is an acute infection of the colon by organisms of the genus *Shigella.* The incubation period is short (24 to 48 hours), and the disease is characterized by the sudden onset of abdominal pain, fever, and diarrhea. The colon shows acute inflammation with ulceration. The feces are fluid and contain blood, mucus, and numerous pus cells.

Bacillary dysentery is limited to human beings and is contracted by the ingestion of contaminated material—generally food. The disease is therefore most common in countries or communities where sanitation is poor, and where flies have ample opportunity to feed on human feces before alighting on human food.

Amebic Dysentery.   See Chapter 15 for a description of this disease.

IDIOPATHIC ULCERATIVE COLITIS

Now the commonest cause of serious bowel disease in North America, idiopathic ulcerative colitis affects all age groups and often starts in young adult life.

The disease generally commences with an acute attack of colicky abdominal pain accompanied by diarrhea and the passage of blood, mucus, and pus in the feces. Fever and malaise are also present. The acute attack generally subsides and is followed by chronic ulcerative colitis with recurrent exacerbation of symptoms. Pain, diarrhea, and the passage of blood, mucus, and pus are intermittent.

The disease generally affects the rectum and distal colon most severely, and in the acute phase it is characterized by intense hyperemia of the mucosa. On proctoscopy the mucosa bleeds at the slightest touch. In due course mucosal ulcers develop, these tending to undermine the mucous membrane so that tags or pseudopolyps are formed. The ulcers are covered by a slough. Deep to this is an inflammatory reaction from which the blood and pus are derived.

In chronic ulcerative colitis the disease tends to remain confined to the mucosa. Because the muscle coat itself and the peritoneal surface of the colon are not generally affected, adhesions do not form between adjacent viscera and there is usually no perforation or fistula formation. In this respect the disease differs markedly from Crohn's disease, which can also affect the colon.

Ulcerative colitis generally pursues a chronic intermittent course, producing misery to the patient and leading to anemia, general debility, and loss of weight. A further complication is the development of carcinoma. It has been estimated that about one third of the patients who suffer from the disease for more than 12 years develop cancer. For this reason, and because of the symptoms of the disease, total colectomy is sometimes performed, and the patient is left with a permanent ileostomy. The ileum is brought to the surface of the anterior abdominal wall, a permanent opening is created, and a suitable container is attached.

Ulcerative colitis is occasionally very acute, either at its inception or at some stage in its development. The colon becomes acutely congested, its muscle becomes atonic, and the bowel dilates enormously. This type of disease follows a fulminating course; generally, the transverse colon is involved, and the patient becomes extremely ill. Multiple perforations develop, and the patient dies of toxemia associated with peritonitis. This variant of ulcerative colitis is called *acute toxic megacolon.*

DIVERTICULAR DISEASE OF THE COLON

The current Western diet, which contains inadequate cellulose (roughage), is believed by some authorities to be responsible for the high frequency of

FIGURE 32–8.   *Diverticular disease of the colon.*

Part of this portion of descending and sigmoid colon has been opened. Numerous diverticula are present. There is no evidence of inflammation, and the condition can be labeled *diverticulosis.*

FIGURE 32–9.   *Colonic diverticula.*

This radiograph following a barium enema shows numerous diverticula that are outlined by the radiopaque barium. (Courtesy of Dr. D. E. Sanders.)

colonic diverticula. This disease is most frequent in the distal part of the colon — particularly the sigmoid part. Apart from the presence of numerous diverticula, the most striking change is muscular hypertrophy and shortening of the colon — presumably due to the muscular overactivity that is necessary to propel the small, hard feces. The diverticula themselves consist of outpouches of the mucosa that penetrate weak points in the muscular coat (Figs. 32–8 and 32–9). Often they are merely covered by a thin layer of peritoneum. Sometimes the orifices of the diverticula become obstructed by fecal material and inflammation ensues. Overlying peritonitis with the formation of adhesions, pericolic abscesses, and fistulae develops. The condition is then called *diverticulitis*. Sometimes a mass of chronic inflammatory tissue forming in the bowel wall is sufficient to cause obstruction and to simulate carcinoma. Occasionally diverticular disease can cause massive bleeding, which is life-threatening.

TUMORS OF THE LARGE INTESTINE

    Adenoma. Adenomas are common and are sometimes multiple (Fig. 32–10). They tend to become pedunculated and bleed. Malignant change can

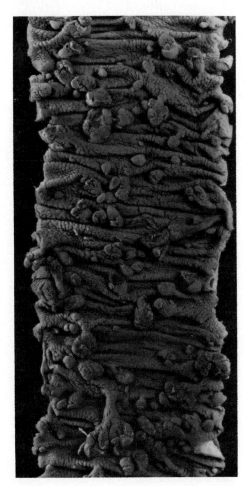

FIGURE 32–10. *Familial polyposis coli.*

The mucosal surface of the colon shows numerous adenomas, many of which are pedunculated and may therefore be labeled *polyps.* (Specimen from the Boyd Museum, University of Toronto.)

FIGURE 32–11. *Carcinoma of colon.*

The specimen shows a typical ulcerating carcinoma. It has a rolled edge where tumor is actively extending.

FIGURE 32–12. *Carcinoma of colon.*

This surgically removed colon has been distended with 4 per cent formaldehyde solution before being opened. Note how the carcinoma encircles the gut and has produced stenosis.

occur but is not inevitable. Nevertheless, in the hereditary condition of *polyposis coli*, there are so many tumors that one invariably becomes malignant and the patient dies of carcinoma.

Carcinoma. The large bowel ranks with the lung and breast as the most common site of fatal malignant disease in Europeans. The rectum and sigmoid colon are most frequently involved. The tumor is usually a well-differentiated adenocarcinoma (Figs. 17–10, 17–11, and 17–12). Initially it may produce a polypoid growth protruding into the lumen, but it generally soon breaks down to produce a typical carcinomatous ulcer (Fig. 32–11). The tumor tends to encircle the gut, and the fibrous stromal reaction that accompanies it produces a stricture (Figs. 32–12 and 32–13). This obstruction produces constipation, but overgrowth of organisms above this soon liquefies the feces so that diarrhea follows. *Alternate constipation and diarrhea are characteristic of partial intestinal obstruction.* When combined with the passage of blood and mucus in the stools, the diagnosis of carcinoma is almost certain. The tumor invades locally, metastasizes to the regional lymph nodes, and finally invades the blood stream to give metastases in the liver, and later, elsewhere. Growth is often relatively

FIGURE 32–13.   *Carcinoma of colon.*

This radiograph following a barium enema shows obvious obstruction in the descending colon. The lesion proved to be a carcinoma similar to that depicted in Figure 32–12. (Courtesy of Dr. D. E. Sanders.)

slow, so that the prognosis following resection is good if the tumor is detected in the early stages of development and correspondingly poor if the tumor is detected in the later stages.

The Appendix

The importance of the appendix as a site of intra-abdominal mischief is not proportional to its size or apparent uselessness. The organ is a hollow cul-de-sac opening into the cecum, and it is seldom more than 7 cm in length. Its major disease is acute inflammation.

ACUTE APPENDICITIS

Incidence. Acute appendicitis is common in persons living in highly civilized societies, but spares the inhabitants of poor and undeveloped areas of the world. The reason for this is not precisely known, but it is presumed to be related to diet—a low roughage/high meat diet apparently predisposing to the disease. Appendicitis is rare in children under two years of age, is more common in children above the age of two years, and has its maximum incidence in young adults between the ages of 20 and 30 years.

Pathology and Pathogenesis. No specific infective agent can be isolated from an acutely inflamed appendix; the organisms present are those normally found in the feces—in particular, *Escherichia coli*. The inflamed organ is red and swollen; its peritoneal coat is dulled by a fibrinous exudate, and the mucosa is ulcerated. Often found blocking the lumen is a hard mass of feces (called a *fecalith*), which may play some part in initiating the disease.

Complications. Acute appendicitis may resolve spontaneously, but often the wall undergoes necrosis, becomes gangrenous, and *perforates.* Pus and fecal material pour into the peritoneal cavity. This material may become walled off by adhesions to produce a *localized abscess,* but often *generalized peritonitis* ensues, and the outlook is poor. It is impossible to predict the course of an individual case, and early removal of the appendix (appendectomy) is the treatment of choice in all cases. If the patient is seen later in the course of the disease when a localized abscess mass is present, it is best to allow the inflammation to subside and to treat the person surgically at a later date. Suppurative thrombophlebitis with portal pyemia is an occasional complication.

Symptoms. The inflamed turgid appendix causes *pain* that is referred to the midline of the abdomen at about the level of the umbilicus. *Nausea* and sometimes *vomiting* follow. As the parietal peritoneum becomes inflamed, the periumbilical pain shifts to the right iliac fossa, and local tenderness can be detected.

If each case of acute appendicitis had this typical history, the disease would present no diagnostic problems. Unfortunately, atypical cases are common, particularly in the very young and the very old, and even the most astute physician can be mistaken and misled. In view of the seriousness of perforation, it is a wise policy to operate if there is a reasonable suspicion of acute appendicitis. Inevitably, some unnecessary operations will be performed and normal appendices will be removed, but the operative mortality is very low. The alternative policy is to risk allowing an acute appendicitis to rupture and to go undetected. In such cases the mortality is high.

Diseases of the Abdominal Cavity as a Whole

The abdominal cavity is lined by a layer of flattened cells that are sometimes classified as epithelial but are actually *modified connective tissue fibroblasts.* Following surgical procedures that have left raw areas of peritoneum, the exposed connective tissues rapidly differentiate into new peritoneal cells; hence, it is unnecessary to attempt to cover these raw areas. To cover them is detrimental, because the required sutures lead to inflammation and the formation of adhesions.

PERITONITIS

Localized Peritonitis. This condition occurs over an inflamed abdominal organ. Examples, which have been described elsewhere in this chapter, include acute appendicitis, Crohn's disease, diverticulitis, and peptic ulceration. The fibrinous component of the exudate tends to wall-off the inflammation and to localize any infection. Aiding in this process is the *greater omentum,* the fibrovascular fatty apron that hangs from the stomach. This structure has been called the "policeman of the abdomen," for it tends to wrap itself around any area of inflammation; by becoming inflamed itself, the greater omentum adds its fibrinous exudate to the adhesions that limit the spread of infection.

Generalized Peritonitis. This occasionally occurs as a primary disease without evidence of infection elsewhere. The route of infection is presumed to be either via the blood stream or, in young women, via the Fallopian tubes. More commonly, generalized peritonitis is the result of rupture of a part of the gastrointestinal tract, *e.g.,* perforated peptic ulcer, appendicitis, toxic megacolon, volvulus, and penetrating injuries to the abdomen.

In generalized peritonitis the large area of peritoneum forms an admirable absorptive area for toxins; the patient rapidly becomes ill and undergoes shock. Even if the person is treated and survives, he may have localized pockets of infection that can form peritoneal abscesses. One such site is the pelvis, owing no doubt to the effects of gravity. Another is the space between the diaphragm and the liver. Indeed, an abscess in the latter situation *(subphrenic abscess)* is of great importance and should always be suspected if the patient develops signs of infection *(e.g.,* malaise, fever, leukocytosis) following an abdominal event *(e.g.,* appendicitis, laparotomy) and the site of infection is not apparent. The old adage "pus somewhere, pus under the diaphragm" is all too often forgotten.

PERITONEAL ADHESIONS

Following acute peritonitis the fibrinous adhesions can organize to fibrous adhesions. Hence, these are not uncommon overlying an appendix or adjacent to a peptic ulcer. Surgery alone can produce adhesions; the irritant talc or starch used as glove powder is an important factor in their production. The gloves used by the surgeon and assistants should be well rinsed before entering the abdomen.

VOLVULUS

Much of the small intestine and parts of the colon are suspended from the abdominal wall by means of a mesentery. The twisting of a loop of bowel about its mesenteric base is called a *volvulus* and is yet another cause of the "acute abdomen." Twisting of the mesentery soon produces venous obstruction, causing the gut to become rapidly congested and edematous. Soon the arterial supply is cut off and infarction results. Urgent surgical intervention is required for volvulus. Sometimes the twist can be undone, but usually the affected gut must be resected.

INTUSSUSCEPTION

In this condition a segment of gut becomes telescoped into the gut immediately distal to it. The trapped portion is pulled in by peristaltic motions so that the segment of gut and its mesentery are steadily advanced towards the anus. The condition is most common in children and appears to arise spontaneously—perhaps being precipitated by an acute enteritis. In adults intussusception is sometimes caused by a benign tumor that is caught by the peristaltic motions of the gut distal to it. Symptoms of intussusception include intestinal obstruction and the sequelae of infarction of the affected bowel. Passage of blood *per rectum* is characteristic.

HERNIAS

A hernia is an outpouching of an abdominal viscus through a weak point of the abdominal wall. An outpouching of parietal peritoneum first occurs, forming the lining of the hernial sac.

The most common site for a hernia to form is the inguinal region; the hernial sac follows the previous path of the descending testis. The sac generally contains small intestine, and in the early stages of development its contents can be reduced by pressure and returned to the abdomen. The formation of adhesions may later result in the intestinal loops being permanently trapped or *incarcerated*. The hernia cannot then be reduced.

An occasional complication of a hernia is that the venous return from its contents is impaired by twisting or kinking at its neck; venous congestion causes edema, with the swelling further endangering the circulation until the arterial supply is finally cut off and the contents of the sac become infarcted and gangrenous. The hernia is then said to be *strangulated*. A strangulated hernia is a serious condition, since it results in intestinal obstruction and is rapidly followed by generalized peritonitis. Immediate surgical treatment is imperative. The detailed anatomy of the various types of hernias to be found in the inguinal region is therefore of great importance to the surgeon who is called upon to operate on them. Other hernias are found at the umbilicus and at the site of a weak laparotomy scar. Occasionally an internal hernia is formed where a loop of bowel is incarcerated between a viscus and a fibrous adhesion. Paraesophageal, or hiatus, hernias have been described in Chapter 31.

INTESTINAL OBSTRUCTION

Intestinal obstruction (or *ileus*, as it is sometimes called) is a serious condition because if it is complete and is not relieved, it terminates in death. Two types, described below, can be recognized:

Mechanical Intestinal Obstruction. There are many causes of intestinal obstruction: strictures, tumors, hernias, volvuli, and intussusceptions are some forms of mechanical obstruction that have already been described. The obstruction may develop gradually, or it may be complete and sudden, resulting in more severe effects. The higher in the intestinal tract the obstruction occurs, the more profound are its effects and the greater is the threat to life.

FEATURES OF MECHANICAL INTESTINAL OBSTRUCTION

Pain. The intestine above the obstruction exhibits increased peristalsis; such effects can be heard with the aid of a stethoscope. The obstruction causes pain that is diffuse, poorly localized, and cramping or colicky.

Failure to Pass Feces or Gas per Rectum. Constipation, which becomes complete, is an important feature of intestinal obstruction.

Vomiting. Vomiting is a prominent feature of high intestinal obstruction. The vomitus soon becomes green in color and eventually has a foul, fecal odor.

Abdominal Distension. The gut above the obstruction ultimately becomes distended with fluid and gas, causing abdominal distention. A radiograph taken with the patient in the standing position has a characteristic appearance with many fluid levels. Abdominal distension is a late event if the site of the obstruction is low in the intestinal tract.

Nonmechanical Intestinal Obstruction. In the absence of a mechanical obstruction, a failure of the intestinal muscle to propel the gut contents forward is commonly called *ileus*. (Strictly speaking, "ileus," from the Greek *eilos*, meaning "intestinal colic," can be applied to any type of obstruction.) Three types are recognized:

ADYNAMIC OR PARALYTIC ILEUS. Peritonitis is the most important cause of paralytic ileus. To a minor degree it occurs after every abdominal operation, but in such cases it does not last more than three days. The fully developed syndrome occurs in acute peritonitis, such as that complicating acute appendicitis or a perforated peptic ulcer. The gut dilates, vomiting occurs, peristalsis is absent, and the abdomen is silent—a silence that leads to the grave. Paralytic ileus sometimes complicates painful conditions, such as renal colic, and it is also a feature of severe hypokalemia (see Chapter 19).

ILEUS DUE TO VASCULAR OCCLUSION. Mesenteric arterial occlusion or mesenteric venous thrombosis leads to focal intestinal paralysis and obstruction. Gangrene often follows.

SPASTIC ILEUS. Spasm is an uncommon cause of obstruction. It is occasionally encountered in uremia.

THE ACUTE ABDOMEN

The sudden onset of acute abdominal pain, often combined with vomiting and fever, is commonly referred to as "acute abdomen." It is usually caused by peritoneal infection derived from a perforated abdominal organ. The task of diagnosis and treatment, which usually falls to the surgeon, is a subject dealt with in texts of surgery. Only a few of the common causes will be listed here: acute appendicitis, acute cholecystitis, perforated peptic ulcer, ulcerative colitis, diverticulitis, mesenteric thrombosis, volvulus, and strangulated hernia. Each of these conditions demands prompt surgical treatment. However, there are a number of other causes for which surgery is not required and, in fact, is often contraindicated. Acute pancreatitis, basal pneumonia, and acute myocardial infarction are good examples of this group. It is evident that the management of the "acute abdomen" requires great skill and considerable experience.

Review Questions

1. A 25-year-old woman is found to be anemic and complains of weight loss, diarrhea, and offensive frothy stools. Her sister had required a special diet from the age of three years because of a failure to thrive. Discuss the diagnosis.
2. What are the causes of diarrhea with the passage of blood and mucus in the feces? Indicate how information in the case history could give a clue to the most likely diagnosis in an individual patient, particularly with respect to the following:
    (a) age
    (b) duration of symptoms
    (c) travel abroad.
3. Compare Crohn's disease with ulcerative colitis in terms of these factors:
    (a) site of disease
    (b) pathological lesions
    (c) complications.
4. Compare the following diseases: bacillary dysentery, amebic dysentery, and cholera.
5. A man with an inguinal hernia complains of sudden pain over the swelling. He is constipated, and his abdominal region is producing loud gurgling noises (borborygmi). The patient begins to vomit; his condition deteriorates; he develops a fever and passes into shock. His abdomen is distended, tense, and silent. He dies. Give an account of the probable events that led to this man's death.
6. Under what conditions is an abnormal amount of fat found in the feces? What are the effects of this excess?
7. Describe the complications of a chronic gastric or duodenal ulcer.
8. Compare the effects of carcinoma of the stomach with those of carcinoma of the colon.

Selected Readings

Christie, A. B.: Infectious Diseases: Epidemiology and Clinical Practice. 2nd ed. Edinburgh, Churchill Livingstone. See, in particular, Chapter 2, "Food Poisoning: Salmonellosis"; Chapter 4, "Bacillary Dysentery"; and Chapter 5, "Infantile Gastroenteritis."

Colcock, B. P.: Benign ulcerative and granulomatous lesions of the bowel. Surgery Annual, 4:285–303, 1972.

Leading Article: Erosive gastritis. British Medical Journal, 3:211–212, 1974.

Morson, B. C., and Dawson, I. M. P.: Gastrointestinal Pathology. Oxford, Blackwell Scientific Publications Ltd., 1972. A reference book in 676 pages.

Sawyers, J. L., and Herrington, J. L.: Short gut syndrome. Surgery Annual, 4:273–284, 1972.

Schwartz, S. I., and Storer, E. H.: Manifestations of gastrointestinal disease. In Schwartz, S. I., Lillehei, R. C., Shires, G. T., Spencer, F. C., and Storer, E. H. (Eds.): Principles of Surgery. 2nd ed. New York, McGraw-Hill Book Company, 1974.

Chapter 33

After studying this chapter the student should be able to:

- Describe the structure of the normal liver and distinguish between the classic liver lobule and the acinus of Rappaport.
- Indicate how the pressure in the portal vein can be measured.
- Describe the effects of portal hypertension.
- Describe the main pathways in the metabolism of bilirubin.
- List the types of jaundice and describe the main features of each.
- Relate the effects of hepatocellular failure to the normal functions of the liver.
- Describe the causes and effects of the following:
    - (a) hepatic necrosis
    - (b) fatty liver
    - (c) chronic active hepatitis.
- Give an account of acute viral hepatitis.
- Define *cirrhosis of the liver*. Discuss the causes, main pathological lesions, and outstanding clinical features of the following:
    - (a) micronodular cirrhosis
    - (b) macronodular cirrhosis
    - (c) biliary cirrhosis.
- Classify the primary tumors of the liver.

528

DISEASES OF THE LIVER

The liver is the largest organ in the body and performs many vital functions. Its blood supply is unique; in addition to receiving arterial blood via the hepatic artery, nearly all the venous blood draining the gastrointestinal tract passes to it via the portal vein. It is therefore not surprising that the liver occupies a key position in relation to the digestive tract and that it performs many metabolic functions—particularly in relation to fat, carbohydrate, and protein metabolism. The secretion of bile is another important function of the liver. Bile contains the bile acids, which aid digestion, as well as the end products of hemoglobin catabolism. The size of the liver is therefore well matched by the multiplicity of its functions. For convenience these functions of liver may be considered under three headings:

(a) The liver in relation to its blood supply; portal hypertension
(b) Bilirubin metabolism; jaundice.
(c) Hepatocellular failure; cholemia.

In disease, each aspect of liver function can be disturbed—either separately or, more commonly, in combination.

The Liver in Relation to its Vascular Supply; Portal Hypertension

The liver has a dual blood supply. Oxygenated blood from the radicles of the hepatic artery as well as blood from the portal veins enters the liver sinusoids; the mixed blood is then collected into tributaries of the hepatic vein. The region supplied by one terminal branch of the hepatic artery is termed an *acinus* (Fig. 33–1). This functional unit differs from the classic hexagonal *liver lobule,* which is pictured as centered on a hepatic venule (Figs. 33–2 and 33–5). The liver receives much of its oxygen from the hepatic arterial blood; a deficiency of this supply results in necrosis. Such a response is seen in heart failure (see "Nutmeg liver," Chapter 28); the area affected is the peripheral part of Rappaport's acinus. Likewise, extensive necrosis is not uncommon in shock and septicemia. Infarction is rare because of the dual blood supply, but it is occasionally seen following accidental surgical ligation of the hepatic artery as well as in the rare event of disease affecting the hepatic artery, *e.g.,* polyarteritis nodosa.

The normal portal blood is of low pressure (3 to 13 mm Hg) but of large volume (some 1000 to 1200 ml enter the liver from this source per minute). The portal pressure can be measured in several ways. If a catheter is passed through an arm vein, past the right atrium of the heart and then wedged into one of the tributaries of the hepatic vein, the pressure measured in the catheter gives a good indication of the pressure in the terminal part of the hepatic sinuses. This reading is called the *postsinusoidal pressure.*

529

FIGURE 33–1. *The liver acinus.*

The liver acinus is depicted as an area supplied by a terminal branch of the hepatic artery arising in a portal triad (labeled P.S.). The cells in zone 1 are closest to their blood supply, whereas those in zone 3 are most remote. Note that the acinus contains cells belonging to two adjacent classical hexagonal lobules. The latter are pictured as being centered on a terminal hepatic venule (T.h.V.). When the blood supply of the liver is impaired (as in congestive heart failure), the cells in zone 3 first undergo necrosis. The damaged area therefore assumes the shape of a sea star (designated by heavy crosshatching). (Courtesy of Dr. A. M. Rappaport. From Rappaport, A. M.: The microcirculatory acinar concept of normal and pathological hepatic structure. Beitraege Pathologie (Stuttgart), *157*:215, 1976.)

FIGURE 33–2. *Normal liver.*

The cut surface shows the characteristic lobular pattern that is slightly accentuated by congestion. Each lobule has a dark center around a hepatic venule and is surrounded by a pale zone. The arrow points to a small subcapsular angiomatous hamartoma ("cavernous hemangioma").

If a needle connected to a manometer is passed through the skin into the spleen, the intrasplenic pressure measured is closely related to that of blood in the portal vein itself. This is called the *presinusoidal pressure.* Splenic puncture may usefully be followed by injection of a radio-opaque substance, the course of which can be followed by radiography. This is one method of demonstrating esophageal varices, a subject discussed later in this chapter.

PORTAL HYPERTENSION

Obstruction of the blood flow through the liver is a common event in chronic liver disease and leads to portal hypertension. The effects, described in the following sections, are serious:

Development of Portal-Systemic Anastomoses. There are many areas where small tributaries of the portal vein anastomose with those of the systemic circulation. When there is portal hypertension, these anastomoses enlarge and become varicose. Around the colon these varicosities are of little consequence. On the other hand, when they are around the lower end of the

FIGURE 33–3. *Radiograph showing esophageal varices.*

The patient was given a suspension of barium sulfate to swallow; the radiograph shows the outline of the esophageal lumen. Instead of appearing as a simple tube, the esophagus shows numerous indentations that are due to bulging veins. This patient had advanced cirrhosis of the liver. (Courtesy of Dr. D. E. Sanders.)

esophagus, the thin-walled dilated veins project into the esophageal lumen, and the overlying mucosa is liable to ulcerate following the trauma of swallowing food or as a result of esophagitis (Fig. 33–3). Massive bleeding is the result, and a pint or more of blood can be vomited (hematemesis).

Portal-Systemic Shunting of Blood.   Portal blood destined for the liver is shunted directly into the systemic circulation. Toxic substances from the intestine pass into the systemic circulation and contribute to the neuropsychiatric manifestations described later. Ammonia is believed to be one of these substances. Others are less well defined, but they may be responsible for the fecal odor of the breath noted in patients with chronic liver disease. Organisms from the gut can also gain access to the general circulation and can cause septicemia. Gram-negative endotoxic shock is sometimes seen as a terminal manifestation of liver disease.

The reduction in hepatic blood flow due to shunting can lead to hepatocellular necrosis but usually only as a terminal event.

Congestive Splenomegaly.   Chronic venous congestion leads to splenic enlargement, an important diagnostic clinical sign of portal hypertension. Occasionally, hypersplenism occurs (see Chapter 26).

Ascites.   This condition is considered later.

Bilirubin Metabolism and Jaundice

Of all the symptoms of liver disease, jaundice, or *icterus*, is the most immediately apparent. It is due to an excessive amount of bilirubin in the plasma and tissues. Virtually all the tissues of the body become a bright yellow; this coloration is apparent in the skin when the plasma bilirubin level reaches 2.5 to 3.0 mg per 100 ml. A sign of early jaundice is yellow discoloration of the sclera. This is a particularly useful sign in dark-skinned individuals in whom jaundice in the skin is less apparent. Jaundice can be understood only in relation to bilirubin metabolism (Fig. 33–4).

When red cells are broken down, the porphyrin moiety of the hemoglobin molecule is converted into bilirubin in the cells of the reticuloendothelial system. Bilirubin is insoluble in water; following its release from the reticuloendothelial cells, it is carried in the blood via attachment to albumin. The liver has three important functions in regard to bilirubin:

(a) *The liver extracts bilirubin from the blood.*
(b) *The liver conjugates bilirubin with glucuronic acid to form bilirubin diglucuronide.*
(c) *The liver excretes the conjugated biluribin into the bile.*

Under normal conditions 15 to 20 per cent of the bilirubin content of bile is derived from sources other than red-cell destruction. Much of this originates from the bone marrow during the *formation* of hemoglobulin (ineffective erythropoiesis). The amount of bilirubin formed in this way may be increased in disease, such as in thalassemia and pernicious anemia, and this increase contributes to jaundice. A small amount of bilirubin results from the metabolism of other porphyrins present in enzymes such as oxidases and cytochromes. Figure 33–4 illustrates the main features of bilirubin metabolism. It should be noted

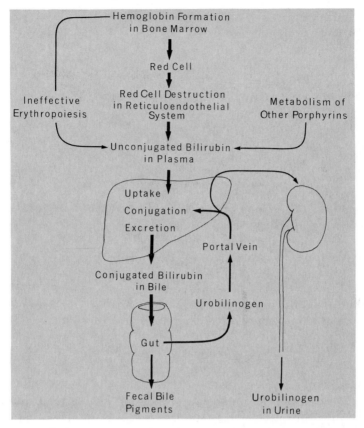

FIGURE 33-4. *Metabolic pathways in the formation and excretion of bilirubin.*

in particular that bilirubin in the intestine is converted into urobilinogen by bacterial action; since some of this urobilinogen is reabsorbed and returned to the liver, there is a very considerable enterohepatic recirculation. A small quantity of urobilinogen is excreted in the urine.

TYPES OF JAUNDICE

Obstructive Jaundice. This occurs when there is an obstruction to the passage of conjugated bilirubin from the liver cells to the intestine. Bilirubin diglucuronide is reabsorbed into the blood, and if the obstruction is complete the patient rapidly becomes deeply jaundiced. The serum bilirubin level may reach 40 mg per 100 ml. Since the conjugated bilirubin is soluble in water and is easily excreted by the kidneys, the urine is dark, contrasting with the feces, which are clay-colored. Urobilinogen disappears from the urine.

Two major types of obstructive jaundice are recognized. In *extrahepatic cholestasis,* the bile duct is blocked mechanically. This condition is commonly caused by a gallstone in its lumen or pressure from outside by a carcinoma of the head of the pancreas. In *intrahepatic cholestasis,* the other type of obstructive jaundice, no obvious mechanical cause can be found in the major bile ducts. Instead, it is assumed that the obstruction is in the canaliculi of the liver itself. This condition can occur under a variety of conditions: It is seen following the administration of certain drugs, such as chlorpromazine and other phenothiazine derivatives; it is an occasional complication of pregnancy; and it is also seen in the acute fatty alcoholic liver and sometimes during the early stages of acute viral hepatitis.

Three other characteristic features of obstructive jaundice should be noted:

(1) *Pruritus.* Often severe, this condition is probably due to retention of *bile salts.*

(2) *Malabsorption.* Due to the lack of bile in the intestine, this is a feature of chronic biliary obstruction.

(3) *Hypercholesterolemia.* This condition is due to increased synthesis by the liver rather than to biliary obstruction. Lipid-laden macrophages accumulate in various organs and may form tumorlike masses termed *xanthomas.* These structures tend to be bright yellow because of their content of carotene; they are most obvious in the skin.

Hemolytic Jaundice. An excessive rate of destruction of red cells causes an increased rate of bilirubin formation; consequently, the liver is unable to deal with the increased load. Increased erythropoiesis adds to this load by contributing additional bilirubin (Fig. 33–4). The bilirubin in the blood in hemolytic jaundice is unconjugated. It is therefore insoluble in water and is not excreted in the urine. Jaundice of this type is therefore said to be *acholuric.* Increased quantities of bile pigments are excreted in the feces, and the amount of urobilinogen returned to the liver is increased.

Hemolytic jaundice rarely reaches the intensity of that seen in the obstructive variety. An exception to this is that seen in erythroblastosis fetalis. Because unconjugated bilirubin is relatively soluble in lipids, in severe hemolytic jaundice of infancy bile pigments pass into the brain tissue and can cause severe damage to the developing central nervous system. This is called kernicterus.

Hepatocellular Jaundice. Jaundice due to liver cell degeneration or necrosis is the result of a number of factors. In part, there is a failure to extract bilirubin from the blood; in part, there is a failure to excrete it. The hepatocellular type of jaundice is therefore of mixed type.

Hepatocellular Failure

The main manifestations of hepatocellular dysfunction are related to the processes of protein and carbohydrate metabolism and to detoxification.

Disturbances of Protein Metabolism. The liver is responsible for the synthesis of most of the plasma proteins, with the major exception of the immunoglobulins. Progressive hepatocellular dysfunction is characterized by hypoalbuminemia. This dysfunction contributes to the formation of edema of the dependent parts in addition to being a factor in the production of ascites.

The liver is responsible for the synthesis of most of the clotting factors, the only notable exception being factor VIII. It is hardly surprising, therefore, that liver disease is often accompanied by tendency to bleed.

The liver is the principal site of deamination of amino acids and is probably the only organ that can convert the ammonia so produced into urea. The other site of ammonia formation is the intestine, where it is formed by bacterial decomposition of protein. Shunting of this ammonia from the portal blood into the systemic circulation has already been mentioned as a possible cause of cerebral dysfunction.

Disturbances of Carbohydrate Metabolism.   Following total hepatectomy in an experimental animal there is profound hypoglycemia. The hepatic reserve is great enough that hypoglycemia is rarely a feature of human disease; occasionally, however, it is seen in acute hepatic necrosis and following an acute episode of alcoholic debauchery. Impaired gluconeogenesis is the mechanism (see Chapter 23). The impaired glucose tolerance encountered in liver disease is due to portal systemic shunting.

Failure of Detoxification.   The liver is responsible for detoxifying many agents — either by conjugating them with glucuronic or sulfuric acid, or by conjugating them with an amino acid. The conjugated products are then excreted in the bile or in the urine: conjugation of bilirubin is a classic example of this type. Many drugs are treated in a similar way, and the administration of depressant drugs such as barbiturates or morphine may induce a coma in a patient with hepatocellular dysfunction. Likewise, some steroid hormones are conjugated in the liver prior to their excretion in the urine. The failure to detoxify aldosterone is a possible factor in the formation of ascites. The gynecomastia, testicular atrophy, and loss of body hair sometimes seen in male patients with cirrhosis have been attributed to estrogen excess resulting from inadequate inactivation.

Neuropsychiatric Manifestations (Hepatic Encephalopathy).   These pathological conditions assume many forms. Patients with chronic liver disease often exhibit steady deterioration in their intellect: forgetfulness and confusion can progress to stupor and finally to coma. Ataxia and a characteristic "flapping" tremor of the outstretched hands are noteworthy accompaniments. The neuropyschiatric manifestations may be chronic, with the patient exhibiting personality changes, mental deterioration, and other neurological symptoms. On the other hand, the syndrome may be acute and terminate in coma with convulsions.

Animals with a portacaval, or Eck shunt,* can be maintained in a reasonable state of health if given a low-protein diet. If given a large protein meal, they develop coma and die rapidly ("meat intoxication"). It is believed that these manifestations are caused by nitrogenous substances; their precise nature is not known, however. Hepatic encephalopathy is seen in patients who have undergone a similar portacaval anastomosis as treatment for cirrhosis of the liver.

Acute encephalopathy is sometimes precipitated by bleeding esophageal varices; the explanation is that the large quantity of protein-containing blood passes into the intestine and amounts to a heavy protein meal. Since bacterial action in the intestine appears to lead to the formation of damaging nitrogenous products, the administration of the antibiotic neomycin is currently recom-

---

*This is an artificial shunt made surgically between the portal vein and the inferior vena cava. Portal blood tends to flow directly into the vena cava rather than through the liver.

mended. It is also of some value in chronic liver disease with impending encephalopathy.

Terminal Manifestations of Hepatic Failure. As the patient's condition deteriorates, certain ill-understood events occur. The plasma sodium level falls, probably because of the intracellular deviation of sodium, and not because of excessive excretion, since administration of salt is not beneficial but, in fact, hastens death by producing circulatory overload. A terminal rise in blood urea nitrogen (BUN) is common and appears to be due to renal failure. This is common in severe hepatic failure, and the combination is known as the *hepatorenal syndrome.* It is debatable whether this is a separate entity. It probably represents renal failure occurring for a variety of reasons in a patient with terminal liver disease.

Degenerative Conditions of the Liver

The liver cells are very susceptible to the effects of many poisons. Poisonous mushrooms, carbon tetrachloride, chloroform, and many drugs (important among which is the anesthetic agent halothane) can all cause severe liver damage, either by a direct action or by some type of hypersensitivity response. Infections, in particular by the viruses of hepatitis, can also produce liver damage.

The effects of hepatotoxic agents can vary from mild, cloudy swelling and fatty change to extensive necrosis (see Chapter 4). There is a variable inflammatory response, and the terms "hepatic necrosis" and "hepatitis" are often used synonymously.

HEPATIC NECROSIS (HEPATITIS)

Types. If the liver cells are severely affected, they undergo necrosis. This usually has a *zonal distribution* — that is, the cells of a particular zone in every lobule undergo necrosis. Centrilobular necrosis is the most common (Fig. 33–5). Sometimes the foci of necrosis are erratically distributed: such a response is termed *focal,* or *spotty, necrosis.* It is typical of viral hepatitis.

Occasionally, the necrosis is more extensive and involves wide tracts of liver. Since whole lobules are destroyed, the term *massive necrosis* is appropriate.

Results. The outcome of necrosis depends upon the severity of the lesions. With *zonal and focal necrosis* the patient may have no symptoms or may suffer from an acute febrile illness with jaundice and gastrointestinal symptoms and then recover. The necrotic liver cells autolyze and are removed; since the sinusoidal structure and reticulin framework of the liver lobules remain intact, there is excellent regeneration as surviving liver cells divide to replace those that are lost. The liver returns to normal.

With *massive necrosis* the patient may die of acute liver failure in the initial phases; this is a feature of acute poisoning and occasionally of viral hepatitis. Some cases of massive necrosis of the liver occur for no known reason. If the patient survives the acute phase, the lobular framework of the necrotic

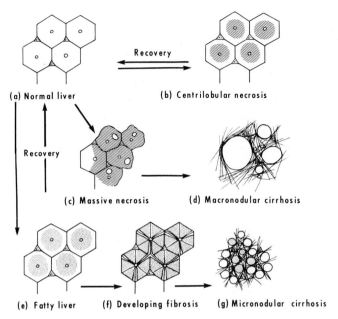

FIGURE 33–5. *The pathogenesis of hepatic cirrhosis.*

a, Depicts four normal liver lobules as hexagonal structures, each with a central hepatic vein. Between the lobules are the portal triads, each containing a branch of the hepatic artery, bile duct, and portal vein. b, shows centrilobular necrosis. When liver cell regeneration occurs, there is complete return to normal. c, Shows massive necrosis with collapse of the affected lobules. When regeneration occurs, a coarsely nodular cirrhotic liver is produced as depicted in d; in some areas normal lobules will be found. e, A fatty liver may return to normal. f, If it persists over a long period, fibrous septa form and these divide up the lobules. Some liver cells degenerate, and others form regeneration nodules. In g, a finely nodular cirrhotic liver develops. No normal lobules remain. (Drawing by Margot Mackay, Department of Art as Applied to Medicine, University of Toronto.)

areas collapses, and the destroyed areas are replaced by scar tissue. Regeneration occurs from the isolated groups of liver cells that remain; since there is no scaffold on which they may be arranged, however, irregular nodules, called *regeneration nodules,* are formed. The final result is a form of cirrhosis of the liver (Fig. 33–5).

FATTY LIVER

Fatty change is an important lesion and can be caused by an inappropriate diet. Starvation and overeating both cause fatty change, but an imbalanced diet results in the most severe change (see "Kwashiorkor," Chapter 23). It is also common in chronic alcoholism.

If the cause of a fatty liver is removed early enough, complete recovery is usual; such recovery is not possible if the condition is allowed to persist indefinitely. Gradually, fibrous tissue forms around Rappaport's acinus. Hepatic cells become isolated as the lobules are split up. Some cells undergo necrosis, whereas others regenerate. This results in a finely nodular cirrhotic liver not fundamentally different from that seen after massive necrosis.

ALCOHOL AND THE LIVER

There can be little doubt that alcohol abuse can adversely affect the liver; whether this is due to a direct toxic action of alcohol on the liver cells or to an effect of the imbalanced diet of the addict has yet to be decided. The liver of the chronic alcoholic often shows fatty change, and in some subjects this progresses to cirrhosis. Acute episodes of alcohol intake result in patchy liver cell necrosis. The cells contain alcoholic hyaline (see Fig. 4–3), and foci of necrosis are accompanied by a polymorph infiltration. This condition, which is called *alcoholic hepatitis,* is a phase in the evolution of alcoholic cirrhosis.

Hepatitis

ACUTE VIRAL HEPATITIS

Two distinct epidemiological types of acute viral hepatitis are known. In *infective hepatitis* due to virus A, the disease commonly occurs in institutions like schools and military camps. It is contracted by the ingestion of contaminated food and has an incubation period of about one month. In *serum hepatitis,* caused by virus B, the disease is usually contracted by an injection of contaminated serum. The nature of the infective agents is described in Chapter 12.

Symptoms of Viral Hepatitis.   The onset is usually insidious with mild fatigue, lassitude, and sometimes fever. Nausea, vomiting, and diarrhea are not uncommon, and an aversion to both food and cigarette smoking is a curious symptom. Such a flulike illness may be the only manifestation of hepatitis, but in other patients the disease progresses and jaundice appears, at first evident in the conjunctivae and later in the skin. Some tenderness over the liver may be noticed, and enlargement of the organ may be detected. Recovery is the usual end-result, but it may take three or four months, or even longer. The two forms of hepatitis have similar clinical features, although serum hepatitis tends to be more severe, and in an appreciable number of cases the disease progresses either to massive hepatic necrosis ending in death or to a chronic form of liver disease culminating in cirrhosis.

CHRONIC HEPATITIS

The term *chronic hepatitis* encompasses a number of different conditions that have three features in common:
(1) Infiltration of liver by inflammatory cells, usually lymphocytes and plasma cells. The infiltrate is concentrated in the portal triads.
(2) Necrosis of liver cells.
(3) Fibrosis of the liver that may terminate in cirrhosis.
The diagnosis of chronic hepatitis is generally made on the liver biopsy. The following types can be recognized:

Chronic Active Hepatitis.   This disease is characterized by recurrent attacks of hepatitis, ultimately developing into cirrhosis, usually of the macronodular type, which is fatal within 10 years. The disease was first described as affecting young people, 75 per cent of the patients being women.

Hypergammaglobulinemia is a characteristic feature, and both antinuclear factor and rheumatoid factors are usually present. Although the disease was originally called *lupoid hepatitis,* there is no evidence that the condition is related to lupus erythematosus itself. Nevertheless, over half the patients also have arthritis. Antibodies that react with smooth muscle are present in most cases, and the disease therefore has a strong autoimmune component.

The syndrome of chronic active hepatitis has now been extended to include other groups of patients. Some are middle-aged women, and others are men who usually have HBAg in their blood. Autoantibodies are usually present, but this autoimmune component is less striking than in the original "lupoid hepatitis."

Other Types of Chronic Hepatitis. There are other types of chronic hepatitis that do not fit into the entity designated chronic active hepatitis. Some are cases of patients who have recovered from an acute attack of viral hepatitis, and yet have evidence of continuing liver damage. Others are asymptomatic and yet are chronic carriers of the hepatitis antigen. Still others have neither HBAg nor demonstrable autoantibodies in their plasma. Viral infection, resolving alcoholic hepatitis, and drug-induced liver damage are suggested as possible causes in this heterogeneous group of conditions labeled chronic hepatitis.

Cirrhosis of the Liver

The term "cirrhosis" (from Greek *kirrhos,* orange yellow + *nosos,* disease) was introduced by Laennec, who was impressed by the tawny color of the liver in this condition, but this is due merely to fatty change of the liver cells. The important structural features of cirrhosis are the *destruction of the liver parenchyma* and its *replacement by fibrous tissue,* thereby disrupting the normal lobular architecture. There is also active regeneration of the liver cells occurring at the same time as this fibrous reparative process. The *formation of regenerative nodules* is the third essential component of cirrhosis.

Cirrhosis is best regarded as an end-stage condition resulting from liver damage due to any cause: poisons, alcohol, inadequate diet, infection, genetic error, and others. Unfortunately, an etiological classification of cirrhosis is unsatisfactory, because the cause is unknown in many cases *("cryptogenic cirrhosis").* For purposes of disease classification, the condition is categorized by descriptions that are based on the gross appearance of the liver. If the nodules are small and of uniform size, the term *micronodular cirrhosis* is applied (Figs. 33–6 and 33–7). This condition commonly, but not always, is due to alcohol abuse. It contrasts with *macronodular cirrhosis* in which the nodules are of varying size, many of them being large (Fig. 33–8). In practice, there is no sharp line of demarcation between these two types of cirrhosis, and many cases fall into a mixed group.

Symptoms of Cirrhosis. Cirrhosis is commonly asymptomatic until some complication makes the condition obvious. The appearance of jaundice, edema of the ankles, or progressive abdominal enlargement may bring the disease to the attention of the patient. Increasing weakness, loss of weight, loss of body hair and testicular atrophy are all features that may appear. Commonly the first

FIGURE 33–6. *Micronodular cirrhosis of the liver.*

The cut surface of the specimen shows complete loss of the normal lobular pattern (compare with Figure 33–2). The liver parenchyma now consists of poorly delineated regeneration nodules that are best seen where light is reflected from the surface on the right-hand side of the picture. In some areas, extensive fibrosis appears as obvious gray-white tissue. The specimen is from a patient who died of bleeding esophageal varices, and who exhibited little clinical evidence of hepatic dysfunction until shortly before death. For a more complete description, see Case History I.

Case History I.   (See Figure 33–6). The patient was a 62-year-old woman with a long history of chronic alcoholism. Six days before admission to a hospital, she noticed black tarry stools (melena). A few days later, she vomited about one pint of blood. On admission, her blood pressure was 95/60 mm Hg, and she was in a state of shock. Her abdomen was distended because of ascites, and her spleen could not be felt. Jaundice was not evident. Laboratory investigations at this time revealed the following:

Serum bilirubin: 1.75 mg per 100 ml (normal, 0.3 to 1.0 mg per 100 ml)
Serum proteins:
  Albumin: 1.8 g per 100 ml (normal, 4.0 to 5.7 g per 100 ml)
  Globulin: 3.9 g per 100 ml (normal, 1.5 to 3.0 g per 100 ml)
  Total: 5.7 g per 100 ml (normal 6.2 to 8.2 g per 100 ml)
Serum potassium: 2.5 mEq per liter (normal, 3.5 to 5.0 mEq per liter)
Hemoglobin: 10.9 g per 100 ml; red cells normochromic and normocytic.

The hypokalemia was attributed to previous diuretic therapy (see Chapter 19). Gastroscopy revealed bleeding esophageal varices, but in spite of transfusion and other supportive treatment, the blood pressure continued to fall, and the patient became more and more confused. She vomited a small quantity of blood on several occasions, but showed no obvious dramatic hemorrhage. Terminally, her urine output diminished, her blood urea nitrogen rose to 65 mg per 100 ml, and the patient suffered a cardiac arrest. She was successfully resuscitated but had a second arrest and was pronounced dead.

Necropsy revealed bilateral pleural effusions and 1500 ml of ascites. There were multiple small acute gastric erosions, and the small hematemeses occurring in the hospital were attributed to them. The kidneys were swollen because of edema, but necrosis was not detectable microscopically (see Chapter 35). The cirrhotic liver, which weighed 1900 grams (normal, about 1500 grams), is shown in Figure 33–6. Esophageal varices were present, but no definite point of bleeding could be identified; this is often difficult, since the veins are emptied of blood after death.

FIGURE 33–7. *Cirrhosis of the liver with fatty change.*

The cut surface of the liver appears very pale; it was greasy to the touch because of severe fatty change. Close inspection reveals loss of the normal lobular architecture and replacement of that structure by small regeneration nodules. This alteration is an example of micronodular cirrhosis; the fatty change gives it a tawny color. For a more complete description, see Case History II.

Case History II. (See Figure 33–7.) The patient was an alcoholic who had died suddenly of a massive pulmonary embolism. He had been treated previously for three separate tumors. In 1963 the patient had a resection of a carcinoma of the colon. In 1968 a carcinoma of the prostate had been resected through the urethra. Estrogen (stilbestrol) had controlled the residual tumor since that time, but the hormone treatments had produced gynecomastia and may have contributed to his heart failure. In 1974 he had an operation for removal of a squamous-cell carcinoma of the lung; he died shortly after the operation. Necropsy revealed residual carcinoma of the prostate, arteriosclerotic heart disease, phlebothrombosis in both leg veins, and massive pulmonary embolism.

FIGURE 33–8. *Macronodular cirrhosis of the liver.*

There is replacement of liver by regeneration nodules that vary greatly in size. The two circular hemorrhagic (dark) nodules shown here consist of hepatoma.

symptom is massive hematemesis and the rapid development of hepatocellular failure with coma and death.

Ascites is a common manifestation of cirrhosis and has several causes. Hypoalbuminemia and aldosterone excess are contributory factors, but the main cause appears to be obstruction of the flow of blood through the liver. This obstruction is postsinusoidal, and results in an increased rate of formation of lymph in the liver. Normally the lymph is drained away by lymphatics into the thoracic duct, but in cirrhosis, the vast excess of lymph produced oozes or weeps from the liver and drips into the peritoneal cavity. The ascites of cirrhosis of the liver is, therefore, a type of lymphedema. Relief of this ascites by removal of the fluid also removes much albumin, often adding to the patient's problems. Also the sudden removal of a large quantity of fluid can lead to hypovolemia and shock.

The other symptoms of terminal cirrhosis—including neuropsychiatric features, coma, and a bleeding tendency—have been described under hepatocellular failure.

BILIARY CIRRHOSIS

Obstruction to the bile duct, particularly if combined with infection (cholangitis) can sometimes lead to such severe liver-cell damage that cirrhosis develops. There is, in addition, a *primary form of biliary cirrhosis.* This is most frequently encountered in middle-aged women. Itching is usually the first symptom, and this is followed by the development of obstructive jaundice. The disease has an autoimmune component, for the blood contains IgM antibodies active against bile-duct components as well as IgG antimitochondrial antibodies. The detection of the latter is a useful diagnostic feature of primary biliary cirrhosis.

Tumors of the Liver

The finding of one or more *vascular hamartomas* (hemangiomas) of the liver is a common event at necropsy, but apart from the very rare occurrence of intraperitoneal bleeding, these are of no significance during life (Fig. 33–4). *Adenomas* are rare, although recently a number of cases have been reported in women on the birth-control pill. The tumors are vascular and clinically can present as a sudden intraperitoneal hemorrhage. This appears to be a rare complication of taking the birth-control pill, but since the event has only recently been recognized, its true incidence has yet to be determined.

CARCINOMA OF THE LIVER

Cancer of the liver can arise in a normal liver, but it is more often encountered in livers that are already the site of some other disease, most commonly cirrhosis (Figs. 33–8 and 33–9). Nevertheless, many other factors are involved, for although in North America and Europe it has been estimated that between

FIGURE 33-9. *Carcinoma of the liver.*

The specimen shows a large, spherical mass of tumor with several small satellite nodules. The tumor has invaded the inferior vena cava, and there is superimposed thrombosis (arrow at lower center). The remainder of the liver shows the characteristic features of micronodular cirrhosis. The nodularity can be seen best on the surface of the liver (arrow at upper left).

The patient had a 13-year history of chronic liver disease and had died following massive bleeding from ruptured esophageal varices. Necropsy revealed tumor invasion of the vena cava and the portal vein. Small pulmonary deposits were the only metastases found. Splenomegaly, ascites, edema of the legs, and testicular atrophy were other findings related to the liver disease.

4 and 10 per cent of patients with cirrhosis eventually develop cancer of the liver, in some parts of Africa and the Orient the figure is closer to 60 per cent. Additional factors that seem to be involved are the ingestion of aflatoxin, an alkaloid derived from a fungus that infects peanuts in African diet and the presence of HBAg antigen, which is present in patients with hepatitis.

Two types of primary carcinoma of the liver are recognized:

Hepatoma. This tumor is composed of atypical hepatocytes and usually occurs in patients with cirrhosis. Quite often portal vein invasion and thrombosis lead to the sudden development of ascites in a patient known to have cirrhosis. Massive hepatomegaly is usually a feature.

Cholangiocarcinoma. About 20 per cent of primary liver tumors are derived from the bile ducts, and histologically they are scirrhous adenocarcinomas. Cirrhosis of the liver is less often a precursor to this type of cancer than hepatoma.

SECONDARY TUMORS OF THE LIVER

It has been estimated that metastatic liver carcinoma is found in about 36 per cent of all cancer patients. It is more common in patients with cancer of the breast, stomach, and colon than in those having primary tumors of other sites. The liver is also a common site for metastatic melanoma.

Review Questions

1. The condition of a man with known chronic liver disease suddenly deteriorates, and he dies. Describe the lesions that you would expect to find at his necropsy.
2. Compare obstructive jaundice with hemolytic jaundice with particular reference to the following:
     (a) the color of the patient
     (b) the color of the urine and feces
     (c) the quantity of urobilinogen in the urine.
3. Why is it dangerous to administer to a patient with advanced liver disease each of the following:
     (a) a large protein meal
     (b) morphine
     (c) intravenous saline?
4. Describe the known factors in the cause and pathogenesis of hepatic cirrhosis.

Selected Readings

Rappaport, A. M.: The microcirculatory hepatic unit. Microvascular Research, 6:212–228, 1973.
Schaffner, F., Sherlock, S., and Leevy, C. M. (Eds.): The Liver and Its Diseases. New York, Intercontinental Medical Book Corporation, 1974, 353 pp. An advanced reference book covering a wide range of topics by 47 contributors.
Sherlock, S.: Diseases of the Liver and Biliary System. 5th ed. Oxford, Blackwell, Scientific Publications Ltd., 1975, 821 pp.
Scheuer, P. J.: Liver Biopsy Interpretation. 2nd ed. London, Baillière Tindall, 1973, 171 pp. An excellent reference book on the morphological aspects of liver disease.
Smetana, H. F.: Cirrhosis of the liver: principles of classification, histogenesis, and pathogenesis. Pathology Annual, 7:107–144, 1972.
Robbins, S. L.: Pathologic Basis of Disease. Philadelphia, W. B. Saunders Company, 1974. Note, in particular, Chapter 22, "The Liver and Biliary Tract."

DISEASES OF THE PANCREAS
AND THE BILIARY TRACT

Chapter 34

After studying this chapter the student should be able to:

- List the secretions of the pancreas.
- Describe the main features of cystic fibrosis as it affects the pancreas, the lungs, and the eccrine sweat glands.
- Describe the known causes, the course, the lesions, and the complications of acute pancreatitis.
- Outline the main features of
    (a) chronic pancreatitis
    (b) carcinoma of the head of the pancreas
    (c) carcinoma of the body of the pancreas.
- Name the structures that constitute the biliary tract.
- List the common types of gallstones.
- Describe the factors that are thought to lead to gallstone formation.
- List the complications of cholelithiasis.
- Describe the clinical and pathological features of the following conditions:
    (a) chronic cholecystitis
    (b) carcinoma of the gallbladder
    (c) carcinoma of the ampulla of Vater.

DISEASES OF THE PANCREAS
AND THE BILIARY TRACT

THE PANCREAS

DEVELOPMENT AND FUNCTION

The pancreas is a dual organ. Its exocrine portion originates from two buds of the primitive gut. The endocrine portion forms the islets of Langerhans, which, despite their small size, are of vital importance because they secrete insulin.

The pancreas lies on the posterior abdominal wall and pours its exocrine secretions into the duodenum. These secretions contain the precursors of three important enzymes: (1) *trypsin*, which digests protein; (2) *lipase*, which splits fat; and (3) *amylase*, which splits carbohydrate. In each case the active enzyme is formed within the contents of the duodenum. The reserve capacity of the pancreas is so great that only severe atrophy of the exocrine elements or blockage of its duct leads to upsets in digestion and absorption. In practice, impairment of fat absorption is the most important disorder; steatorrhea and lack of absorption of fat-soluble vitamins are the predominant symptoms of this condition (see Chapter 32).

CYSTIC FIBROSIS (MUCOVISCIDOSIS)

This disease is inherited as a Mendelian autosomal recessive trait. It is characterized by an abnormality of the exocrine secretory glands and is remarkable for the great variety of its presentations, depending on which glands are affected.

When the pancreas is involved, the gland secretes thick mucus that obstructs the ducts and causes them to dilate. The gland itself atrophies. If the disease develops *in utero*, the absence of pancreatic enzymes leads to such viscosity of the intestinal contents (called *meconium*) that intestinal obstruction and even perforation of the gut ensue *(meconium ileus)*. In the more common type of cystic fibrosis, the infant or child develops a chronic *malabsorption syndrome*, often accompanied by constipation.

When the lung is involved, the thick mucus together with infection produces bronchopneumonia, bronchiectasis, and lung abscesses (see Fig. 30–8). Chronic lung disease is a feature of most cases of cystic fibrosis in patients

547

who survive for several years. Hypovitaminosis A and other effects of malabsorption complicate this clinical picture.

Occasionally the liver and salivary glands are affected. A remarkable feature of the disease is that the eccrine sweat glands secrete a sweat containing a high concentration of salt. *Chemical examination of sweat for the level of salt is a diagnostic test.*

The fundamental defect in cystic fibrosis is not yet known. The secretion of viscid mucus plays an important role in the pancreatic and lung lesions. It does not explain the abnormal sweat-gland function, because sweat contains no mucus.

ACUTE PANCREATITIS

Acute pancreatitis can be mild and can lead to vague abdominal symptoms, but more often it is severe, of sudden onset, and presenting with intense pain often referred to as an "acute abdomen."

Areas of pancreas undergo necrosis and there is an associated acute inflammatory reaction. The pathogenesis is obscure, for although in a few instances the cause is a known infectious agent (*e.g.,* mumps virus) the vast majority of cases are not so related. The disease appears to be due to the sudden release of active pancreatic enzymes within the organ itself. Blood vessels are digested, and in severe cases the whole pancreas is converted into a necrotic, hemorrhagic mass. Released lipases cause necrosis in adjacent peripancreatic fat and omentum; because of their *dystrophic calcification* these areas of fat necrosis are soon evident as chalky white areas. So rapidly may this calcification occur that the patient actually develops symptoms of hypocalcemia (*e.g.,* tetany). The necrotic pancreatic cells release amylase, which can be detected in the blood. A blood amylase determination is a useful test for the diagnosis of acute pancreatitis.

Symptoms of acute hemorrhagic pancreatitis are sometimes difficult to distinguish from those of other causes of acute abdominal pain (*e.g.,* perforated peptic ulcer, acute cholecystitis, and acute appendicitis). Laparotomy is often performed because of the difficulty in arriving at a diagnosis; the surgeon is confronted by blood-stained ascitic fluid containing globules of fat. The detection of amylase in the fluid further confirms the diagnosis. Also characteristic is the presence of many foci of fat necrosis with calcification.

Etiology.   Most patients with acute pancreatitis have chronic gall bladder disease and attacks usually occur *after a large meal* or an *alcoholic spree.* The pathogenesis is not completely understood, but it is thought the entry of a large quantity of acid gastric contents, particularly if it contains alcohol, can lead to excessive stimulation of the pancreas by the hormone *secretin,* which is released from the duodenal mucosa.

Course of Acute Pancreatitis.   Up to 50 per cent of patients die in shock during the first week. Surgery can contribute to this. Complications in those who survive this period are *abscess* and *pseudocyst formation.* The latter consists of a loculated accumulation of fluid in the peritoneum adjacent to the pancreas. Such a cyst usually requires surgical drainage. Another cause of pseudocyst formation is direct injury to the pancreas by a blow to the abdomen.

CHRONIC PANCREATITIS

Chronic pancreatitis—like the acute form of the condition—is also associated with gallbladder disease, overindulgence, and alcoholism. The clinical picture is vague; it ranges from no symptoms at all, to repeated attacks of mild acute pancreatitis that are not severe enough to warrant surgical intervention. Sometimes the major complaint is one of a constant pain in the back.

In its early stages chronic pancreatitis leads to no digestive upset. Later, however, signs of malabsorption may appear, and in a few cases impaired glucose tolerance and diabetes mellitus supervene.

An important feature of chronic pancreatitis is that a surgeon may easily mistake the hard fibrous organ for carcinoma. Even when biopsy or necropsy material is available, the distinction between a fibrosed atrophic pancreas and a scirrhous carcinoma can be very difficult.

CARCINOMA OF THE PANCREAS

Cancer of the pancreas arises from the ducts and is the most important tumor to be considered. About two thirds of the tumors arise in the head of the pancreas. Obstructive jaundice is often the first sign, and characteristically the obstruction is associated with palpable distention of the gallbladder. Carcinoma of the body or tail of the pancreas produces few symptoms until the growth is large, has invaded local structures, or has metastasized. Loss of appetite, loss of weight, vague back pain, and general malaise with depression are the symptoms of this silent killer.

The treatment of carcinoma of the pancreas is extremely unsatisfactory. Occasionally surgical resection is possible, but the inaccessibility of the pancreas and the closeness of important anatomical structures make this disease untreatable in the majority of the cases. Anastomosis of the gallbladder to a loop of intestine relieves the obstructive jaundice with its distressing pruritus.

THE ISLETS OF LANGERHANS

Diseases of the islets are considered in Chapter 24, because their major effects are on glucose metabolism.

THE BILIARY TRACT

INTRODUCTION

Bile is formed continuously by the liver and passes down the *intrahepatic bile ducts* to reach the *common bile duct*. This duct empties into the duodenum, and its orifice is guarded by the *sphincter of Oddi*. Immediately above the sphincter, there is a dilatation called the *ampulla of Vater*. The sphincter of Oddi is normally closed, and bile therefore flows through the *cystic duct* to reach the *gallbladder*, where it is stored and concentrated. When gastric contents—particularly that containing fat—enter the duodenum, the duodenal mucosa secretes a hormone *(cholecystokinin)* that causes the gallbladder to

FIGURE 34–1. *Gallstones.*

The three gallstones shown in the upper part of the picture were solitary stones, each being found in a separate gallbladder. They are composed mainly of cholesterol. One has been cut to show its internal structure. The appearance of lines radiating from the center is due to crystals of cholesterol.

The three faceted stones in the lower part of the picture were found in one gallbladder. One which has been cut, shows a pale center of cholesterol. This is surrounded by rings that contain varying amounts of bile pigments. These stones are considered "mixed."

contract and the sphincter of Oddi to relax. Bile then enters the duodenum.

Diseases of the gallbladder are frequent. Inflammation of this organ *(cholecystitis)* ranks with appendicitis as a cause of abdominal pain requiring surgical exploration. The presence of gallstones *(cholelithiasis)* is often associated with inflammation. This topic is discussed below.

CHOLELITHIASIS

Gallstones may be found in any part of the biliary tract, but they are most frequent in the gallbladder. They are more common in women than in men, in a ratio of about four to one. Pregnancy appears to predispose female patients to stone formation, and the typical sufferer is caricatured as being "female, fertile, fat, and forty." Nevertheless, gallstone disease often affects young adults, and any association with obesity appears to be without foundation.

Types of Gallstones. Gallstones are occasionally composed of pure cholesterol (usually solitary stones) or bile pigments (calcium bilirubinate); most gallstones are *mixed* and consist of cholesterol, bile salts, and calcium salts. Often they are multiple (Figs. 34–1 and 34–2).

Cause of Gallstones. Until recently, *infection* and *stasis* were considered to be the main factors leading to gallstone formation. It is now thought that infection and stasis are the *effects* of cholelithasis, and that the major cause is the *secretion of an abnormal bile by the liver.* The large amount of cholesterol in bile is kept in solution by its being aggregated to form *micelles* having an outer coating of phospholipid and bile salts. A deficiency of bile salt formation appears to be the major factor in producing gallstones.

Complications of Gallstones

OBSTRUCTION.   A stone may become impacted in the neck of the gallbladder or in the cystic duct. Because bile cannot enter the gallbladder, it therefore becomes distended with mucus *(mucocele)*. A stone impacted in the bile duct *(e.g.,* in the ampulla of Vater) causes intermittent obstruction with *obstructive jaundice.* This condition fluctuates in intensity in contrast to the progressive jaundice of carcinoma.

If a gallstone suddenly obstructs one of the bile passages, distention of the wall causes severe pain that is felt in the midline of the abdomen. The common cause is a stone in the cystic duct. The pain is of sudden onset, persists for some hours with unremitting severity, and then abates as suddenly as it began. This is called *biliary colic* and differs from intestinal colic, in which crampy pains recur and remit at intervals.

INFECTION.   The presence of stones in the gallbladder predisposes the patient to the development of cholecystitis. Likewise, a stone in the common bile duct predisposes to infection in the entire intrahepatic biliary system *(ascending cholangitis).* This can be mild and clinically inapparent, or it can cause severe symptoms. Attacks of fever with liver tenderness and jaundice indicate suppurative cholangitis with liver abscess formation.

FIGURE 34–2. *Gallstones.*

One gallbladder contained these small mixed stones. Note how each stone is faceted as a result of contact with its neighbors during its formation. Several "families" of stones are present.

FIGURE 34–3. *Chronic cholecystitis.*

The mucosa is heavily infiltrated by small round cells that under higher power proved to be lymphocytes and plasma cells. The muscular coat has been largely replaced by fibrous tissue and is greatly thickened. The wall contains many glandular spaces, *called Rokitansky-Aschoff sinuses.* These are invaginations of the surface epithelium and must not be mistaken for carcinoma (× 60).

Acute Cholecystitis. Acute cholecystitis is characterized by the sudden onset of pain, fever, nausea, and vomiting. The pain, accompanied by tenderness, is in the right upper quadrant of the abdomen. In over 90 per cent of cases, gallstones are present, and there is often either a history of a previous attack or other symptoms attributable to the stones.

The cause and pathogenesis of acute cholecystitis are not known. Infection is not the cause, since organisms are not present in the bile in the early stages. Impaction of a stone is probably an important factor in initiating an attack. Distention of the gallbladder may imperil its blood supply so that infarction occurs.

Many cases of acute cholecystitis subside spontaneously. The mode of treatment is controversial; some surgeons delay operating until absolutely necessary. In some cases the gallbladder ruptures, leading to a severe peritonitis, which is due partly to an irritating effect of bile and partly to organisms that are found in the later stages of an acutely inflamed gallbladder.

Chronic Cholecystitis. Repeated attacks of acute cholecystitis (either mild or severe) combined with stones results in the gallbladder's becoming greatly thickened, shrunken, and functionless (Fig. 34–3). At this stage the symptoms are vague: flatulence, aversion to fatty foods, indigestion, and ill-defined pain in the upper abdomen.

CARCINOMA OF THE BILIARY TRACT

Carcinoma of the Gallbladder. This tumor is more common in women and the elderly. The prognosis is very poor, since local spread to the liver has generally occurred by the time the diagnosis has been made.

Carcinoma of the Ampulla of Vater. This is an occasional cause of obstructive jaundice.

Review Questions

1. A 70-year-old man has gradually increasing jaundice. He complains of no pain. Discuss the possible causes and indicate the one that is most likely.
2. Describe the clinical features that one should consider in differentiating between an attack of acute pancreatitis and an attack of acute cholecystitis.
3. Courvoisier's law indicates that in obstructive jaundice due to a malignant tumor, the gallbladder is distended and can be palpated, whereas in obstructive jaundice due to gallstones the gallbladder is small and cannot be palpated. Can you suggest why this should be true?

Selected Readings

Leading Article: Dynamics of the common duct. Lancet, 1:236–237, 1968.
Leading Article: Vascular aspects of cholecystitis. British Medical Journal, 2:133, 1968.
Leading Article: Abnormal bile or faulty gall bladder? British Medical Journal, 4:571–572, 1970.
Robbins, S. L.: Pathologic Basis of Disease. Philadelphia, W. B. Saunders Company, 1974. See, in particular, pp. 1038–1055 for a discussion of the biliary system as well as pp. 1056–1077, which is the chapter on the pancreas.

Chapter 35

After studying this chapter the student should be able to:

- Describe the major functions of the kidney.
- Outline the process of urine formation and indicate the relative roles of the various parts of the nephron.
- Define polyuria, polydipsia, nocturia, anuria, and retention with overflow.
- Describe the principles underlying the creatinine clearance test.
- List the methods that are used to examine urine in clinical medicine.
- Describe the important causes and manifestations of acute renal failure.
- Describe the important causes and manifestations of chronic renal failure.
- Describe the important causes and manifestations of the nephrotic syndrome.
- List the types of glomerulonephritis and indicate the outstanding features of each type.

DISEASES OF THE KIDNEYS
AND URINARY TRACT

- Describe the main features and known causes of interstitial nephritis.
- Discuss the pathogenesis of urinary tract infection and describe the clinical features of each of the following: acute urethritis with cystitis, acute pyelonephritis, and chronic pyelonephritis.
- Describe what is meant by the term "end-stage kidney."
- Compare clear-cell carcinoma of the kidney with carcinoma of the bladder.
- Describe the common causes and effects of urinary tract obstruction.
- Classify the types of urinary calculi and list their effects.

THE KIDNEYS

It is a popular misconception that the only major function performed by the kidneys is the excretion of the waste products of metabolism. In fact, the kidneys have many other functions, particularly in relation to maintaining a fixed internal environment. Unless these other functions are appreciated, the features of renal failure cannot be understood.

FUNCTIONS OF THE KIDNEY

1. EXCRETION OF UREA AND CREATININE. These two substances are the nitrogenous end-products of protein metabolism. The normal level of blood urea is between 20 and 40 mg per 100 ml and is often expressed as the blood urea nitrogen (BUN). The normal BUN is 10 to 20 mg per 100 ml. The normal level of blood creatinine is 1.2 mg per 100 ml. Renal failure results in a rise in the level of these two nitrogenous substances in the blood; the resultant condition is called *azotemia.**

2. REGULATION OF EXTRACELLULAR FLUIDS. This is accomplished by controlling the excretion of water and electrolytes—particularly sodium.

3. REGULATION OF ACID-BASE BALANCE. The kidney contributes to the maintenance of a stable blood pH by the excretion of hydrogen ions. This excretion takes place mainly in the distal tubule where hydrogen ions are combined either with phosphate or with ammonia. The synthesis of ammonia by the kidney and its conversion into ammonium ions is an important mechanism in acid-base homeostasis.

---

*The term is derived from *azote*, a name for nitrogen proposed by Lavoisier.

4. REGULATION OF BLOOD PRESSURE.   This aspect of renal failure, which is incompletely understood, is discussed in Chapter 20. There seems little doubt that under some circumstances an ischemic kidney can produce renin, which can then lead to hypertension.

5. REGULATION OF ERYTHROPOIESIS.   Erythropoietin is produced mainly by the kidney and acts as a stimulus to red-cell production. The precise physiological role of this process is not understood; it is known, however, that anemia is very common in renal failure. Occasionally tumors of the kidney result in excessive erythropoietin production, causing polycythemia to ensue.

MECHANISM OF URINE FORMATION: NORMAL AND ABNORMAL

The formation of urine by the normal kidney is described in textbooks of physiology; consequently, only a brief outline of the salient features will be described here.

The glomerular filtrate (approximately 180 liters per day) is derived from blood flowing through the glomerulus and has a similar composition to plasma, except that it has a very low protein content. In the proximal convoluted tubule, 80 per cent of the water and virtually all of the protein and glucose are reabsorbed. If the blood glucose level (and therefore the level in the glomerular filtrate) is high—as in diabetes mellitus—the proximal convoluted tubules are unable to reabsorb all the glucose and this substance thus passes into the urine (a condition called *glycosuria*). Occasionally glycosuria occurs in the presence of a normal blood glucose level; this condition, which is known as *renal glycosuria*, is due to defective tubular function.

In many renal diseases the glomerular vessels become more permeable to protein, and the proximal convoluted tubules are unable to reabsorb the excess protein. The *proteinuria* that results is an important and common finding in renal disease.

Absorption of electrolytes in the proximal tubules is such that the luminal fluid is isotonic with plasma, and the process is therefore called "iso-osmotic absorption." Urea passes freely out of the tubules.

In the ascending limb of the loop of Henle there is considerable transfer of sodium chloride from the lumen to the interstitial fluid of the medulla. Because this part of the renal tubule is impermeable to water, it follows that the modified filtrate within the lumen becomes progressively hypotonic, while the interstitial fluid becomes hypertonic.

In the distal tubule, the pH of the filtrate and its electrolyte composition are finally adjusted. When the hypotonic fluid leaves the loop of Henle and enters the distal tubule, it becomes isotonic with plasma once more, since this part of the nephron is fully permeable to water.

Because the filtrate is surrounded by the hypertonic interstitial fluid of the medulla, in its course through the collecting tubules it tends to maintain osmotic equilibrium by transferring some of its water to the interstitial fluid. The filtrate thereby attains the final composition of urine. The permeability of the distal tubule and collecting tubules is regulated by the circulating level of antidiuretic hormone (ADH) secreted by the posterior pituitary. This hormone, by rendering the tubules more permeable to water, aids the transfer of water from the tubules into the interstitial tissue. A high level of ADH, such as occurs during dehydration, results in the production of a highly concentrated urine. In the absence of antidiuretic hormone, such as occurs in *diabetes insipidus*, a large quantity of dilute urine is produced. Normally 1½ to 2 liters of urine are passed daily; if this quantity is exceeded, the condition is termed *polyuria*. Tubules damaged by hypercalcemia or hypokalemia are less responsive to the action of ADH, and the situation also leads to polyuria. Likewise, the regenerating epithelium of the tubules following tubular necrosis is unresponsive to the action of ADH, and again polyuria results.

If the fluid in the tubules contains an excess of an osmotically active substance such as glucose, water absorption is impeded. It follows that in diabetes mellitus polyuria is a characteristic feature. Since water is lost, thirst is increased, and an excessive quantity of water is drunk *(polydipsia)*. A similar situation occurs in chronic renal failure. The blood urea level is high, and the amount of urea in the glomerular filtrate is also raised, hindering water absorption. Polyuria and polydipsia ensue. It is evident that one of the features of the normal kidney is its ability to produce a highly concentrated or a highly dilute urine according to circumstances. As renal function becomes impaired, this ability is lost and eventually a urine of fixed osmolality is produced.

The continuous production of urine with a specific gravity of about 1.010 regardless of the fluid intake has several important consequences. If the fluid intake is high, then water retention occurs. If the water intake of the body is low, then dehydration results. Finally the normal ability to produce a concentrated urine during sleep is lost, forcing the patient to get up to pass urine during the night, a feature described as *nocturia*.

TESTS OF RENAL FUNCTION

CLEARANCE VALUES. Inulin is a substance that passes freely from the plasma into the glomerular filtrate and is neither absorbed by the tubules nor secreted by them. If U is the concentration of inulin in mg per 100 ml in the urine and V is the volume of urine passed each minute, UV mg is the amount of inulin passed per minute. If the plasma concentration of inulin is P mg per 100 ml, UV mg is contained in $\frac{UV}{P}$ ml, which is the amount of plasma "cleared" of inulin each minute and is equal to the glomerular filtrate (normally 120 ml per min). This forms the basis of a useful clinical test. In practice, the inulin clearance test is difficult to perform, but since creatinine is treated similarly, the *creatinine clearance* is estimated and is a good measure of glomerular filtration rate. The required measurements are: blood creatinine level, the volume of urine passed over a 1-hour period and the creatinine content of a sample of this urine. The normal range is 90 to 130 ml per min. The urea clearance test is also a commonly performed test, but since some urea is reabsorbed by the tubules, the urea clearance is approximately 5/8 of the normal glomerular filtration rate, *i.e.*, the normal range is 60 to 100 ml per min.

BLOOD UREA. The blood urea nitrogen (BUN) is related in part to the protein intake in the diet and in part to renal function. Figure 35–1 shows the relationship between glomerular filtration rate and blood urea. Note that the BUN

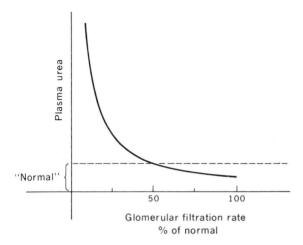

FIGURE 35–1. *Graph showing the relationship between the glomerular filtration rate and the plasma urea concentration.*

Note that the plasma urea concentration remains within normal limits until the glomerular filtration rate has fallen to less than 50 per cent of normal. (From Epstein, F. H.: Approach to the patient with renal disease. *In* Wintrobe, M. M., et al. (Eds.): Harrison's Principles of Internal Medicine. 7th ed. New York, McGraw-Hill Book Company, 1974, pp. 1367–1370. Copyright © 1974 by McGraw-Hill, Inc. Used by permission of McGraw-Hill Book Company.)

is an insensitive indicator of renal function and that at least 50 per cent of kidney substance must be destroyed before an appreciable rise in the BUN is seen. The blood creatinine level is related to muscle bulk and not to dietary intake, and the level of blood creatinine is a more useful indication of renal function.

EXAMINATION OF URINE

Diseases of the kidney and urinary tract are often reflected in abnormalities in the urine and are so common that an examination of the urine *(urinalysis)* is a mandatory procedure with any patient admitted to a hospital or undergoing a routine physical examination. The following methods can be used.

CHEMICAL EXAMINATION. Simple tests are available for detecting protein, glucose, hemoglobin, and ketone bodies. If necessary the amount of protein can be measured; the normal quantity excreted in 24 hours is under 150 mg. Individual proteins can be identified by electroimmunophoresis; for example, Bence Jones protein can be categorized by this method (see page 642).

SPECIFIC GRAVITY. The normal kidney can concentrate urine such that the specific gravity reaches 1.022 or more after a period of dehydration or an injection of vasopressin. Specific gravity readings are misleading if heavy solutes such as glucose or protein are present in the urine. Under these circumstances the freezing point method of detecting osmolarity must be performed.

The normal kidney can dilute urine following a water load, but tests based on this are unreliable and are not used in practice.

MICROSCOPIC EXAMINATION. Much can be learned by an examination of the centrifuged deposit from a sample of fresh urine. A scanty number of red cells, polymorphs, and epithelial cells are normally present. An excess of red cells indicates bleeding. The presence of these cells can usefully distinguish between *hematuria*, which is the presence of red cells in the blood, and *he-*

moglobinuria, which is the existence of free hemoglobin in solution, as in blackwater fever. An increased number of polymorphs indicates inflammation either in the kidney or the urinary tract; generally this condition is due to infection, but it must be confirmed bacteriologically.

Casts are cylindrical structures of precipitated protein that are formed in the renal tubules. Normally a few *hyaline casts* are present, and an increase in their number is found in any condition associated with albuminuria. Casts containing *red cells* indicate bleeding from the glomeruli, whereas casts containing *polymorphs* are found in pyelonephritis. *Granular casts* contain epithelial cells, and their debris indicates renal damage. *Large, broad casts* are formed in the dilated tubules of severely scarred kidneys, and their presence is of grave significance.

BACTERIOLOGICAL EXAMINATION. Urine normally contains some bacteria, but the organisms are too scanty to be seen on a stained smear of *uncentrifuged* urine. A bacterial count of over 100,000 per ml is regarded as abnormal and indicates a renal or urinary tract infection.

General Manifestations of Renal Disease

Renal disease, regardless of its cause, can terminate in renal failure. This may occur acutely or may be of a more chronic nature.

ACUTE RENAL FAILURE

Acute renal failure is characterized by a sudden drop in the output of urine *(oliguria);* this may be followed in due course by complete absence of excretion of urine *(anuria).* Acute renal failure must not be confused with sudden failure to pass urine that is due to the mechanical obstruction of the urinary passages.

Causes of Acute Renal Failure

1. RENAL VASOCONSTRICTION. This is a common event in clinical practice and is seen under the following circumstances:

(a) Whenever there is a sudden decrease in blood volume, such as may occur following hemorrhage, a severe burn, and persistent vomiting or diarrhea. The pathogenesis is considered in Chapter 21, under the heading of "Shock."

(b) Following the escape of free hemoglobin or myoglobin into the circulation, as after an incompatible blood transfusion or a crushing injury to the muscles of a limb.

(c) Following certain complications of pregnancy—notably abruptio placentae.

Renal vasoconstriction results in a diminution in the amount of blood reaching the kidney; in addition, in shock there is a reduction in the blood pressure. Glomerular filtration is therefore severely impaired and oliguria results. The kidney at this stage shows no structural abnormality, and if the condition is adequately treated, complete recovery occurs. However, if the ischemia is not speedily reversed, the condition progresses to acute tubular necrosis.

ACUTE RENAL TUBULAR NECROSIS.   Three major causes of this condition can be recognized:

Ischemia.   Prolonged ischemia as described above soon results in patchy tubular necrosis affecting particularly the terminal portions of the proximal convoluted tubules and the distal convoluted tubules. Characteristically, the basement membrane is disrupted and regeneration is thereby impaired and incomplete.

Poisons.   In particular, necrosis can result if poisoning is combined with prior dehydration. Mercury salts, carbon tetrachloride (used in fire extinguishers), and diethyl glycol (used in antifreeze) are important examples of these poisons.

Infections.   Acute tubular necrosis is seen in Weil's disease and also in yellow fever.

In acute renal tubular necrosis, the glomerular filtrate passes from the tubules into the interstitial tissue of the kidney, which thereby becomes swollen. Little or no fluid is passed as urine. Tubular necrosis is sometimes difficult to distinguish microscopically from postmortem change, but the presence of interstitial edema is one useful histological feature by which one may distinguish between the two. For reasons that are not understood, jaundice and pregnancy when combined with other conditions appear to predispose the kidney to necrosis. Sometimes in pregnancy, the ischemia leads to complete necrosis of the cortex; the condition of *bilateral renal cortical necrosis* results. This affects not only tubules but also the associated glomeruli (see Fig. 21–4).

Other less common diseases that produce acute renal failure include the following:

1. Acute renal diseases, such as acute glomerulonephritis and acute interstitial nephritis.

2. Acute tubular obstruction and subsequent necrosis are sometimes seen following the precipitation of uric acid in hyperuricemia (see Chapter 24).

3. The precipitation of myeloma protein in multiple myelomatosis and the formation of sulfonamide crystals in patients who are treated with these drugs.

Effects of Acute Renal Failure.   During the acute phase, oliguria with the passage of a small quantity of dark urine containing protein, blood products, and cell debris–forming casts is characteristic. In severe cases oliguria is followed by complete anuria. Uremia develops rapidly and is associated with a rise in blood urea nitrogen (BUN), blood potassium, and phosphate levels. Metabolic acidosis occurs, and there is an increase in the volume of the extracellular fluid. If the patient is overhydrated, heart failure may be precipitated and edema develops. Death may be due to overhydration, potassium intoxication, or infection, such as bronchopneumonia. Often, however, the patient sinks steadily into a coma from which he does not emerge; presumably, this is the combined effect of many metabolic upsets.

If the patient survives, he or she passes large quantities of urine for a period of time because the kidneys cannot conserve electrolytes and water. At that point, the patient's life is in jeopardy because of dehydration and electrolyte loss. As the tubular epithelium regenerates, renal function is restored, but complete recovery is unusual.

CHRONIC RENAL FAILURE – UREMIA

Any chronic progressive disease that results in destruction of renal parenchyma leads to chronic renal failure. The diseases include glomerulonephritis, chronic pyelonephritis, nephrosclerosis, lupus erythematosus, diabetic nephropathy, extensive renal tuberculosis, and radiation nephritis. Chronic obstruction of the outflow of urine, such as that caused by prostatic enlargement is a common cause in males.

Effects of Chronic Renal Failure.   The effect of chronic renal failure is uremia that is due to a failure of the kidney to regulate the internal environment. The kidneys can neither concentrate nor dilute, and the urine has a fixed specific gravity of 1.010. This leads to nocturia and easy upset in water metabolism.

Uremia is a clinical state produced by renal failure that is associated with retention of nitrogenous substances in the blood. Some of its features can be explained on the basis of known biochemical anomalies. In many instances we are ignorant of its exact pathogenesis. The features of uremia are enumerated below:

1. GENERAL.   Weakness, easy fatigue, lethargy, insomnia, and malaise are common.

2. CARDIOVASCULAR SYMPTOMS.   Hypertension is common and may lead to heart failure. This contributes to edema both of the tissues in general and of the lung. A terminal pericarditis is often seen.

3. GASTROINTESTINAL SYMPTOMS.   Anorexia, nausea, vomiting, hiccup, and diarrhea are frequent. One explanation of these symptoms is that urea present in the gastrointestinal fluids is broken down to ammonia, which is an irritant and causes *gastritis* and *colitis*. Vomiting and diarrhea can precipitate acute renal failure.

4. NEUROLOGICAL MANIFESTATIONS.   Mental clouding, inability to concentrate, and lethargy are common in advanced uremia. Convulsions and coma may occur terminally. These symptoms may be due to water intoxication and metabolic acidosis. Muscular twitching has been related to hypocalcemia.

5. ANEMIA.   This is characteristic and is unresponsive to treatment.

6. INFECTION.   Advanced renal insufficiency is commonly complicated by infection. Often this is a urinary infection and terminates in septicemia.

7. METABOLIC ACIDOSIS.   This condition leads to a sighing respiration.

8. RENAL OSTEODYSTROPHY.   Retention of phosphate can lead to a lowering of blood calcium and hyperparathyroidism secondary to this.

9. RETENTION OF POTASSIUM.   Hyperkalemia can lead to sudden death (see Chapter 19).

THE PROTEIN-LOSING KIDNEY (NEPHROTIC SYNDROME)

Normally a mere trace of protein escapes into the glomerular filtrate and is almost completely reabsorbed by the proximal convoluted tubules. There are a number of conditions in which the permeability of the glomeruli is increased so that large amounts of protein (mostly albumin) escape into the filtrate and are passed in the urine because the capacity of the tubule to reabsorb protein is limited. This constant loss of albumin results in hypoalbuminemia. The complex of proteinuria, hypoalbuminemia, and edema is called the *nephrotic syndrome*. It may be a complication of many chronic diseases, such as glomerulonephritis, diabetic nephropathy, renal amyloidosis, and lupus nephritis.

The main features of the nephrotic syndrome are listed below:

(a) *Severe Proteinuria*. Normally the 24-hour output of protein is less than 0.15 gram. In the nephrotic syndrome it can exceed 10 grams.

(b) *Hypoproteinemia*. This affects in particular the albumin level of the plasma.

(c) *Generalized Edema*. This condition is due in part to the hypoproteinemia and in part to an increased secretion of aldosterone by the adrenals.

(d) *Susceptibility to Infection*. This condition is due to the loss of immunoglobulins in the urine.

(e) *A Raised Level of Lipoproteins in the Blood*. The blood cholesterol, normally about 250 mg per 100 ml, may exceed 1000 mg per 100 ml. The cause of this increase is unknown.

Diseases of the Kidney

GLOMERULONEPHRITIS

Glomerulonephritis is a term applied to a group of diseases that are not obviously of infective nature, and in which primarily the glomeruli are affected. Although many classifications have been proposed, none has been found to be satisfactory, since in most types of glomerulonephritis neither the cause nor the pathogenesis is known. The types at present recognized have been delineated on the basis of three parameters:

1. CLINICAL FINDINGS. The clinical features of glomerulonephritis vary enormously. The onset may be acute or insidious. Hematuria is common but may range from insignificant to severe: the red cells present in urine may be detectable only by microscopic examination, or the urine may be obviously red. Albuminuria is invariable and if severe leads to the nephrotic syndrome. A patient may recover spontaneously from glomerulonephritis; occasionally the disease is fulminating and leads rapidly to death from renal failure; more often, the damage is progressive and renal failure occurs after a protracted course of many years. Associated clinical features sometimes suggest the cause of glomerulonephritis. For example, some types are associated with infection by *Streptococcus pyogenes*. For the most part, however, the origin of glomerulonephritis is unknown.

2. IMMUNOLOGICAL FINDINGS. Glomerulonephritis is a feature of serum sickness and chronic immune complex disease (see Chapter 9). The renal damage appears to be due to the deposition of immune complexes in the kidney, but the reason for the glomerular localization is not understood. The kidney appears to be damaged as an "innocent bystander," and the pathogenesis of the damage is not understood.

In many types of human glomerulonephritis, deposits of immunoglobulin (IgG or IgA) and complement can be demonstrated by immunofluorescence. The technique used is similar to that illustrated in Figure 9–13. The precise localization of the deposits varies; usually the deposits are granular and are situated in relation to the basement membrane or the mesangium. In a few types—notably the glomerulonephritis of Goodpasture's syndrome—specific antikidney antibodies can be detected in the kidney and in the blood.

3. HISTOPATHOLOGICAL FINDINGS. Light microscopy aided by electron microscopy reveals several types of change. For example, there may be proliferation of mesangial or epithelial cells, and deposits of material (mostly immunoglobulin) are found in the basement membrane or on either side of it. A characteristic electron microscopic finding is fusion of the foot processes of the epithelial cells of the glomeruli (Figs. 35–2 and 35–3). This appears to be an effect of an increased permeability of glomerular vessels to protein and is therefore present whenever there is proteinuria.

The technique of needle biopsy, by which a core of kidney substance can be safely removed during life, has greatly aided the investigation of glomerulonephritis in patients. The material obtained is particularly suited for immunofluorescence studies and electron microscopy as well as for routine light microscopic examination.

Types of Glomerulonephritis

1. MINIMAL-CHANGE GLOMERULONEPHRITIS. The glomeruli appear normal under light microscopy, but under electron microscopy fusion of the foot processes of the epithelial cells is revealed.

FIGURE 35–2. *Normal kidney.*

Survey electron micrograph of a portion of a normal human glomerulus. The capillaries (Cap) are lined by attenuated endothelial cells; the nucleus of one of these is labeled "End." Red cells are easily identified (rbc). A mesangial cell (Mes) is situated between several capillary loops. The capillaries possess a well-marked basement membrane (bm) and are covered by epithelial cells or podocytes (Pod) of the visceral layer of Bowman's capsule. These cells are attached to the basement membrane of the capillaries by numerous foot processes, or *pedicles* (× 3,600). (Courtesy of Dr. Susan Ritchie.)

FIGURE 35–3. *Electron micrograph of glomerulus in lupus erythematosus.*

In some areas, the foot processes (FP$_1$) of the podocytes appear relatively normal, but elsewhere they are swollen and spread over the basement membrane (bm) of the capillary (FP$_2$). This change is commonly described as *fusion of the foot processes*. Prominent subendothelial deposits are present (DEP$_1$). Subepithelial deposits are smaller and less obvious (DEP$_2$). In this patient the deposits were shown by immunofluorescence to contain IgG and components of complement (× 27,500). (Courtesy of Dr. Y. Bedard.)

The majority of the patients are children with the nephrotic syndrome. They respond well to glucocorticoid therapy.

2. MEMBRANOUS GLOMERULONEPHRITIS.   On light microscopy the basement membrane of the glomeruli is shown to be thickened (Fig. 35–4). Eventually this thickening causes obliteration of the vessels, and the glomeruli become functionless. The majority of patients are adults with the nephrotic syndrome. Approximately 30 per cent recover spontaneously and the remainder continue on with their disease and ultimately die of chronic renal failure. Membranous glomerulonephritis and minimal change glomerulonephritis at one time were both classified as types of *nephrosis*. Systemic lupus erythematosus can produce an identical histological picture.

3. PROLIFERATIVE GLOMERULONEPHRITIS.   The glomeruli are enlarged and hypercellular because of mesangial proliferation and infiltration by poly-

morphs (Fig. 35–4). Poststreptococcal glomerulonephritis is the common type of proliferative glomerulonephritis. The illness occurs about three weeks after a streptococcal infection and is characterized by hematuria and edema, particularly of the face. Certain strains of *Streptococcus pyogenes* (nephritogenic strains) are thought to share an antigen with the human glomerulus. Cross-reacting antibodies are assumed to cause the renal damage. About 80 per cent of the patients recover spontaneously and the remainder show permanent damage and ultimately develop chronic renal failure (Fig. 35–5).

4. MEMBRANOPROLIFERATIVE GLOMERULONEPHRITIS (MESANGIOCAPILLARY). The glomeruli show a combination of basement membrane thickening and mesangial proliferation. Several types of membranoproliferative glomerulonephritis are recognized. One type is associated with *Streptococcus viridans* endocarditis; another is associated with a low blood complement level. The location and type of deposits found in immunofluorescent and electron microscopic studies help in delineating these types.

FIGURE 35–4. *Glomerulonephritis.*

A, Normal glomerulus. B, Membranous glomerulonephritis. Note the thickening of the basement membrane of the glomerular capillaries. C, Proliferative glomerulonephritis. The glomerulus is enlarged and shows increased cellularity that is due partly to mesangial proliferation and partly to a polymorph infiltration (× 450).

FIGURE 35–5. *Chronic glomerulonephritis.*

Both kidneys are reduced in size and display a fine granular surface. The patient had developed acute glomerulonephritis following a streptococcal sore throat. Renal failure and systemic hypertension slowly evolved over the next 15 years. Death was due to cerebral hemorrhage. It is not possible to distinguish between the various types of chronic renal disease by a gross examination.

Clinically the patients often present with the nephrotic syndrome. The prognosis is poor.

5. RAPIDLY PROGRESSIVE GLOMERULONEPHRITIS. The glomeruli show proliferative changes and deposits of fibrin. The characteristic lesion, however, is proliferation of the epithelial cells of Bowman's capsule to produce a *crescent*.

Clinically, rapidly progressive glomerulonephritis is associated with the rapid development of renal failure and consequent death. The disease is occasionally encountered in poststreptococcal glomerulonephritis and in polyarthritis nodosa. It is also characteristic of Goodpasture's syndrome, a condition that affects young men and is characterized by pulmonary hemorrhages, hemoptysis, and renal failure. Antibodies are present that react specifically with basement membrane material of the pulmonary and glomerular capillaries.

Focal Glomerulonephritis. Unlike the other types of glomerulonephritis described, this group affects some glomeruli but not others; indeed it may affect parts of only some glomeruli. Two types, which are described below, are recognized:

FOCAL SCLEROSING GLOMERULONEPHRITIS. This disease is progressive and the prognosis is poor.

FOCAL PROLIFERATIVE GLOMERULONEPHRITIS (BERGER'S DISEASE). Focal proliferative glomerulonephritis is associated with IgA deposits in both affected and unaffected glomeruli. The disease is characterized by recurrent attacks of hematuria. Its prognosis is excellent.

Summary.   The diagnosis of glomerulonephritis is the task of the expert who has access to such sophisticated tools as electron microscopy and immunofluorescence. Precise diagnosis is of value in giving the prognosis and in suggesting the best treatment available.

OTHER TYPES OF RENAL DISEASE

Lupus Nephritis.   Glomerulonephritis of either a proliferative or a membranous type is common in systemic lupus erythematosus (Fig. 35–3). It often causes a nephrotic syndrome and ultimately leads to renal failure.

Nephrosclerosis.   Nephrosclerosis is a term used to describe the renal lesions of systemic hypertension (see Chapter 20). In the *benign type*, the arteriolosclerosis causes patchy ischemia. The affected nephrons become atrophic and are ultimately replaced by scar tissue. Hence, the kidneys in benign nephrosclerosis show thinning of the cortex and a granularity of the surface. In malignant hypertension the arteriolar necrosis causes extensive patchy foci of necrosis (*malignant nephrosclerosis*). Renal failure is a common cause of death.

Interstitial Nephritis.   Interstitial nephritis is characterized by an inflammatory reaction in the interstitial tissues. This is associated with tubular damage and the glomeruli are spared until late in the course of the disease. Acute interstitial nephritis can lead to death from acute renal failure; however, the disease is usually chronic. Some cases are caused by drug intake—particularly intake of the penicillin derivative, methicillin. Another group is due to the prolonged intake of large doses of analgesic drugs, particularly aspirin-phenacetin mixtures (*causing analgesic nephropathy*). The condition generally arises from self-medication. Many cases of interstitial nephritis are idiopathic and are difficult to distinguish from chronic pyelonephritis, since the pathological findings of the two diseases are very similar.

Diabetic Nephropathy.   This condition is described in Chapter 24.

RENAL AND URINARY TRACT INFECTION: PYELONEPHRITIS

Bacterial infection of the urinary tract is very common and constitutes a major medical problem. The infecting organisms are usually the gram-negative intestinal bacilli, including *Escherichia coli, Pseudomonas aeruginosa,* and Proteus species. Two routes of infection have been described, but their relative importance has been long debated:

Hematogenous infection.   It is believed that some infection is bloodborne from the colon. Normally organisms that avoid the reticuloendothelial cells of the liver pass into the systemic circulation; they escape into the glomerular filtrate and are expeditiously voided in the urine. If there is an obstruction to the outflow of urine, these organisms flourish and set up acute inflammation of the bladder (*cystitis*), of the renal pelvis (*pyelitis*), or of the kidney and renal pelvis (*pyelonephritis*).

Ascending infection.   There is a rival hypothesis that infection ascends from the perineum and lower urinary tract. Acute cystitis is more common in women (particularly during pregnancy), and it is probable that this is due to the shortness of the urethra and the ease with which vulval organisms can ascend to the bladder. Likewise, urinary infection often follows repeated catheterization. Direct introduction of urethral organisms into the bladder can therefore be implicated. Following acute cystitis "ascending infection" due to reflux of urine up into the ureters can occur.

It is evident that obstruction to the urinary flow is the most important factor predisposing a person toward infection. Pyelonephritis can be unilateral if one ureter is obstructed, such as by a stone. If there has been previous blockage, the hydronephrotic kidney becomes infected to produce a sac of pus known as *pyonephrosis*. Urethral obstruction, such as that due to prostatic enlargement, generally causes bilateral pyelonephritis.

The clinical features of acute urinary tract infection are those of an acute infection: rigors and an acute rise in temperature. Pain is experienced in the loins in pyelonephritis. With cystitis and urethritis the inflammation leads to urgency of micturition together with pain and burning on passing urine. The acute attack generally subsides rapidly either under treatment or spontaneously.

The urine in acute cystitis and acute pyelonephritis contains numerous pus cells; organisms can usually be seen in a stained smear of an uncentrifuged specimen. Hematuria is common.

Chronic Pyelonephritis. In some cases of acute urinary tract infection there are repeated recurrences of the infection and the development of chronic pyelonephritis; this is the commonest cause of chronic renal failure. Its pathogenesis is uncertain, because in some cases there is an obvious cause such as urinary obstruction, whereas in others there is no such obstruction or other reason for urinary stasis. It may be that some intrinsic kidney damage, especially the scars of a previous infection, account for this smoldering infection. Chronic pyelonephritis is characterized by gradual destruction of the renal parenchyma and its replacement by fibrous tissue that is heavily infiltrated by lymphocytes, plasma cells, macrophages, and a varying number of polymorphs. Since the process tends to be patchy, the kidney presents an irregular scarred appearance. Chronic pyelonephritis is often complicated by the development of hypertension, so that hypertensive vascular changes are superimposed. The ultimate result is an end-stage kidney, which is associated with chronic renal failure.

END-STAGE KIDNEYS

Small, scarred, granular kidneys are often found at the necropsy of a patient who died of renal disease. It is difficult—or even impossible—to distinguish between the various types of kidney disease (*e.g.*, chronic glomerulonephritis, chronic pyelonephritis, nephrosclerosis, diabetic nephropathy, and chronic interstitial nephritis (Fig. 35–5). It is in these cases that the overall clinical course and results of previous renal biopsies are of value in arriving at a correct reconstruction of the events leading to death.

TUMORS OF THE KIDNEY

Adenoma. The common benign renal tumor is an adenoma that is usually pinhead-sized and appears as a yellow-white nodule situated beneath the capsule. Its cells are usually arranged in a papillary cystadenomatous pattern and closely resemble those of a carcinoma.

Carcinoma of the Kidney. This is the malignant counterpart of the adenoma and usually appears as a large, soft mass at one or the other pole (see Case History I and Fig. 35–6). A section shows that it has a variegated appearance with some areas being white, others yellow or orange; elsewhere there are foci of bleeding. Microscopically it consists of large spheroidal cells with clear cytoplasm. In well-differentiated tumors these cells are arranged to form tubules. Although the cells resemble those of the normal renal tubules, it was at one time believed that the tumor arose from ectopic adrenal tissue situated on the surface of the kidney. This belief was the origin of the name *hypernephroma*, a term that is still widely used. It has since been discovered that the tumor arises from renal tubular epithelium; all grades of transition can be found between the anaplastic tumors and the benign adenoma.

The clear appearance of the cells is due to their high content of lipid and glycogen, both of which are lost during routine paraffin wax sectioning. The yellow appearance is due to the carotinoid pigments dissolved in the lipid. Probably the best name for this tumor is *clear-cell carcinoma of the kidney.*

Clinically carcinoma of the kidney is often silent for a long time. *Painless hematuria and an abdominal mass are the two common presenting features.*

FIGURE 35–6. *Carcinoma of the kidney.*

The kidney contains a well-circumscribed tumor about 4 cm in diameter. It was yellow in color in the fresh state. Microscopy revealed a clear-cell renal carcinoma. See Case History I for clinical details.

Case History I. (See Figure 35–6). In 1967, at the age of 57 years, the patient presented with a complaint of chronic cough. A radiograph showed ill-defined shadows in both upper lung fields; these were interpreted as being produced by fibrosis. Nineteen years previously, a radiograph was reported to have shown similar shadows, and at that time pulmonary tuberculosis had been suspected. The diagnosis had never been proven, and no treatment had been given.

Several samples of sputum and gastric washings were examined for tubercle bacilli without success. A lymph node biopsy taken at mediastinoscopy revealed noncaseating granulomas. No organisms could be identified in the sections. However, shortly after the procedure, a nodule was noted on the left nostril, and a biopsy again revealed a granulomatous reaction—this time fungi were detected. A repeat biopsy of the nodule was cultured and *Histoplasma capsulatum* was grown. Amphotericin B therapy was instituted, and the patient's condition improved. Nevertheless, he complained of easy fatigue and periodically had attacks of nausea and vomiting. No cause was found.

Two years later, difficulty in passing urine and nocturia led to a transurethral resection of an enlarged prostate. Histopathological studies revealed a benign prostatic enlargement, but a radiograph revealed a translucent area in the first lumbar vertebral body. In spite of the pathology report a diagnosis of carcinoma of the prostate with bony metastases was made. Stilbestrol (a synthetic estrogen) therapy was initiated. Several episodes of painless hematuria were attributed to carcinoma of the prostate. Two years later, however, a cystoscopy failed to detect any bladder or prostatic lesion. Further investigations (an intravenous pyelogram and an arteriogram) showed a lesion in the left kidney. A nephrectomy was carried out for carcinoma of the kidney (see Figure 35–6). Shortly after surgery, the patient collapsed and died in shock.

Autopsy revealed no evidence of carcinoma of the prostate. Both adrenal glands showed almost complete replacement by caseous material due to histoplasmosis (see Figure 39–2). The lesion in the vertebra also showed histoplasmosis. The upper lobes of both lungs were fibrotic and contained scanty granulomas. This case illustrates several points:

(a) Histoplasmosis, like tuberculosis, can become active after remaining dormant for many years.

(b) Attacks of vomiting combined with weakness suggest a diagnosis of Addison's disease.

(c) Major surgery in a patient with Addison's disease is hazardous unless adequate glucocorticoids are given.

(d) In the absence of pathological proof it was unwise to make a clinical diagnosis of prostatic cancer. The significance of the attacks of painless hematuria was not appreciated, causing the diagnosis of carcinoma of the kidney to be delayed for over one year.

Distant and blood-borne metastases are common, with the liver, lungs, and bones being especially involved.

An interesting feature of the tumor is the phenomenon of dormancy. Bony metastases may suddenly erupt many years after the apparently successful removal of the primary growth.

Nephroblastoma, or Wilms' Tumor. This is a tumor of infancy and is described in Chapter 17.

THE LOWER URINARY TRACT

URINARY TRACT OBSTRUCTION (OBSTRUCTIVE UROPATHY)

Ureteric Obstruction. Sudden complete obstruction of one ureter, such as by a calculus, leads to atrophy of the affected kidney and compensatory enlargement of the other. Partial obstruction of a ureter by a stone, tumor, or pressure from an adjacent mass leads to dilatation of the ureter above the obstruction (*hydroureter*) and dilatation of the pelvis of the affected kidney (hydronephrosis).

Urethral Obstruction

The following causes should be noted:

(a) Carcinoma of the urethra. This is uncommon.

(b) Fibrous stricture. This may follow repeated catheterization or may be an after-effect of gonococcal urethritis.

(c) Carcinoma of the prostate.

(d) Benign prostatic enlargement. This is by far the most common and important cause of urethral obstruction and will be considered in detail.

BENIGN PROSTATIC ENLARGEMENT.   It has been estimated that between 30 and 50 per cent of men develop some degree of obstruction after the age of 50 from this cause. A common symptom is a poor stream of urine, and incomplete emptying of the bladder after micturition. This increase in the residual urine predisposes to *infection.* As the bladder refills, the urge to urinate returns and there is *frequency of micturition and nocturia.* The bladder dilates and its muscular wall hypertrophies in response to the increased work needed to expel urine. Its wall becomes trabeculated (see Fig. 36–1). Protrusions of mucosa produce outpouchings, or diverticula, which further predispose to urinary stasis and infection.

Sudden urethral obstruction due to benign prostatic enlargement can occur at any time. The enlarged median lobe of the prostate overlying the urethra can act like a ball valve. Likewise, inflammation (prostatitis) can compress the urethra.

Acute urethral obstruction must be distinguished from anuria. In both conditions no urine is passed through the urethra, but with obstruction the bladder becomes painfully enlarged. Ultimately, the increased pressure may force some urine through the urethra. This *retention with overflow* can deceive the unwary attendant into believing that the obstruction has been relieved.

The treatment of acute urinary obstruction requires expert attention. Either a catheter is passed through the urethra or else a needle is inserted into the bladder through the anterior abdominal wall; in either event, the obstruction is relieved. Urine must not be drained too quickly, however, or the sudden reduction in pressure will lead to bleeding. In addition, sudden decompression can cause an equally sudden diuresis, and this can cause hypovolemic shock.

Effect of Urinary Obstruction on the Kidney.   Obstruction of the outflow of urine produces a back-pressure effect on the kidney that results in tubular atrophy and ultimately in destruction of renal parenchyma. The pelvis dilates and hydronephrosis results (Fig. 35–7). Evidence of chronic renal failure, such as a raised BUN, in an elderly person always suggests the likelihood of obstructive uropathy, particularly if the azotemia (excess of nitrogenous substances in the blood) fluctuates in intensity over a period of a few days.

NEUROGENIC BLADDER

When lesions of the spinal cord damage the corticospinal tracts, there is loss of voluntary control of micturition. As the bladder dilates local reflexes are responsible for automatic evacuation of urine. If the cord lesion is low, or if the nerves to the bladder are directly involved, even this automatic reflex is lost, and the bladder fills and finally overflows. In either event, urinary stasis—particularly when combined with repeated catheterizations—predisposes the patient to urinary tract infection.

FIGURE 35–7. *Hydronephrosis.*

The kidney shows dilatation of the pelvis and severe damage to the renal parenchyma such that the organ is converted into a bag of fluid. The condition resulted from intermittent ureteric obstruction by a low-grade carcinoma of the bladder. See Case History II for clinical details.

Case History II. (See Figure 35–7.)   In 1948 at the age of 44 years, the patient noticed that his urine suddenly became red. Microscopic examination of the urine showed numerous red cells; tests for hemoglobin were positive. Cystoscopy revealed numerous "papillomas" in the bladder and these were *fulgurated* (burned with an electric spark). Because of repeated recurrences the diagnosis was subsequently changed to papillary carcinoma. During the next 25 years the bladder tumors were treated on at least 34 occasions. In 1973 when the patient was 69 years of age, a mass was noted in the left side of the abdomen. This was identified as a nonfunctioning kidney and was removed. There were further recurrences of tumor, and in 1975 a partial cystectomy (removal of part of the bladder) was undertaken. A tumor similar to that shown in Figure 35–8 was found.

URETERIC REFLUX

It is not uncommon to find hydroureter and hydronephrosis in the absence of any organic obstructive lesion. In such cases, it is believed that these are examples of neuromuscular incoordination. Radiographic studies indicate that in some patients urine passes up the ureter by abnormal peristaltic waves traveling in an upward direction.

TUMORS OF THE URINARY PASSAGES

Apart from carcinoma, tumors of the urinary passages are uncommon.

Carcinoma.   Well differentiated tumors of the transitional epithelium are often multiple and appear as noninvasive papillomatous growths with delicate fronds that give the lesions a resemblance to a sea anemone (Fig. 35–8). Histologically, these tumors are papillomatous and appear benign, but unfortunately they tend to recur even after local treatment (see Case History II). In

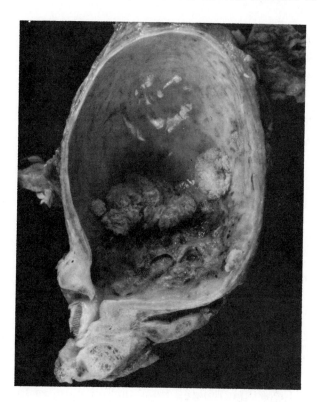

FIGURE 35–8. *Carcinoma of the bladder.*

This radical cystectomy specimen was inflated with formalin solution before being opened. Numerous papillomatous tumors are seen attached to the bladder lining. Microscopy revealed a papillary transitional-cell carcinoma.

practice it is wise to regard them as low-grade carcinomas. Nevertheless, some authorities recognize the entity of benign papilloma of the bladder and attribute recurrence to the formation of new tumors. The less well-differentiated transitional cell tumors are the obvious carcinomas that show invasion of the wall and appear as sessile nodules or papillomatous lesions that break down into indurated malignant ulcers.

Histologically, the tumors are transitional cell carcinomas of varying degrees of differentiation. In some tumors there are areas of squamous cell change, and not infrequently tumors are found in which the entire growth is composed of squamous-cell carcinoma. These cases tend to have a poor prognosis. Cancer of the bladder is particularly common in the Middle East and is associated with schistosomiasis. The increased incidence of bladder cancer in aniline dye workers and in those engaged in the rubber industry has been noted in Chapter 17. There is also an increased incidence in those who indulge in heavy cigarette smoking.

Urinary Calculi

Urinary stones, or calculi, have plagued mankind for centuries; they are particularly common in the hot desert regions of the Middle East. Calculi can be divided into two main groups: primary and secondary.

1. *Primary calculi.*   These are presumed to occur because of a high concentration of chemicals in the urine or because of a defective mechanism for keeping these crystalloids in solution. Three common types are known:

URATE STONES.   These are smooth, consist of uric acid and urates, and are common in patients who suffer from gout.

CALCIUM OXALATE STONES.   These characteristically have a spiky surface that causes hematuria by damaging the mucosa.

MIXED CALCIUM OXALATE AND PHOSPHATE STONES.   This type of stone occurs in the hypercalcemia that accompanies hyperparathyroidism and prolonged periods of recumbency.

2. *Secondary Calculi.*   These stones are composed of calcium and magnesium oxalates and phosphates. They are formed around a focus of necrotic tissue, organisms, fibrin, a foreign body, or a primary stone. They are often secondary to infection. The most common type is found in the renal pelvis; as it grows, it assumes the shape of the pelvis and produces a shape that has been likened to that of a staghorn.

Effects of Urinary Calculi

These may be listed:

(a) INFECTION.   Patients with recurrent urinary tract infection should always be investigated for the possibility of urinary stones.

(b) OBSTRUCTION.   This is frequently intermittent.

(c) HEMATURIA.

(d) PAIN.   A stone formed in the renal pelvis can pass down the ureter and cause severe colicky pain lasting for a time ranging from several minutes to several hours. This *renal colic* is usually accompanied by hematuria.

Review Questions

1. Explain why a deficiency of vasopressin (antidiuretic hormone, or ADH) causes polyuria.
2. Explain how the creatinine clearance test is carried out. What is the significance of a value of 30 ml per minute?
3. Describe the changes that occur in the blood in uremia.
4. Outline the principles involved in the classification of glomerulonephritis.
5. A 65-year-old male patient is in the hospital, having had a myocardial infarction ten days previously. His urine output suddenly diminishes. Suggest reasons for this sudden change.
6. Discuss the abnormalities that would be expected in the urine of a patient with each of the following conditions:
   (a) clear-cell carcinoma of the kidney
   (b) transitional-cell carcinoma of the bladder
   (c) acute pyelonephritis
   (d) severe chronic pyelonephritis
   (e) severe amyloidosis affecting the kidney.

7. List the common causes of hematuria. How may hematuria be distinguished from hemoglobinuria? Outline the investigations that may be carried out to arrive at a correct diagnosis.

Selected Readings

Frazier, H. S.: Renal regulation of sodium balance. New England Journal of Medicine, *279*:868–875, 1968.

Heptinstall, R. H.: Pathology of the Kidney. 2nd ed. Boston, Little, Brown and Company, 1974. A comprehensive reference work in two volumes. See, in particular, Chapters 7 to 14 for information on glomerulonephritis.

Leading Article: Vesico-ureteric reflux. Lancet, *1*:1072–1074, 1968.

Leading Article: Defensive mechanisms of the bladder. British Medical Journal, *3*:486, 1969.

Leading Article: Escherichia serotypes and renal infection. Lancet, *1*:532–533, 1971.

Leading Article: What is chronic pyelonephritis? British Medical Journal, *2*:61–62, 1971.

Merrill, J. P., and Hampers, C. L.: Uremia. New England Journal of Medicine, *282*:953–961, and 1014–1021, 1970.

Chapter 36

After studying this chapter the student should be able to:

- Describe the development of the testis and relate this to the following:
     (a) The occurrence of inguinal hernias
     (b) The blood supply of the testis
     (c) The metastatic spread of testicular tumors
     (d) Spermatogenesis.
- Describe cryptorchidism and its complications
- Give an account of torsion of the testis.
- Classify the common causes of orchitis and epididymo-orchitis.
- Classify the tumors of the testis.
- Describe the clinical and pathological features of benign prostatic enlargement.
- Describe carcinoma of the prostate with regard to the following factors:
     (a) Frequency
     (b) Clinical features
     (c) Spread.

The Testes

The testes develop from a mass of mesoderm in the posterior abdominal wall. While still retaining their original blood supply, they migrate downwards and forwards, traversing the anterior abdominal wall through the inguinal canal until they finally come to lie in the scrotum. A process of peritoneum accompanies this descent, forming the tunica vaginalis, which surrounds the testis

576

MALE REPRODUCTIVE ORGANS; DISORDERS OF STRUCTURE AND FUNCTION

and its epididymis. The sac usually loses connection with the peritoneal cavity, but the inguinal region remains a point of weakness throughout life and is a common site for the development of a hernia. This is the price that has to be paid for having the male gonads in the scrotum where the temperature can be maintained at a lower level than is found in the abdomen from which the testes descended. There is evidence that this cool environment is necessary for the development of sperm (spermatogenesis).

CRYPTORCHIDISM

In *cryptorchidism* one or both testes fail to descend and reach the scrotum. The glands are then situated either within the abdomen or in the inguinal canal. Failure in spermatogenesis results in infertility if both testes are affected. An undescended testis remains immature and is particularly liable to develop a malignant tumor, particularly a seminoma. Unless an undescended testis can be made to descend, either by medical or surgical means, it should be removed, since it remains a permanent hazard.

TORSION OF THE TESTIS

During violent exercise or following trauma the testis can rotate, causing a twist of the spermatic cord and its blood vessels. This rotation causes sudden pain; unless the testis can be untwisted soon (either by manipulation or by open surgery), first the veins and then the arteries become obstructed. The organ becomes intensely congested and subsequently infarcted. Torsion of the testis tends to occur if the testis is abnormally mobile because of a mild developmental defect, which is sometimes bilateral. Hence, following torsion of one testis, the other should be fixed to prevent a similar event occurring on the other side.

INFECTIONS OF THE TESTIS

Acute infections of the epididymis (epididymitis) and testis (orchitis) generally occur secondarily to infection of the urinary tract or prostate. Acute epididymo-orchitis sometimes follows prostatitis and is a well-recognized complication of surgery on the prostate unless the vas deferens and its related lymphatics have been tied previously. Gonococcal epididymo-orchitis is an important complication of this infection. In bacterial infections, the brunt of the damage falls on the epididymis, while the testis is affected secondarily. In mumps orchitis, it is the testis that suffers most. It has been estimated that from 20 to 25 per cent of adult males who develop mumps suffer from acute orchitis about one week following enlargement of the parotid glands. With resolution of the disease some testicular atrophy takes place; if this is severe—particularly if it is bilateral—permanent sterility can result. The testis is enclosed in a dense fibrous coat, the tunica albuginea; in acute inflammation there is a rapid rise in tissue tension. Hence, severe pain is a feature of acute orchitis and epididymo-orchitis.

Tuberculosis of the urinary tract sometimes spreads and affects the epididymis. Years ago, in tertiary syphilis a testicular gumma was not uncommon, but now this lesion is distinctly rare.

TUMORS OF THE TESTIS

Although rare, tumors of the testis are the most common form of cancer to affect males between 20 and 35 years of age. The majority of the tumors are thought to arise from primitive pluripotential germ cells. As might be expected, they give rise to tumors that vary greatly in their differentiation and prognosis. Four major types, which are described below, have been recognized:

Seminoma. This is the most common tumor and occurs in a somewhat older age group than the others. It consists of uniform cells having clear cytoplasm, and it tends to produce a uniform bulky enlargement of the testis. Local invasion beyond the testis is not evident, but the tumor first metastasizes to the lymph nodes. It should be noted that the lymphatics of the testis follow the blood vessels and terminate in lymph nodes around the aorta. Seminoma of the testis, although malignant, is very radiosensitive and with treatment has a good prognosis. A five-year survival of 90 per cent of treated patients can be expected.

Teratoma. This tumor shows a mixed histological picture, having both epithelial and connective tissue elements (see Fig. 17–16). Occasionally, the tumor is well differentiated and cystic, and it resembles the ovarian teratoma. Nevertheless, the vast majority of testicular teratomas are solid and show areas of anaplastic growth—usually of the epithelial element. Teratomas tend to form a discrete nodule in the testis and subsequently invade the capsule. Since there is metastasis to the regional lymph nodes and the blood stream, the prognosis is worse than that of seminoma. The five-year mortality of patients with this tumor is approximately 30 to 50 per cent.

Embryonal Carcinoma. This unsatisfactory term is used to describe a tumor that microscopically resembles a carcinoma and also shows glandular differentiation and considerable pleomorphism. The tumor, which is often quite small, exhibits a more aggressive and lethal behavior than either seminoma or teratoma. The five-year survival rate of patients is about 35 per cent.

Choriocarcinoma. This is the least common and most malignant type of testicular tumor. It metastasizes via the blood stream, and the primary growth is often small. In fact, the growth is sometimes of microscopic dimension, so that the patient presents clinically with multiple metastases—the primary tumor being located only at necropsy after a painstaking search. Histologically, the tumor resembles its counterpart in the female.

Combined Tumors. These tumors show a mixture of the types described above. Their existence supports the concept that these testicular tumors have a common cell of origin. At one time it was thought that seminomas could be regarded as carcinomas of the seminiferous tubules, whereas the others all arose from pluripotential cells. This view is now no longer held.

Other rare tumors of the testis are known. The most intriguing of these is one derived from the stroma: the *interstitial cell tumor,* which like its parent cell, secretes androgens. When this tumor occurs in children, there is precocious sexual development. When it occurs in adult males, estrogen production sometimes predominates so that feminization with gynecomastia results.

HYDROCELE

An accumulation of fluid in the tunica vaginalis is called a *hydrocele.* When the tunica still communicates with the peritoneal cavity, this condition may be found in any case of ascites. Under normal conditions in which the tunica is an isolated sac, the development of a hydrocele suggests either an inflammatory condition of the testis or epididymis, or it suggests the development of a tumor. The presence of fluid can easily be detected by placing a flashlight behind the swelling and observing that it transilluminates. A mass in the scrotum produced by a solid tumor does not behave in this way. Between 25 and 50 per cent of acute hydroceles are due to trauma; in such cases there may be blood present also. Much blood in the sac is termed a *hematocele.*

The Prostate

The prostate gland is situated at the base of the bladder and is traversed by the first part of the male urethra. Its functions are largely unknown, but it contributes its secretions to the seminal ejaculate during intercourse and its enlargement is a source of considerable annoyance in old age.

PROSTATITIS

Acute prostatitis is generally a complication of urinary tract infection and can be a complication of gonorrhea. It is sometimes precipitated by catheterization and cystoscopy. The changes are similar to those of inflammation in other situations and therefore can terminate in suppuration.

Chronic prostatitis is extremely common as an incidental finding at necropsy. It generally accompanies urinary tract infection and may be associated with numerous calculi within the gland. Chronic prostatitis of clinical significance leads to fibrosis, which may give the gland a firmness that can be mistaken for carcinoma.

BENIGN PROSTATIC ENLARGEMENT

This is the most common disease of the prostate and is also called *prostatic hypertrophy* or *nodular hyperplasia.* The disease is extremely common in men over 50, and its incidence increases with age. Consequently, in men over the age of 80 years, about 80 per cent have some degree of involvement. The prostate gland becomes enlarged and nodular. This can be detected clinically by rectal examination. On cross section, cystic nodular areas are found, which can be proved microscopically to be due to foci of glandular hyperplasia. In other areas, there is overgrowth of smooth muscle or fibrous tissue. These elements give the gland a texture that is firm but not usually so hard that it mimics carcinoma. The nodular elements press on local blood vessels so that focal areas of infarction are not uncommon. Bleeding can occur into these areas, and clinically hematuria is a frequent symptom. The other major effect of prostatic enlargement is distortion of the prostatic urethra and its obstruction (Fig. 36–1). The secondary effects of this enlargement on the bladder and kidneys are described elsewhere (see Chapter 35).

The cause of benign prostatic enlargement is not known, but it is presumed to be related to hormonal imbalance of old age. A deficiency of androgens or an excess of estrogenic substances has been suggested but not proven.

The treatment of benign prostatic enlargement is surgical. Prostatectomy can be performed through an abdominal incision or through the urethra using an operating endoscope.

CARCINOMA OF THE PROSTATE

Deaths from carcinoma of the prostate constitute the second most frequent cause of death from carcinoma in men in the United States. It is common to find small foci of carcinoma in elderly patients dying from other causes, but the significance of these has been disputed (see "Latent Carcinoma," Chapter 17). Progressive clinical cancer of the prostate is less common and may present

FIGURE 36–1. *Benign prostatic enlargement.*

This specimen of bladder and prostatic urethra has been opened from the front. The prostate is enlarged, and its nodular median lobe projects into the bladder, acting as a ball valve to obstruct the passage of urine. The bladder wall is greatly thickened. Hypertrophy of muscle bundles is responsible for the ribbed or trabeculated appearance of its lining. (Specimen from the Boyd Museum, Toronto.)

with urinary obstruction or the development of symptoms due to local invasion or metastatic growth. Cancer of the prostate involves such local tissues as seminal vesicles, rectum, and bladder; it also metastasizes to the regional lymph nodes. More significant is the blood-borne metastatic spread; approximately 70 per cent of cases show bony metastases, particularly of the lower spine. These lesions are noteworthy for being osteosclerotic. Metastatic spread to the liver and lungs is also common.

Microscopically, cancer of the prostate is generally a well-differentiated adenocarcinoma, and it tends to excite a considerable scirrhous reaction. A prostate with cancer is stony hard—the salient clinical feature, which can be detected by rectal examination. In any patient suspected of malignant disease, particularly with metastatic bony spread, a rectal examination is mandatory if the patient is over 50 years of age.

The normal prostatic epithelium secretes acid phosphatase. In carcinoma, particularly if the bulk of tumor and its metastases are great, there is an elevation of the blood level of this enzyme. A test of the level of this enzyme is useful diagnostically, but a normal level of acid phosphatase does not exclude early carcinoma of the prostate.

Prostatic massage can express material through the urethra; malignant cells can be found in this fluid. This method is not completely reliable and has been criticized, since malignant cells appear in the blood following massage, and this could conceivably initiate the formation of metastases.

The most satisfactory method of diagnosis following clinical suspicion is a biopsy, which can generally be performed through the urethra.

The normal prostate is dependent upon androgens, and many carcinomas also are dependent upon androgenic hormones. Some degree of hormonal control of cancer of the prostate can be obtained by estrogen administration, castration, or a combination of the two. The results are sometimes quite striking; generally, they are of limited duration. The once-popular high-dosage estrogen therapy is now less favored, since it has been found that patients tend to have a much higher incidence of death from cardiovascular complications. The gynecomastia and skin pigmentation are other disadvantages of estrogen therapy.

Review Questions

1. Discuss the possible causes of a swelling that occupies one side of the scrotum and appears to involve one testis. How would the clinical history and the presence of pain influence the differential diagnosis?
2. Describe the common symptoms and signs of advanced carcinoma of the prostate. What biochemical abnormalities would be expected in the blood?

Selected Readings

Blandy, J. P.: Benign prostatic enlargement. British Medical Journal, 1:31–35, 1971.
Leading Article: Undescended testis. British Medical Journal, 2:248–249, 1970.
Robbins, S. L.: Pathologic Basis of Disease. Philadelphia, W. B. Saunders Company, 1974. Chapter 26, which discusses the male genital system, should be used as a source of further information and references.

Chapter 37

Chapter Outline

After studying this chapter the student should be able to:

● Describe the hormonal changes that are associated with the following:
   (a) the development of the female secondary sexual characteristics
   (b) the menstrual cycle
   (c) pregnancy
   (d) lactation.

FEMALE REPRODUCTIVE ORGANS; PREGNANCY AND ITS DISORDERS

- Give an account of the ovarian tumors that are derived from the germinal epithelium.
- Describe the causes and important effects of salpingitis.
- Differentiate between the exocervix and the endocervix.
- Describe what is meant by a "cervical erosion."
- Give a general account of carcinoma of the cervix with regard to the following factors:
  (a) predisposing causes
  (b) age of onset
  (c) mode of development
  (d) symptoms.
- Define amenorrhea, menorrhagia, metrorrhagia, and dysmenorrhea. Give at least one cause of each condition.
- Describe the outstanding features of each of the following:
  (a) uterine fibroids
  (b) carcinoma of the endometrium
  (c) endometriosis.
- List the features of toxemia of pregnancy
- Describe what is meant by "ectopic pregnancy."
- Define spontaneous abortion and give one common cause of this process.
- Classify the causes of bleeding during pregnancy.
- Contrast placenta praevia with abruptio placentae.
- Describe the outstanding features of hydatidiform mole and choriocarcinoma.

Introduction: Hormonal Aspects of the Female Genital Tract

The hormones secreted by the ovary play a leading part in regulating the major biological events in a woman's life. It is therefore appropriate to describe these before the individual organs and their abnormalities are discussed.

Childhood and Adolescence. During childhood the ovary secretes small quantities of *estrogen;* this secretion is sufficient to inhibit the hypothalamus. Hence, the release of gonadotropins from the pituitary is inhibited (see Chapter 39). After the age of about seven years, the hypothalamus becomes less sensitive to estrogen, its set-point is raised, and this leads to the release of

583

gonadotropin (chiefly *follicle-stimulating hormone,* or FSH) from the adenohy-pophysis. Ovarian estrogen production is thereby stimulated sufficiently to cause the *development of secondary sexual characteristics:* the breasts and uterus enlarge, and the subcutaneous fat is redistributed to produce the charac-teristic female contours. Shortly after this, the "cycling" center in the hypothal-amus comes into operation and menstruation commences.* Under the influ-ence of FSH, the ovarian follicles enlarge and secrete estrogen. At midcycle there is a surge of pituitary *luteinizing hormone* (LH) that causes ovulation. The follicular cells are converted into the corpus luteum, and *progesterone* is secreted.

Endometrial Changes in the Menstrual Cycle.   During the first half of the menstrual cycle the endometrium (both glands and stroma) undergoes hyper-plasia. Following ovulation, progesterone causes the glands to form secretion; the endometrium is thus suitably prepared for implantation of the developing fetus. If conception does not occur, the corpus luteum degenerates, and es-trogen and progesterone levels decline; the endometrium undergoes necrosis and is passed in the menstrual flow as the cycle starts again.

Pregnancy.   The fetal chorionic tissue that forms the placenta secretes *chorionic gonadotropin,*† which maintains the corpus luteum for the duration of pregnancy. In turn the corpus luteum secretes estrogen and progesterone. These inhibit the hypothalamic–hypophyseal system so that ovulation does not occur. Breast development is induced by the combined effects of placental hor-mones (estrogen, progesterone, and placental lactogen). During the latter part of pregnancy pituitary prolactin induces further changes.

Lactation.   Following delivery, lactation is established under the influence of prolactin. The act of suckling causes release of oxytocin — this helps to express the milk.

THE OVARY

DEVELOPMENT

The ovaries develop, as do the testes, in the mesoderm of the posterior ab-dominal wall. Each ovary has three components: (a) a covering of *germinal epithelium* that is modified peritoneal mesothelium; (b) a *stroma* derived from mesoderm, and (c) *germ cells* that later mature into ova. Stromal cells form each *graafian follicle,* and after the release of the ovum they also form the *corpus lu-teum.* Both these structures manufacture sex hormones, as previously de-scribed. It should be noted that the primitive gonad is asexual, being neither male nor female. The primordial germ cells, which are sequestered early in the formation of an embryo and are probably of endodermal origin, migrate to the gonad and there develop into either ova or sperm. The stroma of the gonad has

---

*The rhythmic cycling center that awakens at puberty is peculiar to the female. It is responsi-ble for the coordinated formation of releasing factors that in turn control the adenohypophysis and ultimately the ovarian function. The presence of male hormones in the fetus prevents the develop-ment of a cycling center in the male.

†Human chorionic gonadotropin (HCG) is produced soon after implantation of the fertilized ovum. Its detection in the urine forms the basis for the common pregnancy tests. The test becomes positive at the time of the first missed menstrual period.

the ability to secrete hormones of either female or male type. Hence, it is not surprising that tumors of the ovary sometimes produce an excess of either male or female hormones.

Diseases of the Ovary

CYSTS

Cysts derived from unruptured graafian follicles or from corpora lutei are extremely common. Since they rarely exceed 3 cm in diameter, they are rarely the cause of trouble.

PRIMARY TUMORS

Benign Tumors of Germinal Epithelium. Benign tumors of the germinal epithelium form cystic spaces with papillary epithelial ingrowths. They are therefore called *papillary cystadenomas.* These benign lesions can reach enormous proportions and can occupy much of the pelvic cavity or even the abdominal cavity. The largest one reported weighed 328 pounds!

Malignant Tumors of the Germinal Epithelium. *Papillary cystadenocarcinoma* is the most common primary malignancy of the ovary and is the malignant counterpart of the cystadenoma. As with papillomatous lesions of the bladder, it is difficult to draw a line between benign and malignant lesions. There is a gray area between the two extremes, and in this area individual pathologists will differ in their opinions. The malignant ovarian tumors show profuse papillomatous projections both into the cystic cavities and from the surface. Since peritoneal seeding is common, the other ovary is often involved (Fig. 37–1). Abdominal swelling due to *ascites* may be a prominent and distressing clinical manifestation. The presence of malignant cells in ascitic fluid is a helpful diagnostic finding. Lymph node and widespread blood-borne metastases occur, as with other carcinomas.

Other Primary Ovarian Tumors. The benign teratoma has been described in Chapter 17 (see Fig. 17–15). Occasionally a component of this tumor becomes malignant, such as in the formation of squamous-cell carcinoma or even a choriocarcinoma.

Other ovarian tumors form a complex group, the description of which is beyond the scope of this book. Some tumors secrete estrogens; others secrete androgens. Hence, the possibility of an ovarian tumor must be considered in any woman showing definite signs of masculinization or of excessive endometrial hyperplasia.

SECONDARY TUMORS

The ovary is involved in metastatic growth more often than any other pelvic organ. The common primary sites are the large intestine, the stomach, and the breast.

FIGURE 37–1. *Carcinoma of the ovary.*

The specimen consists of the uterus with both fallopian tubes and ovaries. The left ovary is enormously enlarged by tumor; the right ovary shows a white area that also contains tumor. Numerous peritoneal nodules of metastatic growth were present in this patient. Note the asymmetry of the body of the uterus. When the organ was opened, a septum was found. It divided the cavity into two unequal parts and was the result of imperfect fusion of the two müllerian ducts.

THE FALLOPIAN TUBES

The fallopian tubes, the uterus, and most of the vagina develop from the two müllerian ducts. Normally these ducts fuse completely to form a single midline uterus and vagina, but sometimes this fusion is incomplete. The most extreme example of this is the rare anomaly of a double uterus and a double vagina. Much more frequent is an incomplete fusion of the parts of the primitive uterus, so that this organ develops with two horns or has a septum partially dividing its cavity (Fig. 37–1). The upper, or cephalic, part of the müllerian duct normally remains separate and forms the fallopian tube. Note that the lumen of the fallopian tubes remains open to the peritoneal cavity, because it is through this opening that the ova reach the lower genital tract.

INFLAMMATORY DISEASE OF THE FALLOPIAN TUBES

Pyogenic infections of the female genital tract tend to spare the vagina and endometrium but tend to attack the fallopian tubes severely. The result is *acute salpingitis*. The fimbriated ends of the tubes become sealed over, and the infection enters a chronic phase. The tubes are distended with pus and assume the shape of retort tubes *(pyosalpinx)*. Ultimately the infection subsides, and the tubes remain distended with clear fluid *(hydrosalpinx)*.

Salpingitis is often accompanied by inflammation of the adjacent pelvic structures, including the peritoneum and bowel. It then forms a component of a more widespread *pelvic inflammatory disease (PID)*. When this disease is acute, because of the peritonitis there are manifestations of an acute abdomen.

When chronic, the condition causes pain, dysmenorrhea, and intestinal obstruction secondary to the formation of fibrous adhesions. The *sterility* that results is due to the closure of the fimbriated ends of the fallopian tubes.

The most common type of PID used to be gonorrheal, but this infection responds so well to chemotherapy that the incidence of gonococcal salpingitis has now declined. PID is more often due to other pyogenic organisms—staphylococci, streptococci, and the coliform organisms. PID is now encountered principally as a postpartum or a postabortal infection.

Tuberculous Salpingitis. This was once a disease to consider as a cause of sterility. The disease has fortunately been eradicated.

THE UTERUS

The uterus consists of two parts: the *cervix* and the *body*.

The Cervix Uteri

The cervix (neck) of the uterus consists of two parts: the *endocervix* and the *exocervix*. The endocervix is lined by a mucus-secreting epithelium with associated glands, whereas the vaginal part, or exocervix, protrudes into the vagina and is covered by stratified squamous epithelium.

CERVICAL EROSION

In women who have borne children, the cervix is often scarred and distorted. Sometimes the endocervical mucosa is everted or "turned out" and can be seen on vaginal examination. This is the common type of "cervical erosion" and was so named because it appeared as if the normal squamous epithelium of the exocervix had become eroded and covered by endocervixlike mucosa. This mechanism is not generally accepted, but the term "erosion" is still widely used. The condition is important in two connections:

(a) Cervical erosion is often accompanied by chronic cervicitis and a persistent mucoid or mucopurulent vaginal discharge.

(b) The appearance may mimic that of a carcinoma.

CERVICAL POLYPS

Inflammatory folds, or polyps, of endocervical mucosa are very common and can protrude through the external os into the vagina. Ulceration and bleeding, particularly following intercourse, can arouse suspicion of cancer. Polyps do not, however, predispose to malignancy.

CARCINOMA OF THE CERVIX

Cancer of the cervix is the most common malignant tumor of the female genital tract and is an important cause of death. It may grow as a cauliflowerlike tumor *(exophytic type)* or it may invade the cervix to produce a nodular, hard mass with overlying ulceration *(endophytic type)*. The peak age of incidence is about 50 years, but the *in-situ* stage is present 10 to 15 years before that. Ninety-five per cent of the tumors are squamous-celled, and the remainder are adenocarcinomas. The chief symptoms are a vaginal discharge, intermenstrual bleeding, and postmenopausal bleeding. It must be appreciated, however, that these are the symptoms of advanced (and often incurable) disease. Carcinoma of the cervix spreads to involve local structures (intestine, ureters, and bladder) and later metastasizes to regional lymph nodes. Widespread metastases can occur, but death is often due to the local effects of the tumor or to radiation damage.

Predisposing Causes.   According to statistics, cancer of the cervix is most common in low-income groups, in women who have had sexual intercourse at an early age, and in women who have had frequent intercourse and many sexual partners. It is uncommon in ethnic groups (*e.g.*, Jews and Indian Muslims) that practice male circumcision at an early age. Herpesvirus infection is more common in patients with carcinoma of the cervix than in control groups, but this may be coincidental and have no etiological relationship; both diseases are more prevalent in the promiscuous.

The Development of Cancer of the Cervix.   Cancer of the cervix is believed to develop slowly, from increasingly severe dysplasia, to carcinoma-*in-situ*, and finally to invasive cancer. These stages can be detected by a cytological examination of scrapings from the cervix (see the "Pap Smear," Chapter 17). Regular examination of all adult women should therefore eliminate deaths from this disease, since early lesions can be treated and cured.

When a Pap (from Papanicolaou, who originated the test) test is found to be positive for abnormal cells, it should be repeated to eliminate errors of interpretation or labeling. The precise course of action varies from one center to another. Patients with mild dysplasia can be followed for evidence indicating that their disease is progressing. Severe dysplasia and carcinoma-*in-situ* demand more active treatment. The experienced gynecologist can detect abnormal areas of the cervix by using the colposcope: these areas can be biopsied (to exclude invasive cancer) and treated by local destructive agents, such as extreme cold, as used in cryotherapy. Another course of action is to biopsy a large "cone" of cervical tissue and search for abnormal areas. When invasive cancer is present, the treatment rests between hysterectomy, radiotherapy, or a combination of both. It is evident that the management of carcinoma of the cervix involves technical skills and good judgment. There are few other areas in medicine where the technologist, the pathologist, and the clinical physician must collaborate if their patients are to receive the best treatment. Overdiagnosis and overtreatment can result in unnecessary surgery that can prevent young women from bearing children. Underdiagnosis and undertreatment, on the other hand, can kill the patient.

The Body of the Uterus

The body of the uterus consists of a powerful muscle (the *myometrium*) and a mucosal lining (the *endometrium*).

The changes that take place in the endometrium during the normal menstrual cycle have already been described. Endometrial abnormalities often cause changes in menstruation; these will be described first.

ABNORMALITIES OF MENSTRUATION

Some menstrual irregularity occurs in every woman's life. This section deals only with certain facets of this important and complex problem.

Amenorrhea, or absence of menstruation, is normal before the menarche, after the menopause, and during pregnancy and lactation. *Primary amenorrhea* denotes a failure to commence menstruation and is usually due to ovarian disease (*e.g.*, ovarian dysgenesis) or to hypothalamic-pituitary disorders. *Secondary amenorrhea* is usually defined as absence of menstruation for more than 12 months, excluding pregnancy and the menopause. Hormonal imbalance due to detectable disease of the ovaries, hypothalamus, or endocrine glands is an occasional cause, but amenorrhea is also a feature of numerous general illnesses, including mental disturbances such as worry, emotional disappointments, and depression. The mechanism is presumably related to nervous influences on the hypothalamic cycling center.

Menorrhagia, meaning excessive or prolonged blood loss occurring at menstruation, is extremely common. Sometimes it is due to a failure of ovulation. No corpus luteum is formed, and estrogens acting in the absence of progesterone lead to *endometrial hyperplasia*. Curettage performed during the latter half of the menstrual cycle shows *absence of secretory activity*. The procedure of curettage is therefore a useful way of diagnosing this type of anovulatory bleeding.

Metrorrhagia refers to intermenstrual bleeding or such irregularity that no periodicity is present. Sometimes this condition is due to an irregular endometrial response to normal ovarian hormonal influence. Thus secretory and proliferative areas of endometrium exist side by side.

Abnormalities of menstruation may be symptomatic of local uterine disease—polyps, endometriosis, fibroids, or carcinoma. When no obvious cause can be found, the clinical term "functional uterine bleeding" is sometimes used.

TUMORS OF THE BODY OF THE UTERUS

Leiomyoma. The leiomyoma is a benign tumor of smooth muscle and usually contains an admixture of fibrous tissue (Fig. 37–2). Hence, it is also called a fibroleiomyoma or "fibroid." Fibroids arise in the myometrium and are generally multiple. They vary in size from those that are scarcely visible in the gross to those weighing over 100 pounds! Some fibroids become pedunculated and appear as subserosal or submucosal nodules. Uterine fibroids are the commonest tumor to afflict women and are present in about 25 per cent of the adult female population. They may cause symptoms in various ways. Their presence may be associated with menorrhagia and irregular bleeding. Occasionally they cause mechanical difficulties during labor. Fibroids appear to be estrogen-dependent, because they diminish in size, degenerate, and even calcify after the menopause.

FIGURE 37–2. *Leiomyoma of the uterus.*

The uterus has been opened to show one large well-circumscribed tumor. Several smaller fibroids were also present, but they are not visible in this photograph. This tumor was an incidental finding in a patient who died as a result of carcinoma of the colon. (Courtesy of Dr. A. Vayalumkal.)

Carcinoma of the Endometrium. Adenocarcinoma of the endometrium is a disease of postmenopausal women with a peak incidence in persons between 50 and 60 years of age. It is less common than carcinoma of the cervix, but the incidence is on the increase, partly because of longer life expectancy. The disease is more frequent among childless women than among multiparous ones.

Carcinoma of the endometrium is characterized by irregular vaginal bleeding accompanied by leukorrhea. The disease probably begins with the development of endometrial hyperplasia, dysplasia, and carcinoma-*in-situ*. Nevertheless, this orderly sequence of development is less well documented than the stages of development of carcinoma of the cervix.

ENDOMETRIOSIS

Pelvic Endometriosis (Endometriosis Externa). In this type of endometriosis, ectopic endometrium is present in the pelvic region (ovaries, uterine ligaments, vagina) and in the peritoneal covering of the bladder and uterus. The pathogenesis of this remarkable state has been much debated. Endometrial tissue regurgitated through the fallopian tubes during menstruation could become implanted in the pelvic organs. Alternatively, peritoneal cells could undergo metaplasia. The occasional occurrence of endometriosis in the umbilicus—and even in the lung—has raised the possibility of lymphatic or bloodborne spread. The pathogenesis remains a mystery!

The endometrial tissue undergoes the same changes as the uterine endometrium during the menstrual cycle. Bleeding into the affected areas causes pain and stimulates fibrosis. Pain during the periods (*dysmenorrhea*) is therefore a feature.

Adenomyosis (Endometriosis Interna). This is a common condition in which normal-appearing endometrium invades the myometrium.

COMPLICATIONS OF PREGNANCY

HYPEREMESIS GRAVIDARUM

Nausea and morning sickness are common in early pregnancy but the origin of these symptoms is not understood. Occasionally the vomiting becomes severe enough to cause dehydration, starvation, and death. Wernicke's encephalopathy can develop in fatal cases (see Chapter 44).

TOXEMIA OF PREGNANCY

Although the term "toxemia" is in common use, no specific toxin has ever been identified. The condition occurs during the last three months (trimester) of pregnancy, and its early stages are characterized by three features:

(a) HYPERTENSION.   This is the most constant feature.

(b) ALBUMINURIA.   This occurs in severe cases.

(c) EDEMA.   Some degree of water and salt retention resulting in edema of the legs is common in normal pregnancy and is of no significance. However, edema of the face or arms, and any marked weight increase due to water accumulation immediately suggests toxemia.

Severe toxemia (termed *pre-eclampsia*) is characterized by headache, visual disturbances (ranging from flashes of light to blindness), abdominal pain, and vomiting. It is a serious condition, because it can be followed by *eclampsia*. This is the most severe manifestation of toxemia and is characterized by epileptiform convulsions that start with twitching of the face, are followed by a *tonic phase* lasting one to two minutes, and terminate in a *clonic phase* with violent, convulsive movements during which the pregnant woman may damage herself.

Toxemia is sometimes familial; it is associated with abruptio placentae, twin pregnancies, and the presence of a hydatidiform mole. It is most common in primigravidae (women who are pregnant for the first time). Vascular spasm appears to be the cause of the headaches, cerebral edema, visual disturbances, and convulsions. Necropsy findings include glomerular changes and liver necrosis together with evidence of disseminated intravascular coagulation. Rarely bilateral renal cortical necrosis results in renal failure (see Chapter 21 and Figure 21–4).

These observations have done little to shed any light on the etiology of toxemia. The disease that causes an appreciable fetal and maternal mortality has no known cause other than that it is associated with pregnancy. Nevertheless, with early diagnosis the condition responds well to simple medical remedies, such as bed rest and salt restriction. For this reason, good antenatal care always includes *routine examination of the patient for hypertension, albuminuria, edema, and excessive weight gain.*

ECTOPIC PREGNANCY

By the time the ovum, which is fertilized in the fallopian tube, reaches the uterus, it is at the correct stage for implantation. If its passage is delayed, implantation occurs in the tube; this is the most common type of ectopic pregnancy. The fetus grows for a time, but its growth usually causes the tube to rupture by the sixth week. Pain and severe intra-abdominal hemorrhage are the result. When the fetus dies, the endometrium is shed and vaginal bleeding occurs. This sign helps to distinguish a ruptured ectopic pregnancy from other abdominal catastrophes.

ABORTION

The expulsion of a nonviable fetus* is termed *abortion* or *miscarriage.* Many causes, both fetal and maternal, have been described. Chief among them is fetal abnormality; spontaneous abortion is an important mechanism by which defective fetuses are eliminated (see Chapter 3).

BLEEDING DURING PREGNANCY

Bleeding from the genital tract during pregnancy not only is alarming for the patient but also is often a warning of a serious abnormality. The types of bleeding may be divided into two groups, described below:

1. Bleeding in Early Pregnancy (before 28 weeks' gestation).   Three important causes should be noted and are considered elsewhere in this chapter:

    (a) abortion

    (b) ectopic pregnancy

    (c) hydatidiform mole.

2. Bleeding in the Later Months of Pregnancy.   Bleeding that occurs after the twenty-eighth week of gestation and before delivery is called *antepartum hemorrhage.* Two causes are of paramount importance:

(a) PLACENTA PREVIA.   In this condition, part or all of the placenta is attached to the lower uterine segment. This part of the uterus stretches and thins out in late pregnancy and especially during labor. The more rigid placenta becomes detached, and this provokes external bleeding. The initial bleeding is often slight and painless: it can be followed by massive bleeding that endangers the life of both mother and child. Urgent hospital treatment is necessary and often cesarean section is required.

(b) ABRUPTIO PLACENTAE.   In this condition there is premature separation of a normally situated placenta. Bleeding occurs between the placenta and the uterine wall, and there may or may not be external bleeding. The condition is most common in primigravidae and in patients with toxemia. Abruptio placentae is characterized by abdominal pain, tenderness of the uterus, and the

---

*The age at which a fetus becomes viable is arbitrarily set at 20 weeks gestation by some authorities and at 28 weeks by others.

development of shock. Death is a complication. As with placenta praevia, urgent hospital treatment is necessary.

HYDATIDIFORM MOLE

This lesion may be regarded as a benign tumor of the placenta (Fig. 37–3). No fetus develops, and the mole generally causes more rapid enlargement of the uterus than is normal for the stage of pregnancy. Bleeding occurs during the early course of pregnancy, and the mole may be expelled spontaneously.

CHORIOCARCINOMA

This is a highly malignant tumor of placental tissue. It may arise in a previous hydatidiform mole, or it may follow either an abortion or a normal labor. The tumor is highly invasive and metastasizes widely. Nevertheless, some cases respond dramatically to chemotherapy. Both hydatidiform mole and choriocarcinoma produce large quantities of chorionic gonadotropin. Consequently the detection of chorionic gonadotropin in the urine is a useful test in these conditions, both for initial diagnosis and for the detection of recurrences or metastases.

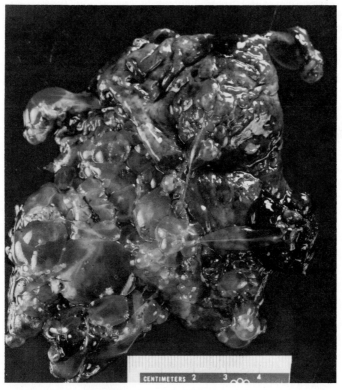

FIGURE 37–3. *Hydatidiform mole.*

The normal placental tissue has been largely replaced by the mole. Note the presence of numerous fluid-filled cysts from which the lesion gets its name. *Hydatis* is from the Greek, meaning "a drop of water."

Review Questions

1. An ovarian mass has been diagnosed by pelvic examination. Speculate on its possible nature. At laparotomy an ovarian tumor was found, and a biopsy revealed that it was a choriocarcinoma. Suggest how the tumor arose and how it might have been diagnosed before surgery.
2. What is the significance of finding no secretory activity in uterine curettings taken 26 days after the first day of the last menstrual period?
3. Explain why carcinoma of the cervix uteri is a preventable disease.
4. Describe the hormonal functions of the placenta.
5. Speculate on the causes of vaginal bleeding in each of the following women:
     (a) a 13-year-old girl
     (b) a 26-year-old married woman who has missed her last two periods
     (c) a woman who is due to give birth in two weeks
     (d) a pregnant woman who is under treatment for toxemia of pregnancy.

Selected Readings

Leading Article: Management of eclampsia, British Medical Journal, 2 1485–1486, 1976.
Leading Article: Screening for cervical cancer. British Medical Journal, 3:659–660, 1976.
Novak, E. R., and Woodruff, J. D.: Gynecologic and Obstetric Pathology. 7th ed. Philadelphia, W. B. Saunders Company, 1974. A comprehensive reference book.
Robbins, S. L.: Pathologic Basis of Disease. Philadelphia, W. B. Saunders Company, 1974. Chapter 27 provides a general overview of the subject.

DISEASES OF THE BREAST

Chapter 38

After studying this chapter the student should be able to:

● Describe the structure and development of the female breast.
● Describe the main features of acute mastitis, plasma cell mastitis, and fat necrosis of the breast.
● List the groups of women who are especially liable to develop carcinoma of the breast.
● Discuss briefly the evidence suggesting that cancer of the breast is due to a viral infection.
● Classify the types of carcinoma of the breast.
● Give an account of the early detection, the prognosis, and the treatment of carcinoma of the breast.
● Describe the routes of spread of breast cancer.
● Define gynecomastia and give three examples of this condition.

DISEASES OF THE BREAST

Structure and Development

The human breast is not a single gland but, on the contrary, consists of about 20 separate glands or *lobes*, each with its own duct opening separately onto the surface of the nipple. The lobes develop, as do the sweat glands, by ingrowths from the surface epidermis; during infancy, they consist only of rudimentary branching ducts surrounded by cuffs of connective tissue that are an extension of the papillary dermis. In the male this state persists throughout life, but in the female during the three- to four-year period before the onset of menstruation, the breasts enlarge and the ducts and the specialized loose periductal stroma that is a characteristic feature of the breast tissue proliferate. During adolescence stromal growth continues, and buds form at the end of the ducts. These are the *lobules*, and they are the beginnings of the secretory gland structure that develops later if pregnancy occurs.

In the adult female the breast shows cyclical changes that parallel those of the endometrium during the menstrual cycle. Under the influence of estrogen there is epithelial proliferation during the first half of the cycle; this proliferation continues as progesterone is added during the second half of the cycle. During this second phase there is abortive secretory activity, and the gland enlarges and feels tense.

The breast attains its maximum development during pregnancy and lactation. The epithelial proliferation and secretory gland formation is such that the organ closely resembles other secretory glands, such as the pancreas.

In the normal resting breast the epithelial component constitutes about 15 per cent of the organ. The remainder consists of lobules of fat contained by fibrous septa that stretch from the dermis to the fascia overlying the pectoral muscles. These septa play a large part in giving the female breast its firmness and configuration. The septa also form an avenue for the spread of carcinoma to the skin and pectoral muscles.

DEVELOPMENTAL ANOMALIES

Supernumerary Breast Tissue. Most mammals develop breast tissue along a milk line. In humans this extends from the anterior axillary fold to the groin; occasionally, accessory nipples are found along this line. When associated with accessory breast tissue in the female, these enlarge and cause pain at puberty and particularly during pregnancy.

Enlargement of the Breast.   It is common to find some enlargement of the breasts in newborn infants in whom some secretion ("witch's milk") may be formed. This enlargement lasts for one to two weeks and is due to the action of maternal hormones. On rare occasions enlargement of one or both breasts takes place during childhood if there is excessive estrogen produced by a functioning tumor of the ovary, adrenal, or pituitary.

The most common type of enlargement of the breast (generally called *hypertrophy*) is seen in girls at adolescence. One or both breasts become so enlarged that partial surgical removal *(reduction mammoplasty)* is required. This *virginal hypertrophy* of the breast is presumably due to hormonal imbalance.

Acquired Disease of the Breast

INFLAMMATION

Acute Mastitis.   Acute bacterial mastitis is generally seen in the breast during the first few weeks of nursing a firstborn child. The offending organism, *Staphylococcus aureus,* appears to gain access through a crack in the nipple. Suppuration requiring surgical drainage generally follows unless early antibiotic treatment is instituted.

Plasma Cell Mastitis.   This is an uncommon condition and generally affects women about 40 years of age. There is often a history of difficult nursing due to inverted nipples, cracked nipples, or infection. In one quadrant of the breast an area of thickening is found that extends beneath the nipple to cause some distortion. There is usually pain and tenderness and sometimes a discharge from the nipple. Pathologically, there is dilatation of the associated ducts; this appears to be the prime lesion. The ducts are filled with a creamy liquid and contain many macrophages with vacuolated cytoplasm. Rupture of this inspissated material into the surrounding stroma causes a chronic inflammatory reaction with many plasma cells and sometimes with tuberculoid granulomas, causing a clinical picture that mimics tuberculosis. Tuberculosis of the breast is, in fact, very rare.

Fat Necrosis.   This condition is generally encountered in fat, pendulous breasts. In about half the patients a history of trauma is obtained. Histologically, there is necrosis of fat cells with an associated inflammatory reaction, at first acute and then progressing to chronicity with foreign body giant cells and a granulomatous reaction. The lesion presents as a lump in the breast, and the histological picture must be differentiated from that of tuberculosis.

MAMMARY DYSPLASIA

This condition has been given many names in the past, the commonest being chronic mastitis. Nevertheless, the condition is not inflammatory and appears to be the end-result of the hormonal changes that take place during women's reproductive life. As noted previously, the breast undergoes cyclic changes of hyperplasia and regression during menstruation. The combined effect of these changes over many years is to produce in some women imbalance between the amount of epithelium and the specialized fibrous tissue. The disease may affect one segment of one breast, commonly the upper and outer quadrant, and produce a relatively localized mass, or it may affect much of the tissue of both breasts, producing a widespread lumpiness. A characteristic feature that helps to distinguish these lesions from carcinoma is that the lumps tend to increase in size and to become more tender before each menstrual period. Several types of mammary dysplasia have been described, but they represent aspects of a single disease rather than constituting separate entities.

1. FIBROSIS OF THE BREAST. This is also known as *mastodynia*, which literally means "pain in the breast." It is an early variant of mammary dysplasia and is characterized by stromal fibrosis with a little epithelial hyperplasia. It generally occurs in women between the ages of 30 and 35 years, and is usually unilateral. Microscopically there is an overgrowth of fibrous tissue, causing the epithelial elements to be surrounded by dense connective tissue rather than by the normal specialized loose stroma.

2. ADENOSIS. This variant is also usually unilateral and affects only a segment of the breast, thereby presenting as a mass. Microscopically there is epithelial overgrowth in the ducts, so that they are lined by a multilayered epithelium. Sometimes intraductal papillomas are formed. Another pattern is the proliferation of ductular and glandular epithelium, so that groups of cells appear to extend into the breast tissue. If there is also surrounding fibrosis, the microscopic picture can closely resemble that of carcinoma. This condition is known as *sclerosing adenosis.*

3. CYSTIC DISEASE. In this variant of mammary dysplasia, epithelial proliferation is combined with cystic dilatation. The cysts are frequently multiple, bilateral, and may at times be large. Cystic disease may be regarded as the end-result of mammary dysplasia, because it presumably occurs following epithelial overgrowth and subsequent involution. Nevertheless, even in cystic disease some evidence of hyperplasia can be found, and occasional papillary ingrowths are seen into the cysts. Another example is the frequent occurrence of spaces lined by epithelium that closely resembles that of apocrine glands (apocrine metaplasia).

Relationship to Carcinoma. Views on the relationship of mammary dysplasia to the subsequent development of carcinoma have varied considerably during the last few decades. At one time it was fashionable to regard the condition as premalignant. Many simple mastectomies were thus performed with a view to averting the development of cancer. Current belief is that although some of the hyperplastic lesions may show increased tendency to become malignant, the overall pattern is that of a disease bearing little direct relationship to cancer. Nevertheless, cancer of the breast is more common in women who also have mammary dysplasia. Since the tumor often arises in the breast not affected by the dysplasia, it is suggested that the hormonal influences leading to dysplasia also predispose to malignant change.

The importance of mammary dysplasia is that it presents as one or more lumps in the breast; these lumps must be distinguished from cancer, generally by biopsy.

Benign Tumors of the Breast

Fibroadenoma.   Fibroadenoma is the commonest tumor of the breast, occurring in women younger than 30 years of age. Although it may be regarded as a localized form of mammary dysplasia, since it is so localized and encapsulated, it is generally classified as a benign tumor. Nevertheless, it responds to hormonal stimulation like the normal breast. The tumor enlarges during pregnancy and regresses after the menopause.

Papilloma.   One or more intraductal or intracystic papillomatous growths are sometimes found in women at or shortly before the menopause. The lesions appear as raspberrylike nodules filling a duct or growing from the wall of a cyst. The lesions frequently bleed and lead to a blood-stained discharge from the nipple. The relationship to carcinoma is disputed, but undoubtedly a number of papillomas do progress to carcinoma, and their removal is a wise precaution.

Malignant Tumors of the Breast

CARCINOMA

In North America cancer of the breast is the most common malignant tumor in women. Breast cancer is responsible for more deaths than any other single tumor. Under the age of 25 years breast cancer is rare; it attains its maximum incidence at about the menopause. The disease is much less frequent in Japan and the Far East. A number of groups in whom the disease is more frequent than in a control population can be singled out:

1. Women of high socioeconomic status.
2. Jewish women
3. Women with a family history of breast cancer
4. Women with a preceding history of breast problems, *e.g.*, mammary dysplasia
5. Single women
6. Women who have had no children
7. Women whose onset of menstruation (the menarche) was early (under 12 years).

The explanation for these observed differences is uncertain. Genetic factors play some part, but environmental factors must be equally important, because in North America the disease is increasing in frequency.

Cause of Breast Cancer
A vast amount of research has been carried out on this subject, and three factors appear to be important.

1. INHERITANCE.   The incidence of cancer of the breast varies greatly in different strains of mice. In humans it has been found if a sister or mother has had cancer of the breast, a woman's chances of developing a similar tumor are increased.

2. VIRUSES.   The Bittner virus causes cancer of the breast in female mice of suitable strains (see Chapter 17). The virus is passed from mother to offspring in the milk, and the high incidence of tumors in a strain, while appearing to be hereditary, is in fact due to neonatal infection.

In an inbred Parsi community living in Bombay there is a group of women who have a very high incidence of breast cancer. Samples of their milk contain particles that resemble the Bittner virus and also contain RNA-dependent DNA polymerase. Evidence is steadily accumulating to incriminate an RNA virus as a factor in the cause of human breast cancer. Whether it is a crucial factor or merely one of many agents acting in concert to cause cancer, remains to be discovered.

3. HORMONES.   Prolonged exposure of breast tissue to the action of estrogen may be important as a factor in causing breast cancer. This would explain the increased incidence associated with advancing age, an early menarche, and those who have not been pregnant.

Types of Breast Cancer

Cancer can arise in either the lobules or the ducts.

LOBULAR CARCINOMA.   The early stage in the development of this cancer is an *in situ* carcinoma. It is only when the malignant cells invade the surrounding tissues *(infiltrating lobular carcinoma)* that a mass can be felt clinically. Although lobular carcinoma is uncommon, it accounts for about 10 per cent of the total number of patients with carcinoma; the tumor is of importance because it often arises multifocally. Since about 20 per cent of patients have a tumor in the opposite breast, it is a common practice to take blind biopsies of the other breast when one performs the mastectomy.

DUCTAL CARCINOMA.   In *in-situ ductular carcinoma* the duct becomes filled with malignant cells. This lesion is difficult to feel but may be detected radiographically. In due course, tumor cells invade the surrounding connective tissues and form one of the varieties of infiltrating carcinoma:

1. *Scirrhous Carcinoma.*   This type accounts for about 75 per cent of all cancers of the breast. The tumor is *stony hard* and nonencapsulated (Fig. 38–1). Microscopically these tumors are adenocarcinomas with varying degrees of differentiation (Fig. 38–2). An outstanding feature is the dense fibrous tissue stroma, which accounts for the hardness of the tumor. It is common to see rows of cancer cells trapped in fibrous tissue and resembling Indians in a file. Clinically, this common type of cancer presents as a hard lump in the breast. As the tumor infiltrates the fibrous septa of the breast, it reaches the skin and pectoral muscle. The lump then becomes *fixed* to both these structures. Contracture of the stroma causes skin dimpling and retraction of the nipple. Invasion of lymphatics and lymphedema give the skin an orange rind appearance (peau d'orange), whereas actual invasion of the dermis converts the skin into a hard mass of tumor like a shield or cuirass *(cancer en cuirasse)*.

2. *Medullary or Encephaloid Carcinoma.*   This tumor is a very cellular adenocarcinoma with little stromal reaction. It is therefore bulky and soft. Ulceration occurs in due course.

3. *Mucoid Carcinoma.*   This uncommon variant is characterized by slow growth and the formation of a bulky, gelatinous, soft tumor.

Metastatic Spread of Carcinoma

Embolic spread is the feature that causes carcinoma of the breast to be so lethal.

LYMPHATIC SPREAD.   Lymphatic permeation and embolism are so common in cancer of the breast that lymph node metastases are present in over 50 per cent of patients when the tumor is first diagnosed. The axillary group are

FIGURE 38–1. *Carcinoma of the breast.*

The figure shows a section through the breast. The carcinoma is deep to the nipple, to which it is firmly attached. Note how the tumor extends along the fibrous septa in the breast. The tumor is not encapsulated, and by gross examination it is impossible to tell how far the growth has extended.

This is an example of an advanced carcinoma of the breast: involvement of the nipple, skin, and axillary nodes results in a poor prognosis. In this particular case, the surgical wound became infected with *Escherichia coli* and *Streptococcus pyogenes*. The patient died as a result of hemorrhage from the wound. This case dates back to 1932; although penicillin had been discovered three years previously by Fleming, it had not yet been introduced into clinical medicine and the sulfonamides had not yet been discovered. For a more complete description, see Case History I. (Specimen courtesy of the Boyd Museum, Banting Institute, Toronto.)

Case History I. (See Figure 38–1.) The patient had noticed a lump in the right breast one year before consulting her doctor. A discharge from the nipple finally convinced her of the need to seek medical advice. On examination the right breast was found to be smaller than the left. A hard mass could be felt deep to the nipple. The nipple itself was indrawn and adherent to the mass. Mobile enlarged axillary lymph nodes contained secondary deposits of tumor.

FIGURE 38–2. *Carcinoma of the breast.*

This photomicrograph shows groups and columns of carcinoma cells embedded in a dense fibrous stroma. In some areas, single columns of cells can be seen (arrows); elsewhere, there is the beginning of tubule formation. The tumor is therefore classified as a poorly differentiated adenocarcinoma. The gross appearance of this tumor was that of a typical scirrhous carcinoma similar to the one depicted in Figure 38–1. The name is derived from the Greek *skirrhos,* meaning "hard" (× 300).

the nodes most frequently involved, particularly from cancers of the upper and outer quadrant. This is the commonest site for cancer. Intrathoracic nodes are involved, especially from tumors in the medial quadrants.

BLOOD-BORNE METASTASES.   Hematogenous spread leads to involvement of the lungs, liver, adrenals, ovaries and bone (Fig. 38–3). These secondary growths are not often detectable at the time of initial diagnosis, but they make their presence known sometimes years later, even after apparently successful treatment. These dormant tumors are common.

Diagnosis of Breast Cancer

Any lump in the breast must be presumed to be malignant until proven otherwise. Usually this determination involves biopsy or local excision. It is useless to rely on detecting the classical signs of cancer—fixation to skin, retraction, and elevation of the nipple, among others. Tumors diagnosed by these signs are often already incurable.

Management of Breast Cancer

The introduction of radical mastectomy (removal of breast, pectoral muscles, and axillary contents with lymph nodes) by Halsted did much to improve the prognosis of breast cancer. Unfortunately, the appearance of late metastases

FIGURE 38–3. *Metastatic breast cancer.*

At the age of 53 years the patient underwent a modified right radical mastectomy for carcinoma of the breast. Seven months later she developed shortness of breath and pain in the right side of the chest. Radiographs revealed evidence of metastases in the lungs and the spine. Nodules of tumor next appeared in the scalp and a biopsy of one of them confirmed the diagnosis of metastatic poorly differentiated adenocarcinoma. She died shortly afterward; necropsy disclosed metastatic tumor in the lungs, bones, adrenals, thyroid, and brain. The liver contained multiple masses of tumor similar in appearance to those depicted in Figure 17–7.

Specimen A shows the cut surface of parts of the three lobes of the right lung. Carcinoma has invaded the lymphatics of the septa as well as the region around the blood vessels and bronchi. This reticulated appearance resulting from extensive lymphatic involvement is common in metastatic breast cancer in lung, and it contrasts with the multiple nodular appearance presented by pulmonary metastases from other tumors and the deposits of growth in the liver found in this case.

Specimen B shows a segment of the bisected thoracic vertebral column. The bodies of two vertebrae show obvious white tumor.

was not influenced by local surgery; alternative, less mutilating procedures have thus been introduced. Radiotherapy (alone or combined with simple excision of the tumor) and removal of the breast alone (simple mastectomy) both have their advocates. The results of treatment seem to be about the same with each of these methods, but there is no agreement as to which is the best. The present trend is to avoid the radical surgery that was once practiced, *e.g.*, radical mastectomy and removal of intrathoracic lymph nodes.

Hormone therapy has its uses as a palliative treatment of metastatic disease. It includes the removal of the ovaries, adrenals, or pituitary in premenopausal women; the administration of testosterone; and, somewhat surprisingly, the administration of estrogens in older patients.

Early Detection of Cancer of the Breast

One would think that the ease with which the breast can be examined and removed would make early diagnosis and effective treatment easy; such is not the case. It seems that spread has often occurred by the time a lump is palpable. Routine physical examination, either by the woman herself or by a medical attendant, might improve the prognosis, but there is no proof of this. Radiography, or mammography, detection of hot spots by thermography (tumors tend to be vascular and hot), ultrasonic studies, and other methods have been introduced, but their value is unproven and their cost is considerable. Undoubtedly, small lesions can be detected, but a small lesion is not necessarily an early one. Prognosis depends on factors other than mere size.

Prognosis of Cancer of the Breast

About two thirds of patients have lymph-node involvement at the time of initial diagnosis, and about 25 per cent of the conditions are inoperable. The overall five-year survival rate is 35 to 40 per cent, but of those treated by radical surgery, about 50 to 55 per cent are alive five years later. The prognosis depends on many factors, including the following:

1. Pregnancy, which sometimes adversely affects prognosis.

2. Histological grade of tumor. Poorly differentiated tumors do poorly compared with well-differentiated ones.

3. The type of tumor in terms of the size of the primary tumor (T), the presence and extent of lymph-node involvement (N), and the presence of distant metastases (M). This is the TNM system of classification. A stage-1 tumor (tumor less than 5 cm in diameter with no lymph-node or distant metastases) has an 80 per cent 5-year survival rate, and a 62 per cent 10-year survival rate, but it can recur even after 10 years, even though the chances diminish with each passing year. For a stage-2 tumor, the 5- and 10-year survival rates are 36 per cent and 22 per cent, respectively, whereas for stages 3 and 4 the outlook is even worse.

The spread and prognosis of breast cancer have been described in some detail because they illustrate the difficulties in assessing the effects of therapy. There are so many types and stages of the disease that unless each medical center uses a similar and comprehensive classification, it is not possible to compare the results of different treatments, or even the same treatment at different centers.

PAGET'S DISEASE OF THE BREAST. This is a chronic eczematous condition involving the nipple, which microscopically shows invasion of the epidermis

FIGURE 38–4. *Paget's disease of the nipple.*

The epidermis is thickened and contains numerous round cells with cytoplasm that stain palely because of their mucin content. The appearances are typical of Paget's disease.

The 74-year-old patient had had a red, scaly area of "eczema" of the left breast for over one year. The lesion was centered on the nipple and was about 4 cm in diameter. It had failed to respond to the application of a variety of steroid creams, which is a response with Paget's disease. The photograph shown is from a 3-mm punch biopsy specimen. Palpation revealed no tumor in the breast, but mammography showed a mass highly suggestive of carcinoma. Mastectomy was performed, and the presence of carcinoma was confirmed.

by large malignant Paget cells (Fig. 38–4). There is almost invariably an underlying ductal carcinoma. Opinions are divided as to whether Paget's disease represents an intraepithelial spread of a breast cancer, or whether epidermis and ductal epithelium are both involved simultaneously in a primary malignant process.

OTHER MALIGNANT TUMORS.   Fibrosarcoma and other malignant tumors occur, but they are rare.

The Male Breast

The diseases of the female breast can also occur in the male, but they are rare. Carcinoma is about 100 times less common in men than in women, but it has a poorer prognosis. Gynecomastia deserves separate consideration.

Gynecomastia is the name given to enlargement of the male breast. As a transient phenomenon it is not uncommon during adolescence and old age, presumably because it is related to hormonal imbalance during these periods of sexual development and decline. Other causes of gynecomastia include

Klinefelter's syndrome (see Chapter 3), heavy dosage of estrogens (*e.g.*, for carcinoma of the prostate), cirrhosis of the liver (see Chapter 33), and estrogen-secreting tumors of the adrenal, the testis, or other site.

Review Questions

1. The super-radical mastectomy, which involves removal of the breast, part of the chest wall, and the axillary, supraclavicular, and internal mammary lymph nodes, was evolved with a view to increasing the cure rate of breast cancer. Explain why you think this operation was designed. Discuss the reasons it has been unsuccessful in attaining its objective.
2. Describe the changes that you would expect to find in an autopsy performed on a woman who had died of carcinoma of the breast.
3. Identify those features that would classify a woman as being at a higher-than-average risk for developing breast cancer.
4. List the conditions that can produce a localized swelling or lump in one breast.

Selected Readings

Leading Article: Treatment of early breast cancer. British Medical Journal, 2:417–418, 1972.
Leading Article: Paget's disease of the skin. British Medical Journal, 1:707, 1972.
Robbins, S. L.: Pathologic Basis of Disease. Philadelphia, W. B. Saunders Company, 1974. Consult Chapter 28 for further details of breast diseases. The figures relating to the incidence and prognosis of cancer quoted in this chapter are from this source.

Chapter 39

After studying this chapter the student should be able to:

- Describe the mode of action of hormones.
- List the hormones that are manufactured in the hypothalamus.
- Give examples of the common manifestations of hypothalamic disorders.
- Describe the components of the neurohypophysis and the adenohypophysis. Indicate how each part develops.
- Outline the features of diabetes insipidus.
- List the hormones manufactured by the adenohypophysis and indicate their main actions.

DISEASES OF THE ENDOCRINE GLANDS

- Describe the common manifestations of hyperpituitarism and hypopituitarism. Give at least two causes of each condition.
- List the hormones produced by the adrenal glands.
- Describe the manifestations of Addison's disease.
- Describe the syndromes produced by adrenal cortical hypersecretion.
- Indicate the value of glucocorticoid therapy and list the important complications.
- Define *goiter* and give four examples of a condition that may cause it.
- Compare hyperthyroidism with hypothyroidism.
- Describe Graves' disease and Hashimoto's disease.

Introduction

Although the nervous system exerts the major controlling influence over the activities of the higher animals, there is an additional mechanism by which one type of cell can influence another—hormone secretion. By the secretion into the blood stream of potent chemicals called *hormones* cells can exert influence at a distant site. Secreting cells that perform this endocrine function may be grouped together to form one of the well-known endocrine glands, such as the thyroid gland, or they may be scattered more diffusely in the tissues. An example of the latter type is the cells in the pylorus that secrete the hormone *gastrin* when stimulated by the presence of food in the stomach. Gastrin stimulates the fundus of the stomach to secrete hydrochloric acid.

This chapter deals only with the common disorders of the major endocrine glands.

Mode of Action of Hormones

The hormones have an extremely potent and highly specific action on their target cells. This selective action is due to the binding of the hormones to specific receptor sites. The water-soluble hormones, such as epinephrine and glucagon, act on receptors on the cell membrane; cyclic AMP is formed, and it acts as a second messenger to stimulate or depress a characteristic biochemical activity (see Fig. 2–9). The lipid-soluble steroid hormones act on receptors within the cell, and the hormone-receptor complex enters the nucleus and then acts by affecting the expression of the cell's genetic material.

HYPOTHALAMUS

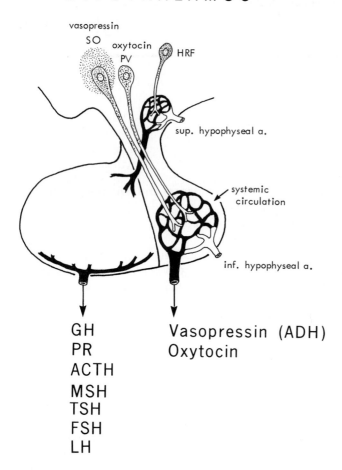

FIGURE 39–1. *The relationship between the hypothalamus and the pituitary gland.*

Vasopressin (antidiuretic hormone, ADH) and oxytocin are manufactured in nerve cells in the supraoptic (SO) and paraventricular (PV) nuclei of the hypothalamus. These hormones are not released into the circulation until they have reached the neurohypophysis. The shaded area surrounding the SO cell body represents the "osmoreceptor" that is responsive to changes in osmolality of the fluid perfusing it. HRF represents an ill-defined group of cells that secrete a series of releasing factors into the primary capillary network of a portal vein. This vein passes in the pituitary stalk to the adenohypophysis where cells manufacture the seven hormones of this lobe of the pituitary: growth hormone (GH), prolactin (PR), adrenocorticotropic hormone (ACTH), melanocyte-stimulating hormone (MSH), thyroid-stimulating hormone (TSH), follicle-stimulating hormone (FSH), and luteinizing hormone (LH). (Drawing by Margot Mackay, Department of Art as Applied to Medicine, University of Toronto. After a drawing by E. Blackstock in Ezrin, C., Godden, J. O., Volpé, R., and Wilson, R. (Eds.): Systematic Endocrinology, New York, Harper & Row, Publishers, 1973.)

THE HYPOTHALAMUS

Although the pituitary gland has been called the "leader of the endocrine orchestra," many of its activities are themselves controlled by the hypothalamus which, although part of the brain, also has many endocrine functions (Fig. 39–1).

The hypothalamus consists of a complex collection of nerve cells and fiber tracts that participate in, and help regulate, many functions of the body. These include regulation of the autonomic nervous system, temperature, blood pressure, plasma osmolality, hunger, thirst, emotions, sexual drive, and sleep. The hypothalamus controls body rhythms; a specific *cycling center* is responsible for controlling the menstrual cycle.

Hypothalamic Hormones. The hypothalamus may be regarded as an endocrine organ, because its cells synthesize two groups of hormones:

1. OXYTOCIN AND VASOPRESSIN. These are discussed later in this chapter.

2. RELEASING AND INHIBITING FACTORS OR HORMONES. These are polypeptides of low molecular weight that pass to the adenohypophysis via a short portal vein and stimulate or inhibit it.

The following releasing factors are recognized:

Corticotropin-releasing factor (CRF).

Thyrotropin-releasing factor (TRF).

Gonadotropin-releasing factors (GRF).

Growth hormone–releasing factor (GHRF).

The action of these hormones may be understood by an examination of the action of CRF. This hormone leads to the release of corticotropin (also known as adrenocorticotropic hormone, ACTH) from the adenohypophysis. ACTH acts on the adrenal cortex to cause the release of cortisol (hydrocortisone). ACTH inhibits the release of CRF, while cortisol inhibits the release of both CRF and ACTH. This inhibition is an example of negative feedback, which is a mechanism encountered in the regulation of other hormone secretions.

The releasing factors are produced in picogram (10^{-12} gram) quantities, the pituitary hormones are produced in nanogram (10^{-9} gram) quantities, and the target cells (*e.g.*, the thyroid) produce hormone in microgram (10^{-6} gram) quantities. Thus, the chain reaction shows a considerable amplification effect.

In addition to forming releasing factors, the hypothalamus forms two inhibiting factors:

1. *Gonadotropin-inhibiting factor*
2. *Prolactin-inhibiting factor.*

DISEASES OF THE HYPOTHALAMUS

Many pathological processes (*e.g.*, encephalitis, vascular lesions, head injury, hamartoma, and tumor) can affect the hypothalamus. The effects differ widely, depending on which function is deranged the most. These effects include the following:

1. Obesity due to overeating
2. Somnolence or increased restless activity.
3. Failure to maintain body temperature.
4. Diabetes insipidus that is due to lack of vasopressin, also known as the antidiuretic hormone (ADH).
5. Delayed puberty due to a failure to form gonadotropin-releasing factor. When combined with obesity this condition is known as *Fröhlich's syndrome.*
6. Precocious, or premature, puberty due to a failure to form gonadotropin-inhibiting factor.
7. Visual disturbances due to pressure on the optic chiasma.

THE PITUITARY GLAND (HYPOPHYSIS)

Although small, the pituitary gland, or hypophysis, secretes an amazing variety and number of hormones. The gland and its stalk consist of two parts: the *neurohypophysis*, which develops as an outpouching from the primitive brain, and the *adenohypophysis*, which originates as a diverticulum from the primitive foregut (Fig. 39–1).

The Neurohypophysis

The neurohypophysis consists of the posterior lobe of the pituitary, part of the pituitary stalk (the *infundibular stem*), and part of the brain adjacent to the hypothalamus (the *median eminence of the tuber cinereum*). Two peptide hormones, oxytocin and vasopressin, are manufactured by cells in the hypothalamus and pass via the cells' axons into the neurohypophysis, where they are stored and subsequently released when needed.

OXYTOCIN. This hormone causes uterine contraction during labor and is responsible for milk ejection when an infant is breastfed. The act of suckling initiates a reflex that causes oxytocin release.

VASOPRESSIN (ANTIDIURETIC HORMONE). This hormone acts on the distal and collecting tubules of the kidney and causes water to be retained. Its release is governed by the action of "osmoreceptors" in the hypothalamus. An increase in plasma osmolality associated with dehydration leads to a release of vasopressin and water retention.

Diabetes Insipidus. This disease is caused by a failure in the development of the neurohypophysis or its destruction by a tumor or inflammation. Huge quantities of very dilute urine are passed (*polyuria*), leading to thirst and drinking (*polydipsia*).

The Adenohypophysis

The adenohypophysis consists of the pars anterior, or anterior lobe, of the pituitary, the pars intermedia (which barely exists in humans), and the pars tuberalis in the pituitary stalk. It consists of several cell types (probably seven) and secretes seven hormones:

1. ADRENOCORTICOTROPIN (also called adrenocorticotropic hormone, or ACTH). This stimulates the adrenal cortex to produce cortisol.
2. MELANOCYTE-STIMULATING HORMONE (MSH). This causes darkening of the skin. MSH is closely related to ACTH.
3. THYROID-STIMULATING HORMONE (TSH). This stimulates the thyroid to form its hormone.
4. GROWTH HORMONE (GH). This is necessary for the growth of many tissues, particularly skeletal tissue.
5. FOLLICLE-STIMULATING HORMONE (FSH). This causes enlargement of the ovarian graafian follicle to the point of rupture.
6. LUTEINIZING HORMONE (LH). This causes ovulation.
7. PROLACTIN OR LACTOGENIC HORMONE. This plays a part in the maintenance of the corpus luteum. FSH, LH, and prolactin act on the ovary and are often grouped together as *pituitary gonadotropins:* their actions are considered further in Chapter 37.

DISORDERS OF THE ADENOHYPOPHYSIS

Hyperplasia or neoplasia of the anterior lobe of the pituitary gland may be associated with hypersecretion of one, or several, of the pituitary hormones. On

the other hand, non–hormone-secreting tumors of the pituitary, or tumors arising in the neighborhood, may press on and destroy the parenchyma, leading to
a diminished hormonal secretion. This also occurs when the pituitary is destroyed by other lesions, *e.g.*, infarction or inflammation. Because the clinical
picture may be complex, only the common types will be outlined. Tumors in
the pituitary region give rise to two additional characteristic effects, owing to
their anatomical situation: *compression of the optic chiasma,* which causes loss
of the temporal visual fields of both eyes (bitemporal hemianopsia), and *enlargement of the sella turcica,* which is detectable radiologically.

Hyperpituitarism. The growth hormone–forming cells are usually involved, and the effects of excessive growth hormone are predominant. If the
condition arises in childhood, the result is *gigantism:* the individual is well
proportioned, but huge. Hyperpituitarism in maturity, *i.e.*, after the epiphyses
have fused, leads to *acromegaly* in which the hands, feet, and lower jaw are
enlarged. There is coarsening of the facial features and a high incidence of impaired glucose tolerance (see Chapter 24). Clinical diabetes mellitus occurs in
10 to 15 per cent of patients.

Hyperplasia or an adenoma of the ACTH-producing cells may be the primary cause of Cushing's syndrome, which is described later in this chapter. The
pituitary secretes an excess of ACTH and MSH, and after adrenalectomy, this
overactivity can be so marked that generalized hyperpigmentation results, as in
Addison's disease (see later in this chapter).

Hypopituitarism. In children, deficiency of growth hormone causes severe
retardation of growth, resulting in a midget. The unopposed action of insulin can
lead to attacks of hypoglycemia (see Chapter 24).

Hypopituitarism with lack of gonadotropins leads to lack of testicular or
ovarian maturation. Puberty does not take place. Fusion of the epiphyses, normally produced by the sex hormones, is delayed. If growth hormone production is normal, these eunuchoid patients develop abnormally long limbs—their
span exceeds their height (normally they are equal). Gonadotropin deficiency
can occur in adults. Males exhibit testicular atrophy and loss of libido; females
develop amenorrhea and regression of secondary sexual characteristics.

In adults, anterior pituitary insufficiency can manifest itself as hypothyroidism; often this is combined with evidence of adrenal cortical and gonadotropic
deficiency.

Acute pituitary insufficiency sometimes occurs after parturition and is due
to infarction of the gland. The condition is then called *Sheehan's syndrome.*
When destruction of the adenohypophysis is complete, the condition, called
Simmond's disease, is characterized by extreme wasting. The patients are apathetic; without treatment they ultimately die of adrenal insufficiency (see later
in this chapter).

CONDITIONS SIMULATING HYPOPITUITARISM

Anorexia Nervosa. This condition, often encountered in psychoneurotic
adolescent girls, is the development of an obsessive aversion to food. Extreme
wasting and amenorrhea are the main features and are due to starvation. The
patients are restless and hostile.

Adiposogenital Dystrophy.   This is the male counterpart of anorexia nervosa. It occurs in emotionally disturbed boys who overeat, are fat, and have delayed puberty. The condition resembles Fröhlich's syndrome, which is also sometimes called adiposogenital dystrophy.

THE ADRENAL GLANDS

The Adrenal Medulla

The cells of the adrenal medulla liberate epinephrine and norepinephrine in response to sympathetic stimulation. These hormones cause a rise in blood glucose, a rise in blood pressure, and a redistribution of blood, such that the individual is better adapted for fight or flight. A rare tumor, the *pheochromocytoma,* which is derived from the medulla, secretes these agents in excess and leads to systemic hypertension.

The Adrenal Cortex

Three major groups of hormones (corticoids) are secreted:

Glucocorticoids, e.g., hydrocortisone (cortisol). In physiological concentrations these steroids accelerate the synthesis of glucose from noncarbohydrate precursors and inhibit the actions of insulin. These hormones also have a mild salt-retaining activity.

Mineralocorticoids, e.g., aldosterone, which primarily affects electrolyte metabolism. It causes sodium retention and increases potassium loss in the urine. Aldosterone production is stimulated by hypertensin II and is therefore regulated by the renal blood flow (see Chapter 20).

3. *Sex hormones, e.g.,* estrogen, androgens, and progesterone.

ADRENAL CORTICAL INSUFFICIENCY—ADDISON'S DISEASE

Idiopathic atrophy (perhaps mediated by an autoimmune process) or destruction (usually by tuberculosis) is the common cause of Addison's disease (Fig. 39–2). A low blood pressure, loss of appetite, loss of weight, weakness, and eventual death are the main features. As would be expected, there is hypoglycemia, a fall in serum sodium *(hyponatremia),* and a rise in serum potassium *(hyperkalemia).* The skin and mucous membranes, including the oral mucosa, show increased melanin pigmentation. This is because the low plasma hydrocortisone level stimulates the excessive production of pituitary ACTH and MSH. Both these hormones, especially MSH, cause a darkening of the skin by an effect on the melanocytes. An acute exacerbation of the disease (acute adrenal insufficiency or Addisonian crisis) may occur at any time and is characterized by hypotension, hypoglycemia, epigastric pain, vomiting, coma, and death.

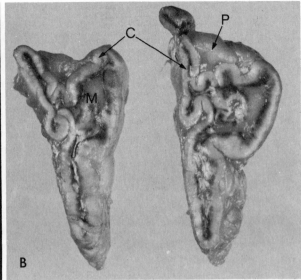

FIGURE 39–2. *Histoplasmosis of the adrenal glands.*

A, The two adrenal glands are enlarged, and the cut surface shows complete replacement of the normal tissue by necrotic, caseous material. *Histoplasma capsulatum* was identified in this specimen. The gross appearance of these specimens is identical with that of tuberculosis, a disease that once accounted for most cases of Addison's disease (today, idiopathic atrophy is now more frequently encountered as a cause of Addison's disease). See also Figure 35–6 and Case History I, page 570 for details of this case.

B, Normal adrenals for comparison. C, cortex; M, medulla; P, periadrenal fat.

ADRENAL CORTICAL HYPERSECRETION

Adrenal overactivity may be secondary to pituitary hypersecretion of ACTH. Usually, however, the overproduction of corticoids is due to idiopathic adrenal hyperplasia, adenoma, or (rarely) a carcinoma. The clinical picture is often mixed, but three main patterns may be discerned.

Adrenogenital Syndrome. In boys, puberty may occur prematurely—even as early as four years ("infantile Hercules"). In girls, male characteristics may develop. In adult women this masculinization, called *virilism,* is manifested as atrophy of the breasts, cessation of menstruation, growth of a beard, and deepening of the voice.

Conn's Syndrome. Excess aldosterone secretion, usually by an adenoma, produces a low serum potassium with sodium and water retention as well as hypertension.

Cushing's Syndrome. The major features of this condition are obesity, hyperglycemia, osteoporosis, systemic hypertension, acne vulgaris, and increased growth of body hair in women.

Cushing's "disease" was originally described as being due to a pituitary tumor. However, the same clinical picture ("Cushing's syndrome) is encountered under other circumstances:

1. With hypersecretion of ACTH due to hypothalamic-pituitary dysfunction.

2. With adrenal hyperplasia or neoplasia.

3. With ectopic ACTH syndrome. An ACTH-like hormone can be produced by some tumors, *e.g.*, oat-cell carcinoma.

4. With glucocorticoid therapy. The syndrome, or mild forms of it, is commonly seen when glucocorticoids are administered in massive doses. Rounding and swelling of the face ("moon face") are particularly characteristic.

GLUCOCORTICOID THERAPY

Replacement glucocorticoid therapy is logical and useful in patients with adrenal insufficiency. However, when used in massive (pharmacological) amounts, the glucocorticoids have two additional actions that can be useful:

1. ANTI-INFLAMMATORY ACTION.   The glucocorticoids (*e.g.*, prednisone) have a suppressive effect on the inflammatory reaction; for this reason they are used in many diseases, *e.g.*, rheumatoid arthritis, herpes zoster, and polyarteritis nodosa. They may be used to advantage when bacterial inflammation might produce serious damage, but antibiotics must also be administered, so that the infection does not spread.

2. LYMPHOID ATROPHY AND DEPRESSION OF THE IMMUNE RESPONSE. This may be used to advantage in treating acute lymphatic leukemia, autoimmune diseases, and hypersensitivity states, such as bronchial asthma. The immunosuppressive action of prednisone is of great use in suppressing the graft rejection reaction, such as in patients with kidney grafts.

Complications of Glucocorticoid Therapy.   The administration of large doses of glucocorticoids over a prolonged period can have serious consequences. Indeed, these may be more serious than the disease for which the treatment was initiated. Important complications are:

1. CUSHING'S SYNDROME.   (See page 615.)

2. OPPORTUNISTIC INFECTIONS.   Overwhelming fungal or viral infections may prove fatal in some patients; it is related to the immunosuppressive effect of glucocorticoids. A quiescent tuberculous focus can be reactivated and can then lead to miliary tuberculosis.

3. OSTEOPOROSIS.   Severe and widespread osteoporosis can lead to fracture formation after trivial injury. Collapse of vertebrae is common.

4. INHIBITION OF WOUND HEALING.   Wound contraction, granulation tissue formation, and collagen formation are inhibited.

5. PEPTIC ULCER.   Peptic ulcer and its complications, especially bleeding, are most common.

6. CATARACT FORMATION.   (See Chapter 42.)

7. DIABETES MELLITUS.   (See Chapter 24.)

8. MENTAL EFFECTS.   An acute mental breakdown (psychosis) may be precipitated. Suicide is an important cause of death.

9. SYSTEMIC HYPERTENSION.   The development of hypertension or the accentuation of existing disease appears to be due to the salt-retaining activity of most glucocorticoids.

10. ACUTE ADRENAL INSUFFICIENCY.   This emergency, characterized by hypotension, shock, and sudden death, occurs if steroid therapy is suddenly withdrawn. It may also occur if a patient who is taking a steroid develops a

severe infection or is subjected to severe injury such as a major surgery and does not have his dose increased. *It is vital that all patients on glucocorticoid therapy as well as their medical attendants be aware of this possibility.*

THE THYROID GLAND

The thyroid gland has the unique ability to trap iodine from the blood and incorporate it as thyroglobulin in the colloid of its vesicles (Fig. 39–3). By the action of a proteolytic enzyme on thyroglobulin the iodine-containing thyroid hormones thyroxine (T_4) and triiodothyronine (T_3) are released. This occurs when the gland is stimulated by thyroid-stimulating hormone (TSH) from the pituitary. TSH secretion is itself stimulated by a low blood level of thyroid hormone both directly and indirectly via thyrotropin-releasing hormone (TRH).

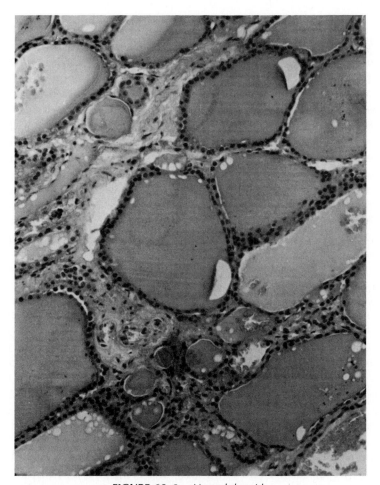

FIGURE 39–3. *Normal thyroid.*

The gland consists of follicles of varying size, lined by a simple flattened or cubical epithelium and filled with homogeneous colloid. The colloid contains thyroglobulin ($\times$ 250).

The inconspicuous C-cells of the thyroid secrete calcitonin; so far, no syndrome has been described in relation to an excess or deficiency of this hormone (see Chapter 40).

Action of the Thyroid Hormones.   In spite of much research, the precise mode of action of the thyroid hormones is not known. However, much has been learned by comparing the normal individual (who is described as *euthyroid*) with those who suffer from excessive or diminished secretion (*hyperthyroid* and *hypothyroid*, respectively.)

A *deficiency* of the thyroid hormones causes any or all of the following conditions: a reduction in metabolic rate; impaired mental and physical growth (most marked in childhood); and anemia, which is less constant.

A hypersecretion of thyroid hormones causes an increase in the metabolic rate and the other changes encountered in thyrotoxicosis that are described later.

GOITER

Any enlargement of the thyroid is called a goiter, and to a minor extent this occurs at times of stress, *e.g.*, during puberty and pregnancy. Indeed, in ancient Egypt the rupture of a thread tied around the neck of a bride was used as an indication of pregnancy. A more potent cause is a diet deficient in iodine. The reason is that the thyroid, being unable to manufacture its hormone, cannot check the secretion of TSH that stimulates it to activity. Before iodine was added to table salt, goiters were common in many parts of the world (*e.g.*, the Great Lakes area of North America, the Andes, the Himalayas, and Derbyshire, England) because the soil carried insufficient iodine for food stuffs to contain even minute quantities of iodine. Repeated phases of hyperplasia followed by involution led to the formation of large, nodular goiters containing many colloid-filled areas, some of which showed necrosis and dystrophic calcification (*nodular colloid goiter;* see Figure 39–4).

The goiters associated with hyperthyroidism, Hashimoto's disease, and neoplasia are described later.

HYPOTHYROIDISM

Hypothyroidism was once frequent in areas of endemic goiter (due to iodine deficiency), but it may also be due to causes other than lack of iodine, such as a congenital absence of the thyroid gland or of one of the enzymes necessary for the synthesis of thyroid hormone. The effects in the child differ from those in the adult.

Cretinism.   An insufficiency of thyroid hormone in the infant leads to cretinism. The child has a bloated face, protruding tongue, a vacant expression, and becomes mentally defective. There is a retardation of growth and dwarfism results.

Myxedema.   This condition is the manifestation of hypothyroidism in the adult. The thyroid generally shows atrophy and lymphocytic infiltration. There is a reduction in mental and physical activity, and the patient exhibits a characteristic bloated appearance because of a curious edema of the skin. This disease is associated with an excessive accumulation of mucoprotein (see Chapter 2).

FIGURE 39-4. *Nodular colloid goiter.*

The specimen consists of the left lobe of the thyroid and shows two nodules, both encapsulated. One is solid, whereas the other is cystic and contains dark, altered blood. Hemorrhage into this degenerate nodule accounts for the sudden swelling experienced by this patient. For further clinical data see Case History I.

Case History I. (See Figure 39-4.) *Nodular colloid goiter.* The patient was a 45-year-old woman who complained of a swelling in the neck. The swelling moved when she swallowed and had the features of an enlarged thyroid (goiter). The patient had had seven pregnancies; it was during the last two that she had noticed some swelling of the neck. However, it was only after the last delivery (one year previously) that the goiter had rapidly become obvious. On examination, several nodules could be felt in the enlarged thyroid. An echogram revealed that one of them was cystic; radioactive studies showed no uptake by this "cold" nodule. T_3 and T_4 levels in the blood were normal. Although a diagnosis of nodular colloid goiter seemed obvious, the fact that the thyroid enlargement had occurred soon after delivery rather than during the pregnancy raised the possibility of malignancy. Cold nodules should always be viewed with suspicion. The left lobe of the thyroid and one nodule in the right lobe were removed.

HYPERTHYROIDISM

This condition is also known as *thyrotoxicosis* and occurs in two forms:

Graves' Disease (Primary Hyperthyroidism). This disease is characterized by a diffuse enlargement of the thyroid gland (goiter) due to a marked hyperplasia of its epithelial elements (Fig. 39-5). There is a raised metabolic rate that manifests itself as a persistent increase in the heart rate; the individual is typically jumpy and nervous. The hands are warm and sweaty; they are seldom at rest and exhibit a fine tremor when the fingers are stretched out. Muscular weakness, which is a common symptom, can be severe. If left untreated, Graves' disease often terminates in heart failure. The eyes have a characteristic appearance: the eyelids are retracted, giving the patient a staring

FIGURE 39–5. *Graves' disease.*

This section shows that the thyroid gland is hyperplastic. The epithelium is columnar and in some small follicles where colloid is deficient, it encroaches upon the acinar spaces. In the large follicles the colloid shows vacuolation where it abuts on the epithelium (× 250).

expression; in severe cases, the globe is actually pushed forward to produce *exophthalmos* (Fig. 39–6). This is produced by edema and lymphocytic infiltration of the contents of the orbit. If severe, these changes can cause loss of sight (*malignant exophthalmos*).

Graves' disease is not due to overstimulation of the thyroid by TSH. The blood contains a thyroid-stimulating substance that is not of pituitary origin. Indeed, it is an immunoglobulin, termed *long-acting thyroid-stimulating factor* (LATS). The disease seems to have an autoimmune component, and it tends to occur in families in which other autoimmune diseases occur (*e.g.,* Hashimoto's disease, myxedema, and pernicious anemia).

Toxic Nodular Goiter (Secondary Hyperthyroidism). This occurs as a secondary phenomenon in a patient who is already suffering from a goiter from some other cause, such as iodine deficiency. The condition is less severe than Graves' disease, and exophthalmos and other ocular manifestations do not occur.

HASHIMOTO'S DISEASE

Like most thyroid disease, this is more common in women than in men. The gland is diffusely enlarged, showing atrophy of its epithelial elements and a

FIGURE 39–6. *Ocular manifestation of Graves' disease.*

This patient noted the development of prominence of both eyes at the same time as the appearance of other symptoms of Graves' disease. The eyelids and periorbital tissues are swollen; the conjunctiva is congested and moist because of excessive lacrimation. The globe itself is pushed forward *(proptosis)* by an accumulation of mucoprotein in the orbital tissues. A similar change is sometimes encountered in the skin of the lower leg and is called *pretibial myxedema*. Note that this occurs in Graves' disease. (Courtesy of Dr. N. Pairaudeau.)

massive infiltration by lymphocytes and plasma cells (Fig. 39–7). A characteristic of the disease is the presence of antithyroid antibodies in the blood. Nevertheless, it is unlikely that these antibodies are responsible for the thyroid damage. A disease similar to Hashimoto's disease can be produced in animals by injections of thyroid tissue with Freund's adjuvant (see Chapter 9); this disease is T-cell–mediated, and it is probable that the same is true of the human disease.

TUMORS

Benign encapsulated nodules in the thyroid gland are common, but the majority are probably focal areas of hyperplasia. These are usually multiple (nodular colloid goiter).

Carcinoma was apparently not uncommon in goitrous districts, but today it is distinctly rare (Fig. 39–8). Carcinoma does not usually take up radioactive iodine and appears as a "cold" nodule on a thyroid scan.

FIGURE 39–7. *Hashimoto's disease.*

Much of the thyroid parenchyma has been replaced by lymphocytes; remnants of thyroid follicles can still be seen (arrows). In the early stages of Hashimoto's disease, the patient may be hyperthyroid, but by the time the gland shows the degree of destruction depicted in this figure the patient is hypothyroid (× 250).

FIGURE 39-8. *Carcinoma of the thyroid.*

The tumor consists of acinar spaces lined by a columnar epithelium. The spaces vary greatly in size and do not contain colloid. Papillary projections fill the larger acini, and the overall pattern differs markedly from that of the hyperplastic gland (compare with Figure 39–5). The cells of the tumor are uniform in appearance and mitoses are not in evidence. On the basis of histological findings it is tempting to label this tumor a papillary adenoma. However, careful search will generally reveal invasion of its capsule; the tumor also regularly metastasizes to lymph nodes. Hence, it should be called a *papillary adenocarcinoma* (× 250).

Review Questions

1. Explain why hormones have a specific action; that is, they affect only their target organs or tissues. Illustrate the answer by using as examples glucagon, insulin, and a steroid hormone.
2. Compare Simmond's disease with anorexia nervosa.
3. A patient with Cushing's disease has both adrenal glands removed and is given hormone-replacement therapy. One year later marked hyperpigmentation of the skin is noted. Can you explain this?
4. It is proposed that a patient be treated with large doses of prednisone (a glucocorticoid). List the items in a patient's medical history and physical examination that would warn you of the possible dangers of this treatment.
5. Give an account of the endocrine disorders that affect the systemic blood pressure.
6. Give an account of the circumstances under which hypothyroidism may occur.

7. Read Case History I on page 570. What investigations might have led to a diagnosis of Addison's disease in this patient?

Selected Readings

Catt, K. J.: ABC of endocrinology. Lancet, *1*:763–765, 827–831, 933–939, 1097–1104, 1383–1389; and *2*:255–257, 353–358, 1970.

Ezrin, C., Godden, J. O., Volpé, R., and Wilson, R.: Systematic Endocrinology. New York, Harper & Row, Publishers, 1973. Chapters 1 to 5 and 7 should be consulted for topics covered in this chapter.

Guillemin, R., and Burgus, R.: The hormones of the hypothalamus. Scientific American, *227*(5):24–33, 1972.

Leading Article: Endocrine exophthalmos. British Medical Journal, *3*:68, 1972.

DISEASES OF THE BONES, JOINTS, AND MUSCLES

Chapter 40

After studying this chapter the student should be able to:

- Describe the formation of bone in the human embryo and distinguish between membrane bone and that formed by endochondral ossification.
- Distinguish woven bone from lamellar bone.
- Give an account of the forms in which calcium occurs in the blood; describe the actions of parathormone and calcitonin.

DISEASES OF THE BONES, JOINTS, AND MUSCLE

- Describe the pathogenesis of acute osteomyelitis and chronic osteomyelitis.
- Describe the features of localized osteoporosis.
- Classify the causes of fracture.
- Describe the stages in fracture healing, and list the causes of fibrous union, nonunion, and delayed union.
- Give a brief account of each of the following conditions:
    (a) osteogenesis imperfecta
    (b) achondroplasia
    (c) osteopetrosis.
- Classify the causes of hyperparathyroidism and indicate the main bony and renal lesions that ensue.
- Compare rickets with osteomalacia.
- Classify the causes of generalized osteoporosis.
- Describe the main features of Paget's disease.
- Give an account of the common tumors of bone.
- Describe multiple myelomatosis.
- Describe the structure of a synovial joint.
- Differentiate between a sprain, subluxation, and a dislocation.
- List three organisms that commonly cause an acute suppurative arthritis and indicate the end-result.
- Contrast rheumatoid arthritis with osteoarthritis.
- Describe how ankylosing spondylitis differs from the classic form of rheumatoid arthritis.

Introduction

During normal embryonic development, condensations of primitive mesodermal connective tissue, called *mesenchyme*, are laid down at the sites of future bone, and by the end of the second month ossification commences. In the development of some bones, notably the vault of the skull, there is a direct conversion of the membranous sheet of mesenchyme to bone. Mesenchymal cells differentiate into osteoblasts, and the bones formed in this way are therefore called *membrane bones*. The long bones develop in a different way: in these, the mesenchyme first differentiates into cartilage, which is subsequently *replaced* by bone. The cartilage cells swell up and die, and the intervening cartilaginous matrix calcifies. This acellular calcified cartilage is eroded by multinucleate osteoclasts, and at the same time osteoblasts lay down lamellar bone (see below). This process, which is called *endochondral ossification*, con-

MARROW SPACE

Compact bone
Cellular layer of periosteum   Endosteum   CANCELLOUS BONE
Fibrous layer of periosteum

FIGURE 40–1. *Lamellar bone.*

Diagrammatic representation of a transverse section through part of the shaft of the long bone to show the arrangement of lamellar bone. The cortex is composed mainly of Haversian systems.

tinues at the epiphyseal ends of the long bones until adult stature is achieved. Proliferation of cartilage at the epiphyses and its subsequent ossification is therefore the way in which the long bones grow in length.

STRUCTURE OF BONE

Bone is composed of calcified osteoid tissue; the latter consists of collagen fibers embedded in a specialized ground substance. Although the precise composition of bone salts is not known, they are generally considered to be composed of hydroxyapatite, a complex molecule of calcium phosphate and calcium hydroxide. Bone also contains small quantities of magnesium, sodium, and potassium as well as carbonate and citrate ions.

Depending on the arrangement of the collagen fibers, two histological types of bone may be recognized:

Woven Bone. This type shows an irregular arrangement of collagen bundles and is the type of bone that is formed under the following three circumstances:

(1) during the initial stages of the formation of membrane bones; (2) when bone forms in the midst of differentiating granulation tissue, as in fracture healing; and (3) in certain bone disorders and tumors.

Lamellar or Mature Bone. In this type of bone the collagen bundles are arranged either in parallel sheets or in concentric laminae around a central vessel, thereby forming Haversian systems (Fig. 40–1).

In the outer dense cortex of the long bones, Haversian systems predominate, whereas flat plates are seen under the periosteum and endosteum. This type of bone is called *compact bone.*

The central portion of the long bones is hollowed out to form the medullary cavity, which contains marrow. Thin struts of bone remain, which are constructed of flat bundles of collagen with few Haversian systems. The central trabeculated part of the bone is called *cancellous;* like compact bone, it is composed of lamellar bone.

Lamellar bone is formed when bone is laid down on a previous scaffolding. This may consist of any of the following: (a) calcified cartilage, as in normal endochondral ossification; (b) woven bone, as in growing membrane bones; and (c) lamellar bone itself, as in the circumferential growth of all long bones.

In the normal adult the entire skeleton is composed of lamellar bone.

METABOLIC FUNCTIONS OF BONE: CALCIUM METABOLISM

Bone serves as a reserve of both calcium and phosphate, containing 99 per cent of the total body calcium and 90 per cent of the total body phosphorus. Nevertheless, the remaining 1 per cent of calcium is a vital fraction, because it is available to the soft tissues, and it is necessary for proper neuromuscular activity, cardiac rhythm, and enzyme activities, such as in blood coagulation.

Calcium in the blood exists in three forms: (1) *ionized calcium,* which is diffusible and constitutes 65 per cent of the total plasma calcium; (2) *protein-bound calcium,* which is nondiffusible, since it is attached to albumin; and (3) *nonionized diffusible calcium,* which exists as citrate. The ionized calcium is the most important fraction and is in equilibrium with the calcium salts in bone. The level in blood is regulated by two hormones. When the blood calcium level falls, *parathormone* from the parathyroid glands is released, stimulating osteoclastic activity, which results in the resorption of bone. The released bone salts cause the serum ionic calcium level to return to normal. Overproduction of parathormone, *(hyperparathyroidism)* results in hypercalcemia. The other hormone of note is *calcitonin,* which is secreted by the C cells of the thyroid. This has the effect of lowering blood calcium, and the stimulus for its secretion is hypercalcemia. Vitamin D plays a minor role in regulating the blood calcium level, since it has a mild parathormonelike activity.

The normal serum calcium is 9.2 to 10.4 mg per 100 ml, and in healthy persons it is remarkably constant because of the efficiency of the regulating mechanisms. The serum calcium and phosphate together maintain a reciprocal relationship. Thus, if there is a rise in the serum level of either calcium or phosphate, there is a corresponding fall in that of the other. However, if the level of one substance is low, the other does not necessarily rise.

Alkaline Phosphatase. This enzyme is manufactured by the osteoblasts, but its precise role in bone formation is not understood. It is known that some of the enzyme escapes into the blood, and the serum level is a good index of the overall osteoblastic activity within the body. For example, in Paget's disease, which is discussed later, it is high. The enzyme produced by bone differs from that formed in the liver. Recall that a high level of alkaline phosphatase is also seen in obstructive jaundice, and it is sometimes necessary to estimate these two isoenzymes separately to distinguish between bone disorder and hepatic disease.

Although bone appears rigid and inert, it is as susceptible as the soft tissues to adverse circumstances. Indeed, the effects on bone are often more severe and permanent.

There is a continuous process of remodeling of bone throughout life, with bone resorption by osteoclasts and bone deposition by osteoblasts, each keeping pace with the other. If either predominates, osteoporosis or osteosclerosis results. *Osteoporosis* is a condition in which the organic matrix (osteoid), although reduced in amount, is normally mineralized. The bone trabeculae are greatly thinned, and as a whole, the bones are fragile and liable to fracture. The radiographic appearance is therefore one of rarefaction. Osteoporosis may be brought about either by excess destruction of bone or by defective formation.

In *osteosclerosis* there is excessive formation of osteoid; being calcified, the osteoid makes the bones appear dense on a radiograph.

Infections of Bone

PYOGENIC INFECTIONS

The term "osteomyelitis" is applied to pyogenic infections because both bone marrow cavity and the bone itself are involved.

Acute Osteomyelitis. This infection occurs most often in childhood; generally it develops at the end of one of the long bones of the lower limbs. The explanation for this localization is that this is an area commonly traumatized; furthermore, if an injury occurs during the course of a bacteremia associated with a skin infection, the organisms, commonly *Staphylococcus aureus*, become localized and set up a metastatic lesion. An acute inflammatory reaction ensues, and this is accompanied by rigors, fever, and acute tenderness of the region. Owing to the rigidity of the bone, the increased tension produced by the exudation leads to compression of blood vessels and ischemia. Necrosis of marrow and bone consequently follows; pus is formed, and it tracks under the periosteum, thereby further imperiling the blood supply to the cortex. In this way, quite extensive necrosis of bone can occur; indeed, the whole shaft can eventually become involved. *During the early stages,* however, no necrosis may be evident on radiography, and if a child has an illness suggestive of acute osteomyelitis, treatment is begun before time has occurred to produce radiographic changes.

With modern therapy, acute osteomyelitis frequently resolves. This was not so in the preantibiotic days. The dead bone, called a *sequestrum,* acts as a foreign body and provides a focus for continued growth of organisms. Together with the trapped collections of pus, the conditions are ideal for the development of chronic inflammation.

Chronic Osteomyelitis. Pus ruptures through the periosteum into the muscular and subcutaneous tissues and ultimately escapes to the skin surface through one or more sinuses. The vascular periosteum attempts to re-form the shaft of bone by producing new bone that encases the sequestrated shaft, and is called an *involucrum* (Fig. 40–2). Osteoclasts slowly erode the sequestrum and detach it at each end, but this process may take many months or years to ac-

FIGURE 40–2. *Osteomyelitis of the tibia.*

This amputation specimen shows the typical appearances of extensive chronic osteomyelitis. The dead shaft of the bone forms a sequestrum and is surrounded by thick, irregularly shaped new bone that constitutes the encasing involucrum. The sequestrum can be seen through a hole in the involucrum at the lower end of the specimen. (HS44.1, Reproduced by permission of the President and Council of the R.C.S. Eng.)

complish; in practice, spontaneous healing does not occur. If the condition is not treated, it may lead to death as a result of pyemia, toxemia, or amyloid disease.

Chronic suppurative osteomyelitis is fortunately very rare these days. However, a description of it is useful because it illustrates the typical features of a chronic suppurative inflammation. It demonstrates the combination of the following factors: (1) *acute inflammation* with fluid exudation and pus formation; (2) *demolition* by macrophages and osteoclasts; (3) *regeneration* of bone by osteoblasts; and (4) *repair* with granulation tissue and extensive scar tissue formation.

OTHER INFECTIONS

Tuberculosis of Bone. Unlike pyogenic osteomyelitis, tuberculosis of bone is generally insidious in its onset and is characterized by bone destruction with very little reactive new bone formation. One of the common sites of infection is the vertebral column *(Pott's disease)*. The affected vertebrae frequently collapse and produce an angulation of the spinal column; forward deviation is called a *kyphosis* and lateral deviation is called a *scoliosis*. As with tuberculosis elsewhere, caseous tissue is formed. When this softens, it becomes a "cold abscess" that tracks along the line of least resistance and is ultimately discharged to the exterior. In tuberculosis of the spine, the pus tends to enter the psoas sheath, track down in it beneath the inguinal ligament, and present as a fluctuating mass that subsequently discharges to the surface. Fortunately, tuberculosis of bone is now a rarity.

Syphilis.   Syphilis of bone is now extremely uncommon. It is generally seen in the later stages of the disease, with periostitis predominating. The bone tends to become osteosclerotic, in contrast to becoming osteoporotic in tuberculosis.

Bone Disorders Caused by Physical Disturbances

LOCALIZED OSTEOPOROSIS

Effects of Immobilization.   Whenever a joint is immobilized, either by a cast or by disease, the neighboring bones develop osteoporosis. This effect is a form of disuse atrophy—the greater the degree of immobility, the more marked is the osteoporosis. Thus, if there is paralysis of a whole limb (*e.g.,* in poliomyelitis), osteoporosis affects all the bones of that limb.

PRESSURE ATROPHY.   Any expanding lesion that exerts pressure on bone causes local ischemia and pressure atrophy. Recall that cartilage—being avascular—does not show this pressure atrophy. Thus, an aneurysm of the aorta that presses on the vertebral column causes pressure atrophy of the vertebrae, but the intervening discs remain unaffected.

Benign tumors arising in bone cause pressure atrophy; the adjacent periosteum responds by producing new bone around the lesion. Thus, a benign tumor gives the appearance of expanding the bone.

FRACTURES

Causes
EXCESSIVE MECHANICAL FORCE
Direct Violence.   A good example is a blow that causes a depressed fracture of skull or a broken scapula.

Indirect Violence.   A fracture of the clavicle caused by falling on an outstretched arm is an example.

Muscular Action.   Sudden, unexpected strains during violent exercise can cause fractures in normal bones (*spontaneous fractures*).

FRACTURES OF ABNORMAL BONE.   A fracture in a diseased, weakened, bone that has been subjected to a normal strain is called a *pathological fracture.* Secondary carcinoma must always be borne in mind as a cause of this. Indeed, a pathological fracture may be the first indication of malignancy, *e.g.,* carcinoma of the lung.

Stages in Fracture Healing. The stages in fracture healing are illustrated in Figure 40–3. Notice that the hematoma between the bone ends is organized, and that the granulation tissue so formed matures either to woven bone or cartilage. This hard material, which initially unites the bone ends, is called *callus.* The woven bone or cartilage of which it is composed is gradually replaced by mature lamellar bone. Thus, during regeneration of bone the two embryological methods of bone formation—endochondral and intramembranous—are faithfully repeated in later life.

Abnormalities of Fracture Healing

REPAIR OR FIBROUS UNION. Although the cells of the granulation tissue of a healing fracture are called osteoblasts, they are capable of differentiation along several lines. If immobilization is not satisfactory, the cells behave like fibroblasts, and the bone ends become united by ordinary fibrous scar tissue that cannot be converted into bone.

Fibrous union is particularly common in situations in which the blood supply is impaired or immobilization is difficult. Thus, it occurs in fractures of the carpal scaphoid bone; when fibrous union has occurred, surgical intervention is

FIGURE 40–3. *Stages in the healing of a fracture.*

a, Hematoma formation. b, Acute inflammation followed by demolition. Loose fragments of bone are removed, and the bone ends show osteoporosis. c, Granulation-tissue formation. d, The bone ends are now united by woven bone, cartilage, or a mixture of the two. This hard material is called *callus.* e, Lamellar bone is laid down; calcified cartilage and woven bone are progressively removed. f, Final remodeling.

necessary to remove the fibrous tissue and to create thereby a new fracture in which bone formation can occur.

NONUNION.   Complete lack of union between the fracture ends results from the interposition of soft parts. Muscle or fascia can separate the two bone ends, and because there is no continuous hematoma between them, union of any sort is impossible. This phenomenon is sometimes utilized deliberately in order to form a new false joint.

DELAYED UNION.   In the presence of a continuous hematoma, any cause of delayed healing retards bone regeneration. In practice the following causes are most important:

Movement.   Movement of any sort is harmful to the healing process, because it excites an inflammatory reaction, damages the delicate granulation tissue, and inhibits the formation of bone. In surgical practice every effort is made to reduce movement to a minimum. If the bone ends are impacted, union is usually rapid; indeed, one method of treating a fracture is to bring the ends of the broken bone together under high compression. This provides rigid immobilization and speeds healing. If the bone ends are not impacted, the fracture is either stabilized by external splints or casts. Alternatively, an operation is performed, and then screws, nails, or plates are inserted to minimize movement between the ends of the broken bone.

Infection.   Infection produces osteomyelitis and can lead to extensive ischemic necrosis with sequestrum formation. Infection is particularly liable to occur if the fracture is compound, *i.e.*, if one of the bone ends has penetrated the skin and is exposed to the exterior.

Poor Blood Supply.   Whereas complete loss of blood supply results in necrosis of bone, poor blood supply leads to slow granulation-tissue formation and to slow healing. Certain sites (*e.g.*, fractures of the neck of the femur, the shaft of tibia, and the carpal scaphoid bone) are notorious for this complication. In these situations it is particularly important to avoid other possible causes of delayed healing, such as movement. Some form of internal splintage is commonly used with these fractures. For example, a pin is passed into the head of the femur so that rigid immobilization is immediately obtained. This technique is particularly useful in old people. If an elderly person falls and fractures the neck of the femur, the injury can be treated by external immobilization in a plaster cast. Unfortunately, the patient is confined to bed for many weeks and is liable to develop many complications: venous thrombosis, pulmonary embolism, bronchopneumonia, and urinary-tract infection. Pinning the head, on the other hand, can allow the person to get up immediately and to escape these hazards of recumbency.

Myositis Ossificans.   If there is an extravasation of fracture hematoma into surrounding muscles, its subsequent organization and ossification results in the condition called *traumatic myositis ossificans*. Sometimes the large masses of bone formed around a joint can seriously interfere with movement.

GENERALIZED BONE DISORDERS

There is no very satisfactory classification of generalized bone disorders, but in practice the disorders can be considered under three headings:

(1) *Developmental anomalies*

(2) *Abnormalities due to metabolic disorders*

(3) *Abnormalities occurring in the adult; these are generally of unknown cause.*

Developmental Abnormalities

Many developmental abnormalities are known, but these are rare, for the most part. Three examples will be considered below:

OSTEOGENESIS IMPERFECTA

This disease is inherited as an autosomal dominant trait with incomplete penetrance. Probably because of a failure in bone formation, the entire skeleton consists of thin, weak bones. In the congenital form of this condition the prognosis is poor because multiple fractures occur *in utero* and during birth. The disease can first appear after birth. The child's bones are thin and brittle, so that fractures are common, and considerable deformity develops in due course.

ACHONDROPLASIA

This disease is also transmitted as an autosomal dominant factor. The essential feature appears to be defective endochondral bone formation, and the long bones of the limbs are therefore short. A person who expresses this condition is called an *achondroplastic dwarf*. The trunks and head are of normal size, although the middle of the face tends to be depressed because the base of the skull is formed of cartilage and is therefore affected. The person with this condition has a normal intelligence and is very muscular and agile.

OSTEOPETROSIS (ALBERS-SCHÖNBERG DISEASE)

In this condition there is increased formation of bone so that the skeleton is hard and inelastic. However, the bones are particularly liable to fracture because of their inelasticity. Bone encroaches on the marrow cavity and this can result in leukoerythroblastic anemia (see Chapter 26). The disease is inherited as an autosomal recessive trait.

Abnormalities of Bone Due to Metabolic Disorders

Endocrine Disturbances. Skeletal changes associated with pituitary and thyroid disease are considered elsewhere. By far, the most important hormone in relation to bone metabolism is parathormone, which is derived from the four parathyroid glands.

HYPERPARATHYROIDISM

An excessive secretion of parathormone leads to bone resorption (either generalized or patchy in distribution) to produce osteitis fibrosa cystica, which is discussed later.

The main action of parathormone is to regulate the equilibrium between the ionic calcium in the blood and the calcium in the bones. An increased secretion of the hormone causes resorption of bone, a rise in the level of plasma calcium *(hypercalcemia)*, and an increased excretion of calcium in the urine *(hypercalciuria)*. Parathormone secretion itself is regulated by the level of calcium in the blood perfusing the glands. Some investigators believe that parathormone can lead directly to the removal of calcium ions from bone by a process of diffusion, but this view is not generally accepted. It is more likely that osteoclastic activity is always necessary before calcium salts can be removed. The two views are not in fact irreconcilable; if calcium salts are first removed by diffusion, the exposed osteoid may be removed by osteoclastic activity. Whatever the mechanism, *in hyperparathyroidism there is excessive osteoclastic activity*, and as bone is removed, it is replaced by fibrous tissue.

Hyperparathyroidism can be divided into two groups:

PRIMARY HYPERPARATHYROIDISM. This condition is due to the excessive production of parathormone either as a result of idiopathic hyperplasia or as a result of neoplasia (generally benign). The level of *serum calcium is raised.*

SECONDARY HYPERPARATHYROIDISM. Hyperplasia and hypersecretion of the glands can be induced by a persistently *low level of serum ionized calcium.* This is seen most frequently in two groups of conditions: (1) *rickets and osteomalacia*, which are described later; and (2) *chronic renal disease.*

The relationship between chronic renal disease and parathyroid function is complicated. In chronic renal disease there is retention of phosphate and a raised serum level (hyperphosphatemia). There is also a depression in the level of serum calcium, which in its turn acts as a stimulus to the parathyroids, leading to their hyperplasia and hypersecretion. Calcium is mobilized from the bones, which become progressively demineralized. The calcium is excreted by the kidney, but this excretion can lead to further renal damage by metastatic calcification and stone formation. Chronic renal disease produces its most severe effects on the growing skeleton of children. Growth is stunted (causing renal dwarfism), and the bones show the changes of rickets and osteitis fibrosa.

Osteitis Fibrosa Cystica* *(von Recklinghausen's Disease of Bone).* In the early stages of this disease there is generalized bone involvement. The outstanding features are pains in the bones and weakening of the bones that can result in bending, deformity, and spontaneous fracture. Since there is an increased excretion of calcium via the kidneys, renal stones are not uncommon and can be responsible for the initial symptoms — that is, hematuria, pain, and urinary infection. Metastatic calcification is common (see below). In some instances of hyperparathyroidism, the bones contain tumorlike masses composed of osteoclasts together with localized blood-filled cysts. These *brown tumors,*

---

*The term is a poor one, because the disease is not inflammatory, and the cysts are not always present.

as they are called, closely resemble histologically the giant-cell tumors of bone but are considered to be merely focal areas of hyperplasia.

Metastatic Calcification.   Metastatic calcification is the deposition of calcium salts in normal tissues other than osteoid or teeth; it is due to a derangement of calcium or phosphate metabolism. The most common cause is hypercalcemia due to hyperparathyroidism or extensive destruction of bone that can occur with multiple osteolytic tumors. It is also a feature of chronic renal disease.

Calcification can occur in many sites, but in the kidney the results are the most serious, because combined with the effects of calculi, progressive renal damage leads to progressive renal failure.

Inadequate or Excessive Amounts of Vitamins.   Vitamins C and D are most concerned with formation of bone. See Chapter 23 for a more complete discussion of vitamin C.

VITAMIN D DEFICIENCY: RICKETS AND OSTEOMALACIA

The body obtains vitamin D partly from food and partly by synthesizing it from steroids in the skin by the action of ultraviolet light. An inadequate diet (particularly in those countries where there is not much sunlight) and the malabsorption syndrome will lead to its deficiency. Vitamin D aids in the absorption of calcium and phosphorus from the intestine, and in addition it has a slight parathormonelike action. Very high doses given therapeutically lead to hypercalcemia and hypercalciuria. The main effect in vitamin D deficiency is an *impaired calcification of cartilage and osteoid.*

Rickets.   In rickets there is a failure of the calcification of cartilage that normally occurs at the growing epiphyses. Cartilage is therefore neither removed nor replaced by osteoid. Continued growth of the cartilage causes a considerable enlargement of the bone ends. Similarly, the costochondral junctions are enlarged, producing the clinical deformity called the "rachitic rosary." Because the overall growth of bone is diminished, the child becomes dwarfed. Even the osteoid that is formed is poorly calcified, and the weakened bones are liable to bend and become deformed. Knock-knees, kyphosis, and other deformities are common.

Osteomalacia.   The counterpart of rickets in adults is osteomalacia. It is most common in women, because pregnancy imposes an additional drain on the supplies of calcium and vitamins.

The normal adult bone is continually being remodeled; as bone is removed by osteoclasts it is replaced by osteoid layed down by osteoblasts. In healthy persons the osteoid promptly calcifies, but in people with vitamin D deficiency this calcification fails to occur and the bones ultimately consist largely of osteoid. This is the condition of osteomalacia (softening of the bone): although there is an abundance of osteoid, it is poorly calcified. In osteoporosis, by contrast, the matrix is normally calcified but is reduced in quantity.

In osteomalacia all bones are affected, but it is in the weight-bearing areas that the effects are most severe. Gross pelvic distortion occurs and causes complications in subsequent pregnancies. Collapse of the vertebrae gives rise to pain resulting from compression of the spinal nerves as they leave the intervertebral foramina.

FIGURE 40–4.   *Normal vs. osteoporotic vertebral bodies.*

A, Normal vertebral bodies. *B,* Moderate osteoporosis. *C,* Severe osteoporosis. The vertebral bodies have been sectioned to show their internal structure. Note the well-formed cancellous bone of the normal vertebral bodies in *A* as well as the structure of the intervertebral discs. One small focus of degeneration can be seen (white arrow). In *B* the specimen shows well-developed osteoporosis, but the overall shape of the vertebrae is preserved. The discs show severe degenerative changes (black arrows). In *C* the specimen shows severe osteoporosis. The vertebrae have been compressed by the bulging discs.

Abnormalities of Bone Occurring in the Adult

GENERALIZED OSTEOPOROSIS

Disuse Osteoporosis. Prolonged recumbency leads to increased osteoclastic activity and resorption of bone. There is excessive mobilization of calcium, resulting in hypercalciuria and a tendency for renal stones to form. The blood calcium level remains normal, since the process is gradual.

Idiopathic Osteoporosis. Osteoporosis—especially of the pelvis, spine, and ribs—is not uncommon in old age *(senile osteoporosis)*, and compression of the vertebrae causes backache that can be severe (Fig. 40–4). There is also some diminution in height, but since the condition occurs so slowly the patient rarely notices this. Osteoporosis is particularly common in women past the menopause *(postmenopausal osteoporosis)*; this has been attributed to lack of estrogens. Occasionally osteoporosis occurs in a younger age group for no obvious reason. The condition is also a feature of the malabsorption syndrome and can be produced by the prolonged administration of glucocorticoids.

PAGET'S DISEASE OF BONE (OSTEITIS DEFORMANS)

This disease is not an inflammatory one, although it was so considered by Sir James Paget in the nineteenth century. The cause is not known, and the disease seems to be more common in males, particularly those over the age of 40 years.

In the early stages of the disease the bones become softened because of osteoclastic resorption, and the weakened bones tend to bend. Since this is particularly noticeable in the weight-bearing bones, bowing of the femora is characteristic. In the later stages of the disease, irregular subperiosteal bone formation occurs, causing bones to become thicker and hardened. Serum calcium and phosphate levels remain within normal limits, but the serum alkaline phosphatase is greatly raised because of the rapid turnover of bone.

The skull is frequently affected, and as it becomes increasingly thickened, the patient notices a need for an increased hat size. Blindness, deafness, headaches, and facial paralysis are complications that may result from compression of nerves in their bony canals. An occasional complication is the development of osteosarcoma, a tumor that is uncommon in adults except in association with this disease.

Tumors

TUMORS OF BONES

The tumors of bone form a complex group in spite of the apparent simplicity of bone structure. Indeed, the histogenesis of some of the tumors is quite obscure. The occurrence of tumors arising from the marrow and the frequency of skeletal metastases add further to the confusion.

Benign Tumors. Osteoma, chondroma, fibroma, and other tumors all occur but are uncommon.

FIGURE 40–5. *Giant cell tumor of bone.*

This radiograph shows the "soap bubble" appearance of a tumor that occupies the upper end of the tibia. Note how the joint space is not encroached upon by the growth. Cartilage cannot exhibit pressure atrophy because it is avascular. (Courtesy of Dr. D. E. Sanders.)

Intermediate Tumors

GIANT-CELL TUMOR OF BONE.   This tumor characteristically occurs in the ends of one of the long bones in young adults. Pain and swelling soon after are the predominant symptoms. The radiograph generally shows a characteristic appearance; because the tumor destroys areas of bone, these appear as a series of translucent areas that have been likened to a mass of soap bubbles (Fig. 40–5). Microscopically, the tumor consists of fusiform cells and abundant multinucleate giant cells that resemble osteoclasts. On this account the tumor has also been called an *"osteoclastoma,"* but since the precise nature of the cells is not settled, *giant-cell tumor* is now the current name.

The behavior of giant-cell tumors is generally that of a benign tumor. Nevertheless, local invasion can occur, and between 10 and 15 per cent of the tumors metastasize.

Malignant Tumors

CHONDROSARCOMA.   This tumor is composed of atypical cartilage cells, and it is often difficult to distinguish histologically from a benign chondroma. Local invasion and later metastasis to the lungs are the main features.

OSTEOSARCOMA.   Osteosarcoma is the most common and most malignant of this rare group of primary bone tumors. It affects males more frequently than females, and it is most commonly seen in persons between the ages of 10 and 25 years. Pain is the usual presenting symptom (see Chapter 1, Case History I).

The tumor is composed of malignant osteoblasts that exhibit considerable pleomorphism; giant cells are often abundant. In well-differentiated tumors there is a considerable amount of osteoid produced, which may or may not calcify to form bone. When there is much bone formation, the tumor is described as *osteosclerotic*. Tumor spreads beneath the periosteum, elevates it, and produces a fusiform swelling. Spicules of new bone radiate from the periosteum (Fig. 40–6). On radiography this gives a characteristic "sun ray" appearance. In tumors producing little calcified material the lesion is described as *osteolytic;* the radiograph shows an irregular bony defect and a surrounding soft tissue shadow as growth elevates the periosteum and finally penetrates it.

The outlook for a patient with osteosarcoma is extremely poor, because pulmonary metastases appear early.

FIGURE 40–6. *Osteosarcoma.*

The lower end of the femur is greatly expanded by this malignant tumor. The original cortex of the shaft, which can still be discerned, is indicated by the dotted line. Tumor, in addition to replacing the marrow cavity, has extended beneath the periosteum.

TUMORS OF BONE MARROW

Myeloma.   This tumor is derived from cells that show a marked tendency to differentiate into plasma cells. Because the neoplasia is usually multicentric, the condition is known as *multiple myelomatosis.* It occurs predominantly in persons over 40 years of age and produces multiple osteolytic, punched-out lesions of bone, particularly in the bones in which red marrow is normally found, *i.e.*, the skull, the vertebrae, and the ribs (Fig. 40–7). This widespread involvement of the skeleton can produce so much demineralization that hypercalcemia, metastatic calcification, and renal failure occur. The bony lesions often produce severe pain; a pathological fracture is sometimes the first evidence of the disease.

The tumor cells form large amounts of a homogeneous immunoglobulin called *myeloma protein.* In addition, some tumors produce an excess of light chains, and this polypeptide produced (*Bence Jones protein*), having a molecular weight of about 22,000, is excreted by the kidney and can be recognized by heating a sample of urine. It precipitates when the urine is heated to between 60 and 80° C. and redissolves on further heating or cooling. Bence Jones protein may precipitate in the tubules of the kidney, cause obstruction, and lead to renal failure. Metastatic calcification and renal stone formation add their quota to kidney damage.

Metastatic Tumors.   Secondary tumors of bone are much more common than the primary ones. They develop from blood-borne metastases of carcinoma, and the primary site is generally the prostate, breast, bronchus, kidney, stomach, or thyroid (Fig. 40–8). Metastatic tumors are generally multiple and destroy bone locally to produce rarefaction on radiography *(osteolytic secondaries).* Exceptions to this tendency to destroy bone occur with carcinoma of the prostate and occasionally carcinoma of the breast or other site (Fig. 40–8). In these instances the tumor stimulates new bone formation, and the tumors are hard and radiopaque *(osteosclerotic).* A pathological fracture or pain is the usual presenting symptom. In addition, if the disease is extensive, a leukoerythroblastic anemia can result.

DISEASES OF JOINTS

A synovial joint consists of two or more opposing *cartilage-covered bone ends* that are united by a sleeve of connective tissue called the *capsule,* the innermost layer of which is modified into a secreting membrane called the *synovium.* The synovium consists of one or more layers of flattened or cubical cells that secrete a clear, pale, viscid fluid *(synovial fluid)* containing mucoprotein. The synovial fluid not only lubricates the joint but is also the main, if not the only, source of nourishment of the hyaline cartilage covering the bone ends.

ARTHRITIS

Arthritis is an inflammation of a joint. There is usually an increased amount of synovial fluid present because of a concomitant inflammation of the synovial

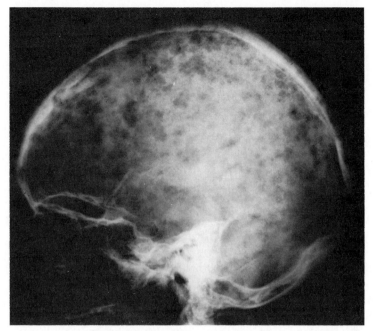

FIGURE 40–7. *Multiple myelomatosis.*

This radiograph of the skull shows numerous osteolytic tumor deposits that produce a typical moth-eaten appearance resulting from numerous punched-out areas where bone has been destroyed. An appearance similar to this can sometimes be seen in secondary carcinoma. (Courtesy of Dr. D. E. Sanders.)

FIGURE 40–8. *Secondary carcinoma in bone.*

A, This section of bone is from a patient who died of carcinoma of the prostate. The cancellous bone in the vertebral bodies shows patchy white tumor deposits that are densely hard because of new bone formation. *B,* Solitary osteolytic metastasis from a carcinoma of the kidney.

643

membrane (*synovitis*). Arthritis may be traumatic, as after the forcible twisting, hyperextension, or hyperflexion of a joint. Such an injury may lead to a
minor tear (called a *sprain*) in the capsule, but if the injury is more severe, the
capsule may rupture and allow partial or complete displacement of the bone
ends to occur. A partial displacement is called a *subluxation,* and a complete
one is called a *dislocation.* Simple sprains heal well, but the weakness that
follows capsular rupture predisposes to recurrent dislocation. Arthritis may be
infective in nature. It may follow a penetrating joint injury when the infection
is introduced from outside. The infection may be blood-borne; thus, a suppurative (septic) arthritis may complicate gonorrhea, lobar pneumonia, or
staphylococcal septicemia. Unless energetically treated in the early stages with
antibiotics, infective arthritis leads to rapid destruction of the articular cartilage; the whole joint cavity fills with inflammatory exudate that organizes and
obliterates the joint space. In this way the joint is destroyed, and the bone ends
are united first by fibrous tissue (*fibrous ankylosis*) and later by bone (*bony
ankylosis*).

Tuberculous arthritis may occur as an isolated lesion or may complicate an
adjacent tuberculous osteomyelitis. The disease is now uncommon.

The common types of chronic arthritis are rheumatoid arthritis and osteoarthritis.

Rheumatoid Arthritis.   This disease occurs most frequently in young
women and is characteristically polyarticular (affecting many joints) and symmetrical. The small joints of the hands and feet are most severely affected, but
the elbows and knees also suffer badly. Rheumatoid arthritis is a systemic
disease, and in its active phases there are malaise, anemia, pyrexia, weight loss,
and bouts of sweating. The onset of the disease is occasionally acute, but
usually it is insidious as swelling, pain, and stiffness of the joints develop.

The affected joints are swollen, tender, and painful. In the early stages the
synovial membrane is acutely inflamed; later, there is proliferation of its connective tissue component together with a heavy infiltration by lymphocytes
and plasma cells. The proliferating synovium steadily encroaches upon the articular margins, and a layer of inflamed granulation tissue, called a *pannus,*
spreads over the cartilage of the joint surface and destroys it. The joint space is
gradually obliterated by fibrous adhesions, and eventually fibrous ankylosis
occurs. In this late stage there is severe disuse atrophy of the adjacent bones
and muscles, and the overlying skin is smooth and shiny. The results of advanced rheumatoid arthritis are tragic to see: progressive contractures lead to
flexion deformities that are found in particular in the hands, which have a characteristic ulnar deviation of the fingers (Fig. 40–9). The flexed, ankylosed larger
joints render the patient immobile and bedridden.

The nature of rheumatoid arthritis is unknown, but the basic lesion seems
to be fibrinoid necrosis of collagen. It has therefore been classified as a
collagen disease (see Chapter 27). The widespread nature of the process is
evidenced by the development of lesions in places other than the joints. The
most characteristic of these is the subcutaneous nodules that develop over
pressure points. They consist of a large area of necrobiotic collagen surrounded
by a palisaded layer of fibroblasts and epithelioid cells. Similar nodules are encountered elsewhere; thus, in the sclera of the eye a rheumatoid nodule can

FIGURE 40–9. *The hand in rheumatoid arthritis.*

This patient had had rheumatoid arthritis for many years and was severely incapacitated. The hand shows marked swelling of the metacarpophalangeal joints and extreme deviation of the fingers toward the ulnar side. Apart from movement of the thumb, very little movement was possible. The hollowed appearance between the metacarpal bones is due to atrophy of the small muscles of the hand. This patient was in a hospital because a rheumatoid nodule had developed in the sclera of her left eye. To prevent perforation of the globe and loss of the eye, a fascia lata graft was applied and was successful in saving her sight.

break down and cause perforation of the globe. A destructive process with fibrosis can involve the aorta; the condition then has the appearance of syphilitic aortitis. Generalized enlargement of the lymph nodes and splenomegaly may also be present. Amyloidosis is an important complication; indeed, it is the only significant fatal lesion in rheumatoid arthritis, which may otherwise smolder on for many years and produce complete crippling.

The sera of most patients with rheumatoid arthritis contain an autoantibody that reacts with human immunoglobulin. This antibody is called the *rheumatoid factor*. Although its detection is useful in diagnosis, its significance in the pathogenesis of the disease is not known. The rheumatoid factor is not present in psoriatic arthritis; this is a useful distinguishing point between the two diseases which in other respects closely resemble each other.

ANKYLOSING SPONDYLITIS

This condition is related to rheumatoid arthritis and is believed by some authorities to be a variant of that disease. Nevertheless, there are some rather striking differences:

(a) The disease generally affects young men.

(b) The vertebral joints and large peripheral joints, such as the hip, are generally affected, whereas the small distal joints are spared.

(c) There is bony ankylosis of the affected joints in the later stages of the disease. The spinal ligaments and margins of the intervertebral discs undergo ossification and in due course the spinal column is converted into a composite bony mass, the so-called *bamboo spine.*

(d) Subcutaneous nodules are not formed, and the rheumatoid factor is not present.

OSTEOARTHRITIS

Osteoarthritis, despite its name, is not an inflammatory, but rather a degenerative, disease of joints. It is one of the commonest human afflictions, because it is essentially an accentuation of the inevitable aging process of articular cartilage. The nourishment of the hyaline cartilage of joints is normally rather precarious and depends on the synovial fluid. The constant wear and tear of the joints after many years' activity leads to a gradual deterioration of the central part of the articular cartilage. This process is greatly aggravated by injury; thus, a joint injured in some athletic activity can be complicated by osteoarthritis several years later—even when the patient is still young. Nevertheless, osteoarthritis is generally a disease of later life and affects the spine and large weight-bearing joints, especially the hips.

The smaller joints, however, do not escape entirely. Osteoarthritis, unlike rheumatoid arthritis, is not a systemic disease. The general health remains unaffected, and life is not shortened.

Osteoarthritis begins with softening and fraying of the articular cartilage, which becomes progressively thinner. Ultimately, the underlying bone is exposed, and its surface becomes hard, worn and polished (a change called *eburnation*). Meanwhile, there is proliferation of the cartilage cells of the margin of the articular area. This new cartilage soon ossifies. The result is that the periphery of the articular cartilage is raised and bossed (a process called *lipping*); this is an important radiological finding. The projecting nodules of new bone at the margins of the joint are called *osteophytes*. These not only interfere with the range of the joint's movement but also may become nipped off to form *loose bodies* ("joint-mice"). These loose bodies are a constant nuisance, because they tend to be caught between the opposing bone ends during movement. The result is locking of the joint, which can be excruciatingly painful if a fringe of synovium is also included. A prominent site for osteophytes is the terminal interphalangeal joints of the fingers of elderly people. These painless bony swellings are extremely common and are called *Heberden's nodes*.

In osteoarthritis the joints do not become ankylosed, but the destructive process and the osteophyte formation seriously limit movement, which may become very painful. In such cases the replacement of the joint by an artificial metallic prosthesis has been most useful.

Review Questions

1. Describe the circumstances under which woven bone is formed.
2. Explain how a knowledge of the embryological development of bone helps to account for how a fracture can unite.
3. A patient with a persistent urinary tract infection is found to have a serum calcium of 17 mg per 100 ml and a blood urea nitrogen (BUN) of 80 mg per 100 ml. How may these observations be related?

4. Compare metastatic calcification with dystrophic calcification, giving examples of each type.
5. Predict the effect of a prolonged, excessive intake of vitamin D.
6. Compare generalized osteoporosis with osteomalacia.
7. Describe osteosarcoma in terms of the following factors:
    (a) known predisposing causes
    (b) age incidence
    (c) radiographic features
    (d) clinical presentation
    (e) prognosis.
8. Explain why renal failure is common in patients with multiple myelomatosis.
9. Patients with rheumatoid arthritis sometimes have the following condition:
    (a) osteoporosis of the spine
    (b) renal failure
    (c) aortic valve insufficiency.
Explain the pathogenesis of these extra-articular lesions.
10. Comment briefly on each of the following:
    (a) serum alkaline phosphatase
    (b) serum calcium
    (c) the rheumatoid factor
    (d) Bence Jones protein
    (e) brown tumors of bone.

Selected Readings

Ham, A. W.: Histology. 6th ed. Philadelphia, J. B. Lippincott Company, 1969. Note, in particular, Chapter 18, "Bone," for an account of the structure of bone, its growth, and the healing of a fracture.
Lichtenstein, L.: Diseases of Bone and Joints. St. Louis, The C. V. Mosby Company, 1970, 228 pp.
Lichtenstein, L.: Bone Tumors. 4th ed. St. Louis, The C. V. Mosby Company, 1972, 441 pp.
Robbins, S. L.: Pathological Basis of Disease. Philadelphia, W. B. Saunders Company, 1974. See pp. 1431–1477 for an account of the diseases of bones and joints.
Walter, J. B., and Israel, M. S.: General Pathology. 4th ed. Edinburgh, Churchill Livingstone. Note especially pp. 116–119 for an account of fracture healing.

Chapter 41

Chapter Outline

After studying this chapter, the student should be able to:

- Define the following words: erythematous, macule, patch, papule, plaque, vesicle, bulla, pustule, squamous, telangiectasia, excoriation, and pruritic.
- Differentiate among acute, subacute, and chronic dermatitis.
- List the clinical types of dermatitis and describe the outstanding features of each type.

648

DISEASES OF THE SKIN

- Describe the main features of psoriasis, pityriasis rosea, urticaria, toxic erythema, and erythema multiforme.
- Describe the types of skin reaction that drugs can cause.
- Classify the vesiculobullous diseases and describe the main features of each type.
- Describe the pathogenesis and lesions of acne vulgaris.
- Describe the common melanotic and vascular hamartomas of skin.
- Classify the types of squamous-cell papilloma of skin.
- Describe the lesions that can precede the development of squamous-cell carcinoma of skin.
- Give an account of squamous-cell carcinoma of the skin and compare it with keratoacanthoma.
- Classify the types of malignant melanoma and relate the types to the prognosis.

INTRODUCTION

It has been estimated that between 15 and 20 per cent of patients who consult their doctor do so because of some skin disorder. Nevertheless, the teaching of dermatology is usually sadly neglected in medical education. Perhaps this is due to the complexity of the subject because the number of diseases of the skin that have been described in the literature far exceeds that of any other individual organ. There are several reasons for this. First, the skin is exposed to many insults from the external environment. Second, it is a complex composite organ, because in addition to having a surface epithelium called the *epidermis*, it has associated *hair follicles* with their *sebaceous glands*, *eccrine* and *apocrine sweat glands*, and a specialized connective tissue called the *dermis*, itself composed of dense collagenous bundles and elastic fibers. Third, the skin can be examined and biopsied easily. Fourth, throughout the ages, people have considered the appearance of skin to be very important; this fact has added to the complexity of dermatology. This chapter describes some of the common skin diseases and also a few which, although uncommon, are so serious that they must be recognized early if adequate treatment is to be given.

TERMINOLOGY

There are few areas in medicine that can compete with dermatology for hiding truth with complex names. Nevertheless, with some basic facts and a minimal knowledge of Latin, it is possible to master this terminology.

An area of skin that is altered, usually red (*erythematous*), flat, and not palpable (*i.e.*, cannot be felt) is called a *macule* if it is less than 1.0 cm in diameter;

if it is larger, it is called a *patch*. Similar areas that are palpable are called *papules* if they are small (less than 1.0 cm in diameter) and *plaques* if they are over that size. A blister is called a *vesicle* if small, and a *bulla* if large. *Pustules* contain pus. If flakes of keratin are seen obviously adherent to a lesion, this lesion is called *squamous*. Since most such lesions can be felt, they are therefore called *papulosquamous*. The presence of visible abnormally dilated vessels is called *telangiectasia*. Shallow ulcers or erosions are termed *excoriations* if they are produced by scratching. The observation and description of each individual skin lesion is important, because certain types are characteristic of certain diseases. For example, psoriasis is characteristically papulosquamous, is occasionally pustular, but is never vesicular.

The distribution of the lesions seen in any skin disease is important. A localized rash often indicates a localized cause. Thus, a dermatitis on only one wrist is probably due to sensitivity to a wrist band or a watch strap. Some diseases, *e.g.*, smallpox, characteristically affect the distal parts, such as the hands, feet, and face, whereas others, *e.g.*, chickenpox, tend to affect the trunk rather than the extremities. In a consideration of any skin disease, it is important therefore to include the distribution of the rash and the individual characteristics of its lesions.

The presence of itching is characteristic of certain skin diseases, such as scabies, neurodermatitis, and atopic dermatitis. The term *pruritus*, which is commonly used, is synonymous with itching. Note that the presence or absence of itching is as dependent upon the make-up of the individual as it is on the nature of his lesions. Some people itch easily, others do not.

DERMATITIS AND ECZEMA

Dermatitis and *eczema* are synonymous terms used to describe a particular skin reaction pattern that primarily involves the epidermis. Three histological types are recognized: acute, subacute, and chronic.

Histopathological Types of Dermatitis

ACUTE DERMATITIS. The epidermis shows intercellular edema *(spongiosis)* that terminates in the separation of epidermal cells and in the formation of vesicles or bullae (Fig. 41–1). The dermis shows an acute inflammatory reaction with edema and, surprisingly enough, a perivascular lymphocytic infiltrate. The absence of polymorphs is noteworthy but is not understood. The vesicles formed in the epidermis rupture, and clinically this produces a "weeping" or crusted surface.

SUBACUTE DERMATITIS. Spongiosis and vesicle formation are still evident, but the epidermis reacts by increasing mitotic activity so that it becomes thicker *(acanthosis)*. Keratinization is disturbed, with the result that in places the keratin layer retains cellular nuclei. This condition is called *parakeratosis*.

CHRONIC DERMATITIS. Spongiosis is scanty, and veiscles are not formed. Chronic dermatitis is characterized by acanthosis (thickening of the epidermis) together with the formation of excessive keratin *(hyperkeratosis)* and, in places, parakeratosis (Fig. 41–2). Clinically, chronic dermatitis appears as indurated, scaly papules or plaques, and the skin markings tend to be accentuated. This latter feature is known as *lichenification*.

FIGURE 41–1. *Acute dermatitis.*

The epidermis shows some thickening *(acanthosis)* that is due mainly to the separation of the cells by edema *(spongiosis)*. In several places the cells have torn apart to produce intraepidermal vesicles. The largest of these spongiotic vesicles is on the left-hand side and contains coagulated exudate. There is a sparse infiltration of the dermis by lymphocytes. The biopsy was taken from a patient with acute allergic contact dermatitis due to exposure to poison ivy (× 240).

Clinical Types of Dermatitis. The clinical types of dermatitis are many and various. They cannot be distinguished from each other histologically but differ in their causes and clinical presentation.

PRIMARY IRRITANT DERMATITIS. Externally applied chemical irritants are a frequent cause of dermatitis *(contact dermatitis)*: a common example is the chronic lichenified hand eczema seen in housewives whose hands are brought repeatedly into contact with water, detergents, and other household agents. Alkalis, acids, and many industrial chemicals can act as primary irritants, and if applied over a long period they lead to a refractory chronic dermatitis. Elderly individuals with dry skin may develop a dermatitis that is due to exposure to agents such as water, soap, and detergents that would be harmless in a younger person.

ALLERGIC CONTACT DERMATITIS. The development of cell-mediated sensitizing antibodies toward chemicals results in the production of *allergic contact dermatitis*. Iodine, formaldehyde, dyes, plants (*e.g.*, poison ivy), and nickel (used in costume jewelry) are among the many agents that can cause this type of allergic dermatitis (Fig. 41–3). It is noteworthy that certain parts of the skin are more sensitive to irritants than others. Thus, allergic contact dermatitis is more common on the backs of the hands than it is on the palms. Likewise, the face is particularly sensitive and may react to agents that elsewhere cause little

FIGURE 41–2. Chronic dermatitis.

There is marked acanthosis and hyperkeratosis (Hyp) together with one focus of parakeratosis (Para). These changes should be compared with the normal skin present on the right-hand side of the specimen in Figure 41–1 (× 240).

trouble. Dermatitis around the eyes can be due to nail polish, which causes little trouble when applied to the hands or feet.

PHOTODERMATITIS.   Ultraviolet light can act on chemicals (either applied topically or taken systemically) present in the skin and so alter them that direct irritant effects *(phototoxic dermatitis)* or new antigen formation and subsequent sensitization *(photoallergic dermatitis)* results. Agents that are well known to cause this sensitizing effect when applied topically are perfumes, coal-tar derivatives, and halogenated salicylanilides (used in deodorant soap).

Many drugs taken internally can have a similar affect. Common examples are chemotherapeutic agents such as sulfonamides and tetracyclines, diuretics *(e.g.,* chlorothiazide), and tranquillizers *(e.g.,* chlorpromazine), to name a few.

INFANTILE ECZEMA AND ATOPIC DERMATITIS.   These two conditions occur in atopic (allergic) individuals, but the pathogenesis is obscure, for although the associated respiratory diseases such as hay fever and bronchial asthma appear to be caused by IgE sensitization, the skin lesions are more complex and the damage is probably cell-mediated.

NUMMULAR ECZEMA.   This condition tends to occur in atopic individuals and is characterized by the formation of localized, coin-shaped plaques of subacute or chronic dermatitis. Itching is usually marked.

STASIS DERMATITIS.   Stasis dermatitis is common on the legs and is related to chronic venous stasis. It occurs following venous thrombosis in the

FIGURE 41–3. *Acute dermatitis.*

This patient sustained a sprain of the left ankle, and adhesive tape was applied for support. Thirty-six hours later an acute vesicular dermatitis appeared and subsequently became bullous. Note how the rash is limited to the region previously covered by tape (lines of demarcation are obvious). Areas where the skin was folded are spared.

lower limbs and in patients with varicose veins. In addition to the usual features of a dermatitis, stasis dermatitis is characterized by a brown discoloration of the skin. This is produced by hemosiderin secondary to petechial hemorrhages. Chronic ulcers are a common complication and are usually initiated by trauma, caused either accidentally or by scratching. Such *stasis ulcers* (see Fig. 7–4) are often situated over the medial malleolus and heal slowly because of the poor blood supply to the skin.

SEBORRHEIC DERMATITIS.   A type of chronic dermatitis is frequently seen in the scalp and results in the formation of greasy scales or dandruff. This condition is termed *seborrheic dermatitis;* although it is extremely common, its precise nature is not understood. The dermatitis can extend beyond the scalp and affect the face. Occasionally there is involvement of the trunk, particularly the front of the chest, and the flexural regions such as the axilla or under the breasts. This type of dermatitis can be encountered in all age groups, ranging from infants (cradle cap) to old people.

NEURODERMATITIS.   A feature of some forms of dermatitis, including the atopic variety, is marked itching. This leads to scratching and self-perpetuation because of the continued physical trauma. The condition is then referred to as *chronic neurodermatitis* (Fig. 41–4). Localized plaques of neurodermatitis, which frequently occur on the back of the neck and the front of the ankles, are called *lichen simplex chronicus.*

FIGURE 41–4. *Neurodermatitis.*

This patient had a chronic lichenified dermatitis on the front of both ankles. *A* shows a close-up of the hyperkeratosis and accentuation of the crease lines that are typical; they are fancifully likened to lichen on a tree trunk. Constant scratching and rubbing, often with the opposite heel, perpetuated the condition. The nodules shown higher on the leg in *B* are also self-induced. They consist of dense scar tissue with overlying acanthosis and depigmentation. The lesions are called *prurigo nodularis* (from the Latin word *prurigo,* meaning "to itch") and are produced by the patient continually picking at them.

PAPULOSQUAMOUS ERUPTIONS

A group of diseases, of widely differing origins, is characterized by papulosquamous lesions. Common examples are chronic dermatitis, psoriasis, pityriasis rosea, secondary syphilis, and ringworm.

Psoriasis. This is a chronic disease that fluctuates in intensity both spontaneously and under the influence of treatment. It occurs as sharply demarcated erythematous plaques with a dry, silvery scale. Common sites are the elbows, knees, and other extensor surfaces. The palms, soles, and scalp are also frequently affected (Fig. 41–5). Psoriasis is not usually itchy, and vesicles are never formed. This distinguishes it both clinically and histologically from dermatitis.

Pityriasis Rosea. Pityriasis rosea is a common, self-limiting eruption of young adults. It affects the trunk primarily and resembles secondary syphilis. A viral cause is suspected but has never been proved. The disease clears spontaneously in six to eight weeks and does not recur.

FIGURE 41–5. *Psoriasis.*

The characteristic psoriatic plaque is sharply delineated, red, and covered by a silvery scale. The lesions, particularly when on the soles of the feet, can easily be misdiagnosed as ringworm.

DISEASES CHARACTERIZED BY A DERMAL INFLAMMATORY REACTION

An inflammatory reaction in the dermis is present in many skin diseases, including those that affect primarily the epidermis (*e.g.*, dermatitis, psoriasis, and pityriasis rosea). A localized area of dermal inflammation is a feature of many infections (*e.g.*, tuberculosis and erysipelas), but there is a group of conditions in which the primary event is a widespread vascular inflammatory reaction within the dermis. The most mild example of this group is urticaria.

Urticaria. Urticaria, or *hives,* is a common disease that afflicts many individuals at some time or another in their life. Symptoms include an acute inflammatory reaction in the dermis that is characterized by vasodilatation, scanty polymorph accumulation, and marked edema. Clinically urticaria commences with marked itching, which is followed by the appearance of erythema and swelling. The lesions tend to develop a pale center, or *wheal,* surrounded by an erythematous edge. They thereby resemble the common mosquito bite and the triple response (see Chapter 5).

Acute urticaria is sometimes a type I hypersensitivity reaction mediated by IgE, but it is also seen in immune-complex reactions. It may follow the ingestion of a particular food or drug, and as in other hypersensitivity reactions, small quantities of the agent are sufficient to induce an attack. Thus, the menthol in a cigarette or toothpaste can precipitate acute urticaria in a sensitized person.

FIGURE 41–6. *Erythema multiforme.*

The lesions have a bright red border and a pale center produced by the subepidermal edema. In places, the papules have joined together; the lesions have an arcuate outline.

Each urticarial lesion of urticaria lasts only a few hours, but repeated attacks of urticaria may occur over a period of many months or even years *(chronic urticaria).* In patients having such attacks the cause is rarely found.

Urticaria affects the dermis. When the subcutaneous tissues are involved, the condition is termed angioedema. In both urticaria and angioedema, the mucous membranes (including that of the tongue) can be involved. In one type of hereditary angioedema there is a deficiency of C_1 esterase inhibitor. This is a serious condition, because lesions occur not only in the intestine, causing colic, but also in the larynx, in some cases leading to death from asphyxiation (the lesions obstruct the passage). In some families many members ultimately die in this way.

Toxic Erythema.   This general term is applied to many conditions in which the epidermis is normal, at least in the early stages, but in which there is a dermal inflammatory reaction showing vasodilatation and a perivascular accumulation of cells, particularly lymphocytes. Viral exanthems (*e.g.,* measles) fall into this group. Toxic erythema is one manifestation of an adverse drug reaction.

Erythema Multiforme.   This is an acute disease that may be regarded as a severe variant of toxic erythema. The onset is usually sudden, and the patient rapidly develops symmetrical lesions of varying types—urticarial, erythematous macular, papular, and sometimes vesicular (Fig. 41–6). The characteristic lesion is an erythematous papule with a central hemorrhagic area, so that the lesion tends to resemble a target or iris. The dermal inflammatory reaction is sometimes so marked that fluid accumulates beneath the epidermis, and a *subepidermal vesicle* forms. The dermal reaction causes secondary degeneration of the epidermis. The severity of the dermal inflammatory reaction and the degenerate appearance of the epidermal roof serve to distinguish the lesions from those of bullous pemphigoid, which is described later. Erythema multiforme is often idiopathic, but it is sometimes precipitated by a variety of factors, including the following: previous herpes simplex of the lips, vaccination, drug intake, exposure to sunlight, and internal malignant disease. Erythema multiforme tends to affect the extremities, but in some instances it causes mucosal lesions. Severe cases of erythema multiforme that affect mucous membranes in addition to the skin are termed the *Stevens-Johnson syndrome.* This form of the disease can be extremely severe and can lead to death.

DRUG ERUPTION

Drug eruptions are so common and produce such a wide variety of lesions that they must be considered in the differential diagnosis of any skin eruption.

The common type of drug eruption is erythematous, papular, of widespread distribution, and very itchy. Severe cases become vesicular and constitute one variety of erythema multiforme. Petechial lesions are not uncommon, and severe cases exhibit a definite vasculitis and lead to the formation of hemorrhagic and necrotic lesions. Sometimes the lesions closely resemble well-recognized dermatoses, such as measles and lupus erythematosus. The pathogenesis of drug eruptions varies. Those of an urticarial nature appear to be the result of a type I hypersensitivity reaction. Others are mediated by immune complexes. In most, the pathogenesis is obscure.

VESICULOBULLOUS DISEASES

The formation of vesicles or bullae is an outstanding feature of this group of diseases. For accurate diagnosis, a biopsy of an early lesion is often necessary, because the region of origin of the vesicle is of vital importance in differential diagnosis. Some vesicles are formed within the epidermis, whereas others are formed beneath the epidermis.

Intraepidermal Vesicles. The superficial subcorneal vesicles and pustules of impetigo and candidiasis can generally be diagnosed so easily clinically that a biopsy is not necessary. Likewise, the spongiotic vesicles of acute and subacute dermatitis rarely need pathological confirmation. There are, however, two groups of intraepidermal vesiculating diseases in which biopsy is often useful. These are pemphigus and the vesiculating viral diseases. In both, the vesicles are formed by acantholysis.

THE PEMPHIGUS GROUP OF DISEASES. *Pemphigus vulgaris* is a chronic blistering disease that tends to occur in middle- and old age, particularly in Jews of Eastern European ancestry. Blisters frequently involve the mouth and lead to soreness, inability to eat, and great incapacity. The blisters tend to break easily, leaving eroded painful surfaces. Pathologically, the vesicles are formed by separation of the epidermal cells above the basal layer (Fig. 41–7). The cells appear to lose their cohesiveness and to become detached. This process is termed *acantholysis,* and the free or acantholytic cells are found lying in the fluid of the vesicle. The vesicles are generally flaccid, and on pressure can be made to extend laterally. Once the disease commences, it tends to

FIGURE 41-7. *Pemphigus vulgaris.*

Acantholysis has produced the characteristic suprabasal blister. Note how the papillary dermis is covered by a row of basal cells, which have been likened to a row of tomb stones, and are still adherent to the basement membrane. Compare this acantholytic vesicle with the spongiotic vesicles of acute dermatitis (× 500).

progress and to be fatal after a variable course lasting, on the average, about 18 months. This poor prognosis was the rule before the advent of modern therapy. Nevertheless, even with systemic prednisone and other immunosuppressant drugs, pemphigus is still serious, because while the disease itself may not be fatal, the complications of the treatment sometimes are.

A number of other acantholytic blistering diseases are known; some are variants of pemphigus, but others are rare and will not be considered.

THE VESICULAR VIRAL DISEASES. The vesicles formed in zoster, chickenpox, smallpox, vaccinia, and herpes simplex closely resemble each other histopathologically. The invaded epidermal cells show degeneration, tend to fuse to form multinucleated masses, and exhibit acantholysis. The intraepidermal vesicle so formed contains degenerate and multinucleate acantholytic cells. Distinction between the various types of virus vesicles is not possible histologically, but the clinical features combined with electron microscopy of vesicle fluid and other virological investigations can distinguish one disease from the other.

A biopsy of the lesions of a typical case of chickenpox, herpes simplex, or zoster is not generally warranted. Sometimes, however, atypical cases are encountered, and if a virological service is not available, a biopsy is useful in distinguishing such cases from other localized vesiculating diseases, such as a patch of acute contact dermatitis or a bullous drug reaction.

Subepidermal Vesicles. Subepidermal vesicles are formed in severe erythema multiforme and in certain drug eruptions, as previously described. They are also characteristic of bullous pemphigoid.

BULLOUS PEMPHIGOID. Bullous pemphigoid is a chronic blistering disease that resembles pemphigus vulgaris clinically but has a much better prognosis. Unlike the lesions of pemphigus, the vesicles and bullae of this condition are usually tense rather than flaccid. Mucous membrane involvement is less common and less severe.

Microscopically, the vesicles are found to be subepidermal. A useful diagnostic test is the demonstration of autoantibodies to skin basement membrane, both free in the serum and fixed in the skin (see Fig. 9–13). Patients with pemphigus vulgaris also produce an autoantibody, but its specificity is directed against epidermal intercellular substance. Hence, the two diseases are quite distinct from each other both histologically and immunologically.

ACNE VULGARIS

This familiar disorder of teenagers affects those areas in which sebaceous glands are plentiful—face, back, and upper chest. The primary lesions are due to the plugging of pilosebaceous follicles with adherent keratin. Oxidation of the surface of the plugs produces a dark-colored substance, and results in the familiar *"blackhead,"* or *comedo.* The affected follicles dilate and become filled with the lipid secretions of sebaceous glands. In these the anaerobic saprophyte *Corynebacterium acnes* proliferates and splits the lipids to produce irritating fatty acids. When the follicle ruptures, there is an inflammatory reaction, causing papules and pustules to be formed. Tetracycline therapy, which is now so much in vogue, is designed to inhibit the growth of *C. acnes.*

Hamartomas of the Skin

The hamartomas of the skin are termed *nevi.* The common examples are the melanotic and angiomatous varieties.

MELANOTIC HAMARTOMAS

Melanotic hamartomas are commonly called *moles.* Almost every person has at least a dozen or more of them. The parent cell is the melanocyte, which develops from the neural crest and migrates to the epidermis with the peripheral nerves. The melanocytes here become incorporated into the basal layer of the epidermis and appear as cells with clear cytoplasm (Fig. 41–8). A focal abnormal proliferation of these cells leads to a mass that soon invades the dermis. The proliferating cells lose their ability to produce melanin and are then termed "nevus cells." Early in the formation of a nevus, melanin-producing cells are formed at the dermoepidermal junction, and the lesion is called a

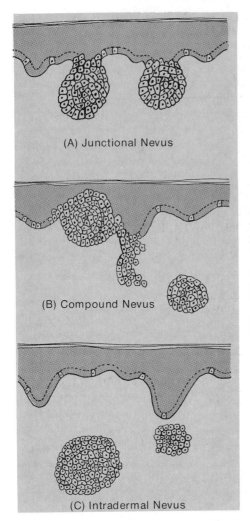

(A) Junctional Nevus

(B) Compound Nevus

(C) Intradermal Nevus

FIGURE 41–8.   *Melanotic nevi of skin.*

Sketches showing the development of melanotic nevi: The only cells drawn are melanocytes and nevus cells. *A,* Junctional nevus. Focal proliferation of melanocytes in the basal layer of the epidermis produces nests of cells that become nevus cells. *B,* Compound nevus. Some nevus cells have invaded the dermis. *C,* Intradermal nevus. The junctional activity has ceased and all the nevus cells are in the dermis. The epidermis is normal and contains scattered melanocytes that appear as clear cells in the basal layer of the epidermis. (Drawing by Margot Mackay, Department of Art as Applied to Medicine, University of Toronto.)

junctional nevus. This is deeply pigmented and barely palpable. As the nevus develops, a dermal portion is formed, and ultimately a nonpigmented intradermal nevus results (Fig. 41–9). Nevi are seldom present at birth, but they develop during childhood.

Once the nevus cells have entered the dermis, they rarely show any further proliferation. The junctional element, however, can exhibit spurts of proliferation (junctional activity), and although this proliferation is of little significance during the years of development in childhood, in adult life any marked growth is regarded with suspicion, because it may be the first indication of malignant change.

Nevocellular nevi, unlike many other hamartomas, do occasionally become malignant. *Any change, such as an increase in size, bleeding, ulceration or change in degree of pigmentation, should suggest the possibility of malignancy.* Excision or biopsy is then indicated.

FIGURE 41–9. *Compound melanotic nevus.*

This brown lesion had been present on a 56-year-old woman's back for many years. She had detected a slight increase in size over the preceding year, and she had it excised for cosmetic reasons. The nevus has a lobulated smooth surface, is not ulcerated, and shows no evidence of malignancy.

VASCULAR HAMARTOMAS OF SKIN

Various types of vascular anomalies are encountered in the skin. Sometimes at birth or shortly afterwards a red, vascular, spongy nodule develops in the skin: this grows rapidly for a while, but regresses after a few years and leaves an area of scarring. This type of nevus is composed of capillary-sized blood spaces and is often called a *capillary hemangioma* or strawberry nevus. Another type of nevus is composed of a few dilated capillary channels. Such a lesion appears as a flat, erythematous patch that is colloquially called a *port-wine stain.* Vascular nevi are of little importance apart from their cosmetic appearance. Sometimes they are multiple, and on occasion they are associated with similar lesions in deeper organs. When vascular nevi involve the face, for instance, angiomatous lesions of the central nervous system or eye are sometimes found and a number of characteristic syndromes can be recognized. Small hemangiomas commonly develop in elderly people and appear as bright red papules, 2 to 4 mm in diameter on the trunk *("cherry angiomas").*

Benign Tumors of the Skin

SQUAMOUS-CELL PAPILLOMA

This is generally used as a descriptive term that includes a number of separate entities. The common types are described below:

Epithelial Nevus. This type of papilloma is generally present at birth and appears as a warty lesion, sometimes of linear distribution. It tends to recur after simple curettage and can then be mistaken for a malignant tumor. Only excision of the local area can effect a cure.

Seborrheic Keratosis. Papillomas, frequently with considerable melanin pigmentation and overlying hyperkeratosis, are extremely common on the backs of the hands, on the trunk, and on the face of elderly people. The lesions

FIGURE 41–10. *Seborrheic keratosis.*

The neck of this elderly woman was covered by numerous pigmented seborrheic keratoses. The largest lesion shown in the center of the picture had been bleeding recently because of the mechanical irritation of clothing. The lesion was easily removed by curettage. Histopathogical studies confirmed the diagnosis.

seem to be stuck onto the surface of the skin and appear as flat or roughened pigmented warty nodules or plaques (Fig. 41–10). Such lesions are easily eliminated by curettage. The lesions never become malignant, but when heavily pigmented they are liable to be confused with other pigmented lesions of the skin, such as melanotic nevus, pigmented basal-cell carcinoma, or malignant melanoma.

Verruca Vulgaris.   The *common wart* is a type of papilloma that is due to an infection by one of the papovaviruses (Fig. 17–2). In some situations the same virus causes a somewhat different lesion. On the soles of the feet the epidermal overgrowth and hyperkeratosis produce a painful lesion known as a *plantar wart.* Sometimes the virus produces multiple small, flat lesions called *plane warts.* In moist areas, such as on the penis and in the female genital region, pedunculated cauliflowerlike lesions are produced and are known as *condylomata acuminata.*

Malignant Tumors of the Skin

The most common malignant tumor of the skin in whites is the basal cell carcinoma. This is illustrated in Figure 41–11 and is described fully in Chapter 17. As with squamous-cell carcinoma the major predisposing cause is prolonged exposure to ultraviolet light.

FIGURE 41–11. *Basal-cell carcinoma.*

A basal-cell carcinoma of the right side of the forehead of a 56-year-old man is shown. The lesion has the typical appearance, with a depressed center and a raised, rolled edge over which dilated blood vessels can be seen traversing. The dome-shaped swelling just above the medial aspect of the right eyebrow has the features of an epidermoid cyst, commonly called a *sebaceous cyst,* or *wen.* The lesion is formed by cystic dilatation of a plugged pilosebaceous follicle.

SQUAMOUS-CELL CARCINOMA

This tumor commonly arises on the sun-exposed skin in a pre-existing actinic keratosis (Figs. 41–12 and 41–13). Actinic keratoses are areas of epidermal dysplasia caused by prolonged exposure to ultraviolet light They appear as scaly erythematous areas on the face, ears, backs of hands, or forearms. In

FIGURE 41–12. *The effect of sunlight on human skin.*

Although a deep suntan is regarded by many as a status symbol indicative of health, the effect of sunlight on human skin is predominantly detrimental. Prolonged exposure leads to damage to the dermal collagen fibers, and this contributes to the wrinkled appearance of the aging skin. Good advice is that if you want to look young, keep out of the sun! Epidermal damage leads to actinic keratoses and ultimately to cancer. These changes are most marked in individuals with fair skin. They have pale blue eyes and are of northern European stock (e.g., Celts and Scandinavians). (Drawing by Susie Shin.)

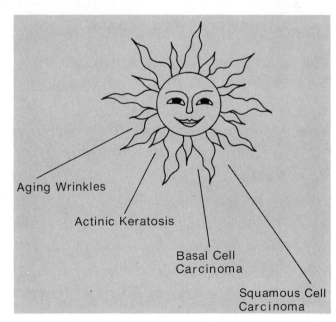

contradistinction to seborrheic keratoses, they must be regarded as precancerous. Squamous-cell carcinoma arising in an actinic keratosis is invasive, but metastases are late and the prognosis is relatively good. It should be stressed that the transition to malignancy frequently takes many years, and quite simple treatment is adequate for the cure of most actinic keratoses.

Squamous-cell carcinoma may also arise in normal skin or in persons with Bowen's disease. The latter is a type of carcinoma-*in-situ* that can occur on any part of the body and appears as a circumscribed, erythematous, slightly indurated, scaly patch or plaque. This type of squamous-cell carcinoma is more malignant than that arising from an actinic keratosis. It tends to metastasize to regional lymph nodes and ultimately to the blood stream.

Squamous-cell carcinoma must be differentiated both clinically and pathologically from a keratoacanthoma, which it closely resembles, and which also occurs on the sun-exposed skin.

KERATOACANTHOMA

In this lesion there is a localized exuberant overgrowth of atypical squamous epithelium that appears to invade the dermis and to surround a central keratotic plug. Around the lesion is an inflammatory reaction. Keratoacanthoma

FIGURE 41–13. *Actinic keratoses.*

The left ear of this elderly man shows several erythematous, hyperkeratotic lesions. He had spent much of his working life out-of-doors.

has been regarded by some as a type of self-healing carcinoma. The shape of the lesion is characteristic clinically, because it appears as a volcanolike lesion with a central keratotic depressed plug. The natural history also is quite characteristic: the lesion grows rapidly for two or three months, remains stationary, and then involutes spontaneously. Healing results in considerable scarring, and the treatment of choice is therefore simple excision, since this gives a good cosmetic result.

MELANOMA

Malignant melanoma of the skin can arise in four ways (Fig. 41–14):

(a) *In a pre-existing nevus.* Considering the number of nevi present in all individuals, one sees that this is a very rare event. About 20 per cent of malignant melanomas arise in this way.

(A) Lentigo Maligna

(B) Superficial Spreading Melanoma

(C) Nodular Melanoma

FIGURE 41–14. *Types of malignant melanoma.*

A, Lentigo maligna. Proliferation of atypical melanocytes in the basal layer of the epidermis is accompanied by a lymphocytic response in the dermis. After many years dermal invasion can occur. B, Superficial spreading melanoma. Proliferation of atypical, malignant melanocytes occurs over a wide area of the basal layer of the epidermis. The melanoma cells invade the epidermis, and in one area they also invade the dermis. C, Nodular melanoma. The lesion is more localized than in the case of the superficial spreading variety. Melanoma cells invade the epidermis and extend deep into the dermis. This type of tumor has the worst prognosis. (Drawing by Margot Mackay, Department of Art as Applied to Medicine, University of Toronto.)

FIGURE 41–15. *Nodular malignant melanoma.*

This black lesion had recently appeared and showed superficial ulceration. The clinical diagnosis was malignant melanoma. Before radical treatment of such a lesion is undertaken, it must either be biopsied or (if small enough) be completely excised locally. Histopathological diagnosis is essential before one undertakes definitive treatment of any malignant lesion. (Photograph courtesy of Dr. Wallace H. Clark, Jr.)

(b) *As a nodule in previously normal skin* (Fig. 41–15). This type of tumor *(nodular melanoma)* has a very bad prognosis, since it soon spreads to the regional lymph nodes and then to the blood stream.

(c) *As a flat, variably pigmented lesion on previously normal skin (superficial spreading melanoma)* (Fig. 41–16). The prognosis is better here than with nodular melanoma.

(d) *In a lentigo maligna.* A malignant lentigo is a flat, pigmented lesion that occurs on the face of elderly patients. It may be regarded as a melanoma-*in-situ.* After many years, dermal invasion occurs, but even then the prognosis is good.

The types of melanomas have been described in some detail because they illustrate a very important point. Tumors that closely resemble each other microscopically sometimes have quite different prognoses. Thus, the lentigo maligna melanoma has a very good prognosis, whereas that of the nodular melanoma is appalling. This subdivision of melanoma has come about by a combined clinicopathological study of the structure and behavior of a large number of tumors.

OTHER TUMORS OF THE SKIN

Many different types of tumors are known, but they are described in detail in specialized texts. Their diagnosis depends on histological examination – a

FIGURE 41–16. *Superficial spreading type of malignant melanoma.*

Two black nodules of tumor are surrounded by superficial, barely palpable growth. Some areas are pigmented, whereas others show erythema. The pale areas of depigmentation are due to foci of tumor regression. Features leading to a diagnosis of melanoma in this lesion are the nodules, the irregular pigmentation, the changing clinical appearance, and the erythema. (Photograph courtesy of Dr. Wallace H. Clark, Jr.)

fact that emphasizes the necessity for submitting all excised tissue for pathological examination. The experienced clinician is not surprised to find that an occasional lesion that is "typical" of a wart or mole turns out to be something quite different.

Review Questions

1. A young woman develops a subacute dermatitis of both earlobes, the neck, and the left wrist. Suggest the possible causes and indicate how you would confirm the diagnosis.
2. Give an account of the possible causes of a widespread vesiculobullous rash.
3. Compare pemphigus vulgaris with bullous pemphigoid.
4. Give an account of the black tumors of the skin and indicate the treatment of each.
5. Describe the development of the common mole, or melanotic hamartoma.
6. Compare and contrast basal-cell carcinoma with squamous-cell carcinoma of the skin.

Selected Readings

Behrman, H. T., Labow, T. A., and Rosen, J. H.: Common Skin Diseases. 2nd ed. New York, Grune & Stratton, Inc., 1971. A simple, well-illustrated account of skin diseases.

Fitzpatrick, T. B., et al.: Dermatology in General Medicine. New York, McGraw-Hill Book Company, 1971. One of the three standard texts on dermatology. A good reference.

Lever, W. F., and Schaumburg-Lever, G.: Histopathology of the Skin. 5th ed. Philadelphia, J. B. Lippincott Company, 1975. The standard reference work on skin pathology.

Milne, J. A.: An Introduction to the Diagnostic Histopathology of the Skin. London, Edward Arnold (Publishers) Ltd., 1972. An excellent introduction to the subject.

Moschella, S. L., Pillsbury, D. M., and Hurley, H. J. (Eds.): Dermatology. Philadelphia, W. B. Saunders Company, 1975. One of the three standard texts on dermatology. For reference only.

Rook, A., Wilkinson, D. S., and Ebling, F. J. G. (Eds.): Oxford, Blackwell Scientific Publications Ltd., 1972. One of the three standard texts on dermatology. For reference only.

Chapter 42

After studying this chapter the student should be able to:

- Describe the development of the eye.
- List the common causes of conjunctivitis.
- Define cataract and give six causes of this condition.
- Classify the types of glaucoma and describe the outstanding clinical and pathological features of each type.
- Describe the pathogenesis and effects of retinal detachment and indicate the treatment.
- Classify the types of uveitis and describe the main features of acute iritis.
- Describe the important features of malignant melanoma of the choroid and retinoblastoma.

    A knowledge of the complex structure of the eye and the manner of its formation is essential for a proper understanding of ocular disease. This information is summarized in Figures 42–1 and 42–2.

    Many human eye disorders are poorly understood because they are difficult to investigate adequately. Because it is not practicable to take biopsies of the eye, the early morphological changes of disease cannot be examined. Sight is so valuable an asset that the eye is preserved at all costs, and its removal is considered only when there is the threat of malignant disease, or when advanced disease has destroyed all useful function.

Development of the Eye

    A hollow bud of the forebrain (the primary optic vesicle) develops at the future site of the eye, and as it approaches the surface ectoderm, the vesicle

668

becomes invaginated to form the optic cup (Fig. 42–1A and B). The outer layer of this cup remains thin and forms the pigment layer of the retina; the inner layer thickens to form the sensory layer. This complex structure contains the highly specialized rods and cones, which are sensitive to light, as well as nerve cells, whose long axons converge on the optic disc and constitute the optic nerve. It will be appreciated that the retina and the optic nerve are really part of the central nervous system, and if they are damaged, regeneration is impossible.

The two layers of the retina never fuse firmly; it is in the plane between these layers that separation can occur in the condition known as *retinal detachment*. The optic vesicle induces the overlying ectoderm to thicken, invaginate, and form a vesicle that matures to form the lens (Fig. 42–1B and C). Meanwhile, mesoderm around the globe differentiates to form the choroid; which is a vascular connective tissue coat containing pigmented melanocytes and helps to nourish the retina. Anteriorly, mesoderm contributes to the formation of the ciliary body and the iris. These mesodermal components of the uvea: the ciliary body, the iris, and the choroid are conjointly called the *uveal tract* (Fig. 42–2). The ciliary body contains muscle that is attached via the suspensory ligaments to the lens. Contraction of this muscle changes the shape of the lens and therefore alters its focal length. The ciliary body has one other important function: its epithelium-covered processes secrete a clear fluid, *the aqueous humor*.

The ectoderm and mesoderm overlying the developing eye form the cornea. The bulk of this structure consists of orderly, parallel bundles of collagen embedded in a specialized ground substance and so arranged that the cornea is transparent (Fig. 42–3). It forms the major lens component of the eye because refraction of light is greater at a tissue-air interface than at a tissue-fluid interface. The anatomical lens of the eye, surrounded by fluid, is of lesser importance in this regard. However, because the lens can change its shape under the influence of the muscles of the ciliary body, it provides a fine-adjustment mechanism by which one can focus quickly from distant to close objects. With advancing age the lens becomes more rigid and less capable of adjustment; the person with this lens rigidity finds it difficult to focus on close objects and requires a simple magnifying glass in order to read. This condition is called *presbyopia*.

The formation and disposal of aqueous humor are important because derangements of the mechanisms involved are a major cause of glaucoma and therefore of blindness. The fluid is secreted into the posterior chamber, flows forward between the iris and the lens, and then flows through the pupil and into the anterior chamber (Fig. 42–2). This cavity is bounded anteriorly by the

669

FIGURE 42–1. *Development of the human eye.*

See text for description. (Drawing by Margot Mackay, Department of Art as Applied to Medicine, University of Toronto.)

FIGURE 42–2. *Structure of the human eye.*

See text for description. (Drawing by Margot Mackay, Department of Art as Applied to Medicine, University of Toronto.)

FIGURE 42-3. *Normal cornea.*

This electron micrograph shows collagen arranged in orderly bundles called *lamellae*. Parts of two flattened connective tissue cells are also shown. (Photograph courtesy of Dr. M. Ghosh, Department of Ophthalmology, University of Toronto.)

cornea and posteriorly by the iris. Absorption of aqueous humor occurs at the angle of the anterior chamber. Fluid passes through a meshwork of connective tissue bundles, termed the *trabecular meshwork*, and ultimately drains into the canal of Schlemm, which encircles the globe at the corneosclerotic junction. From this canal, aqueous humor passes into the venous plexuses at the corneosclerotic junction.

DISEASES OF THE EYE

CONJUNCTIVITIS

Acute conjunctivitis can occur as a result of many irritants. Dust and chemicals can cause an acute primary irritant effect. There may be an allergic reaction such as in patients who are hypersensitive to components of eyedrops (*e.g.*, atropine). Acute inflammation may be a component of the exanthem of an acute viral disease such as measles, or it may be caused by a direct infection—either bacterial, chlamydial (see Chapter 11), or viral (*e.g.*, herpes simplex and zoster). Mild attacks of acute conjunctivitis show a typical catarrhal inflammation, but severe infections are purulent and more serious, because there is a constant danger of corneal involvement (keratitis), ulceration, and subsequent scarring. Infections by streptococci, staphylococci, and gonococci are usually purulent. Ophthalmia neonatorum (acute conjunctivitis occurring during the first ten days of life) is generally gonococcal.

Injuries and ulcerations of the cornea heal by scar tissue formation, and although the scar is made of collagen, it does not resemble the normal cornea because it is not transparent. Hence, involvement of the pupil area leads to blindness. Homografts from the eyes of cadavers are useful in treating this type of blindness. Similarly, they are of value in replacing the distorted, deformed corneas that are the result of maldevelopment (*corneal dystrophy*).

CATARACT

If the lens changes its physical characteristics and becomes opaque, the condition is called a *cataract*. The lens is a unique structure; it is of epithelial origin, is completely surrounded by a capsule that is in fact a basement membrane, and it has no blood supply. The hyaloid artery that nourishes it during development does not persist. Ionizing radiation, systemic administration of glucocorticoids, uveitis, trauma, hypocalcemia, galactosemia, and diabetes mellitus are numbered among the numerous factors that can adversely affect the metabolism of the lens and result in its degeneration and opacification. Nevertheless, the most common cause of cataract formation is old age, and some degree of senile cataract is present in all persons over 70 years of age. Removal of these cataracts produces a welcome return of sight. Glasses can compensate for the loss of accommodation that an absent lens decrees. Contact lenses are also successfully used by the cataract patient following surgery.

GLAUCOMA

The term *glaucoma* is applied to any condition in which the intraocular pressure is increased. It is an important condition because it causes blindness. The raised intraocular pressure impairs the blood supply to the sensory retina; in particular, the sensitive nerve cells and their long processes that form the optic nerve undergo degeneration. Two major types of glaucoma are recognized: primary and secondary.

Secondary Glaucoma.   In secondary glaucoma, which is usually unilateral, the increased pressure occurs as a complication of some other disease and results in mechanical obstruction of the flow of aqueous fluid from the ciliary body to the venous channels into which it ultimately drains. Generally, the obstruction is in the trabecular meshwork, which may become blocked by inflammatory exudate, fibrin, blood, or degenerate tumor. Uveitis, trauma (particularly if it is accompanied by bleeding), advanced cataracts, and tumors are other causes of secondary glaucoma.

Primary Glaucoma.   This disease is typically bilateral and is not accompanied by any other obvious intraocular disease. Two types can be distinguished:

OPEN-ANGLE OR CHRONIC SIMPLE GLAUCOMA.   This form of glaucoma is a slowly progressive disease of the elderly and is usually painless and symptomless until late in its development. An observant patient may notice a reduction in peripheral vision, but often the person's only complaint is that of difficulty in reading. The patient probably seeks eye care simply to request a stronger pair of reading glasses. For this reason it is imperative that all patients older than middle age should have tests to detect glaucoma during the course of periodic examinations for a change in glasses. The intraocular pressure can be measured quite simply, and an ophthalmoscopic examination will often reveal another sign of glaucoma called *optic nerve cupping*. This is a name given to enlargement of the central depression normally seen in the optic disc. It is due to the pressure-induced atrophy of the optic nerve fibers. Untreated, this type of glaucoma results in blindness, whereas a patient whose glaucoma is detected early has a good prognosis for retaining vision. The pathogenesis of open-angle glaucoma is not known. The filtration angle of the anterior chamber is open, and subtle abnormalities in the trabecular meshwork are assumed to be present.

CLOSED-ANGLE OR CONGESTIVE GLAUCOMA. This disease typically affects women between 40 and 60 years of age. The anterior chamber is shallow and this anatomical variation is responsible for the obstruction of the outflow of aqueous fluid at the angle of the anterior chamber.

This form of glaucoma is characterized by a series of episodes of raised intraocular pressure. In a subacute attack there is blurring of vision and the patient sees *halos around lights* because of the edema of the cornea. Later if an attack of acute glaucoma occurs, there is *pain* (so severe that it can cause vomiting), edema and congestion of the eyelids and conjunctiva, clouding of the cornea, and rapid loss of vision. Vision may be saved if an acute attack is treated early, but persistent high pressure leads to a state of absolute glaucoma. The eye is painful, blind, and stony hard. The eye ultimately shrinks and softens when the ciliary body stops producing aqueous.

RETINAL DISEASE

Retinal Detachment. A retinal detachment is the result of a separation of the sensory retina from the pigmented layer; it can be produced by inflammatory exudate, hemorrhage, or tumor, *e.g.*, a malignant melanoma (Figs. 42–4 and 42–5). Nevertheless, the commonest type of retinal detachment occurs in elderly persons, particularly those who are near-sighted. Thinning of the retina leads to the formation of a hole that is usually situated anteriorly and is identified by careful ophthalmoscopic examination. Often, the first symptoms of a detachment are flashing lights and "floaters," followed by the appearance of a dark shadow in the visual field. It is essential for the physician to make a correct diagnosis, to locate the site of the tear, and subsequently to seal this tear, either by directing a photocoagulating beam into the eye or by applying diathermy to the scleral surface. If the hole is sealed, the retina reattaches and usually no further trouble occurs. However, if the hole is not sealed, the detachment will extend. Since the retina loses its blood supply from the underlying choroid, it soon undergoes degeneration and irreversible loss of function.

Retinopathy Due to Small-Vessel Disease. The sensory retina, which is

FIGURE 42–4. *Normal retina, choroid, and sclera.*

Note the following layers: (1) Sclera, composed of dense collagen. (2) Choroid, more cellular and containing blood vessels. (3) Pigment epithelium, formed from the outer layer of the optic cup. (4) Rod and cone
layer consisting of processes of the photoreceptors. (5) Layer containing the nuclei of the photoreceptors.
(6) Nuclei of the bipolar cells; processes of these cells connect with the photoreceptors externally and with
the ganglion cells internally. (7) Ganglion cell layer; the long axons of these cells enter the layer of nerve
fibers and ultimately form the optic nerve. (8) Layer of nerve fibers ($\times$ 250).

the most important functional part of the eye, derives its major blood supply
from the central artery of the retina. Disease of this vessel and its branches
leads to degenerative changes in the retina itself.

HYPERTENSIVE RETINOPATHY.   In systemic hypertension there is thickening of the small retinal arterioles. As these vessels become occluded, areas of
the retina become infarcted. These lesions are called "cotton-wool spots"
because of their fluffy appearance. Because the weakened vessels rupture,
hemorrhages are frequent, and in the acute malignant phase of hypertension
there is edema of the optic disc *(papilledema)* owing to raised intracranial pressure.

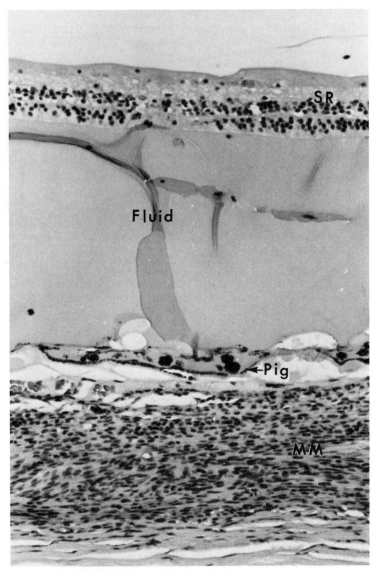

FIGURE 42–5. *Retinal detachment in melanoma.*

The sensory retina (SR) is atrophic (compare with Figure 42–4) and is separated from the pigment epi-thelium (Pig) by coagulated protein-containing fluid. The choroid is invaded by spindle-shaped cells of malignant melanoma (MM) (× 250).

DIABETIC RETINOPATHY. Diabetic retinopathy is the second leading cause of adult-onset blindness in North America. This form of retinopathy, along with the renal lesions, constitutes the most important change produced by small-vessel disease in diabetes mellitus. Diabetic retinopathy usually occurs in diabetics whose disease began in youth and who have been treated for many years with insulin. Now that these diabetics are able to survive into middle age, diabetic retinopathy is becoming much more common than in the days when the patients died while still young. The characteristic finding is saclike aneurysmal dilatation of some of the capillaries. The abnormal vessels proliferate and bleed. Vision is lost because of vitreal scar tissue formation, which leads eventually to retinal detachment. As in hypertensive retinopathy, areas of infarction and inflammation also occur.

Retinoblastoma.   This is the commonest intraocular tumor of childhood. It is often present at birth and invariably manifests itself before the age of four years. In some patients the disease is inherited as a Mendelian dominant trait; this is one of the few human malignant tumors in which heredity has been proved to be important. Inherited cases are often bilateral.

DISEASES OF THE UVEAL TRACT

The uveal tract, which is the principal vascular connective tissue component of the eye, is the part most severely affected by inflammatory disease. The iris, ciliary body, or choroid may be affected separately (termed *iritis, cyclitis,* and *choroiditis,* respectively) or in combination. Iridocyclitis or anterior uveitis is a common combination. Choroiditis or posterior uveitis often occurs alone.

Both acute and chronic uveitis may be caused by known infective agents—bacterial, viral, protozoal, and helminthic. Nevertheless, many examples have no known cause and present a grave problem both in diagnosis and treatment.

Acute Uveitis

ACUTE SUPPURATIVE IRIDOCYCLITIS.   This disease is usually a complication of a penetrating injury; rarely, pyogenic organisms reach the eye during the course of a septicemia or a pyemia. The condition is serious because the infection can easily involve the entire eye *(panophthalmitis)* and can lead to loss of sight.

ACUTE NONSUPPURATIVE IRIDOCYCLITIS.   This is a poorly understood condition. Probably it is not caused by simple infection but rather results from some immune mechanism. It is a complication of many systemic diseases, *e.g.,* syphilis, sarcoidosis, lupus erythematosus, rheumatoid arthritis, and particularly ankylosing spondylitis.

EFFECTS.   In acute iritis the eye becomes painful and red and there is hyperemia of the deep vessels of the conjunctiva. The pupil is contracted, and the iris may be difficult to see clearly because of inflammatory exudate in the anterior chamber. This response causes the aqueous fluid to become hazy or milky and to produce a "flare" in the narrow beam of light from a slit lamp. Clumps of white cells and fibrin stick to the posterior surface of the cornea as white *keratic precipitates* ("KP"). Fibrinous adhesions, which later organize to fibrous tissue, form between the iris and the lens posteriorly and between the iris and cornea anteriorly. These anterior adhesions (called *synechiae*) obliterate the filtration angle and can lead to glaucoma. To prevent these adhesions from forming and to break down any that are already present, atropine drops are used to dilate the pupil. Note that this treatment is diametrically opposite to that of congestive glaucoma in which the pupil is made to constrict by the application of pilocarpine drops. Therefore, it is of vital importance to be able to distinguish between acute glaucoma and acute iridocyclitis.

Chronic Uveitis. This is a condition that may be caused by a known infective agent, *e.g.*, *Treponema pallidum* or *Mycobacterium tuberculosis*, but it is often idiopathic. Visual defects are also a feature because with choroiditis the external layers of the sensory retina undergo degeneration.

TUMORS OF THE UVEAL TRACT

The important tumor of the uveal tract is the *malignant melanoma* derived from the melanocytes that are normally present. It is a disease of white adults and is therefore rare in most parts of Africa and in the Orient.

Over 80 per cent of ocular melanomas arise in the choroid and are often symptomless in the early stages. Elevation and detachment of the retina occur when the tumor breaks through the pigment epithelial layer of the retina and causes subretinal fluid to accumulate (Fig. 42–5). The patient's seeing a flash of light may be the first indication of an underlying tumor. A large tumor may cause glaucoma or may bleed into the vitreous. Malignant melanoma of the choroid is known to metastasize widely, but after the eye has been removed about 60 per cent of the patients survive longer than 10 years. Even so, it is not uncommon for metastases to appear many years later. The classic, but uncommon, picture is that of a man with an artificial eye, who 30 years after enucleation presents with an enlarged liver that is due to secondary deposits from an intraocular melanoma.

Review Questions

1. Relate the development of the eye to the following factors:
   (a) retinal detachment
   (b) the concept of the uveal tract as a distinct entity
   (c) the ability of the optic nerve to regenerate following damage.
2. Compare the symptoms, clinical findings, and treatment of acute anterior uveitis with those of acute congestive glaucoma.
3. Describe the eye changes which can complicate these conditions:
   (a) systemic hypertension
   (b) diabetes mellitus
   (c) ankylosing spondylitis
   (d) sarcoidosis treated with prednisone (a glucocorticoid).

Selected Readings

Cairns, J. E.: Corneal disease. British Medical Journal, 2:33–35, 1970.

Duke-Elder, S.: Parsons' Diseases of the Eye. 15th ed. Baltimore, The Williams & Wilkins Company, 1970, 597 pp. This well-tried textbook can be consulted for clinical details of diseases of the eye.

Hogan, M. J., and Zimmerman, L. E.: Ophthalmic Pathology. 2nd ed. Philadelphia, W. B. Saunders Company, 1962, 797 pp. The standard reference book for pathology of the eye.

Leading Article: Cotton-wool spots. British Medical Journal, 4:1474, 1966.

Leading Article: The changing pattern of retinoblastoma. Lancet, 2:1016–1017, 1971.

Paton, D., and Craig, J. A.: Cataracts. Clinical Symposia (Ciba), 27:1–32, 1975.

Perkins, E. S., and Hansell, P.: An Atlas of Diseases of the Eye. 2nd ed. Edinburgh, Churchill Livingstone, 1971, 86 pp. A well-produced color atlas of eye diseases.

Chapter 43

After studying this chapter the student should be able to:

● List the common diseases of the external ear.
● Describe the clinical features, pathology, and complications of acute otitis media and chronic otitis media.
● Describe otosclerosis and Ménière's disease.
● Compare and contrast conductive deafness with sensorineural deafness.

The sense of hearing is comparable to the sense of sight in that it is of immense practical and psychological value to humans. The vital sensory component of the ear in the cochlea, like the retina of the eye, is highly specialized; it cannot regenerate and cannot be biopsied without irreparable damage to the sense organ. Even at necropsy the ear is technically extremely difficult to examine. Both the cochlea and the vestibular apparatus, which subserves the functions of balance and positional sense of the head, are deeply embedded in one of the hardest bones of the human body. It is therefore of little wonder that our knowledge of the pathology of these sense organs is fragmentary.

The ear is conveniently divided into three separate parts: external, middle, and internal (Fig. 43–1).

The External Ear

The external ear, with its pinna and external auditory meatus, terminates medially at the eardrum, or tympanic membrane. In general, diseases of the ex-

678

ternal ear closely resemble those of the skin. Inflammation, called *otitis externa*, is common and has many causes. It may be a component of seborrheic, atopic, or contact dermatitis. Mechanical irritation by the overzealous use of cotton swabs, hairpins, matchsticks, and other foreign bodies introduced by the patient is a common cause, because itching is a frequent symptom. The chemical irritation produced by an accumulation of earwax is another cause; disease is sometimes perpetuated by the ill-advised use of prescription ear-drops containing irritating or sensitizing chemicals (*e.g.,* neomycin). Bacterial, viral, and fungal infection, particularly by *Aspergillus* species, can sometimes be incriminated. A chronic otitis externa should also lead to the suspicion of an underlying chronic otitis media associated with a perforated drum.

The specialized ceruminous glands can produce so much secretion that the earwax blocks the auditory canal. This is a common cause of conductive deafness, and one that can be easily relieved with gratifying results.

TUMORS OF THE EXTERNAL EAR

Squamous-cell carcinoma is the commonest malignant tumor of the external ear and generally begins with an actinic keratosis. Basal-cell carcinoma is not uncommon; occasionally, tumors of the ceruminous glands are encountered.

The Middle Ear

The middle ear is a cavity filled with air and lined by a flattened epithelium. The vibrations of the eardrum in its lateral wall are relayed by the *malleus* and *incus* to the *stapes* (these are the three auditory ossicles), which fits into the oval window and transmits impulses to the inner ear. Anteriorly, the cavity of the middle ear communicates with the pharynx via the *auditory* (Eustachian or pharyngotympanic) *tube,* whereas posteriorly there is connection with the air spaces in the mastoid process of the temporal bone.

ACUTE OTITIS MEDIA

Acute infections of the middle ear (acute otitis media) are usually bacterial in origin with *Streptococcus pyogenes,* the pneumococci, *Hemophilus influenzae,* and *Staphyloccus aureus* being the common causative organisms. The disease is most frequent in children and is often a complication of an upper respiratory streptococcal or viral infection. At this age the shortness of the auditory

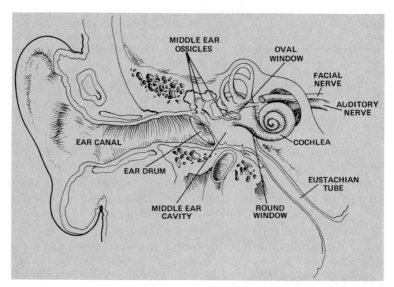

FIGURE 43–1. *Diagrammatic section through the human ear.*

The ear canal or external auditory meatus terminates at the ear drum. From the ear drum vibrations are transmitted by the three ossicles to the oval window. The round window is covered by a membrane and is designed to equalize pressures between the middle ear and the inner ear. Thus, when the stapes is pushed inward the membrane of the round window bulges outward into the middle ear. (From Beadle, K. R.: *In* Bleck, E. E., and Nagel, D. A. (Eds.): Physically Handicapped Children. New York, Grune & Stratton, Inc., 1975, p. 93. Reproduced by permission of Grune & Stratton, Inc.)

tube and blockage produced by swelling of the nasopharyngeal lymphoid tissue ("adenoids") are factors that encourage organisms in the nasopharynx to ascend into the middle ear and to cause infection. Lack of the immunoglobulin IgA in the secretions has been suggested as another predisposing factor. The disease is characterized by severe pain in the ear combined with hearing loss. The inflammatory exudate that collects in the cavity of the middle ear is at first clear but can later become purulent. The eardrum becomes inflamed and may rupture. This event is often averted by surgical incision of the tympanic membrane (a procedure called *myringotomy*), because a well-placed surgical wound heals better than one produced by spontaneous perforation.

Acute otitis media usually resolves with modern chemotherapy aided by surgical drainage, but the following complications should be noted:

1. *Adhesions.* These can affect the tympanic membrane and form between the three ossicles. Fibrinous at first, they are later replaced by scar tissue.

2. *Chronic Otitis Media.*

3. *Spread of Infection.* Involvement of meninges, brain, and mastoid air cells is described later.

CHRONIC OTITIS MEDIA

This condition may occur insidiously or may follow an acute attack, especially if the treatment has been inadequate. Persistent ear discharge and deafness are the main features of chronic otitis media.

The chronic inflammatory reaction in the mucosa is sometimes characterized by the formation of inflammatory granulation tissue containing cholesterol crystals surrounded by foreign-body giant cells. The condition is called a *cholesterol granuloma*. Fibrous adhesions can form in the cavity of the middle ear, and by involving the eardrum and the ossicles, these adhesions can lead to deafness. The lining mucosa may show metaplasia and become replaced by a respiratory type of epithelium with ciliated cells and goblet cells—the latter producing much sticky mucus. Since there is often a permanent hole in the eardrum, a persistent discharge of thick, mucoid material follows (often called the "glue ear").

COMPLICATIONS OF OTITIS MEDIA

"Epidermoid Cholesteatoma." This misleading name is applied to a cyst within the middle ear that is filled with keratin and lined by epidermis. The cyst is thought to be derived from squamous epithelium that migrates into the middle ear through a perforated eardrum. This condition is a serious complication of otitis media, because the cyst enlarges and produces local pressure effects as well as perpetuating a chronic infection. Surgical treatment is necessary for its cure.

Spread of Infection. In both acute and chronic otitis media, infection can spread to involve adjacent structures. The conditions resulting are described below:

MASTOIDITIS. Involvement of the mastoid air cells is a particularly serious condition, since suppuration occurs and further spread of infection is a serious hazard. The disease is characterized by generalized signs of an acute suppurative process (causing malaise and fever) together with pain, redness, and swelling of the bony mastoid prominence behind the ear.

SIGMOID SINUS THROMBOSIS. The sigmoid sinus, which is one of the large venous sinuses within the skull, lies in close proximity to the mastoid air cells. Thrombosis itself is serious, but when a thrombus is invaded by pyogenic organisms, the result is *pyemia*. Infected thrombi break off and lead to pulmonary pyemic abscesses.

MENINGITIS. Organisms either from the mastoid air cells or from the middle ear can penetrate the thin bone to reach the meningeal space and lead to meningitis.

BRAIN ABSCESS. If infection reaches the meninges, adhesions may limit the spread of infection and yet allow bacteria to continue their onward march into the brain, causing either a cerebellar or a temporal-lobe abscess.

SEVENTH-NERVE PARALYSIS. The seventh, or facial, nerve pursues a complex course through the middle ear and can be damaged either by otitis media or by surgery performed on a diseased ear.

LABYRINTHITIS. Infection can spread to involve the inner ear.

OTOSCLEROSIS

In this disease of unknown cause, parts of the petrous temporal bone are replaced by woven bone. The disease is probably quite common, but it becomes clinically apparent only if the stapes is involved. When this bone becomes ankylosed in the oval window, deafness ensues. The disease is particularly distressing, since it is generally bilateral. It has been estimated that approximately 2 per cent of all white persons suffer from deafness from this cause. The plight of these victims of otosclerosis has indeed been the inspiration for the development of microsurgery in which the surgeon operates by using a binocular microscope.

CONDUCTIVE DEAFNESS

This term is applied to any form of deafness in which there is a failure of conduction of sound impulses from the external environment to the internal sensory organ of the inner ear. Blockage of the external auditory meatus, lesions in the middle ear, and otosclerosis are the main causes.

The Inner Ear

This region of the ear is situated in the dense, petrous temporal bone and consists of a bony labyrinth containing the intercommunicating channels of the membranous labyrinth—the cochlea with its complex sensory auditory organ and the semicircular canals, whose main function is concerned with balance and sense of position of the head. The cochlear nerve arises from the sensory end-organs in the cochlea, joins with the vestibular nerve, and transmits to the brain-stem impulses that are then relayed to the cortex.

SENSORINEURAL DEAFNESS

Deafness due to a defect of the sensory organ or the cochlear nerve is termed *sensorineural.* It is beyond the scope of this chapter to describe this in any detail, but the following causes are noteworthy:

LESIONS IN THE RECEPTOR SENSORY ORGAN IN THE LABYRINTH. It is well recognized that certain drugs can damage the eighth nerve, and that most of these drugs belong to the streptomycin family. Loud noise, whether from an industrial source or from pop music, is capable of causing permanent damage. Other causes are fractures, vascular occlusion, and viral infections—particularly mumps and intrauterine rubella.

NERVE DAMAGE. Schwannoma of the vestibulocochlear (eighth cranial, or auditory) nerve is an important cause.

BRAIN DAMAGE. Injury to the temporal bone, in particular, is an important cause of sensorineural deafness.

MÉNIÈRE'S DISEASE

The auditory component of the inner ear is closely connected with the organ of balance. This association is illustrated by the symptomatology of *Ménière's disease.* The disease affects the membranous labyrinth as a whole and is characterized by paroxysmal attacks of intense vertigo (giddiness) associated with unilateral deafness and tinnitus (buzzing in the ears). The disease is not uncommon, and Shakespeare's mention of the "falling sickness" in *Julius Caesar* is generally regarded as a reference to this disease.

Review Questions

1. Describe the complications and dangers of having otitis media and a perforated eardrum.
2. A patient develops signs of an intracranial space-occupying lesion together with deafness in one ear. Discuss the possible causes of this condition and the examinations that might be performed to arrive at a diagnosis.
3. In spite of medical treatment a patient has persistent otitis externa. Suggest some reasons for this persistent inflammation.

Selected Readings

Friedmann, I.: Pathology of the Ear. Oxford, Blackwell Scientific Publications Ltd., 1974, 607 pp.

Friedmann, I.: The apparently barren regions of the temporal bone. International Pathology Bulletin, *16*:9–32, 1975.

Konigsmark, B. W., and Gorlin, R. J.: Genetic and Metabolic Deafness. Philadelphia, W. B. Saunders Company, 1976, pp. 24–26, 45.

Chapter 44

After studying this chapter the student should be able to:

- Describe the overall structure of the central nervous system and the meninges. Distinguish between neurons and neuroglia.
- Describe the formation and fate of cerebrospinal fluid (CSF).
- Describe the effects of a raised intracranial pressure and list the common causes.

DISEASES OF THE CENTRAL NERVOUS SYSTEM

- Distinguish between subdural hemorrhage and extradural hemorrhage in terms of of these factors:
    - (a) site of bleeding
    - (b) source of bleeding
    - (c) causes
    - (d) clinical effects.
- Describe the cause and effects of subarachnoid hemorrhage.
- Outline the causes and effects of cerebral hemorrhage, cerebral thrombosis, and cerebral embolism; describe the differences between these three types of stroke.
- Define the following terms:
    - (a) hemiplegia
    - (b) positive Babinski sign
    - (c) pseudobulbar palsy.
- Describe pyogenic meningitis with respect to the following factors:
    - (a) causes
    - (b) clinical effects
    - (c) CSF findings
    - (d) complications.
- List the causes of cerebral abscess.
- List the agents that cause aseptic meningitis and encephalitis.
- Discuss the pathology of multiple sclerosis and describe its clinical features.
- Give examples of poisons that cause permanent central nervous system damage.
- List the neurological complications of the following conditions:
    - (a) thiamine deficiency
    - (b) pellagra
    - (c) pernicious anemia
    - (d) alcoholism and liver disease.
- Outline the important features of
    - (a) Alzheimer's disease
    - (b) Parkinson's disease
    - (c) Huntington's chorea
    - (d) motor neuron disease.
- List the known causes of epilepsy and describe the outstanding features of the following:
    - (a) psychomotor epilepsy
    - (b) petit mal epilepsy
    - (c) grand mal epilepsy
    - (d) Jacksonian fit
- Describe the types and effects of the common tumors that arise in the brain and in the meninges.

685

Structure and Function

The central nervous system consists of nerve cells *(neurons)* and a supporting matrix of neuroglia in which they are embedded. It is richly supplied by blood vessels and is formed as a hollow tube during development, lined on the inside by *ependyma,* and covered on the outside by a layer of *pia mater.*

The neurons are the essential cells of the nervous system. They are formed by the differentiation of primitive neuroblasts during embryonic life and are unable to divide at a later time. Neurons possess the specialized property of excitability. They may be excited by a variety of stimuli to produce an impulse that is propagated throughout the cytoplasm of the cell. Since the axon of a nerve cell is often several inches or even feet in length, the impulse is conducted from one part of the body to another. *Excitability* and *conduction* are thus two characteristic properties of the nerve cells. Under abnormal circumstances, there may be changes in their excitability and conductibility. In the case of motor neurons, the effects may be obvious enough and may take the form of paralysis or convulsions. With sensory neurons, the equivalent effects can be anesthesia or pain and paresthesia (abnormal spontaneous feeling such as tingling).

The brain cannot be regarded as a simple organ comparable to the liver. Each cell is not equivalent to its neighbor and cannot be regarded as performing a similar function. In fact, the brain acts as a series of systems, and the elaborate inter-relationship between the vast number of neurons is responsible for the complex function and behavior of the nervous system of the higher animals. Not only is the nervous system responsible for receiving and transmitting all sensory stimuli from its peripheral receptor organs, but also its central organization is designed for interpreting all stimuli. At its highest level, the nervous system is responsible for consciousness, memory, and intelligence. Abnormalities in function in these areas produce diseases that at present are mainly in the realm of the psychiatrist and have no known morphological features. This aspect of the abnormalities of the nervous system cannot be dismissed lightly, since it has been estimated that approximately one half of all patients occupying hospital beds do so because of psychiatric disease.

With regard to its efferent properties, the nervous system controls or influences all muscular activities in the body, including beating of the heart, contraction of the walls of blood vessels, function of skeletal muscle, ventilation of the lungs, and motility of the gastrointestinal tract. Furthermore, much glandular secretion is influenced by the nervous system. Indeed, there is scarcely any bodily structure or function that is not in one way or another under nervous control. It is therefore of little wonder that abnormal nervous function can produce many diverse effects. When no obvious structural change is present, these effects are classified as functional diseases. Two examples of such diseases may be quoted. First, hysterical hyperventilation can be so marked that it causes respiratory alkalosis and tetany. Second, impotence in the male and frigidity in the female are most commonly related to psychological causes. Whether abnormal nervous function can produce structural abnormalities in other organs is a much debated point. Anorexia nervosa in humans and pseudocyesis (false pregnancy) in animals are good examples. In the first instance, individuals (usually young women) refuse to eat, become emaciated, and may ultimately die of starvation or one of its complications. In the second instance, the animal's hormonal balance is so changed that pregnancy is closely simulated. Whether a psychosomatic explanation is responsible for other disease states is less well substantiated. Nevertheless, diseases such as primary thyrotoxicosis, peptic ulcer, urticaria, and psoriasis seem to be aggravated by mental stress.

To understand the behavior of the nervous system in disease, one must first have knowledge of its normal structure and function. The student is therefore advised to consult the standard texts on neuroanatomy and physiology. It is necessary to have an overall picture of the organization of the major motor tracts before many diseases can be understood.

THE MOTOR SYSTEM

The large neurons of the frontal cortex give rise to long axons that constitute the corticospinal, or pyramidal, tract. This tract crosses to the opposite side in the medulla, and its axons control the anterior horn cells of the spinal cord. Damage to the pyramidal tract results in an *upper motor neuron paralysis.* Voluntary movement is lost, but the muscles retain their tone. The arms assume a flexed position, whereas the legs are extended. The tendon reflexes are brisk, and the Babinski sign is positive.* If the anterior horn cells (or their cranial equivalents) or their axons in the peripheral motor nerve are damaged, a *lower motor neuron lesion* results. There is paralysis, but the muscles are flaccid, and the reflexes are absent.

THE MENINGES

There are three coverings, or meninges, of the central nervous system: (1) the *pia mater,* (2) the *dura mater,* and (3) the *arachnoid.* Their functions are described briefly.

1. The *pia mater* closely envelops the brain and spinal cord.

2. The *dura mater* is closely adherent to the bony and ligamentous protective housing provided by the skull, vertebral column, and connecting ligaments. The *falx cerebri* forms an extension of the dura mater that assumes a sickle shape and separates the two cerebral hemispheres. A similar extension of the dura mater forms the *tentorium,* which separates the cerebrum above from the cerebellum below.

3. The third layer of the meninges is the *arachnoid,* which forms a thin, translucent covering like a spider's web lying between the pia mater and the dura mater.

The space between the arachnoid and the pia is called the *subarachnoid space* and contains cerebrospinal fluid (CSF). This fluid originates in the choroid plexuses of the ventricles and finally escapes through the foramina in the roof of the fourth ventricle to reach the subarachnoid space. Ultimately, the fluid is absorbed in the arachnoid granulations of such major sinuses as the superior sagittal sinus.

---

*A positive Babinski sign means that when the sole of the foot is stroked, the big toe dorsiflexes. Normally the toe moves down (plantarflexes).

INCREASED INTRACRANIAL PRESSURE

Effects. The rigid, bony enclosure of the brain is a necessary protective shield; its presence, however, has some attendant disadvantages. Any lesion that causes the brain to expand tends to cause a rise in intracranial pressure, which in turn increases the pressure in the veins. Initially CSF and venous blood are displaced, but as venous obstruction is produced, there is soon a marked rise in intracranial pressure and an increase in CSF pressure. This rise in pressure tends to reduce cerebral blood flow, but it activates reflexes that counteract the effect by raising the systemic blood pressure. An increase — sometimes to very high levels — in blood pressure is an important sign of raised intracranial pressure. In its turn, it reflexly slows the heart rate. *Routine care of a patient with a suspected intracranial lesion therefore involves monitoring of the blood pressure and the heart rate.*

Raised intracranial pressure is characterized by *headaches,* often severe, that are probably caused by stretching of the meninges. *Vomiting* is common and is due to stimulation of the medullary centers. Progressive mental impairment may also occur. The pressure on the veins returning blood from the retina causes edema of the optic disc *(papilledema),* which can be seen with an ophthalmoscope. This edema is an extremely important sign of increased intracranial pressure. Edema of the optic disc is also serious, because if allowed to persist it causes atrophy of the optic nerve and, ultimately, blindness.

Causes

1. EDEMA OF THE BRAIN.   Generalized edema of the brain is a feature of a raised arterial PCO_2 and of encephalitis. Localized edema is a feature of injury and infarction of the brain.

2. OBSTRUCTION OF THE FLOW OF CSF.   Any obstruction to the flow of CSF from the choroid plexuses in the ventricular system to the superior sagittal sinus causes an increase in the intracranial pressure. Blockage of the aqueduct of Sylvius, obstruction of the foramina in the roof of the fourth ventricle, and adhesions in the subarachnoid space (such as may occur following meningitis) are examples of such obstruction.

3. MENINGITIS.   Any form of meningitis causes an increase in exudation of fluid into the CSF. In addition, there is obstruction due to the formation of fibrinous and subsequent fibrous adhesions, particularly at the base of the brain.

4. SPACE-OCCUPYING LESIONS.   *Hemorrhage* into the brain, the formation of a *hematoma* (whether within the brain, subdural space, or extradural space) and the formation of an *abscess* or *tumor* are all examples of space-occupying lesions that ultimately cause an increase in intracranial pressure.

Apart from the generalized consequences of raised intracranial pressure, space-occupying lesions have additional effects. A lesion of one cerebral hemisphere causes such swelling that part of the hemisphere is pushed beneath the falx cerebri to the other side. *This is an example of herniation* (see Fig. 44–6). Furthermore, in such a supratentorial lesion, the expanded brain pushes downward through the orifice of the tentorium cerebelli in such a way that the midbrain is forced downward and part of the cerebrum (the unci of the temporal lobes) herniates. This has several effects, which are described in the following paragraphs.

(a) There is pressure on the third nerve. The nerve affected first is on the same side as the lesion, and this leads to dilatation of the pupil. *A fixed, dilated pupil is an important sign of the herniation and occurs first on the same side as the cerebral lesion. Careful and frequent examination of the eyes is therefore an important part of the care of patients with suspected cerebral lesions, e.g.,* a head injury.

(b) Downward movement of the brainstem tears small blood vessels. Compression of, or bleeding into, the midbrain and pons causes serious effects. When the upper brain stem is affected, there is loss of consciousness. With lower brain-stem damage, there is respiratory arrest and death.

(c) An expanding lesion of one cerebral hemisphere may force the midbrain to one side in such a way that a cerebral peduncle is pressed against the tentorium. This causes damage to the pyramidal fibers on the side opposite the cerebral lesion; since these fibers cross over in the medulla, there is *an upper motor-neuron paralysis of the body on the same side as that of the cerebral lesion.*

Increased intracranial pressure can force the medulla into the foramen magnum together with the tonsils of the cerebellum. *Cerebellar herniation compresses the medulla, causing respiratory arrest and death. It can be precipitated by performing a lumbar puncture on a patient with a markedly raised intracranial pressure.* This procedure is therefore contraindicated under these circumstances.

TRAUMATIC LESIONS OF THE CENTRAL NERVOUS SYSTEM

An injury involving the jaws is sometimes accompanied by a much more important injury to the brain. Blows on the head produce damage to the region beneath the injury and to the brain at the opposite pole; this is the so-called *contrecoup injury.* Minor injuries cause petechial hemorrhages and traumatic inflammatory edema, whereas more severe injuries may actually tear *(lacerate)* the brain, and hemorrhage may be of sufficient magnitude to cause death.

Subdural Hemorrhage. Sometimes a venous sinus or vein is torn, and blood escapes into the loose subdural space, producing a subdural hematoma. If the collection of blood is small, it is of little importance. If it is large, the hematoma organizes at the periphery, and remains fluid at the center. The cyst that is formed imbibes fluid and enlarges to form a *chronic subdural hematoma* that acts as a space-occupying lesion. The injury that causes this type of lesion is often relatively mild, and in an elderly or alcoholic patient it may be completely overlooked. Weeks later, headaches and other signs and symptoms of raised intracranial pressure appear.

Extradural Hemorrhage. This form of hemorrhage occurs when the *middle meningeal artery* is torn; it is usually in association with a fracture of the skull involving the temporal region. Unconsciousness may occur immediately after the injury, but the patient often recovers and feels well for a few hours. This *lucid interval* is deceptive. Presently, as the bleeding proceeds, increasing signs of raised intracranial pressure appear; this is followed by coma and death. It is evident that *all cases of head injury, except the most trivial, should be observed carefully for 24 hours.* This word of caution applies particularly to

FIGURE 44–1.   *Berry aneurysm.*

An unruptured aneurysm (An) is seen to be arising from the left vertebral artery. Note the following normal structures: FL, frontal lobe; TL, temporal lobe; Olf, olfactory nerve; Opt, optic nerve; MB, mamillary body; P, pons; M, medulla oblongata; SC, spinal cord; Cb, cerebellum; CbT, cerebellar tonsil; and Uncus. (Courtesy of Dr. N. B. Rewcastle.)

persons suspected of being drunk—a state that may be mimicked by the combination of medicinal brandy given by a well-wisher and an extradural hemorrhage.

NONTRAUMATIC CEREBROVASCULAR DISEASE

Subarachnoid Hemorrhage.   This condition is not uncommon in persons between the ages of 20 and 50 years. The hemorrhage stems from a ruptured aneurysm of one of the major cerebral arteries in the area of the circle of Willis. The aneurysms lie in the subarachnoid space and are from 0.5 to 1.0 cm in diameter; because of this size, they are often called *berry aneurysms* (Figs. 44–1 and 44–2). They are thought to arise at the site of congenital defects in the elastic coat of the arteries. Sometimes they are multiple.

Cerebral Hemorrhage, Thrombosis, and Embolism.   Atherosclerosis and hypertension both predispose to *cerebral hemorrhage* (sometimes called *cerebral apoplexy*). Commonly, the site is from a branch of the middle cerebral artery. The area of brain affected is in the region of the basal ganglia, the external and

FIGURE 44–2. *Berry aneurysm.*

This is the same specimen as in Figure 44–1, but the aneurysm has been lifted up to show its connection with the vertebral artery. (Courtesy of Dr. N. B. Rewcastle.)

the internal capsule. The immediate effects of hemorrhage tend to be more severe than those produced by thrombosis. In both there is the clinical picture commonly called a "stroke."

With hemorrhage there is usually sudden loss of consciousness. As blood disrupts the substance of the brain, coma deepens and death ensues. This course is not inevitable, however, and the bleeding may stop.

With thrombosis the patient may experience prodromal or warning signs (*e.g.,* transient hemiplegia, blindness in one eye, speech defect, or confusion) before the onset of the stroke. The stroke itself often occurs during sleep; although consciousness may be lost, this effect is not invariable. Sometimes evidence of progressive damage may be apparent over a period of several days. Apparently, this is due to spread of the thrombosis and hence is called a *thrombotic stroke in evolution.* Thrombosis causes *infarction,* which can itself lead to later hemorrhage in the damaged area (Fig. 44–3).

The infarct caused by thrombosis is usually pale; in those patients who survive, the area softens (a process called *colliquative necrosis*). The microglial cells enlarge, become phagocytic, and appear as large, foamy macrophages. The damaged nerve fibers are not replaced, and the area heals by proliferation

Right   Left

FIGURE 44–3. *Cerebral softening and hemorrhage.*

The brain has been sectioned horizontally and is viewed here from below. There is severe damage. On the right-hand side there is extensive softening (Sof). Note the shrunken appearance of the affected area, which extends outward to involve the gray matter of the cerebral cortex. The internal capsule (Int Cap) is severely affected. It lies between the lentiform nucleus (L) and the caudate nucleus (C) anteriorly and between the lentiform nucleus and thalamus (T) posteriorly. Loss of its corticospinal fibers leads to an upper motor neuron lesion of the opposite side of the body. The patient had had a stroke three months before death. This attack, which had been attributed to a cerebral thrombosis, left the patient with a left hemiplegia. She subsequently had another stroke involving the opposite side. Note the extensive hemorrhage (Hb) that has occurred into the area of softening on the left side. (Courtesy of Dr. N. B. Rewcastle.)

of astrocytes, which produces a *glial scar.* The area of brain thus collapses, and sometimes a central cyst remains where once there was brain tissue. Note that any nerve cells destroyed are not replaced.

Infarcts are sometimes found in the absence of detectable thrombosis of a cerebral artery. The explanation is generally to be found in the extracranial arterial supply to the brain—the carotid and vertebral arteries. Severe stenosis of these vessels can seriously imperil the blood supply to the brain. Under these circumstances, infarction is to be found in the "water-shed" areas that are at the boundary zones where the vascular territories of two cerebral vessels join.

Cerebral embolism is the least common cause of a stroke. The embolus generally originates from the heart, and the onset of the stroke is sudden.

CLINICAL FEATURES OF STROKE. In cerebral hemorrhage, thrombosis, and embolism, the clinical picture depends on the size and location of the area of brain affected. With a severe stroke, consciousness is lost, but recovery gradually sets in, and consciousness then returns. At first, speech is often impaired, but as time passes, it returns to normal. The neurological findings depend upon the area of brain affected. Commonly, the long cerebrospinal tracts in the internal capsule are destroyed, and the picture is that of hemiplegia—loss of voluntary movement on the side of the body opposite to that of the cerebral lesion (upper motor neuron lesion). Destroyed neurons are never replaced and lost axons are never regenerated. Nevertheless, considerable clinical recovery can be expected following a stroke. Good nursing and physical therapy can do much to tide the patient over the severe initial period. For example, during this time bedsores and urinary tract infections should be prevented. Good oral hygiene and maintenance of adequate fluid and food intake are also important. Finally, encouragement and physical exercises can do much to minimize the effects of the ultimate paralysis or other neurological losses.

Quite apart from acute episodes of thrombosis or infarction, cerebral atherosclerosis can lead to multiple, bilateral, ischemic lesions in the brain. The characteristic mental deterioration of old age is one effect of the lesions, but if they are extensive, there may be severe bilateral damage to the corticospinal tracts. When bilaterally innervated muscles such as those of the tongue and pharynx are affected, the condition is called *pseudobulbar palsy.*

Infections of the Central Nervous System

PYOGENIC BACTERIAL INFECTIONS

Pyogenic bacteria may produce a diffuse infection of the subarachnoid space, a condition that is called *meningitis,* or they may produce a localized suppuration in the brain substance, a condition called *cerebral abscess.*

Pyogenic Meningitis

MODE OF INFECTION. Two routes are common:

Blood-borne. Hemophilus influenzae and the meningococcus gain entry to the blood, presumably from an infection in the upper respiratory tract. The route is probably via the choroid plexuses, where the organisms are filtered out of the blood during the course of a septicemia. The infection spreads through the ventricular system and reaches the subarachnoid space in the region of the basal cisterns. It is here that the most severe effects are seen. The pia mater and the arachnoid are acutely inflamed, and there is a massive polymorphic and fibrinous exudate into the subarachnoid space. With modern chemotherapy the patients often survive, but even then the exudate may undergo organization, and the foramina in the roof of the fourth ventricle may become blocked. Cerebrospinal fluid accumulates in the ventricular system, which expands accordingly; this is one mechanism by which *hydrocephalus* develops. In the young child the pressure exerted on the developing bones leads to a tremendous enlargement of the vault of the skull.

Local Spread. Meningitis may follow the spread of infection from the middle ear or mastoid air cells—sites of infection that are common in child-

Right   Left

Abscess

FIGURE 44–4.   *Cerebral abscess.*

Sagittal section of the brain showing a large abscess in the right temporal lobe. When the brain was sectioned, pus drained from the abscess, which now appears to be empty. Owing to chronic otitis media, the patient had a chronic discharge from his right ear. He developed headaches and stiffness of the neck but was moribund by the time he reached the hospital. Necropsy revealed an extradural abscess overlying the roof of the right middle ear. Infection had spread into the brain. (Courtesy of Dr. N. B. Rewcastle.)

hood. It is also a complication of a fractured skull in cases in which the wound is exposed to the exterior or to the nasal cavity. Fracture of the cribriform plate of the ethmoid bone is followed by an escape of cerebrospinal fluid into the nose (a condition called *cerebrospinal rhinorrhea*). Meningitis may follow.

CLINICAL FEATURES.   Fever, severe headache, disorder of consciousness, and convulsions (particularly in children) are the outstanding symptoms. Stiffness of the neck and resistance to forward bending are the outstanding signs. The diagnosis is made by performing a lumbar puncture (recall the dangers of this procedure in a patient with raised intracranial pressure). The pressure of the fluid is increased, as is its protein content. The glucose level is low, because the organisms ferment the sugar. Numerous polymorphs are present, and organisms can be demonstrated either directly on a smear or by culture.

Cerebral Abscess

MODE OF INFECTION.   As with meningitis, there are two modes of infection.

Blood-borne. Patients with chronic chest infections (empyema, lung abscess, and bronchiectasis) sometimes develop a cerebral abscess. Presumably, the infection is blood-borne; an alternative explanation is that spread occurs from an infected nasal air sinus—a common accompaniment of chronic chest suppuration.

Local Spread. As with meningitis, local spread occurs from an infected middle ear or nasal air sinus (Fig. 44–4).

VIRAL INFECTIONS

Viral Meningitis (Aseptic Meningitis). Poliovirus, coxsackie viruses, ECHO viruses, and mumps virus are among the many agents that can cause meningitis. The symptoms are similar to those of pyogenic meningitis, but they are less severe. The cerebrospinal fluid contains lymphocytes rather than polymorphs. An important point of differentiation is that *the glucose level is normal.*

Viral Encephalitis. The syndrome of encephalitis resembles that of aseptic meningitis, but to it is added evidence of cerebral damage: coma, cranial nerve paralysis, and hemiplegia, for example. Some of the causative agents are described in Chapter 12.

Diseases Affecting the Myelin Sheath

The major nerve fibers both within the central nervous system and in the peripheral nervous system have the myelin sheath, which acts as an insulating covering, thereby aiding in transmission of impulses in the axon. Damage to the myelin sheath leads to impaired conduction, even though the axon itself remains intact. Two groups of disorders are recognized:

1. The *demyelinating diseases,* of which multiple sclerosis is by far the most frequent.

2. The *dysmyelinating diseases, or leukodystrophies,* in which myelin formation is impaired.

MULTIPLE SCLEROSIS

Multiple sclerosis, or disseminated sclerosis as it is also called, is a chronic disease characterized by exacerbations and remissions that often extend over many years. The brain and spinal cord show the development of well-circumscribed foci (plaques) of demyelination (Fig. 44–5). These plaques occur in all parts of the central nervous system, but they are more frequent in certain areas. During the acute phases there is an inflammatory reaction and severe impairment of nerve conduction. The nerve axons are generally preserved, and a considerable degree of functional recovery occurs after each phase. Depending on the site of damage, multiple sclerosis first manifests itself as sudden impairment of vision, inability to speak clearly (dysarthria), cerebellar dysfunction, or paralysis due to pyramidal tract damage. Alteration in emotional state and bladder dysfunction also occur. Each acute episode is followed by recovery, occasionally complete. More frequently, however, there is some residual damage so that with the passage of years the patient ultimately becomes quite disabled.

FIGURE 44–5. *Multiple sclerosis.*

Horizontal section of the brain showing many areas of demyelination (arrows). Since it is the myelin sheaths of nerve fibers that give the white matter its color, areas of demyelination appear gray and superficially resemble the gray matter. (Courtesy of Dr. N. B. Rewcastle.)

OTHER DEMYELINATING DISEASES

Several diseases are known that resemble multiple sclerosis but are more acute. Demyelination is also a feature of the encephalitis that occasionally follows certain viral infections, such as following vaccination for smallpox and rabies, as well as following certain naturally occurring viral diseases such as rubella.

THE LEUKODYSTROPHIES

The leukodystrophies constitute a group of rare diseases in which there is a defect in the formation of myelin. Usually manifested during infancy or childhood, they are familial.

TOXIC, DEFICIENCY, AND METABOLIC DISORDERS

The brain is a very active metabolic organ. Although it represents about 2 per cent of the body weight, it is responsible for 20 per cent of the body's resting oxygen consumption. It is not surprising, therefore, that it can easily be affected adversely by many agents that interfere with metabolism. A few of these are listed below.

1. *Poisons.* Lead and arsenic are examples of agents that can cause permanent brain damage. Likewise, poisoning by carbon monoxide can cause necrosis of the basal ganglia and can lead to extrapyramidal syndromes, which are described later.

2. *Deficiency of Oxygen (Hypoxia).*   The brain is extremely sensitive to oxygen deprivation. Even short periods of hypoxia can produce permanent damage.

3. *Vitamin Deficiencies*

VITAMIN B₁ (THIAMINE) DEFICIENCY.   In some patients vitamin B_1 deficiency causes focal areas of necrosis. Several syndromes can occur. For example, in Wernicke's encephalopathy there is paralysis of eye muscles and unsteadiness. It may be combined with loss of memory and confabulation (this is Korsakoff's psychosis that is associated with alcoholism combined with vitamin B_1 deficiency).

PELLAGRA ENCEPHALOPATHY.   This condition is described in Chapter 23.

SUBACUTE COMBINED DEGENERATION OF THE SPINAL CORD.   This condition is due to vitamin B_{12} deficiency and accompanies pernicious anemia.

4. *Metabolic Encephalopathies*

HEPATIC ENCEPHALOPATHY.   Degeneration of neurons is responsible for the mental deterioration encountered in chronic liver disease (see Chapter 33).

CHRONIC ALCOHOLISM.   The pathetic state of some chronic alcoholics is a combined effect of alcohol, vitamin deficiency, and liver damage.

HYPOGLYCEMIA.   Poisoning with insulin causes hypoglycemia, coma, convulsions, and death. Permanent neuronal loss can occur in those who survive; the changes resemble those of hypoxia. At one time, insulin convulsions were used as a treatment for certain psychiatric conditions; this practice has now been abandoned.

DEGENERATIVE NERVOUS DISEASES

There are many diseases of the nervous system in which neuronal degeneration occurs for no known reason. In some of these conditions there is a strong hereditary factor, whereas in others the degeneration is probably due to slow virus infection (*e.g.*, in kuru and Creutzfeldt-Jakob disease; see Chapter 12). A few common examples of degenerative nervous diseases will be described.

1. *Senile Dementia.*   Cerebral atrophy with compensatory dilatation of the ventricles is a common event in old age.

2. *Alzheimer's Disease.*   This disease resembles senile dementia but occurs at an earlier age and is more severe.

3. *Parkinson's Disease.*   This common disease is due to selective degeneration of parts of the basal ganglia. The patient's muscles become rigid, the face is expressionless, and movement becomes difficult. A fine tremor completes the picture; "pill rolling" movements of the fingers are characteristic. This *extrapyramidal syndrome* is also seen following encephalitis, vascular ischemic episodes, and poisoning with carbon monoxide.

4. *Huntington's Chorea.*   Patients with this disease exhibit basal ganglia degeneration as well as cortical neuronal loss. Bizarre grimacing and uncontrolled irregular jerking movements (chorea) are combined with progressive dementia in this disease, which is inherited as a mendelian dominant trait.

5. *Motor Neuron Disease.*   Primary degeneration of the pyramidal tracts, the anterior horn cells, and their cranial equivalents can occur either singly or in combination to produce a variety of syndromes.

FIGURE 44–6. *Glioma of cerebral hemisphere.*

Sagittal section through the brain to show a large tumor in the right cerebral hemisphere. The center of the tumor is necrotic, and it shows dark areas that result from bleeding. Note that the tumor is not encapsulated and that its growh has distorted the lateral ventricles, particularly the one on the right-hand side. The expanding tumor has caused herniation of the hemisphere beneath the falx cerebri (arrow). The falx itself has been removed. (Courtesy of Dr. N. B. Rewcastle.)

EPILEPSY

Epilepsy consists of a sudden, uncoordinated outburst of impulses from a group of nerve cells. The seizure that results may be sensory and can lead to a sudden abnormal feeling, smell, or other sensation (the *dreamy state* or *psychomotor epilepsy*). There may be rapidly repeated brief lapses of consciousness *(petit mal),* or there may be a motor seizure that results in a generalized convulsion *(grand mal),* which is often followed by a period of unconsciousness.

Seizures may be a manifestation of an acute disease, ranging from fever in young children to alcohol withdrawal in adults. Repeated seizures suggest an organic cause such as a post-traumatic scar. When seizures begin in childhood, however, no cause can usually be found and the disease must be labeled *idiopathic.* Epilepsy commencing in adult life always suggests a detectable organic cause. The possibility of a tumor must always be considered (Fig. 44–6).

Case History I. (See Figure 44–6.)   The patient had had no previous history of epilepsy; he suffered his first attack at the age of 58 years. It started with twitching of the left foot, and then the involuntary movements spread to involve the whole leg, the left arm, and finally the whole body. With the onset of a generalized convulsion, the patient lost consciousness. This type of focal motor seizure that steadily extends to involve adjacent areas is called *Jacksonian epilepsy*. Examination of the patient at this time revealed no abnormal neurological signs. Radiography and electroencephalography showed no evidence of a focal brain lesion. Although a diagnosis of carcinoma of the lung was considered, sputum examination was negative for malignant cells, and a chest radiograph was normal. Nevertheless, the epileptic attacks continued. On several occasions the patient bit his tongue and was incontinent. Three months after the first attack, the patient suddenly developed a left-sided hemiplegia. Carotid artery thrombosis was considered but arteriography failed to confirm the diagnosis. Radiographs, however, showed deformity of the right lateral ventricle. The patient died suddenly. A necropsy revealed a glioblastoma multiforme (see Fig. 44–6).

The wide variation in the clinical features of an epileptic attack is a reflection of the complexity of the brain itself. Our frequent inability to find the cause of these attacks is a reflection of our state of knowledge.

Tumors of the Central Nervous System

Primary Tumors. The tumors are called *gliomas*; several types are described, the common one being derived from astrocytes (Fig. 44–6). Well-differentiated astrocytomas invade slowly, but the poorly differentiated tumors (Grades III and IV astrocytoma, or glioblastoma multiforme) are more malignant and kill rapidly. Although all gliomas are locally invasive and may metastasize within the central nervous system, one curious feature of these tumors is that *none of them ever produces distant metastases*. In spite of this, the prognosis is usually poor, because gliomas are difficult to remove surgically.

The *meningioma* is a benign tumor arising from the arachnoid granulations of the dura; it is therefore not a tumor of the brain itself. It is included here because the effects produced are very similar to those of a cerebral tumor. It produces pressure atrophy of the underlying brain; unless removed, a meningioma kills the subject by its local effects or because of an increased intracranial pressure.

Secondary Tumors. These are more common than primary growths. Carcinoma of the lung in males and carcinoma of the breast in females are the common primary tumors in these cases.

Review Questions

1. A patient is suspected to have an intracranial lesion such as a tumor or brain damage following a head injury. Explain why it is important to monitor each of the following:
     (a) the level of consciousness
     (b) the blood pressure
     (c) the pulse rate
     (d) the size of the pupils.
2. Classify the causes of increased intracranial pressure. Explain why it can be dangerous to perform a lumbar puncture.

3. Compare the causes and effects of a subdural hemorrhage with those of an extra-dural hemorrhage.
4. List the common causes of a stroke. Distinguish them according to the differences in clinical presentation.
5. A child has fever and convulsions. Describe the symptoms that would suggest a diagnosis of meningitis. Discuss how the diagnosis may be confirmed.
6. What is the most common malignant tumor of the brain in males over the age of 40 years? Outline the possible effects of a tumor situated in the right frontal lobe.

Selected Readings

Escourolle, R., and Poirier, J.: Manual of Basic Neuropathology. Translated and adapted by L. J. Rubinstein. Philadelphia, W. B. Saunders Company, 1973.

Foley, J. M.: The nervous system. *In* Robbins, S. L. (Ed.): Pathologic Basis of Disease. Philadelphia, W. B. Saunders Company, 1974, Chapter 32.

Simpson, J. A., and Mawdsley, C.: Diseases of the nervous system. *In* Macleod, J. (Ed.): Davidson's Principles and Practice of Medicine. 11th ed. Edinburgh, Churchill Livingstone, 1974, pp. 793–910.

INDEX

Numbers in *italics* denote illustrations; t denotes tables.